Eberhard Löhr · Lutz-Dietrich Leder (Eds.)

Renal and Adrenal Tumors

Pathology, Radiology, Ultrasonography, Magnetic Resonance (MRI), Therapy, Immunology

With Contributions by
R. Ackermann, K.-D. Bachmann, H. Behrendt, P.E. Billimoria, H.Chr. Dominick, M.D. Gross, R. Hartung, W. Havers, R. Heckemann, J.V. Kaude, R.E. Kinard, E.K. Lang, L.-D. Leder, E. Löhr, A.A. Moss, R.-D. Müller, H.J. Richter, E. Scherer, M. Serdarevic, B. Shapiro, W.P. Shuman, J.L. Williams, C. Wirtz

Second, completely revised Edition

With 229 Figures (17 in Colour) in 406 Separate Illustrations

Springer-Verlag Berlin Heidelberg NewYork
London Paris Tokyo

Professor Dr. Eberhard Löhr
Röntgendiagnostisches Zentralinstitut
Klinikum der Universität Essen
Hufelandstraße 55
D-4300 Essen

Professor Dr. Lutz-Dietrich Leder
Institut für Pathologie
Klinikum der Universität Essen
Hufelandstraße 55
D-4300 Essen

ISBN-13: 978-3-642-71209-8 e-ISBN-13: 978-3-642-71207-4
DOI: 10.1007/978-3-642-71207-4

Library of Congress Cataloging in Publication Data
Renal and adrenal tumors. Bibliography: p. Includes index. 1. Kidneys – Tumors. 2. Adrenal glands – Tumors. I. Ackermann, R. (Rolf) . II. Löhr, E. (Eberhard) . III. Leder, Lutz-Dietrich. [DNLM: 1. Adrenal Cortex Neoplasms. 2. Kidney Neoplasms. WJ 358 R393] RC280.K5R44 1987 616.99′261 86-31555

2127/3145-543210

Preface

After the positive response which followed the first edition of this book 6 years ago, the editors were encouraged to prepare a completely reworked second edition that includes the modern advances in this field. There has been a complete change of diagnostic procedure in the detection of renal tumors, which is now based on sonography, computed tomography, and nuclear magnetic resonance imaging, pushing intravenous urography and angiography completely into the background. Also, new methods of treatment with radionuclides using embolisation are incorporated.

The description of morphological structures forms the basis for understanding and recognising pathology of the kidneys and adrenals. The contents of pathological morphology could be extended, as we are of the opinion that the detection and therapy of renal and adrenal tumors are derived from different areas of diagnostic science.

We are indebted to Springer-Verlag for the excellent book production. On bchalf of all thc authors, wc would likc to thank our collcagucs and associates for their cooperation in the realisation of this project.

The editors hope that this volume will be of interest to radiologists, pathologists, urologists, pediatrists, and also radiotherapists.

Essen, April 1987

Eberhard Löhr
Lutz-Dietrich Leder

Table of Contents

Pathology of Renal and Adrenal Neoplasms
LEDER, L.-D., RICHTER, H.J.

Immunologic Aspects of Malignant Renal Disease
ACKERMANN, R.

List of Contributors

ACKERMANN, R., Medizinische Einrichtungen der Universität Düsseldorf, Urologische Klinik, Moorenstraße 5, D-4000 Düsseldorf 1

BACHMANN, K.-D., Universitätskinderklinik Münster, Vredenweg 19, D-4400 Münster

BEHRENDT, H., Urologische Klinik, Universitätsklinikum der Gesamthochschule Essen, Hufelandstraße 55, D-4300 Essen

BILLIMORIA, P.E., Loma Linda University, Medical Center, Department of Radiology, Loma Linda, CA 92354, USA

DOMINICK, H.CHR., St. Anna-Stift, Kinderklinik, Karolina-Burger-Straße 51, D-6700 Ludwigshafen

GROSS, M.D., Division of Nuclear Medicine, University of Michigan, Medical Center, Veterans' Administration Hospital, 2215 Fuller Road, Ann Arbor, MI 48105, USA

HARTUNG, R., Urologische Universitäts-Klinik Rechts der Isar, D-8000 München

HAVERS, W., Klinik und Poliklinik für Kinder- und Jugendmedizin, Universitätsklinikum Essen, Hufelandstraße 55, D-4300 Essen

HECKEMANN, R., Augusta Krankenanstalt Bochum, Abteilung Radiologie, Bergstraße 26, D-4630 Bochum

KAUDE, J.V., Department of Radiology, University of Florida, College of Medicine, Box J-374, JHMHC, Gainesville, FL 32610, USA

KINARD, R.E., Department of Radiology, University of Florida, College of Medicine, Box J-374, JHMHC, Gainesville, FL 32610, USA

LANG, E.K., University of New Orleans, Medical Center, Department of Radiology, 1542 Tulane Avenue, New Orleans, La., USA

LEDER, L.-D., Institut für Pathologie, Universitätsklinikum Essen, Hufelandstraße 55, D-4300 Essen 1

LÖHR, E., Röntgendiagnostisches Zentralinstitut, Universitätsklinikum Essen, Hufelandstraße 55, D-4300 Essen 1

MOSS, A.A., University of Washington, School of Medicine, Department of Radiology SB-05, Seattle, Wash. 98195, USA

MÜLLER, R.-D., Radiologisches Zentrum, Universitätsklinikum Essen, Hufelandstraße 55, D-4300 Essen 1

RICHTER, H.J., Pathologisches Institut, Universitätsklinikum Essen, Hufelandstraße 55, D-4300 Essen 1

SCHERER, E., Strahlenklinik, Universitätsklinikum Essen, Hufelandstraße 55, D-4300 Essen 1

SERDAREVIC, M., Röntgendiagnostisches Zentralinstitut, Universitätsklinikum Essen, Hufelandstraße 55, D-4300 Essen 1

SHAPIRO, B., Division of Nuclear Medicine, University of Michigan, Medical Center, Veterans' Administration Hospital, 2215 Fuller Road, Ann Arbor, MI 48105, USA

SHUMAN, W.P., University of Washington, School of Medicine, Department of Radiology SB-05, Seattle, Wash. 98195, USA

WILLIAMS, J.L., Department of Radiology, University of Florida, College of Medicine, Box J-374, JHMHC, Gainesville, FL 32610, USA

WIRTZ, C., Strahlenklinik, Universitätsklinikum Essen, Hufelandstraße 55, D-4300 Essen 1

Pathology of Renal and Adrenal Neoplasms

L.-D. LEDER and H.J. RICHTER

1 Tumors and Tumorlike Lesions of the Kidney in the Adult

1.1 General Remarks

To understand and correctly interpret the morphology of tumors of the kidneys, and in the case of malignancy the morphology of their metastases, it is important to know that the kidney of man is a true metanephros. This means it is of mesodermal origin [165]. On the other hand, there is no doubt of the epithelial character of the tubular cells, which are of mesodermal origin. Thus it is understandable that in renal neoplasms both epithelial and nonepithelial, e.g., mesenchymal, elements may be found, for instance in Wilms' tumor and adenocarcinoma of the kidney.

1.2 Heterotopic Tissue

1.2.1 Adrenal Tissue

It is very seldom that one finds heterotopic tissue in bioptic material. Such observations are usually confined to autopsy studies. APITZ [12] found accessory adrenal tissue in 261 of 4309 individual autopsies. There are no differences between sexes [338]. In most of the cases, the adrenal tissue is located near the upper pole of the kidney.

Macroscopically, one sees a subcapsular nodular plaque with a roundish shape and a yellow-orange color. Some of these nodules may reach a size of up to 2 cm in diameter. Up to now ectopic adrenal tissue has never been found in the medulla.

Microscopically, the lesions look very much like normal adrenal cortical tissue, sometimes mimicking the normal zones [338].

1.2.2 Endometriosis

There are rare and occasional reports describing involvement of the urinary tract by endometriosis [1, 24]. Histologically, typical endometrial glands surrounded by endometrial stroma are found. Since endometrial glands follow the normal cycle, mitoses may occur during the proliferation phase. This must be kept in mind in order to avoid misinterpreting the condition as primary or metastatic adenocarcinoma of the kidney.

1.2.3 Cartilaginous Islands

Cartilaginous islands are designated by some as true benign tumors, namely chondromas [238]. However, cartilage is found within renal parenchyma, usually together with renal dysplasia [37]. Also, there are histogenetic relationships among renal dysplasia, nodular renal blastema, mesoblastic nephroma, and nephroblastoma, which are discussed in Sect. 2. Macroscopically and histologically the lesions present the typical appearance of mature cartilaginous tissue. It should be stressed here that neither heterotopic adrenal tissue in the kidney nor endometrial tissue (if confined to the kidney) nor cartilaginous islands appear to produce any symptoms during life.

1.3 Benign Mesenchymal Tumors

1.3.1 Leiomyoma and Lipoma

Leiomyomas and lipomas are discussed together here because it is known that both kinds of tumors may be found side by side in the same kidney and, furthermore, adipose tissue may be mixed up with smooth muscle cells to form leiomyolipomas [12, 333].

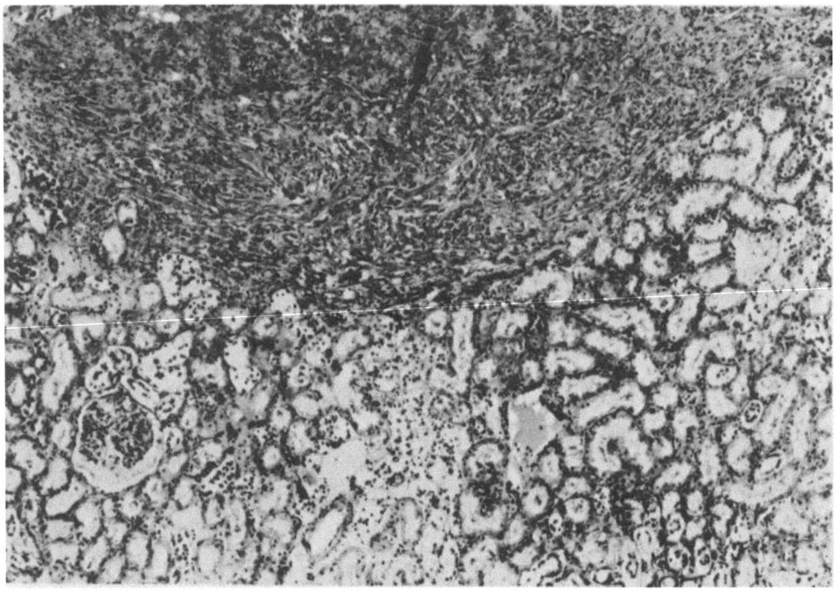

Fig. 1. Renal cortical nodule (leiomyoma) consisting predominantly of smooth muscle cells. H & E, × 56

Benign mesenchymal tumors are much more common in women than in men. This holds true for both leiomyomas and lipomas as well as for myolipomas. The lesions are very rare and most of them are found in the elderly. Usually, they are detected incidentally at autopsy, since they are in general too small to cause clinical symptoms. Their origin is not quite clear. If tumor-terms are used, then a neoplastic origin is implied; however, this has not yet been proved. A hamartomatous origin may also be taken into consideration [161]. BENNINGTON and BECKWITH [31] think that the term choristoma, which denotes tumorlike formations of displaced tissues, is much more appropriate.

Generally, the lesions have little diagnostic importance in comparison to primary malignant neoplasms of the renal parenchyma. BENNINGTON and BECKWITH [31], for instance, mention that before 1975 fewer than 50 leiomyomas and lipomas had been described that were large enough to produce clinical symptoms during life, and DINEEN et al. [100] found only 17 cases of renal lipomas in the literature that were large enough to be of surgical significance. It may be mentioned in this connection that leiomyomas and lipomas are found relatively often in patients with tuberous sclerosis [198], which was first described by FISCHER [122].

Macroscopically, most of the lesions represent only small nests of fatty tissue and/or smooth muscle and are usually found in the cortex. Many range from 0.1–1.0 cm in diameter. They are relatively sharply circumscribed.

Microscopically, they consist of mature adipose tissue or smooth muscle cells (Fig. 1) or both.

1.3.2 Angiomyolipoma

This lesion should also be regarded as a choristoma [31]. It is known that about 80% of patients with tuberous sclerosis bear angiomyolipomas [79, 186, 108, 116]. On the other hand, a considerable number of cases is not related to tuberous sclerosis.

Angiomyolipomas are not extremely rare. Whereas FARROW et al. [116] reported only 32 cases out of 2409 surgically excised tumorous kidneys observed over a period of 50 years, MA and CHAN [260] noted 57 cases including five personal observations, and BUSCH et al. [57] found in the literature as many as 200 cases not associated with tuberous sclerosis.

According to FARROW et al. [116], the lesions are usually solitary and unilateral. Size and clinical symptoms vary considerably from case to case. Fever or hypertension may be the first and only clinical symptoms [135, 61]. Interestingly enough, YUM et al. [432] identified juxtaglomerular cells with typical rhomboid and spheric granules within an angiomyolipoma.

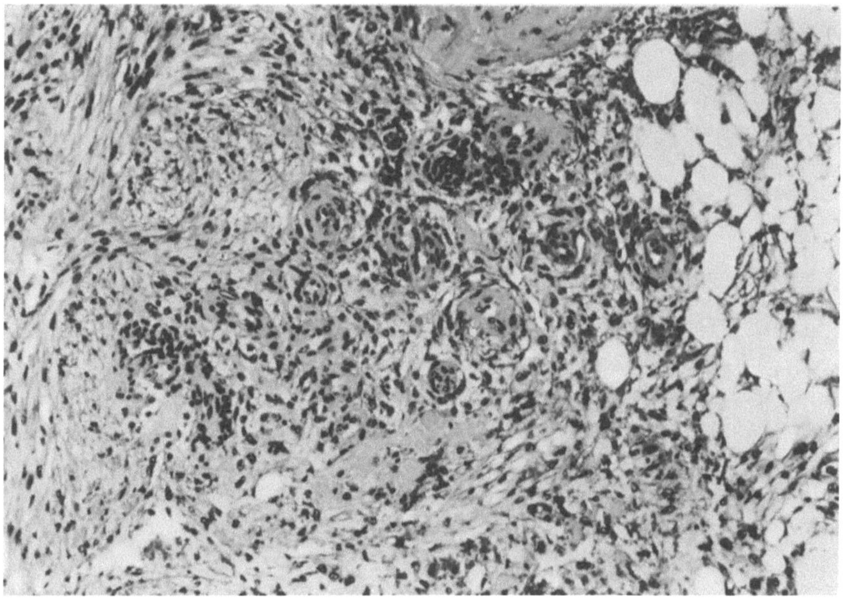

Fig. 2. Angiomyolipoma. The lesion consists of adipose tissue, spindle-shaped smooth muscle cells, and prominent blood vessels. H & E, × 140

It is very important to recognize this lesion as reports in the literature show that angiomyolipomas may be confused with a variety of malignancies such as sarcomas or malignant mesenchymomas [323, 161]. FARROW et al. [116] showed very clearly that symptomatic angiomyolipoma may consist of many nodules of different sizes penetrating and destroying large parts of the renal parenchyma, thereby mimicking malignant behavior. It is, therefore, quite possible that some cases of angiomyolipoma of the kidney may be confused with liposarcoma, for instance, or considered variants of nephroblastoma.

Occasionally the tumor vessels may spontaneously rupture, causing massive retroperitoneal bleeding [416, 409]. Such cases are usually not associated with tuberous sclerosis.

Macroscopically, angiomyolipomas may range in size from 3–20 cm in diameter. Larger nodules may cause anatomic alterations of the kidney structure which, if detected by clinical methods such as angiography, may closely mimic a malignant process. In addition, expansive growth, locally invasive growth, extension to perirenal structures, and extension beyond the capsule have all been reported. Thus, the grade of destruction of the kidney may be marked.

Microscopically (Fig. 2), one finds a mixture of mature fat cells, strands and sheets of smooth muscle cells, and relatively thick-walled blood vessels that are characteristically devoid of elastic fibers [175]. Mitotic figures have been reported, and moderate pleomorphism of the nuclei can also be found. The muscle cells of the thick-walled vessels often form imperfect walls and gradually merge with extravascular interlacing fascicles of smooth muscle cells (Fig. 3).

Biologically, the lesion is benign. Therefore, surgical treatment is followed by a nearly 100% cure rate [323, 116, 161]. However, several authors recently reported regional involvement of lymph nodes [41, 89, 266], inferior vena caval tumor thrombus [52], massive recurrence with perforation of the colon and invasion of the diaphragm [235], and involvement of the spleen [197]. Therefore, some few cases of angiomyolipoma may be considered potentially malignant, although at least part of the above mentioned manifestations may simply reflect multicentricity of the disease rather than metastases.

1.3.3 Hemangioma

Hemangiomas are relatively uncommon in the kidney; up to 1951, only 72 had been reported [274]. STANLEY et al. [368] described three cases of cavernous hemangioma, which are particularly rare. Many of the tumors are seen around the 3rd and 4th decade. If these tumors produce clinical symptoms, then hematuria is usually

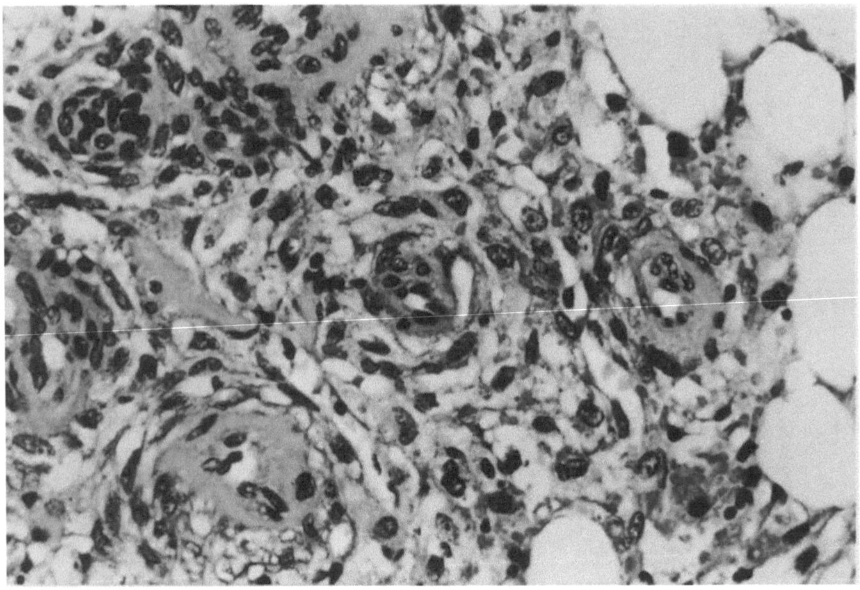

Fig. 3. Same case as Fig. 2. At higher magnification the characteristic intimate relationship between smooth muscle cells of the vessel walls and the interstitial tissue is readily demonstrated. H & E, ×350

present [21, 119]. As the blood coagulates, blood clots may produce colicky pains [132].

Hemangiomas of the kidney may be very small. In consequence, they may easily be missed in clinical explorations, for example, on excretory urograms, as well as on macroscopic and microscopic examination by the pathologist.

Macroscopically, hemangiomas appear as prominent blood-filled areas or spaces on the cut surface.

Microscopically, they may be of the capillary type or may represent cavernous hemangiomas. There is no difference in their microscopic appearance when compared to hemangiomas of other localizations.

1.3.4 Juxtaglomerular Tumor

Juxtaglomerular tumor was first described by Robertson et al. [340]. They reported on a young male patient with hypertension and hypokalemia that was due to a renin-secreting renal tumor. The tumor resembled hemangiopericytoma and contained large amounts of renin. At least eighteen additional reports have established this entity and its histologic characteristics [346, 90, 139, 166, 293, 254, 22, 361]. Thus, altogether about 20 cases are known so far.

Macroscopically, juxtaglomerular tumors are small, encapsulated or at least well-circumscribed lesions, located in the renal cortex. No macroscopic criteria of malignancy can be seen. On the cut surface, they reveal a grey color in contrast to renal adenocarcinomas, which usually are yellowish.

Microscopically, the tumor is composed of cells resembling epithelioid histiocytes. Many small blood vessels may be interposed. The main feature that enables one to identify the lesion are the many cytoplasmic renin-containing granules that can be readily demonstrated by methods such as immunofluorescence with anti-human-renin.

Electron-microscopic investigations revealed that these granules are identical to those of the normal granular epithelioid cells of the juxtaglomerular apparatus [20, 35, 115]. Since the tumor cells resemble smooth muscle cells or pericytes or tumor cells of hemangiopericytoma, it is thought that the juxtaglomerular tumor of the kidney is a peculiar variant of hemangiopericytoma [31].

1.3.5 Lymphangioma

Lymphangiomas are benign mesenchymal tumors that usually occur in children and are exceedingly rare in the kidney [187, 425].

Macroscopically, they are described as large, unencapsulated tumors. From the cut surface one sees that the lesion is multicystic. The tumors may be so large as to replace considerable parts of the kidney.

Histologically, they represent a convolute of wide, thin-walled vessels with smooth muscle cells in their walls, lined by a single layer of flattened cells. The cystic spaces contain a more or less eosinophilic fluid.

Biologically, no malignancies have been reported, and no metastases have been observed after nephrectomy.

1.3.6 Fibroma (Renomedullary Interstitial Cell Tumor)

Fibromas are usually mentioned in every pathology textbook as the classic example in which the characteristics and features of a benign mesenchymal tumor are explained. This gives the impression that fibromas are very common, not only generally but also among benign mesenchymal tumors of organs, such as the kidney. COLVIN [76] reported and cited a number of such lesions. However, when XIPPEL [429] examined multiple sections of both kidneys in 250 autopsies, he noted leiomyomas, lipomas, and myolipomas, but not one case of cortical fibroma. A similar result was found earlier by REESE and WINSTANLEY [333]. BENNINGTON and BECKWITH [31] also have never seen fibromas of the renal cortex.

Medullary fibromata have been reported by ZANGEMEISTER [434], REESE and WINSTANLEY [333], and XIPPEL [429].

Grossly, these fibrous nodules are very small, ranging from 0.1–0.3 cm in diameter. They compress the surrounding renal parenchyma.

Histologically, they are composed of slender cells lying between a dense and often hyalinized matrix. Since renal tubules may be entrapped, these lesions do not seem to represent true benign neoplasms.

Electron-microscopic investigations of such nodules have shown that their cells do not resemble normal fibroblasts but are derived from medullary interstitial cells [251]. Therefore, it was proposed to term them "renomedullary interstitial cell tumors."

In summary, it must be accepted at present that there are no lesions in the kidney that can be proven to be true "fibromas." This agrees very well with the view of experts in fibroblastic disorders: STOUT [376] stated that it is exceedingly difficult to decide whether or not there is a true benign neoplasm composed of fibroblasts, and MACKENZIE [263] considers the fibroma a doubtful entity with regard to both its identification as such in a particular case and its existence in general.

1.3.7 Neurogenic Tumors

Up to now we have not been able to find reports in the literature on benign neurogenic tumors such as neurinomas or neurofibromas involving the renal parenchyma.

1.4 Malignant Mesenchymal Tumors

1.4.1 Leiomyosarcoma

BENNINGTON and BECKWITH [31] think that leiomyosarcoma is the most common sarcoma of the kidney. This conclusion is drawn from the observation of FARROW et al. [117] who found over a 60-year period at the Mayo Clinic that 15 of 26 renal sarcomas were leiomyosarcomas. To the best of our knowledge, this tumor has not been described previously in children. Most of the cases have been reported in females [23, 156, 257]. HELMBRECHT and COSGROVE [181] described two cases and reviewed the literature. They found a total of 69 reported cases.

Macroscopically, the tumors afflict the right and left side with equal frequency. Often there is a local relationship to the renal capsule. As is the case with hemangiopericytoma, it may be difficult to assess whether a leiomyosarcoma is primary renal or has arisen in the retroperitoneum with secondary extension to the kidney. The cut surface shows a firm, elevating, slightly whitish mass. The tumors are lobulated, and whorled configurations may be conspicuous. One may see areas of hyalinization, necroses with the formation of cysts, and calcifications as well as focal hemorrhages.

Microscopically, the lesions are composed of spindle-shaped cells. Typically, these possess an eosinophilic cytoplasm with very fine longitudinal fibrils. The nuclei are rod-shaped and elongated with plump ends. The cells are usually arranged in bundles of different thickness. Tumor cells that have been cross sectioned reveal a typical microscopic feature, namely centrally placed nuclei surrounded by a clear cytoplasm. The cell borders stand out very distinctively in such cross sections. Mitoses can be found in varying numbers. Myofilaments can be demonstrated on electron micrographs [390].

Biologic behavior. As is the case with leiomyosarcomas of the uterus and other sites, the histologic picture does not offer reliable criteria that can be used as prognostic indicators. By and large, the number of mitotic figures seems to be the best criterion. The tumors tend to recur locally, and blood-born metastases may appear in the lungs. However, liver, regional lymph nodes, peritoneum, and mesentery may also show metastases. At present radiation therapy and chemotherapy seem to be of little value. Nephrectomy is presently the treatment of choice.

1.4.2 Rhabdomyosarcoma

As is generally known, malignant striated muscle occurs in many nephroblastomas. However, there are some reports of pure rhabdomyosarcoma of the kidney [285, 185, 354, 117]. In spite of these reports, it must be seriously considered whether or not apparently pure rhabdomyosarcomas of the kidney are only overgrowths of malignant muscle in nephroblastoma. There are, however, no convincing arguments in favor of this view. Thus, the objection that perhaps rhabdomyosarcomas are actually nephroblastomas because in normal renal parenchyma cross-striated muscle does not occur is not very striking: rhabdomyosarcomas have been reported in many sites that are devoid of striated muscle, for instance, the paranasal sinuses, the extrahepatic biliary duct, the ureter, the bladder, the prostate, and the subcutaneous tissue of the genital region [114, 97].

Macroscopically, the tumors present the typical aspect of a malignant mesenchymal tumor.

Microscopically, a very accentuated pleomorphism may be conspicuous. The crucial feature is the demonstration of cross-striated muscle cells, which sometimes can be found only after a very prolonged search. It is worthwhile emphasizing that in every undifferentiated spindle cell tumor with malignant features cross-striation must be searched for, especially with a mucoid or myxomatous matrix which can often be found in conjunction with rhabdomyosarcomas irrespective of their location.

1.4.3 Liposarcoma

Liposarcoma is a very rare malignant renal tumor. It is said that the frequency of this tumor was formerly overestimated [427], and indeed, in the series of Farrow et al. [117], renal liposarcoma was rare. On the basis of the present literature, we estimate no more than about 35–40 published cases in the world.

Macroscopically, renal liposarcomas are described as occurring usually in the outer cortex or subcapsular where they form large masses. On the cut surface they are multilobular and yellow, greyish, or pink. As with liposarcomas of other localizations, the cut surfaces are often strikingly slimy, and the coincidence of fatty tissue and slimy material is a very valuable clue to diagnosis.

Microscopically, the tumors may exhibit all grades of differentiation beginning with features corresponding to "proliferating lipoma" and ending with frankly sarcomatous patterns made up of cells that cannot easily be identified as malignant fat cells. Often, there is a marked myxomatous component (Fig. 4). In many cases special fat stains have to be applied to identify malignant fat cells.

The *biologic behavior* depends on the differentiation, as is the case with liposarcomas of other localizations.

1.4.4 Angiosarcoma (Hemangioendothelioma)

True hemangiosarcoma or malignant hemangioendothelioma of the kidney seems to be extremely rare. Bennington and Beckwith [31] found many references to malignant vascular

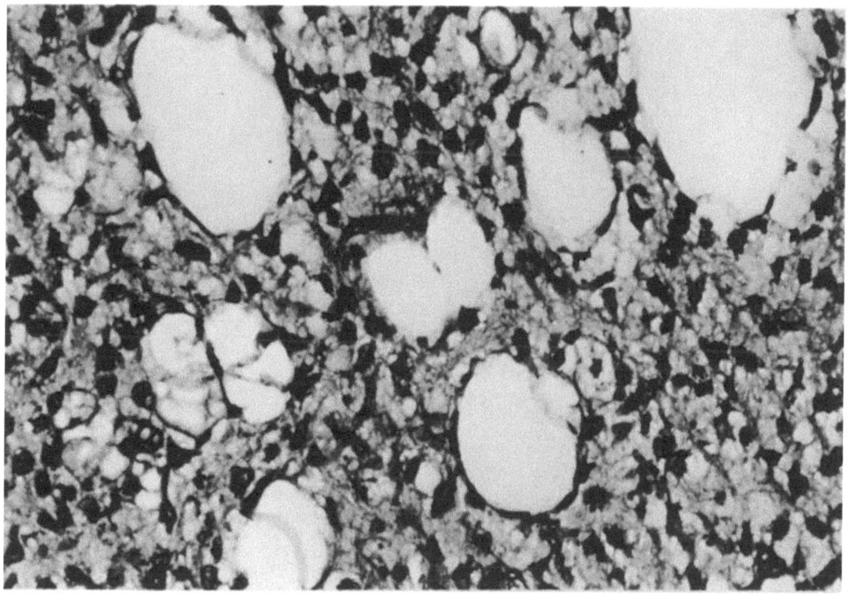

Fig. 4. Liposarcoma. Atypical fat cells of varying maturity with admixture of many stellate cells that form the typical myxomatous background. H & E, ×350

tumors of the kidney, but on close examination such cases often proved to be adenocarcinomas with prominent vascularity or angiomyolipomas. Indeed, it is common experience that adenocarcinomas of the kidneys are sometimes so extremely well vascularised that they closely mimic hemangioendothelioma or some other vascular tumor. Only one single report could be found by BENNINGTON and BECKWITH [31] that may be accepted as a true renal hemangiosarcoma [324]. In reviewing the literature, we have met with a similar experience. An excellently documented case is described by ALLRED et al. [9]. CHATTERJEE and POWELL [66] found six acceptable cases.

1.4.5 Hemangiopericytoma

Hemangiopericytoma, a very uncommon tumor, was first described by STOUT and MURRAY [377]. The tumor may be found anywhere in the body. Nine reports of it involving the kidney have been noted by BENNINGTON and BECKWITH [31]. Only a few additional cases have been reported since then [292, 419]. The macroscopic and microscopic features are exactly the same as in other regions.

Macroscopically, the growths are located eccentrically, perhaps because they arise from capsular tissue elements. The cut surface shows multinodularity and different shades of grey-pink, reddish brown, and yellow. A tumor capsule may be present. Because of the eccentric location, it is difficult to decide whether or not there is a retroperitoneal origin with secondary extension to the kidney, thereby producing compression of the renal parenchyma.

Microscopically, there are many vascular spaces lined by endothelial cells. These are surrounded by tumor cells that closely mimic pericytes, having pale cytoplasm and round or oval nuclei. The tumor cells are separated from the endothelial cells by a distinct basement membrane that can be demonstrated by one of the reticulin stains. The neoplastic pericytes usually form collarettes or whorls around the vessels. Each tumor cell is surrounded by reticulin fibers (Figs. 5 and 6). Mitoses can be found in varying numbers.

Biologic behavior. Hemangiopericytomas are difficult to interpret with regard to their biologic outcome. Of eight patients four died, one had metastases 7 months after operation, and in three no metastases were found [31]. It must be stressed that the histologic picture does not permit prognostic predictions.

1.4.6 Fibrosarcoma

In the older literature most malignant tumors composed of spindle-shaped cells were called fi-

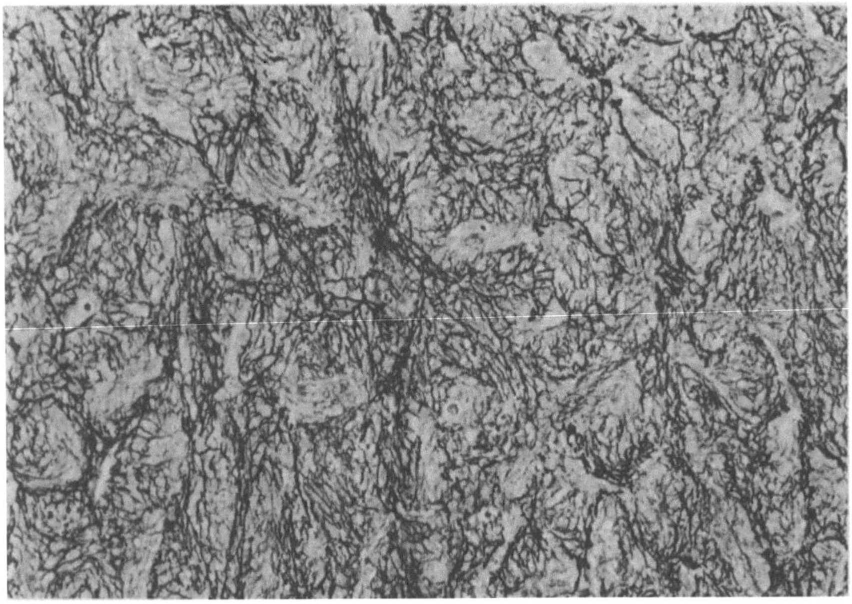

Fig. 5. Hemangiopericytoma. The reticulin stain reveals a typical pattern consisting of large collarette-like accumulations of tumor cells around small, centrally placed blood vessels. H & E, ×140

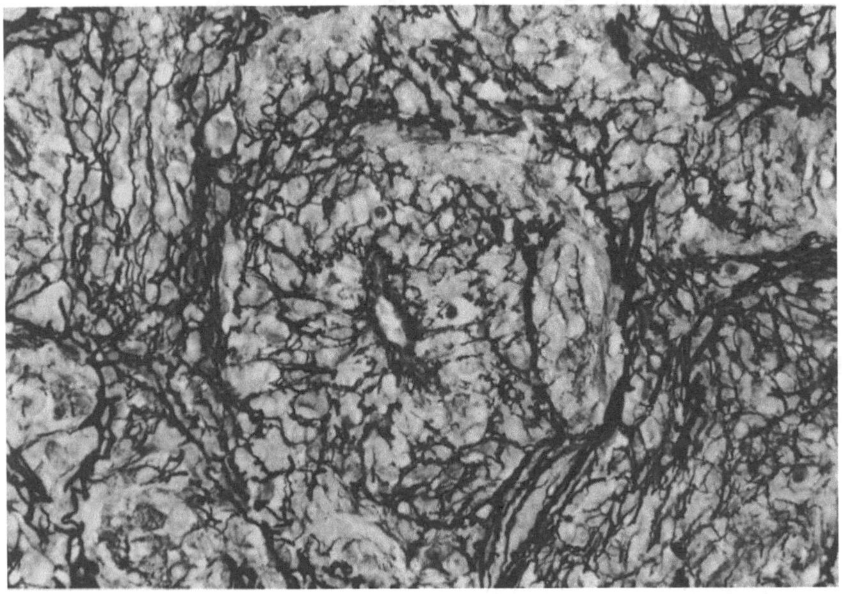

Fig. 6. Same case as Fig. 5. At higher magnification the typical structure becomes evident: a small vessel is surrounded by thick layers of perithelial cells in a meshwork of reticulin fibers. H & E, ×350

brosarcomas. This was especially true for those adenocarcinomas of the kidney with a sarcomatous growth pattern. With the improvement of knowledge and investigative techniques, including histochemical methods, the diagnosis of fibrosarcoma of the kidney has become more and more rare. Thus, it is understandable that nowadays no reliable figures concerning the frequency of fibrosarcoma of the kidney and no information about its macroscopic, microscopic, and biologic behavior is available.

1.4.7 Fibroxanthosarcoma and Malignant Fibrous Histiocytoma

Bennington and Beckwith [31] have seen one case of fibroxanthosarcoma of the kidney, and currently, only five well documented cases have been reported [53]. The tumor consists of spindle cells within a collagenous stroma. Atypical histiocytes containing variable amounts of lipid may be admixed. There are also bizarre giant cells. A prominent mitotic activity with abnormal mitotic figures may be present. Biologically, the tumors are said to be aggressive with a high frequency of recurrences and occasional metastases [303, 221]. The differential diagnosis has to consider xanthogranulomatous pyelonephritis, malakoplakia, and renal adenocarcinoma.

According to OJEDA et al. [306], nine cases of primary renal malignant fibrous histiocytoma have been described, and one additional case is reported by CHEN [68]. Histologically, the tumors show the very same picture as that known from other sites [106]. The tumors tend to recur and may give rise to distant metastases. Their response to chemotherapy and irradiation may be relatively poor [328, 353]. The descriptions of fibroxanthosarcoma and malignant fibrous histiocytoma are very similar to each other, so it is possible that both terms cover the same lesion.

1.4.8 Osteogenic Sarcoma and Chondrosarcoma

The occurrence of osteogenic sarcoma in the kidney probably reflects the mesodermal origin of the renal parenchyma, which might be also true for other benign and malignant mesenchymal tumors of this organ. Osteogenic sarcomas were reported by HAINING and POOLE [160], HAMER and WISHARD [164], HUDSON [194], SOTO et al. [363], JOHNSON et al. [212], BIGGERS and STEWART [36], MICOLONGHI et al. [287], and TUTTLE et al. [400]. Interestingly enough, the patients' ages ranged from 52–82 years, whereas osteogenic sarcomas of the bones tend to occur in the first and second decade [84]. All had an abdominal mass, and there was evidence of calcification in the roentgenograms. All developed metastases and died of their tumors.

Histologically, the tumors show extreme pleomorphism with many spindle-shaped cells. There are occasional multinucleated giant cells and unequivocal calcifying osteoid tissue. In other words, tumor osteoid with respective malignant cells can be found throughout the neoplasms. It may be added here that we found two reports of primary chondrosarcoma of the kidney [265, 299]. In consequence, large renal tumorous masses containing calcified and bony structures may represent osteogenic sarcoma or chondrosarcoma in extremely rare cases.

1.4.9 Hemoblastoses

It is widely known that in hemoblastoses, especially in leukemia, the kidneys may be heavily infiltrated. For example, STERNBY [372] investigated 108 leukemic patients for renal infiltrates: 42% of the cases with lymphatic leukemia and 24% of those with myelogenous leukemia were positive. It is our own experience that on close examination renal infiltrates can nearly always be found with leukemias. However, very often these infiltrates are only of microscopic size.

Macroscopically, the infiltrates may be diffuse or nodular (Fig. 7). Usually the infiltration is limited to the outer cortex giving the kidney parenchyma a pale grey-pink or grey-white color.

Microscopically, the infiltrating cells may severely destroy the renal parenchyma. The identification of the leukemic cells with respect to the various subgroups of leukoses may be extremely difficult if conventional histologic stains alone are used. However, the naphthol AS-D chloroacetate esterase reaction [248] may serve as an aid in identifying myelogenous leukemia, since this enzyme histochemical method stains myeloid cells bright red. The main advantage of the method is that it can be applied routinely to formalin-fixed, paraffin-embedded tissue, which is not the case with all other enzyme cytochemical methods (Fig. 8).

Malignant lymphomas not uncommonly also involve the renal parenchyma. RICHMOND et al. [337] have reported that in patients with malignant lymphoma there was a lymphomatous infiltration of the kidneys in 33.5% of the cases. Concerning the various forms of malignant lymphoma, the authors found renal involvement in 13% of the cases of Hodgkin's disease, 63% of lymphocytic lymphoma, and 46% of histiocytic lymphoma (large cell lymphoma). MARTINEZ-MALDONADO and RAMIREZ DE ARELLANO [272] reviewed 49 patients with malignant lymphoma including Hodgkin's disease. They found renal involvement in 42% of the autopsy cases.

There are some reports that show that multiple myeloma is not necessarily confined to the bones but may well involve the kidneys [71, 314]. Most of the cases are secondary spreads,

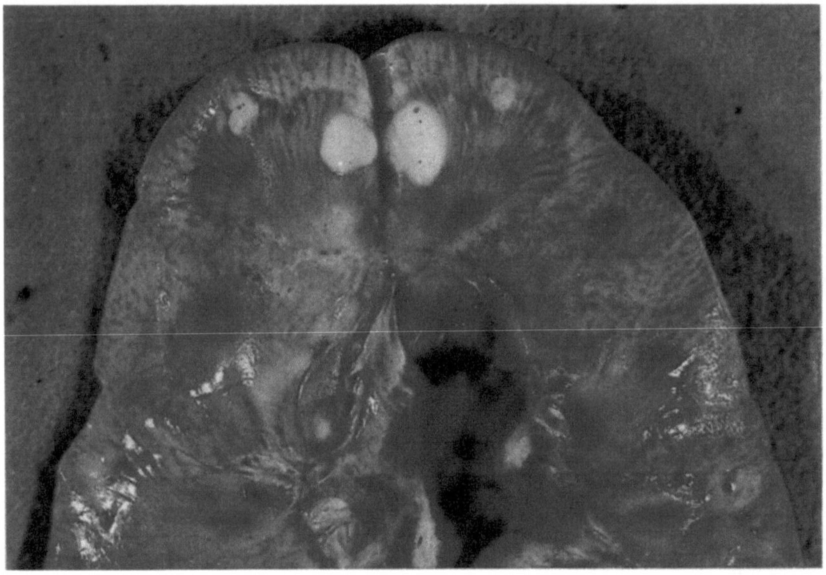

Fig. 7. Nodular renal cortical infiltrate in a case of myeloid leukemia (myelosarcoma)

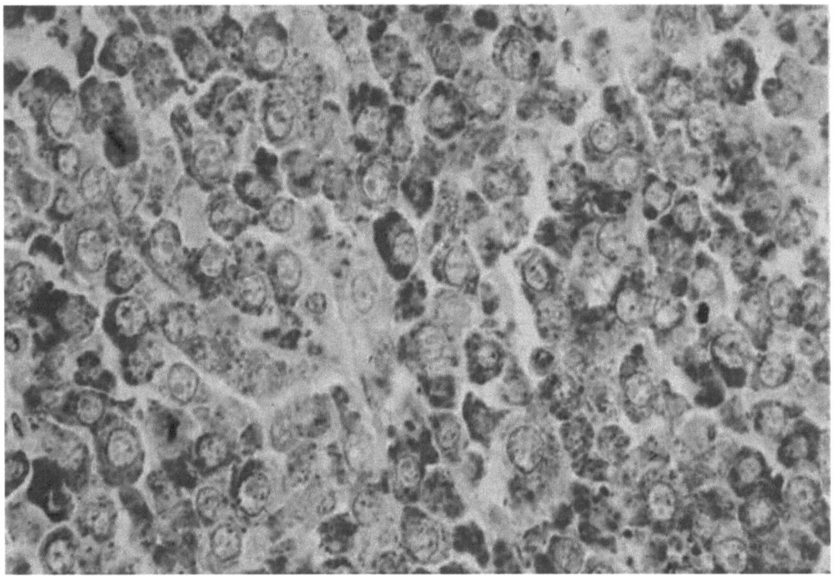

Fig. 8. Nodular growth in a myeloid leukemia subjected to the chloroesterase reaction. The cells disclose an intense activity indicating their myeloid nature that otherwise can hardly be established for certain. × 560

but there are very rare reports of primary multiple myeloma of the kidney [101]. KANDEL et al. [217] found eight cases in the literature and added one further case.

The histologic diagnosis of secondary or primary multiple myeloma usually presents no problem to the experienced pathologist. However, there may be two difficulties. Firstly, if the tumor cells are dedifferentiated so that their plasmocytic nature is obscured, diagnosis may be missed. Secondly, a heavy focal infiltrate of reactive normal plasma cells may resemble plasmocytoma.

In such cases the appliance of immunoperoxidase methods for detecting immunoglobulin components, e.g., κ- and λ-chains, can be recommended (Fig. 9). Myeloma cells will show monoclonality, whereas reactive plasma cells will not. The methods have been well developed, but their use may remain confined to pathology institutes of larger tumor centers [for details see 392].

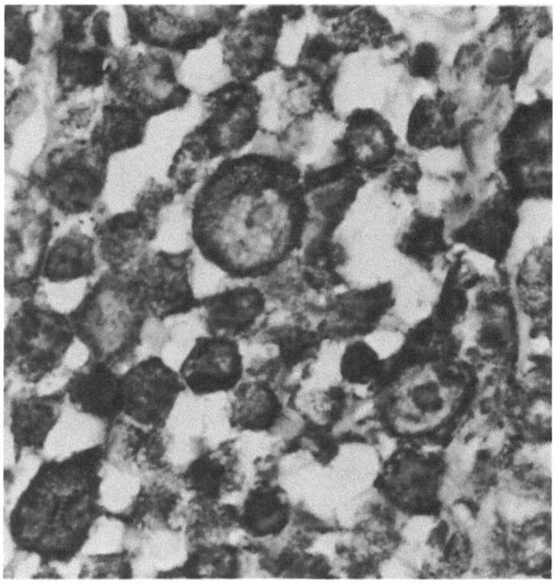

Fig. 9. Pleomorphous plasmocytoma subjected to the immunoperoxidase technique for the detection of λ-chains. All cells are heavily positive disclosing their plasma cell character and the production of a monoclonal paraprotein both of which cannot be reliably established on H & E-stained sections. ×880

1.5 Epithelial Tumors

1.5.1 Renal "Adenoma"

Renal adenomas and adenocarcinomas cannot be clearly separated because they virtually overlap one another without any sharp, definite, or definable boundary. These facts had been expressed by several authors very early, and many of them noticed that the similarities between cells of true adenocarcinomas of the kidney on the one hand and cells of so-called adenomas of the kidney on the other are so intimate that the description of one is almost the description of the other [124]. However, the term "renal adenoma" became very popular through constant usage in spite of the fact that nobody was able to define "renal adenoma" sufficiently well as to separate it from a small adenocarcinoma. Later on, as it was observed that tumors less than 3 cm in diameter usually did not metastasize, size became the main criterion. Thus, tumors that were larger than 3 cm in diameter were considered malignant.

However, there is a defect in this concept. It must be born in mind that BELL [27] in his series described two tumors less than 2 cm in size that had metastasized and quite a lot of tumors larger than 10 cm in diameter that had not. This clearly pointed out that size alone is not sufficient to decide whether a given node is an adenoma or an adenocarcinoma. This was supported by a review of 180 "adenomas" performed by MURPHY and MOSTOFI [297].

Meanwhile we know that there is no gross, histologic, histochemical, or immunologic criterion that allows us to reliably distinguish adenocarcinoma from adenoma. Electron-microscopic observations have also shown that separation of renal adenoma and adenocarcinoma is absolutely arbitrary and definitely impossible, since their features are essentially the same [304, 356, 355, 390, 123, 30, 77, 322]. For detailed information about the problem the reader is referred to the excellent discussion given by BENNINGTON and BECKWITH [31].

In summary, we generally support and accept the view that many of the so-called adenomas may be better interpreted as small adenocarcinomas that have not yet produced metastases [275, 78, 32, 114, 123]. If, however, the lesions are extremely small (Fig. 10), one must admit that the term "adenoma" is reasonable and preferable.

This view has important practical consequences with biopsy cases. For example, an equivocal tumor less than 3 cm in diameter may be found incidentally at surgery. In such a doubtful case, it is very important how the lesion will be termed by the pathologist. In agreement with BENNINGTON and BECKWITH [31], we feel it better to diagnose such a nodule as a potential adenocarcinoma. Following their proposal the patient can be told then that such a small nodule rarely leads to metastases. In consequence, the psychological harm will not be too extensive, and the surgeon is able to plan, together with the patient, a suitable follow up that will be understood and accepted.

1.5.2 Renal Cell Oncocytoma

Renal cell oncocytoma was first reported by ZIPPEL [436] but the lesion remained unrecognized for a long time. It had been regarded as a renal cell carcinoma in the past, until KLEIN and VALENSI [228] presented a series of 14 cases and demonstrated convincingly their benign na-

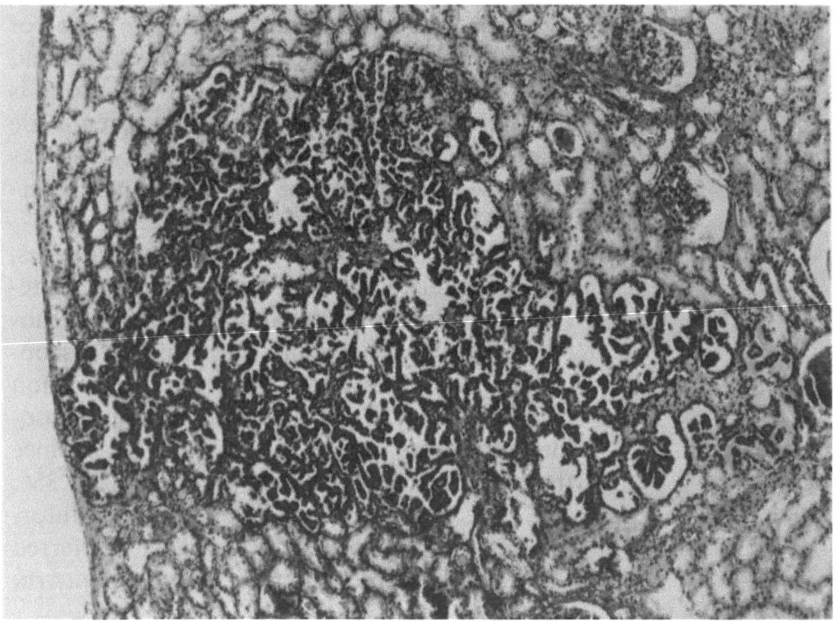

Fig. 10. Very small renal cortical adenoma disclosing a papillary pattern. Incidental finding at autopsy. Such a small lesion may well be labeled "adenoma" in spite of the fact that definite criteria are lacking that clearly separate adenoma from carcinoma. H & E, ×56

ture. Subsequently, many reports appeared confirming the results of KLEIN and VALENSI [228]; up to 1983, more than 50 cases had been published [70]. Oncocytoma cells probably derive from the epithelium of the distal tubule [105], although other authors have maintained their origin from proximal tubule cells. The tumor affects predominantly males (2:1) and occurs usually in the elderly with a peak incidence in the 7th decade. The incidence of these tumors varies between 4% and 7% of all renal neoplasms [7, 70] and its frequency tends to increase [374].

Macroscopically, the tumors can attain large sizes, some may be as large as 20 cm in diameter with a weight of 2300 g [70]. They are usually well circumscribed with a characteristically lobated cerebriform surface. The cut surface exhibits a tan-brown color, and large tumors may contain a stellate scarry center. Cystic changes and hemorrhage may occasionally be encountered. Six cases of multicentric oncocytoma are described in the literature so far [67, 405]. Bilateral oncocytomas, some of which were multicentric, have also been observed [435].

Microscopically (Figs. 11 and 12), the neoplasms consist exclusively of uniform polygonal cells with abundant cytoplasm replete with eosinophilic granules due to a greatly increased number of mitochondria. The nuclei are usually round or oval and very regular with a finely dispersed chromatin; the nucleoli are mostly small and inconspicuous. Mitotic figures are absent. There are no necroses. In some cases occasional oncocytes may be greatly enlarged with huge pleomorphic nuclei that may contain cytoplasmic inclusions. Multinucleation may be seen [431].

The cells are arranged in small- to medium-sized clusters and nests that sometimes contain centrally placed abortive lumina. Elaboration by the cells of distinct tubules is rare. The cell clusters are surrounded by delicate strands of a vascular stroma or by broad, edematous, loosely structured septae.

Renal oncocytomas must be distinguished from granular cell renal carcinoma. It is recommended that many samples from a single given tumor should be examined in order not to miss the clear cells of adenocarcinoma. If parts of the tumor contain clear cells, the diagnosis of a renal carcinoma has to be made.

Claims of metastasizing renal oncocytomas are in all probability based on unduly limited sampling. The presence of metastases, mitotic activity, prominent atypia, prominent papillary architecture, necroses, vascular invasion, and obvious local invasion favor the diagnosis of a renal cell carcinoma rather than that of an oncocytoma.

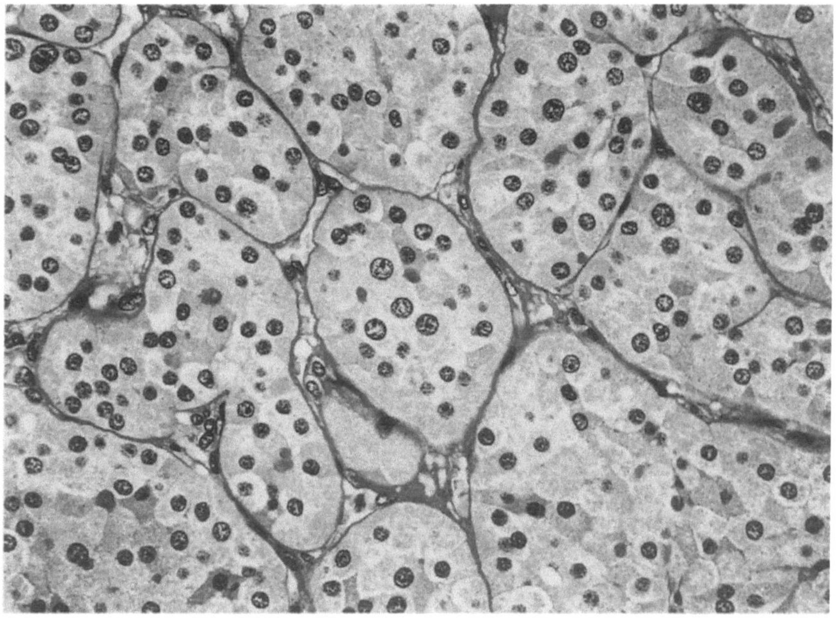

Fig. 11. Renal cell oncocytoma consisting exclusively of polygonal, finely granulated cells arranged in solid clusters. Mitoses are absent. H & E, ×350

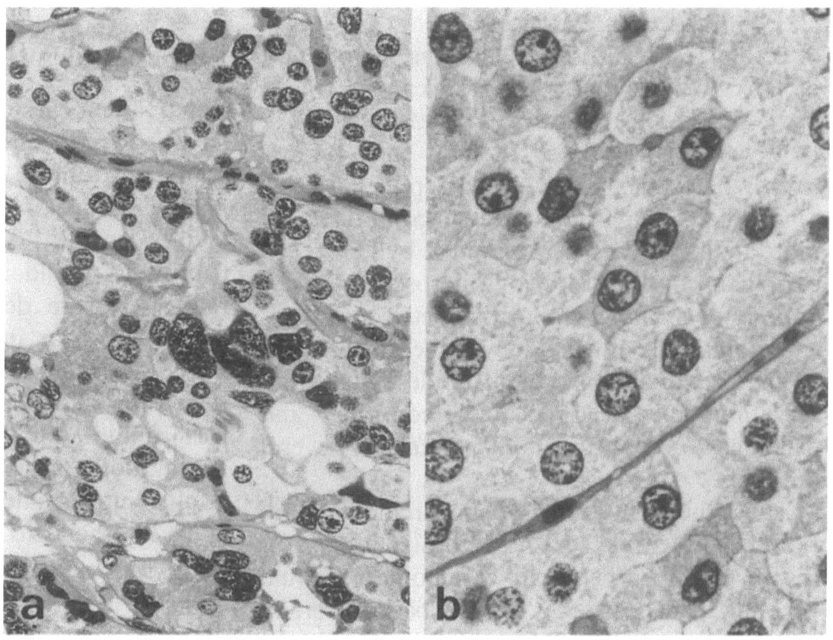

Fig. 12 a, b. Same case as Fig. 11. **(a)** In this area greatly enlarged cells with atypically appearing, multiple hyperchromatic nuclei are present. H & E, ×350. **(b)** At high magnification the characteristic eosinophilic granulation of the oncocytes can readily be demonstrated. H & E, ×880

The prognosis is excellent as has been documented by several authors in long-term studies [228, 284, 70]. Removal of the tumor is curative.

1.5.3 Renal Carcinoid

Primary carcinoid tumor of the kidney is a curiosity. At least eight examples are documented in the literature [277, 433]. They may occur in pure form [365] or in association with teratoid lesions [120]. Whereas the latter will not pose serious differential diagnostic problems, the pure form may be confused with granular adenocarcinoma of the kidney.

1.5.4 Renal Adenocarcinoma

1.5.4.1 Introduction

As the term hypernephroid carcinoma shows, adenocarcinoma of the kidney was formerly considered to be derived from occasional rests

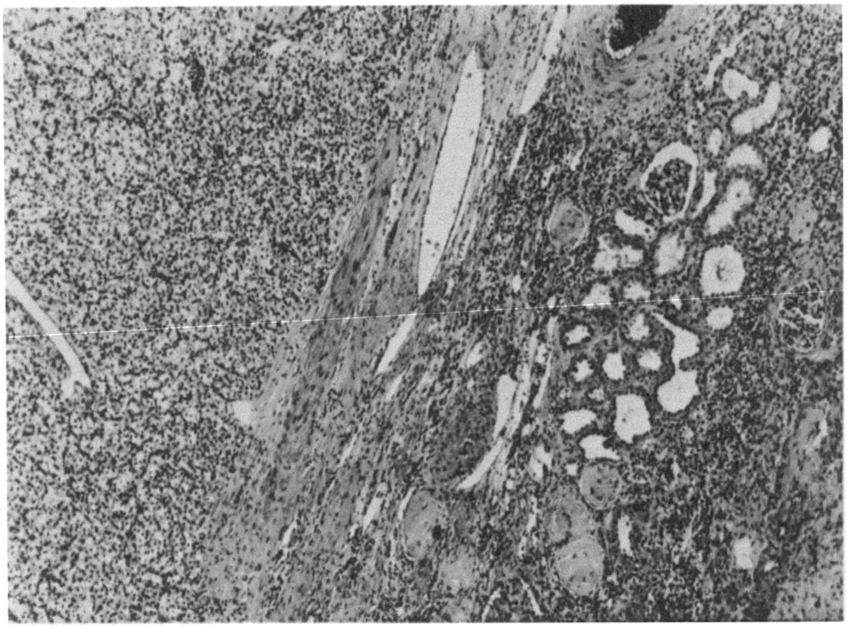

Fig. 13. Renal adenocarcinoma (*left*) in a kidney with severe chronic interstitial nephritis (*right*) due to abuse of phenacetin. H & E, × 56

of ectopic adrenal tissue. This was the opinion of GRAWITZ [149] and his view can be traced back to the cell rest theory of COHNHEIM [73]. However, SUDECK [382] thought such tumors to originate from renal tubular epithelial cells. Since then, heavy controversy continued for more than 70 years. It was ended by OBERLING et al. [304] by their electron-microscopic observations of striking similarities between adenocarcinoma cells of the kidney and epithelial cells of the proximal convoluted tubules. These observations have been repeatedly confirmed and extended to renal tumors of animals by several authors.

Thus, the term "renal adenocarcinoma" has become preferable. All other designations, for instance, "hypernephroid carcinoma," should be omitted because they do not pay due credit to the now well-established origin of renal adenocarcinoma from renal tubule cells. In addition, WALLACE and NAIRN [414] have shown that antibodies to brush border antigens specific for cells of the proximal convoluted tubules react uniformly with cells of renal adenocarcinomas and also with cells from so-called renal adenomas.

It may be mentioned here that there are some reports in the literature [80, 159] in which atypical carcinomas of the kidney are described that are thought to originate from the collecting duct epithelium.

1.5.4.2 Epidemiology

Renal adenocarcinoma is not very common, having a frequency of approximately 2% of all malignant tumors in the adult [114]. Most adenocarcinomas of the kidney occur in the 5th or 6th decade; however, the age range is from 6 months to old age [352, 27]. The incidence rate rises from decade to decade. The tumor may well occur in children as several reports have shown [302, 39, 92, 313, 322, 330]. On review of the literature, WALTER and VETTER [415] found 82 cases concerning children below the age of 16 years. Both in children and in adults, more males than females are afflicted [370, 39], the ratio being about 2:1.

1.5.4.3 Causes

Very little is known about the causes of renal adenocarcinoma. Small "adenomatous" growths usually develop in arteriosclerotic or contracted kidneys, that is to say, in the vicinity of scarring processes [56], or in kidneys "showing evidence of previous disease" [97]. In such cases small multiple adenomatous nodes that cannot be clearly separated from small renal adenocarcinomata are not rare. We have seen one case of renal adenocarcinoma within a kidney from a patient abusing phenacetin (Fig. 13). This case probably reflects a causative relationship between scars and adenocarcinoma rather than a direct relationship to phenacetin itself. The same may be true for the increased occurrence of renal cell tumors in endstage kidneys [196, 308].

There are several reports of adenocarcinoma originating in polycystic renal disease [49, 193, 278, 339, 74]. Tobacco users are said to show an increased frequency of renal adenocarcinomas [33]. Thus, the conditions above mentioned may be considered possible predispositions. However, no reliable data on this hypothesis are available as yet.

1.5.4.4 Paraneoplastic Syndromes

Patients commonly show fever, anemia, and an elevated sedimentation rate. It is not known whether or not or to what extent these features are due to regressive changes or are paraneoplastic syndromes. Interestingly, clear cell adenocarcinomas are reported to be more often associated with fever than are granular cell cases [43]. RAWLINS et al. [332] succeeded in extracting pyrogenic substances from tumor tissue.

Some cases show hypercalcemia not associated with skeletal metastases, and the calcium level decreases to normal after removal of the tumor [320, 143, 305, 395]. A salt-losing syndrome due to unilateral renal adenocarcinoma [239] has been described.

Polycythemia, possibly due to secretion of erythropoietin by the tumor [231], can be observed in about 3% of cases [183, 131, 103, 141, 220]. It disappears after nephrectomy [153, 85] but reappears with the advent of metastases [309], which clearly proves a definite relationship rather than a fortuitous combination. Moreover, it has been established statistically that erythrocytosis accompanies renal adenocarcinoma more frequently than other tumors [245]. Some cases may show an otherwise unexplainable hypertension [246]. Furthermore, leukemoid reactions, polyneuromyopathy, gastrointestinal disturbancies, and gynecomastia, as well as Cushing's syndrome and other endocrinologic disturbances have been reported.

STAUFFER'S syndrome comprising hepatomegaly and hepatic dysfunction has been observed in quite a number of renal adenocarcinomas [369, 205]. Liver biopsy usually discloses nonspecific findings such as "reactive hepatitis." Since the syndrome seems to be relatively frequent in renal adenocarcinoma [403], it may be a diagnostic aid in detecting hypernephroma. At any rate, unexplainable liver dysfunctions accompanied by "reactive hepatitis" should lead to an intensive search for occult renal adenocarcinoma.

Some patients develop amyloidosis. BERGER and SINKOFF [34] found an incidence of 2.9% amyloid deposits in renal adenocarcinoma. The deposits were located either in the tumor-bearing kidney or throughout the body in a distribution typical of secondary amyloidosis. DEYHLE [98] reviewed the literature and compiled 30 cases. Among all cases of amyloidosis that occur in association with malignant neoplasms, about 10%–25% concern adenocarcinomas of the kidney [44, 316].

1.5.4.5 Cytologic Diagnosis

Cytology may be successfully applied for the diagnosis of bladder cancer. It is also possible to demonstrate carcinomatous cells that stem from neoplasms of the renal pelvis or the ureter. However, the procedure is essentially of little value if one attempts to establish or to rule out the presence of adenocarcinoma of the renal parenchyma. This has been clearly shown by UMIKER [401] who found positive cytology only when the adenocarcinoma was far advanced. He detected malignant cells in 4 of 15 patients with known renal adenocarcinoma. FOOT et al. [127] saw tumor cells in only 5 of 60 cases with carcinoma of the kidney, and EVANS et al. [113] reported no positive cases among 55 patients. In the view of KOSS [232] tumors of the renal parenchyma away from the pelvis offer only a very slim chance of cytologic detection in the early stages. He, therefore, finds the urinary sediment to be of questionable value in diagnosing primary renal parenchymal cancers.

1.5.4.6 Renal Biopsy

In nonneoplastic kidney diseases, renal biopsy has become a routine method, but is usually not applied to patients with the clinical diagnosis of renal adenocarcinoma because of the possibility of tumor dissemination and hemorrhage. However, if a patient is at high surgical risk, renal biopsy may be required to achieve a cor-

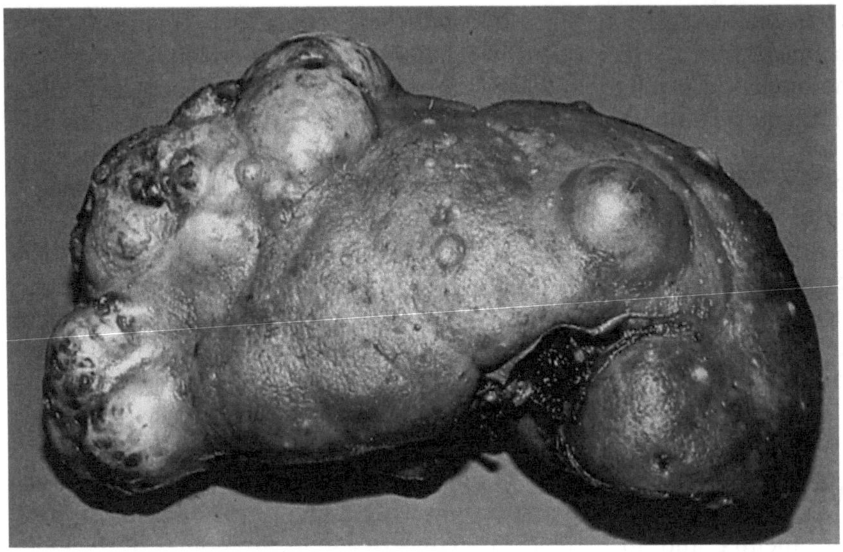

Fig. 14. Kidney of a 70-year-old female showing multiple nodules of different sizes some of which are cystic. Histologically, all nodes disclosed the same plant cell-like cells typical for renal adenocarcinoma. It could not be decided which of the nodes was primary and which were secondary

rect tissue diagnosis that can serve as a basis for palliative radiation therapy or chemotherapy.

1.5.4.7 Gross Pathology

Renal adenocarcinoma affects both kidneys with equal frequency [151]. There are some writers who reported a predilection for the upper part of the kidney. However, comparison of many articles shows that the localization is most likely random, or perhaps the middle portion is somewhat more commonly affected [138]. In about 1% of cases bilateral tumors are found. Approximately 5% of patients have multiple tumors (Fig. 14) in the same kidney [291]. Certainly one could argue that bilateral tumors as well as multiple tumors might be metastases and secondary to one single adenocarcinoma. This problem cannot be solved as yet because there are no histologic criteria that help in differentiating between metastases to the same or opposite kidney and multiple independent primary carcinomas.

The size of the tumors varies greatly. As has already been pointed out, there are tumors less than 3 cm in diameter. However, the largest tumors may reach a size of much more than 10 cm, and a few attain giant proportions. There is no firm relationship between the size of the tumor and the presence and duration of symptoms. This is shown by the observation of NEWMAN and SCHULMAN [301]. These authors found that in a series of 22 renal adenocarcinomas discovered incidentally, half of the tumors were already greater than 9 cm in diameter at the time of diagnosis.

The gross aspect of adenocarcinoma of the kidney is usually quite the same irrespective of size. In most cases one finds a protruding tumor that represents an irregular mass consisting of several irregularly formed nodes evoking a lobular appearance (Fig. 15). The cut surface is characteristically variegated, but the tumors are predominantly yellowish orange. Very often one finds hemorrhages, and the cut surface bulges because of proliferation pressure. If the tumor contains large amounts of lipid, a pale yellow or orange hue will be pronounced. If, on the other hand, the tumor is more sarcomatoid, the cut surface will have a grey or whitish color. Necrotic parts are dry, yellow, or grey. Old necroses will change to cystic spaces with fibrous walls. Old hemorrhages will contain hemosiderin, which adds a brownish tinge. There may be extensive scarring and foci of calcification.

Usually, the tumors compress the renal parenchyma at their peripheries. This results in the formation of a flimsy pseudocapsule, consisting of a condensed thin layer of connective tissue replacing the atrophic renal parenchyma. Dissection of the calyces may demonstrate tumor infiltration along these channels. Invasion of the main renal vein can be commonly seen, and sometimes cast-like masses of a tumor-throm-

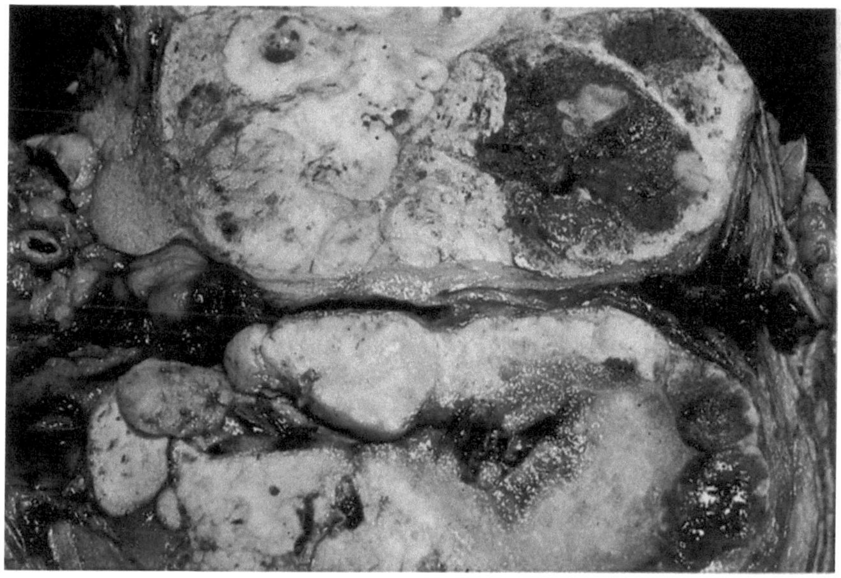

Fig. 15. Cut surface of a typical renal adenocarcinoma with whitish or slightly tan areas and large necroses with hemorrhage. There is but a small rest of renal parenchyma to the *right*. Adrenal tissue can be seen to the *left*. The tumor weight was 580 g. There was infiltration of the perirenal adipose tissue and renal pelvis (56-year-old female)

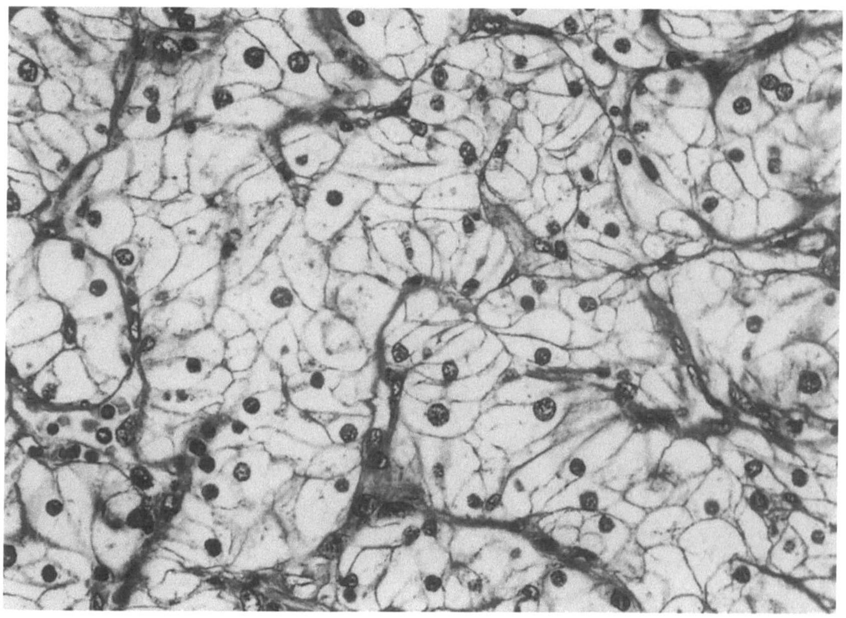

Fig. 16. Renal adenocarcinoma with a solid growth pattern formed by sheets of polygonal clear cells interrupted by a delicate fibrous stromal tissue containing thin-walled blood vessels. H & E, ×350

bus may extend into the lumen of the inferior vena cava.

In summary, the gross appearance of renal adenocarcinoma shows a large variety of macroscopical criteria, and it is this variety that makes a renal adenocarcinoma so grossly characteristic.

1.5.4.8 Histopathology

There is a very wide range of structural variations in renal adenocarcinomas. Not only do the microscopic features vary from case to case but also to a greater or lesser degree from area to area in the same growth. This can be readily shown when large sections or multiple sections are prepared from the same neoplasm. Many histologic classifications have been proposed that, of course, have brought about nothing but confusion and have obscured the unifying features of renal adenocarcinomas.

The classic form is a growth made up of relatively large cells with a clear "empty" cytoplasm due to a high content of lipids and glycogen (Fig. 16). Since both of these substances are

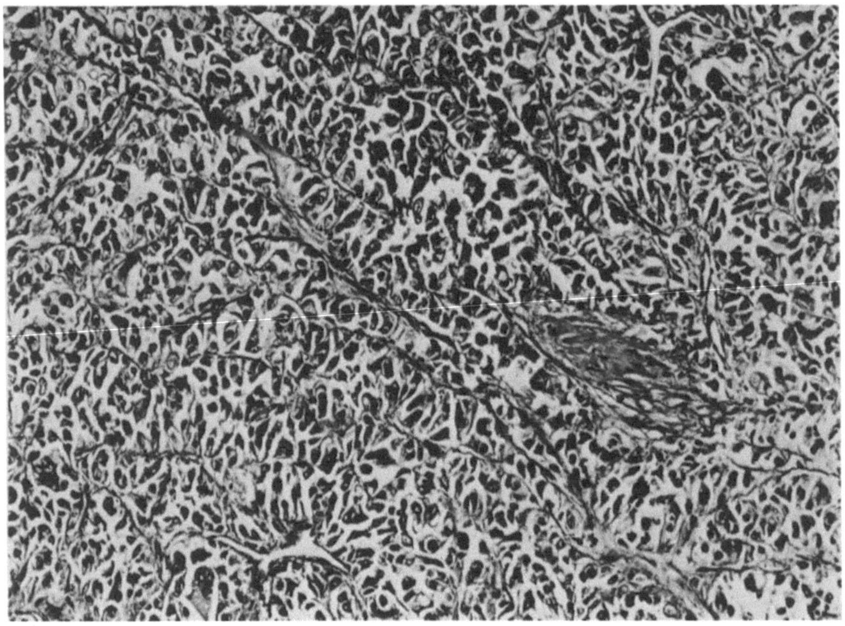

Fig. 17. In this renal adenocarcinoma a trabecular pattern can be seen made up of cylindroid cells with moderate anaplasia. H & E, ×140

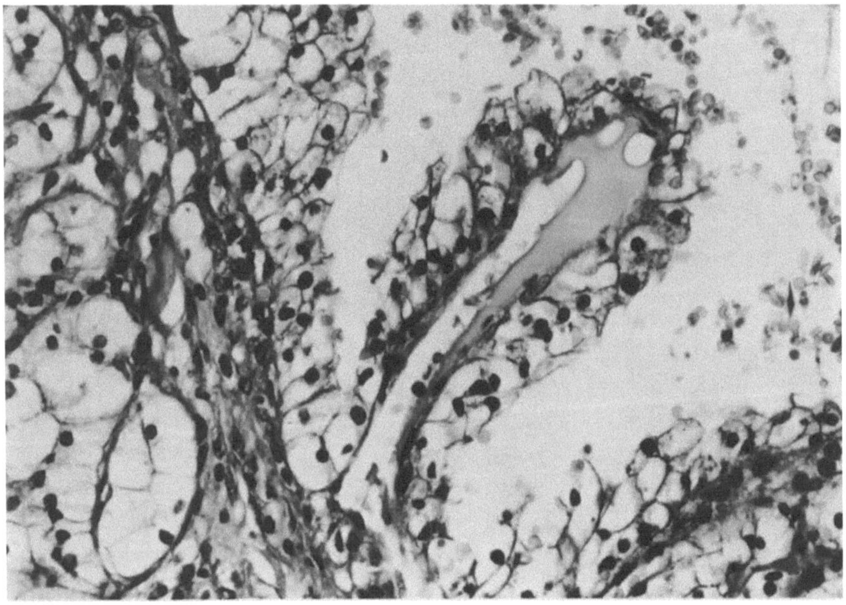

Fig. 18. Adenocarcinoma of the renal cortex with clear cells covering papillary processes. H & E, ×350

dissolved during the histologic embedding process, the microscopist will find clear plant cell-like cells with fairly well recognizable cell borders that, of course, are not cell membranes but represent small rims of cytoplasmic components other than glycogen and lipids. The cells are arranged in a solid alveolar fashion, a lace-like manner, sheets, trabeculi (Fig. 17), and papillary processes (Fig. 18), and sometimes there are even tubules. The form of the cells is usually polygonal, cuboidal, or columnar, and the cytoplasm is relatively broad. The nuclei are usually and characteristically small. They have a dense chromatin and stain uniformly. Their shape is relatively regular and round. There are rarely giant cells (Fig. 19). Mitoses can hardly be found.

The stroma is often very delicate and scanty, consisting only of a few fibers that are found together with many thin-walled capillary ves-

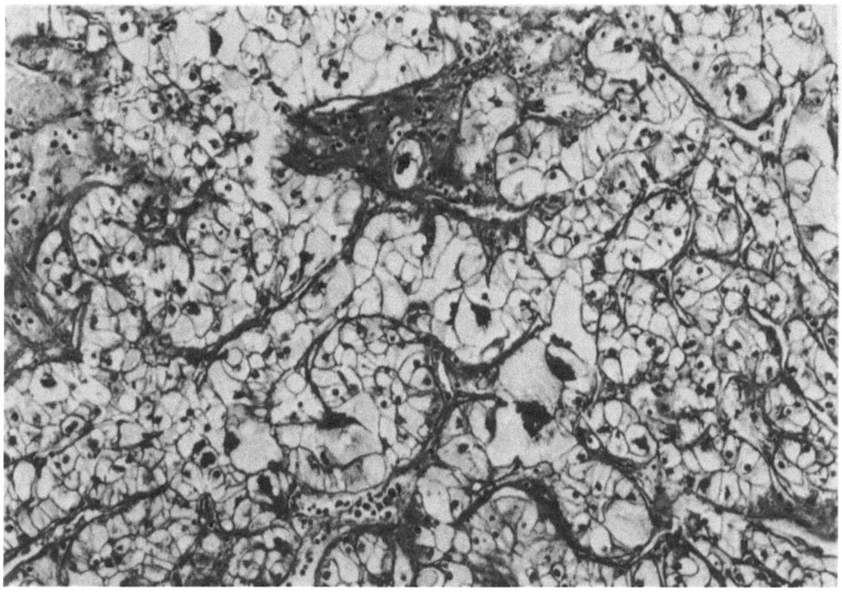

Fig. 19. Renal adenocarcinoma with large, clear, plant cell-like cells some of which have attained giant proportions and are multinucleated. H & E, ×140

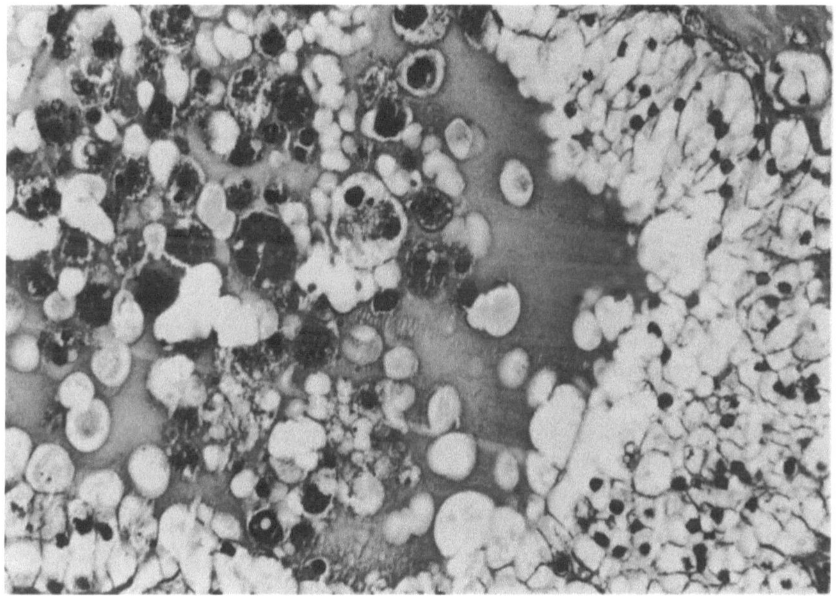

Fig. 20. Cystic renal adenocarcinoma. The cyst walls are covered by clear cells. The lumen contains a colloidlike mass together with many hemosiderin-laden macrophages indicating previous hemorrhage. H & E, ×350

sels. Sometimes these appear as dilated sinusoids. Since the vessels within the tumor are very thin-walled, blood will leak relatively often into the tumor tissue. This accounts for the many hemosiderin-containing macrophages that can be constantly found within histologic sections of renal carcinoma (Fig. 20). However, not only may macrophages contain hemosiderin but the tumor cells themselves also take up this substance (Fig. 21). Hemosiderin-laden tumor cells, therefore, can be observed relatively frequently in this kind of cancer.

While in many cases clear cells make up the bulk of the tumor, there are examples in which the cells have a finely granular eosinophilic cytoplasm (Fig. 22). This appearance is due to large numbers of mitochondria. On close examination one will find granular cells in nearly every renal cancer. Often tubules, trabeculi, or papillary processes are lined by a mixture of clear and granular cells. Transitions between clear cells and granular cells can readily be found. EVANS [114] felt that neoplasms predominantly composed of granular cells would grow

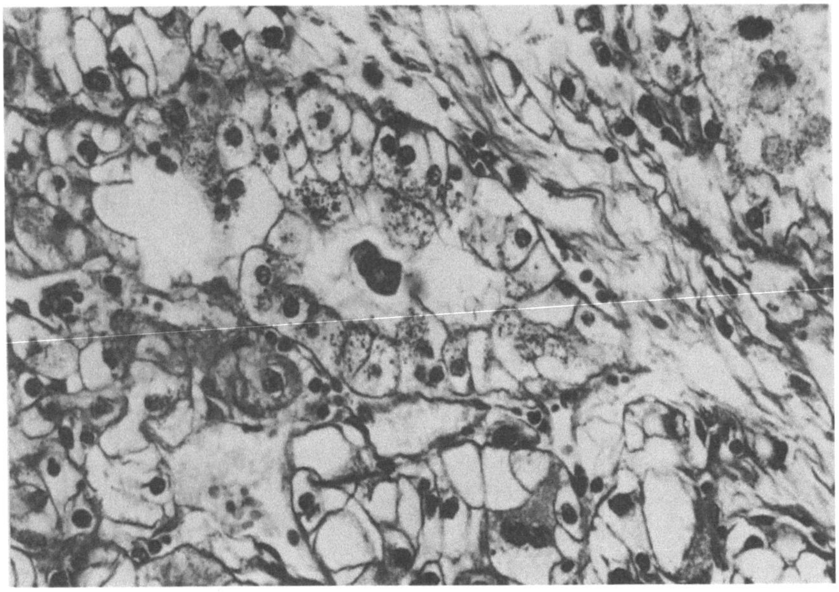

Fig. 21. Renal adenocarcinoma with a slight tendency of tubule formation. The clear cells around the *center* of the photograph contain finely granulated deposits of hemosiderin due to preceding hemorrhage. H & E, ×350

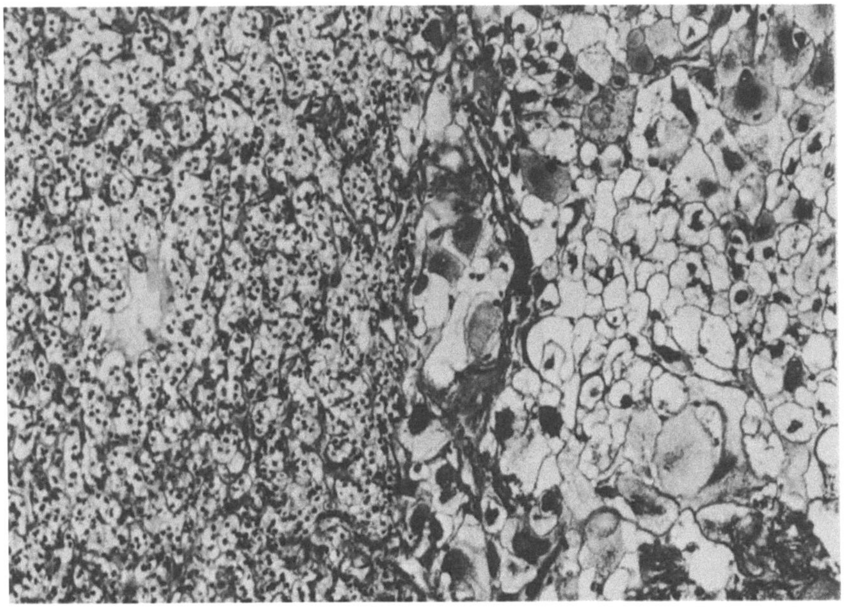

Fig. 22. Renal adenocarcinoma with two distinctively different tumor cell populations: small clear cells to the *left* and huge anaplastic, partly granulated cells to the *right*. H & E, ×140

more rapidly than those consisting of clear cells. However, he believed this to be only a general rule with many exceptions.

If an adenocarcinoma of the kidney histologically consists of a mainly papillary growth, then the stroma of the papillary processes may contain foam cells. These are histiocytes that have phagocytized lipid material.

Very rarely a compact tubulopapillary pattern or even a pronounced tubular pattern is observed which in a way mimics the convoluted tubules of the normal kidney. There may be a colloidlike eosinophilic mass within such tubular spaces (Fig. 23).

In some very malignant cases, sarcoma-like structures may predominate (Fig. 24). Here papillary, tubular, or clear cell elements, in other words typical features of adenocarcinoma of the kidney, can be found only after prolonged search. If, in such cases, only a few samples of tumor tissue are histologically investigated, the correct diagnosis may be missed and the tumor may be erroneously interpreted as sarcoma. Sarcomatoid renal carcinomas are very

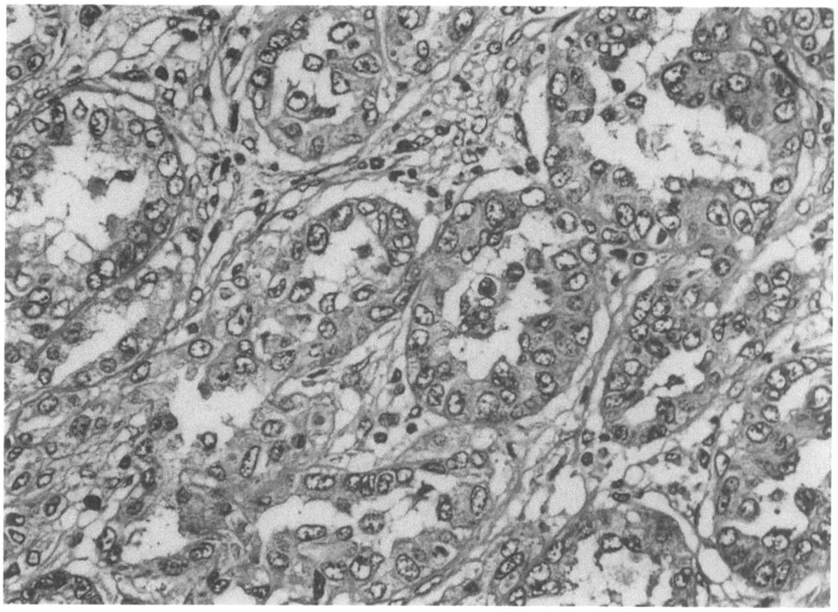

Fig. 23. Renal adenocarcinoma with pronounced formation of tubular structures resembling convoluted tubules. This differentiation occurs extremely rarely. H & E, ×350

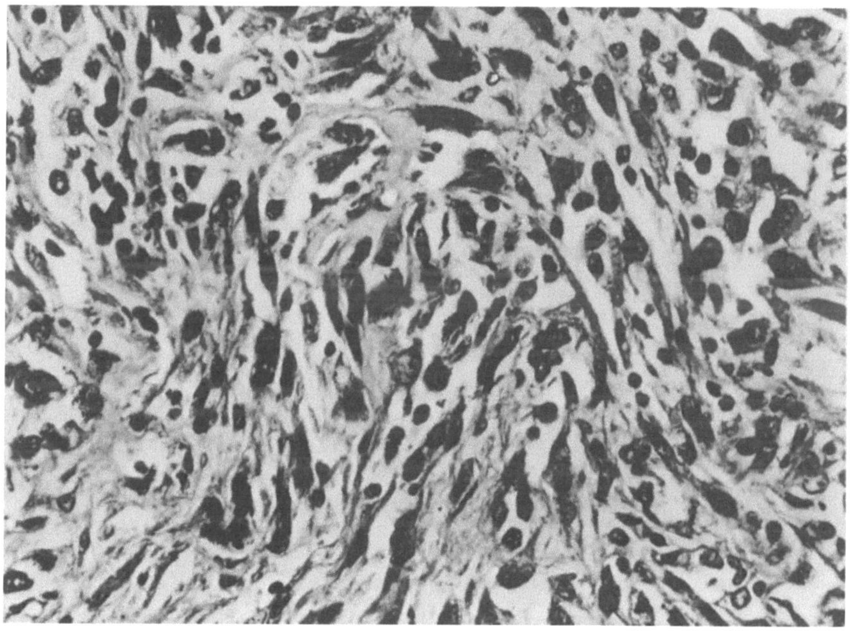

Fig. 24. Typical sarcomatoid renal adenocarcinoma. H & E, ×350

aggressive and have a poor prognosis. Therefore, they may be treated vigorously by adjuvant chemotherapy and/or irradiation [396].

Interestingly enough, Hou and Willis [191] found areas in very poorly differentiated adenocarcinomas of the kidney that simulated osteosarcoma. This makes the occurrence of primary osteosarcoma in the kidney very questionable, as has been explained above. Whatever the case, since the kidney is of mesodermal origin, it must principally be expected that epithelial growths as well as sarcomatous growths can develop and that both kinds of differentiation may appear together as described. It may be added that the publications on primary osteosarcoma of the kidney cited above involved without exception the elderly; this fact also favors the view that these neoplasms originate from renal mesodermal structures and have nothing to do with primary osteogenic sarcomas of the skeleton.

Not rarely, one finds foci of calcification (Fig. 25), sometimes in the form of scattered psammoma bodies. There may be a cartilaginous or osseous metaplasia of the stroma. In

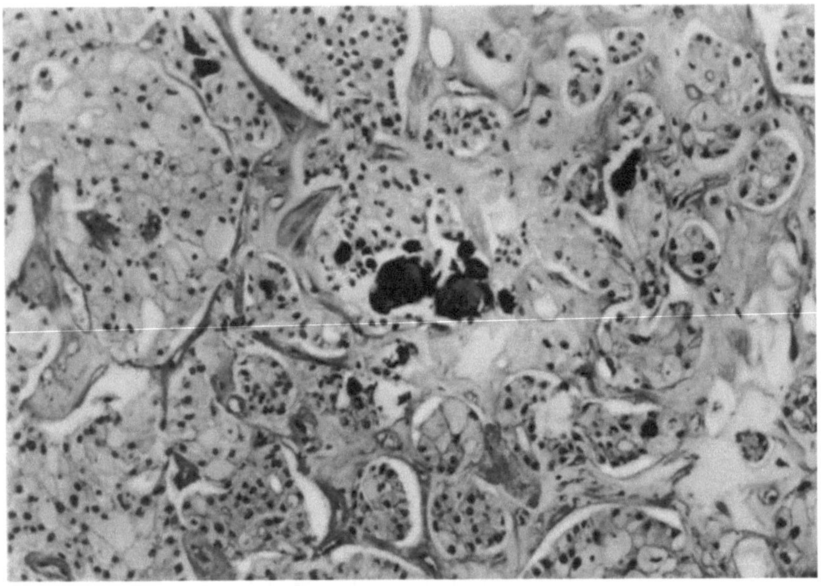

Fig. 25. Renal adenocarcinoma with slightly granulated tumor cells and microcalcifications. H & E, ×140

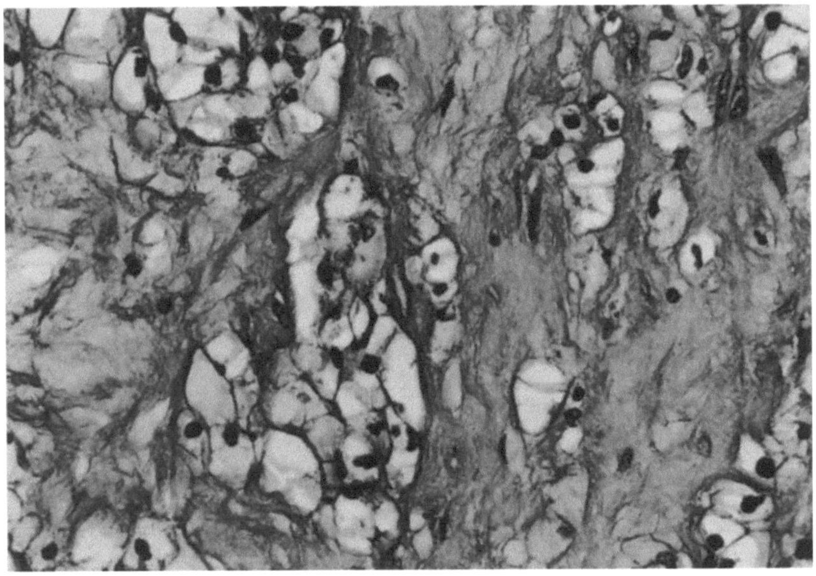

Fig. 26. Dense hyalinized stroma entrapping clear cells of renal adenocarcinoma. H & E, ×140

older necroses, cholesterol crystals may be formed due to the high lipid content of the tumor cells. Since cholesterol crystals will be dissolved by the usual histologic preparation, only crystalloid clefts are seen. These are usually surrounded by foreign body giant cells. Necroses and hemorrhage produce marked fibrosis and the formation of dense hyalinized collagenous tissue (Fig. 26).

A rare macroscopic variant is termed "multilocular cystic renal adenocarcinoma" characterized by particularly thick-walled cysts that are lined by carcinomatous cells; TAKEUCHI et al. [388] found 12 cases in the literature. The lesions probably represent carcinomas with pronounced cystic degeneration rather than cysts with secondary malignant transformation [349].

1.5.4.9 Histologic Differential Diagnosis

Renal adenocarcinomas may be very uniform in their histologic appearances and, moreover, are often characterized by their typical cells, which resemble plant cells. However, there are many deviations from this average histologic picture: some cases may resemble a variety of other conditions.

A histologic differential diagnosis is given below that can be used to differentiate renal adenocarcinoma from other renal neoplasms or disorders and from metastatic renal disease. The following conditions are included: true renal sarcoma, histiocytic tumors, nephroblastoma, secondary carcinoma including pleomorphic transitional cell carcinoma as well as clear cell carcinoma of the renal pelvis, malakoplakia, and xanthogranulomatous pyelonephritis.

Sarcomas and Renal Adenocarcinomas. If spindle cells and multinucleated giant cells can be found, then rhabdomyosarcoma must be considered. In this case myofibrils or cross-striation must be searched for. If intracellular lipids can be demonstrated by appropriate fat stains, a sarcomatoid renal adenocarcinoma is more probable than a true sarcoma. In such a case more material should be investigated to find areas in which the tumor may be clearly differentiated in the way of a typical adenocarcinoma. As has been proposed by TANNENBAUM [390], electron-microscopic investigations may assist in the differential diagnosis of difficult cases; this is possible even with cases in which only wet formalin-fixed material is available because sarcomatoid-appearing epithelial cells do retain certain epithelial ultrastructural features.

In any case, before the diagnosis of primary renal sarcoma is made, irrespective of the subtype, an exhaustive investigation of the whole tumor for foci of adenocarcinoma with the preparation of many blocks and sections should be performed. BENNINGTON and BECKWITH [31] have found that the majority of tumors called "renal sarcoma" were really sarcomatoid adenocarcinomas after very thorough examinations had been carried out on review.

Histiocytic Tumors and Renal Adenocarcinomas. It is very seldom that tumors of the histiocytoma group involve the renal parenchyma. They may be separated from carcinoma by the tendency to form compact cellular masses consisting of histiocytic cells, giant cells, and fibrous cells and by the lack of any tendency to form tubular or papillary structures.

Nephroblastomas and Renal Adenocarcinomas. Usually nephroblastomas and renal adenocarcinomas can be distinguished very easily because nephroblastoma is characterized by its typical triphasic histologic pattern, which is made up of (1) a background of mesenchymal spindle cells that surround (2) focal collections of renal blastema and (3) epithelial components (see Sect. 2).

Secondary Carcinomas and Renal Adenocarcinomas. Carcinoma of the renal pelvis may infiltrate the renal parenchyma. If the pelvic carcinoma is of the clear cell type, then it may be very difficult to separate this tumor from adenocarcinoma of the kidney. However, we believe that if enough sections of a given tumor have been investigated, typically differentiated areas will usually be found that disclose its origin. Nevertheless, there may be some isolated cases in which the differential diagnosis cannot be made.

Carcinomas of other organs such as breast, lung and intestine metastasize to the kidney with varying frequency. WAGLE et al. [413] reviewed 81 cases of secondary carcinoma of the kidney that were detected in a survey of 4413 autopsies, indicating an incidence of about 2%. Lungs, stomach, breast, and the contralateral kidney were the common primary locations of the parental growths in approximately 43% of the 81 cases. BENNINGTON and BECKWITH [31] have pointed out that patients with carcinoma at autopsy disclose metastases to the kidney in about 5% of cases, and BRACKEN et al. [51] found metastatic disease of the kidney in 7.2% of 11328 autopsies performed on patients who died of malignant disease. This is approximately two or three times as frequent as the incidence of renal adenocarcinoma. Therefore, the possibility of a secondary neoplasm in the case of a renal tumor should be kept in mind.

Malakoplakia and Renal Adenocarcinoma. Malakoplakia is a relatively rare condition that may involve a variety of organs. There are some reports of malakoplakia of the renal parenchyma [81, 31] and of the renal pelvis. The condition may mimic carcinoma very closely, especially macroscopically.

The typical feature of malakoplakia is the occurrence of Michaelis-Gutmann bodies (Fig. 27a). These are deposited within proliferating macrophages that possess broad and sometimes clear cytoplasms, so that confusion with renal carcinoma may be made by the unwary: malakoplakia is very rare and not every pathologist may have experience with this condition [237].

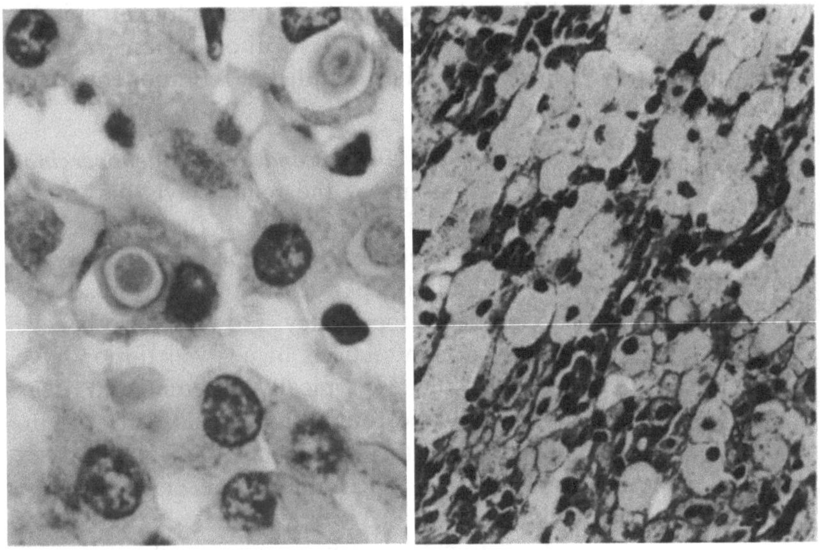

a b

Fig. 27. (a) Malakoplakia. Note the large macrophages that contain Michaelis-Gutmann bodies one of which can be seen very clearly at the *center*. H & E, ×1200. **(b)** Xanthogranulomatous pyelonephritis with many foam cells. Note the typical stippling of the cytoplasm that cannot be found to this extent in cells of renal adenocarcinoma. Many lymphocytes and plasma cells are located in between the foam cells. H & E, ×140

Xanthogranulomatous Pyelonephritis and Renal Adenocarcinomas. This differential diagnostic possibility is mentioned in most textbooks of pathology. We consider the probability of confusion of these two conditions of minor importance because in xanthogranulomatous pyelonephritis inflammatory changes predominate sufficiently as to prevent its misinterpretation as a renal adenocarcinoma. In xanthogranulomatous pyelonephritis many foam cells may be found that occasionally may resemble clear cells of renal adenocarcinoma. However, under close examination the finely vacuolated macrophages of pyelonephritis bear little resemblance to the carcinomatous clear cells (Fig. 27b).

1.5.4.10 Grading

Most authorities believe that microscopic features do not help very much in assessing prognostic statements concerning renal adenocarcinoma. Usually, the tumors are remarkably well differentiated.

MOSTOFI [294] stated that extensive grading is both difficult and of very little value. He, therefore, distinguished only two kinds of renal adenocarcinoma, namely well-differentiated cases and poorly differentiated cases. The prognostic significance of microscopic features other than differentiation has also been investigated with poor results. The prognosis of renal adenocarcinoma can be much better assessed if tumor size, extent of local invasion, vascular involvement, and metastases are taken into consideration [125, 318].

We would like to emphasize here the relative value and the statistical character of grading procedures. In the individual case all consequences must be based on a thoroughly prepared pathology report that includes the grade of malignancy as only one of a host of prognostic parameters. Thereby, the clinician is informed both about the grade of malignancy *and* about all the other no less important particular findings. It is only the synopsis of the total of these criteria that should serve as a therapeutic and prognostic guideline. An isolated use of the grading cipher alone is unwise: according to JONAS et al. [214], the histological degree of malignancy as a single prognostic parameter is of little informational value. At any rate, grading results should not be used without reflection and should by no means be viewed as a comfortable substitute for the thorough study of a surgical pathology report.

Two examples of grading proposals will be given here. According to HERMANEK et al. [184], all "adenomas," together with carcinomas composed of clear cells and presenting a solid growth pattern, should be labelled "grade I," which expresses a good prognosis. Cases with exclusively granular pattern or papillary growths as well as sarcomalike cancers should be labelled "grade III," indicative of a bad outcome. All other cases represent "grade II" malignancies.

However, there is nothing new about this, since FOOT and HUMPREYS [126] stated already that renal tumors of a low grade of malignancy are well encapsulated and consist of clear cells that are regularly arranged and possess uniform nuclei devoid of mitotic activity. Principally, the same was found by SKINNER et al. [362] who studied 329 patients with renal carcinoma, applying a grading procedure based mainly on nuclear morphology: in grade I, nuclei are indistinguishable from those of normal tubular cells; in grade II, there are slightly irregular, often pyknotic nuclei without abnormal nucleoli; in grade III there are moderately enlarged, irregular, pleomorphic nuclei with large nucleoli; in grade IV one finds numerous bizarre giant nuclei. The result was that pure clear cell carcinomas have a better prognosis than have granular and mixed forms, and that spindle cell types have the worst prognosis, which, in addition, worsens with increasing nuclear grade of malignancy. AMTRUP et al. [11] also found the best prognosis for clear cell tumors without necroses and a poor prognosis for granular cell carcinomas.

In summary, it is clear that the more undifferentiated, the more pleomorphic, and the greater the mitotic activity of a given adenocarcinoma, the more likely it will behave as highly malignant: but only in terms of statistics, which need not apply to the individual patient!

1.5.4.11 Staging

There are various staging systems that describe the spread of a given tumor at nephrectomy simply by means of Roman numerals. Staging procedures can thus be defined as an attempt to transform very complicated individual situations that vary considerably from case to case into a simple and handy, but unfortunately unbiologic and crude system. One must see clearly the disadvantages of such systems, which lie in the substitution of thoroughly prepared pathologic and histologic reports that include all necessary details by terms like "stage I" or "stage IV," etc. "Stages" are abstracted experience and, therefore, appropriate first of all for statistical analyses. Nevertheless, each of these stages implies differing therapeutic consequences and may be used as guidelines in this respect. However, the statistical character of stages certainly obscures the individual state of a given case, which must always be kept in mind.

The staging system of ROBSON et al. [342] is given here. In stage I the tumor is confined to the kidney and located within the capsule. Stage II includes invasion of the perinephric fatty tissue, while stage III is more advanced as the regional lymph nodes and/or the renal vein and the inferior vena cava are affected. Stage IV is applied when adjacent organs are infiltrated or distant metastases can be diagnosed.

Understandably, the prognosis worsens from stage to stage. VARKARAKIS et al. [407] found the following 5-year survival figures: stage I, 55%; stage II and stage III, 21%; and stage IV, 10%. It must be stressed once more that these figures are only valid in terms of statistics and need not be true in the individual case. The introduction of staging for renal carcinoma is only an abbreviation of a pathology report but no progress in itself. Hence, it can give no more and indeed provides less information than a thoroughly prepared surgical pathology report that, however, the clinician must be willing to read and be able to understand.

1.5.4.12 Spread

At autopsy most patients with renal adenocarcinoma show widespread metastases. The most commonly involved organ is the lung; lymph nodes, liver, bones, adrenals, opposite kidney, brain, heart, spleen, intestine, and skin follow with decreasing frequency in this order [32].

Usually, spread of renal adenocarcinoma follows three main routes: direct extension into the surrounding tissue, lymphogenous spread chiefly to the regional lymph nodes, and hematogenous spread in which embolic cells will pass through the renal veins. MACDONALD and PRIESTLEY [275] found an incidence of 54% venous invasion by the tumor in a study of 509 adenocarcinomas.

Since the para-aortic lymph nodes are located near the cysterna chyli, tumor cells may gain access to the thoracic duct. Then they may enter the vena cava superior via the thoracic duct and reach the pulmonary circulation. Still another route of spread is important, i.e., via the paravertebral venous plexus. The proximity of the kidney to this plexus seems to be the cause of the high frequency of vertebral metastases in patients with renal adenocarcinoma.

It has long been known that adenocarcinoma of the kidney produces metastases of very unusual location and presentation [for review see 417]. For example, metastases in the scalp may mimic hemangioma or a sweat gland tumor [167]. Metastases to the breast occurring many years after nephrectomy may simulate primary mammary carcinoma. Metastases to the tonsils [60], vagina [296], orbit [208], tongue [94], larynx, and heart have all been reported.

An exhaustive and excellent description of the differential diagnosis of metastases of renal adenocarcinoma is given by BENNINGTON and BECKWITH [31] to which the reader is referred. In this context it may be mentioned that tumors such as sebaceus carcinoma, nodular hidradenoma, occasional cases of malignant melanoma, mucoepidermoid carcinoma, acinic cell carcinoma of the salivary glands, some types of oligodendroglioma, clear cell carcinomas of the ovary and thyroid, and, of course, tumors of the adrenal gland may all exhibit considerable similarity to renal adenocarcinoma and vice versa.

1.5.4.13 Prognosis

Despite the fact that renal adenocarcinoma usually grows slowly, the prognosis is poor with an overall survival rate of approximately 20%–25% 10 years after nephrectomy [218]. However, if the cancer is confined to the kidney a 60% 5-year and a 50% 10-year survival rate can be achieved; venous invasion or perirenal extension halves the survival rate [219]. This was not fully confirmed by SKINNER et al. [362], who found no significant prognostic influence of involvement of the renal veins, whereas involvement of the perirenal fat or regional nodes gravely influenced prognosis. They observed an overall survival rate of 44% at 5 years and of 33% at 10 years. If no metastases were present when first seen for treatment, the 5-year survival was 57% and the 10-year survival was 44%.

While one must say that the overall 10-year survival rate of about 25%–33% makes the prognosis for the patient himself poor, these survival rates are remarkably high if one takes into consideration that most patients have had symptoms for a period as long as 1.8 years before they seek medical aid [147]. The survival rates are even more remarkable if one considers that the average size of renal adenocarcinomas is between 5–7.5 cm at nephrectomy [336, 380]. From these facts, BENNINGTON and BECKWITH [31] drew the conclusion that the survival rates in renal adenocarcinoma are not at all discouraging but should lead to considerable efforts to develop techniques that will aid the diagnosis of renal adenocarcinoma at an earlier and, thus, more curable stage.

No significant relationship exists between prognosis and age, sex, and presence of calcification. Local invasion, e.g., extension of the tumor beyond the renal capsule, in contrast, influences the prognosis negatively. The same is true for size of the tumor and presence of regional lymph node metastases, while the influence of renal vein invasion is not quite clear (see above).

MANCILLA-JIMENEZ et al. [267] reported on 34 papillary variants of 224 renal carcinomas. They found by angiography a tendency to avascularity. Most of the cases (85.3%) were in stage I, and many of them were massively necrotic. The survival rate was higher than that for nonpapillary tumors. However, such a positive connection between papillary differentiation and a favourable prognosis remains debatable, since the number of the cases was much too small for statistically significant statements concerning this question. Nevertheless, BOCZKO et al. [42] confirmed the better prognosis of papillary variants, although their series comprised only 6 cases.

If distant metastases exist at the time of nephrectomy, which is reported to be the case in approximately 40% of patients [336, 294], the prognosis is naturally poor. However, exceptions to this have been reported, for instance with surgically resectable solitary metastases [379, 335]. In other cases, metastatic activity may not be forthcoming until 10–15 years following the removal of the growth. Thus, TAKATS and CZAPO [387] reported on a case in which fatal metastases developed only 37 years after diagnosis, and KRADJIAN and BENNINGTON [234] published a case that recurred 31 years after nephrectomy. Rarely, pulmonary metastases may regress after removal of the primary tumor [207, 162]. MATHIAS [273] compiled 20 such cases from the literature and added one further.

2 Renal Neoplasias of Infancy and Childhood

2.1 Nephroblastoma

2.1.1 General Remarks

Nephroblastoma (Wilms' tumor) is a malignant embryonal tumor of the kidney that originates from metanephrogenic blastema. Since metanephrogenic blastema consists of mesoblastic stroma and primitive nephrogenic epithelia, abnormal proliferation of this blastema will produce a mixed tumor (adenosarcoma, carcinosarcoma). The differentiation of the two components will result in epithelial and mesenchymal structures that are found in various stages of maturation in a given tumor. In consequence, each of the tumors will elaborate almost an individual pattern. One may find adipose tissue, cartilaginous tissue, bony tissue, smooth and cross-striated muscle, together with undifferentiated blastema, and rosettelike or tubular differentiated epithelial carcinomatous structures. Altogether, the classical Wilms' tumor is triphasic and consists of (1) epithelial cells in various stages of differentiation, (2) undifferentiated parts of the blastema, and (3) a mesenchymal stromal component.

In rare cases, a given tumor may be composed mainly or exclusively of one of these structural components. Such monophasic nephroblastomas differ from the classical Wilms' tumor not only morphologically but also clinically; they are much more aggressive if sarcomatous and less aggressive if epithelial. Accordingly, these special forms are nowadays separated from the "classical" nephroblastomas.

2.1.2 Epidemiology

Of all malignant neoplasms in children below the age of 15 years 6% are Wilms' tumors. Nevertheless, the incidence of Wilms' tumors in this population is relatively low, namely six to seven cases per million of children per year [430].

The morbidity is very constant: the tumor appears approximately in 1 of 200000 children below the age of 14 years in every nation and race, which has made it possible to use Wilms' tumor as the classical "index cancer" [202, 288]. The peak incidence is found in the second year of life, 50% of cases manifest themselves before the third year, and approximately 80% before the fifth year [190]. According to LEMERLE et al. [250], the average age at the time of diagnosis is 35 months.

An analysis of 1106 cases of Wilms' tumors showed that 13.4% concerned children who where younger than 1 year, and 49 cases (4.4%) were found in adults [227]. However, Wilms' tumor in adults is definitely rare, and its true incidence is hard to determine. BABAIAN et al. [17] found 167 cases in the literature between 1878 and 1980. Wilms' tumors do not show a significant sex preponderance.

2.1.3 Cause

The cause of Wilms' tumor is not known. However, the worldwide constancy of its frequency suggests that environmental factors, racial differences, viral endemic or epidemic causes, and carcinogenic substances probably do not influence its development. Rather, genetic factors may play an important etiologic role, since nephroblastomas occur together with several kinds of malformation syndromes such as aniridia, trisomy 18, hemihypertrophy, and Beckwith-Wiedemann syndrome, as well as together with anomalies of the urinary tract [31, 145]. In cases of bilateral Wilms' tumor, genetic anomalies are observed approximately ten times more frequently [46].

Furthermore, genetic influences are indicated by the occurrence of this tumor in siblings, in monozygous twins, and in consecutive generations of one family [137, 55, 280]. The role of nodular renal blastema as a forerunner of Wilms' tumor must be seriously considered, since renal blastemas occur fifty times more frequently in patients with nephroblastoma than in patients without this lesion [46].

2.1.4 Gross Pathology

Unilateral Wilms' tumors affect the left kidney slightly more frequently than the right [249]. Bilateral tumors can be found in approximately 4% of cases. Sometimes bilateral nephroblastomas show a multifocal or multicentric origin (Fig. 28).

Extrarenal nephroblastomas have been observed, but are extremely rare. AKHTAR et al. [8]

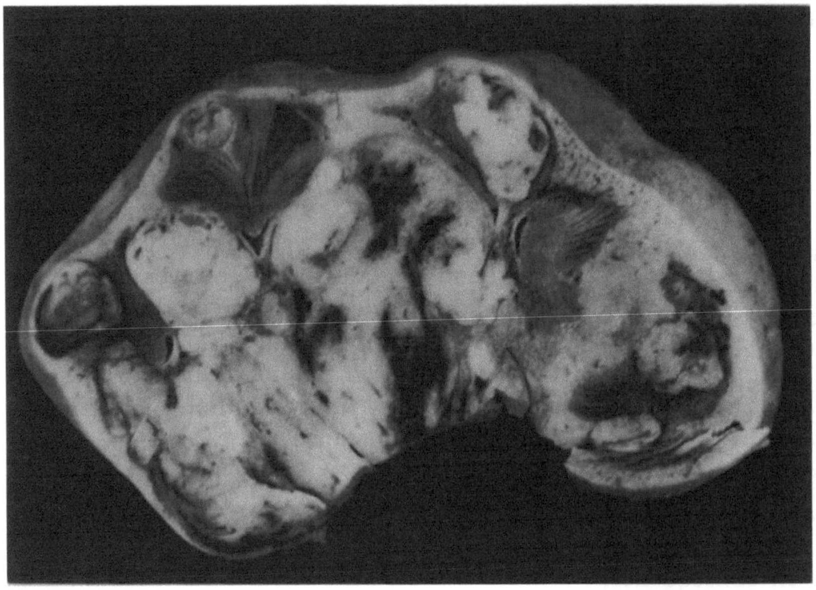

Fig. 28. Multicentric nephroblastoma with several tumor nodes in the cortex and in the medulla

found ten such cases, four of which originated from a teratoma whereas the remainder may have taken their origin from displaced embryonal rests of the mesonephros. Since then, some additional cases have been documented [171, 310, 393, 38, 188].

Nephroblastomas grow often very large before they are detected. Thus, a huge abdominal mass may be the first clinical symptom. In most cases one finds a relatively large tumor (average weight 500 gm) together with a small kidney that is often displaced and considerably compressed by the tumor. Occasionally, the kidney may not be recognizable at all.

The tumor and the intact renal parenchyma are almost always sharply separated from each other by a pseudocapsule made up of parts of the atrophic renal parenchyma or parts of the renal capsule and the perirenal fatty tissue.

The cut surface (Fig. 29) often shows a distinct lobulation and displays grey-white, nodular, slightly bulging, soft areas. In addition, there is necrosis, hemorrhage, and cystic degeneration, especially in very large tumors. The cystic component may be so pronounced that the neoplastic nature of the lesion may be disguised, and the macroscopy may suggest polycystic renal disease. In those tumors in which the mesenchymal stromal component predominates, the cut surface may be very similar to or undistinguishable from that of soft tissue sarcomata.

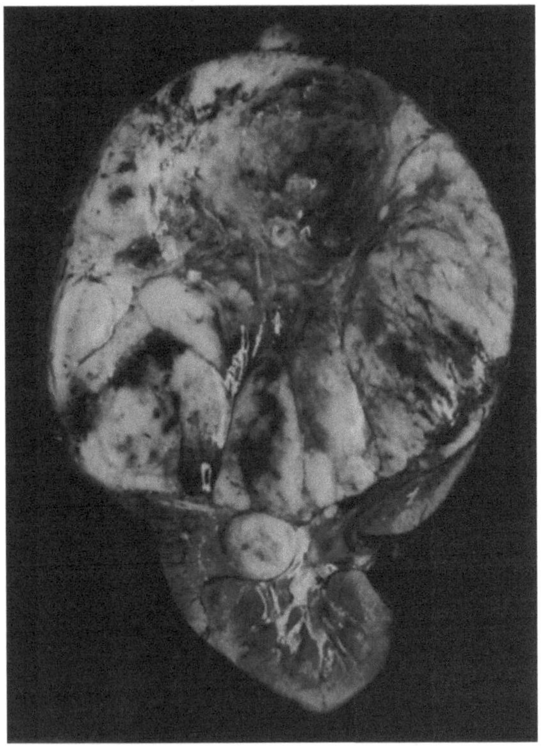

Fig. 29. Nephroblastoma with multinodular greyish-white, bulging areas, hemorrhages, and necroses

Calcification is exceptional and is not an important macroscopic feature. According to the literature, the frequency of calcification, including microcalcifications, varies between 3%–14% [268, 317].

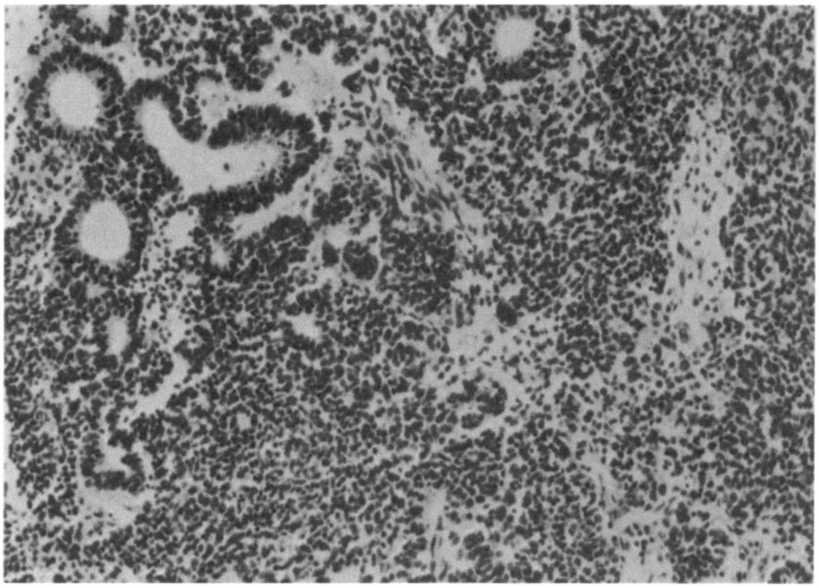

Fig. 30. Triphasic nephroblastoma. There are epithelial-tubular structures, areas of undifferentiated blastema consisting of small densely packed cells, and a mesenchymal stromal component. H & E, ×140

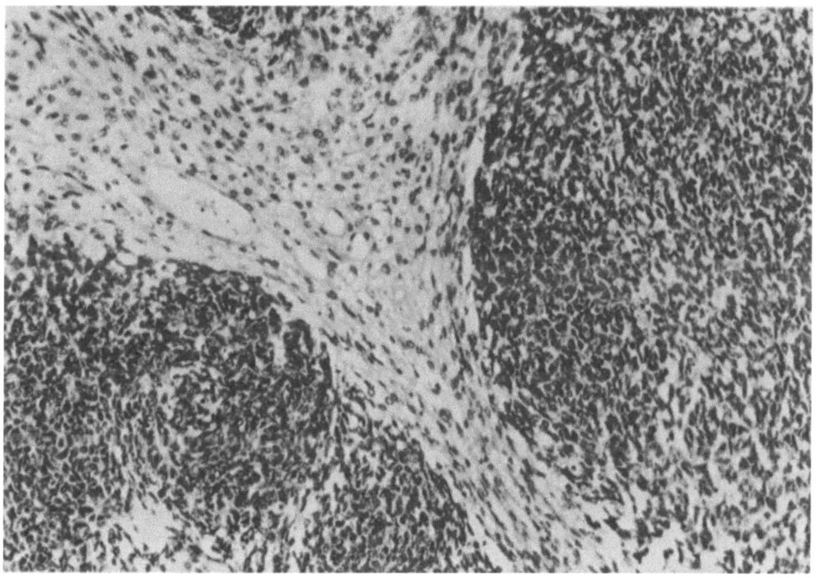

Fig. 31. Nephroblastoma with blastomatous areas separated by broad bands of embryonal mesenchymal stroma. H & E, ×140

Although the nephroblastomatous tissue is usually sharply delineated, in some cases an infiltrative growth is already detectable macroscopically. The pyelon or some calices, respectively, may also be infiltrated. In such cases the pyelon may be completely filled with tumor masses and the tumor tissue may reach the ureter. Finally, an infiltration of the peripelvic adipose tissue or an invasion of the renal veins may be present. Metastases to the regional lymph nodes (15% of cases) are not very frequently encountered [209].

2.1.5 Histopathology

Classic cases contain an epithelial, a blastomatous, and a sarcomatous component (Fig. 30). Independently from each other, these may attain varying stages of maturity. There are often transitional zones between the blastomatous and epithelial and/or sarcomatous areas.

Blastomatous areas are composed of densely packed, slightly oval shaped cells with scanty cytoplasm and intensely hyperchromatic nuclei. These areas are very often separated by inter-

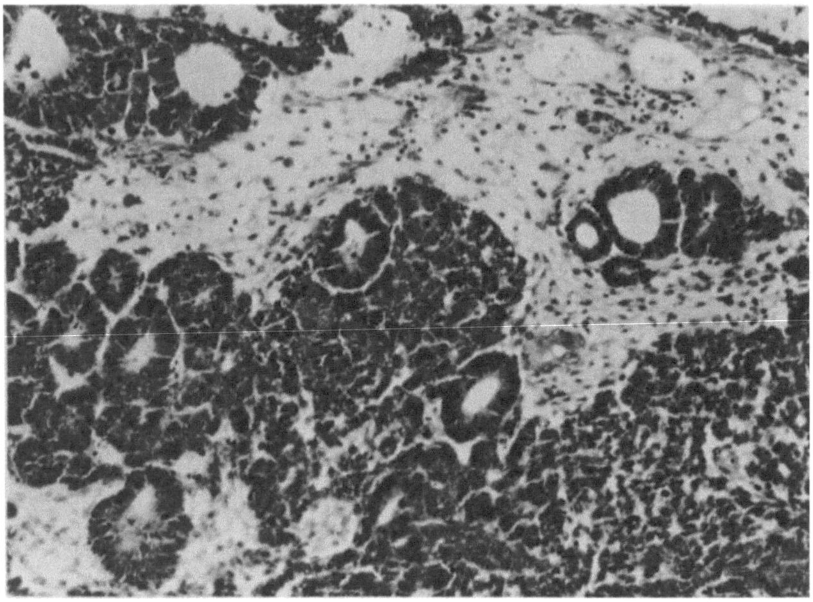

Fig. 32. Epithelial-tubular formations at the margin of blastomatous areas in a nephroblastoma. H & E, ×140

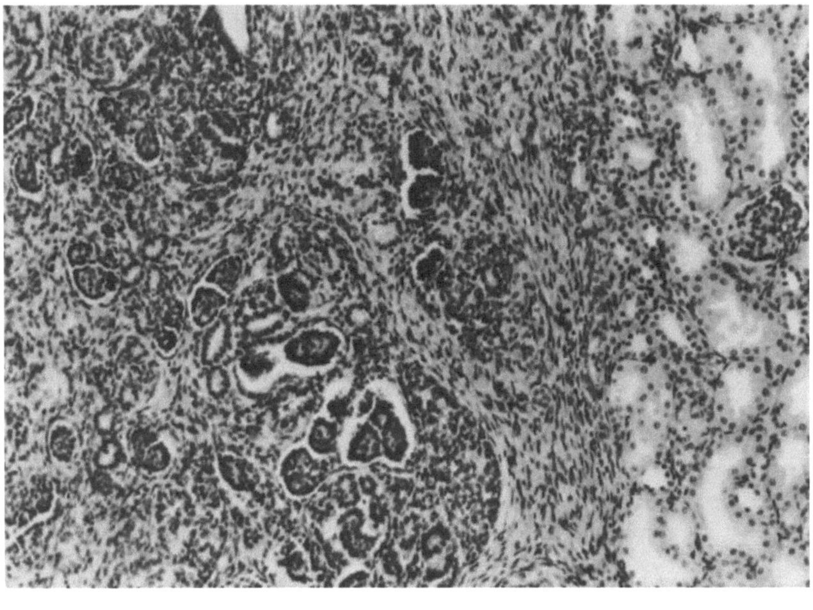

Fig. 33. Well-differentiated nephroblastoma with tubular and glomeruloid formations. Normal renal parenchyma to the *right*. H & E, ×140

posed strands of stroma of varying density (Fig. 31). They may disclose rosettes or single tubules. Their outer zones may have cells arranged in a basaloid pattern or in palisades. There is no constant histotopographic relationship between the various structures of the blastomatous areas. Instead, there may be considerable variations from area to area in the same case and from case to case. Some tumors develop only one pattern, for instance only blastomatous areas with peripherally placed epithelial tubules (Fig. 32).

Within larger blastomatous areas, pseudocysts may form by degenerative changes. True cysts of different sizes may also occur, and these may occasionally contain papillary tumor projections.

The differentiation of the *epithelial elements* shows a rather broad spectrum. Very immature epithelial differentiations may be present in the form of rosettes. On the other hand, formation of tubules with a well-developed basement membrane may be seen together with glomeruloid structures (Fig. 33). All stages of embryonal

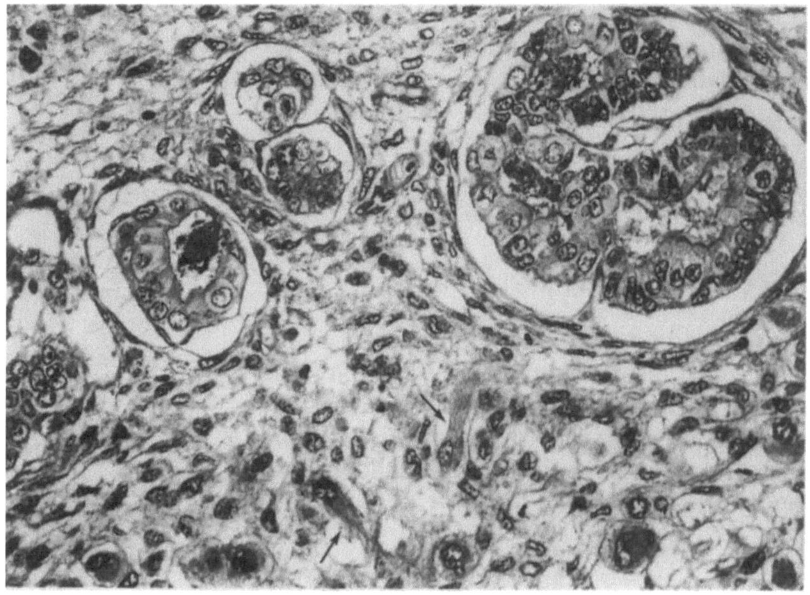

Fig. 34. Nephroblastoma with atypical cross-striated muscle cells (*arrows*) and embryonal tubules. H & E, ×350

nephronogenesis may be imitated. In some cases, the primitive epithelial neoplastic cells may develop into cells that normally cannot be found in the kidney. For example, tumors have been described with squamous epithelial cells or islands of mucoid glands.

The *stromal component* contains basically fibroblastic and myxoid areas with a wide variation both of cellularity and frequency of mitoses. Atypical bizarre mitoses can be found, particularly within the stromal compartments. Occasionally, there are groups of smooth muscle cells or strains of spindle cells whose nature cannot be identified properly by light microscopy.

Cross-striated muscle is a frequent stromal component of nephroblastoma (Fig. 34). The number of such cells varies considerably from case to case. Other structural components such as cartilage, bone, or adipose tissue may also be present or even predominate. In such extremely rare cases one may speak of osteocartilaginous or lipomatous nephroblastoma.

Metastases of nephroblastoma usually exhibit the same histologic pattern as do the primary tumors. If radiation therapy has been applied to the metastases, well-differentiated stromal components may predominate because they are much more resistant to radiation than epithelial structures.

Ultrastructural investigations often allow a more precise characterization of the various cells and their differentiation products. From studies by electron microscopy, there appears to be great similarity between the epithelial cells of nephroblastoma and the cells of the normal immature embryonal blastema [423]. The main difference between these two consists in an asynchronous development of the cytoplasmic organelles in the tumor cells [203]. The same is true for the primitive mesenchymal cells of nephroblastoma. Here, all stages and grades of maturation into the different forms of connective tissue cells can be observed [18, 390, 398, 343].

The extraordinary variation of the histologic patterns that can be found with Wilms' tumors has stimulated many authors to classify them on the basis of histologic features in order to elaborate correlations to their biologic behavior. Beckwith and Palmer [26] separate four basic types according to the quantity of the various nephroblastoma components present. They differentiate between (1) the classic triphasic Wilms' tumor (mixed type), (2) the predominantly epithelial type that contains more than 65% epithelial cells, (3) the predominantly blastemic type that contains more than 65% blastema components, and (4) the stromal type with predominance of sarcomatous or nonsarcomatous stromal structures. Each of these types is again divided into those with and those without anaplastic changes. Anaplastic changes are diagnosed when particularly large nucleoli, pronounced hyperchromasia of the nuclei, and atypical mitoses are present. Finally, a distinction is made between focal and diffuse anaplasia.

2.1.6 Special Histologic Variants

2.1.6.1 Tubular Nephroblastoma

According to CHATTEN [64] monomorphous tubular nephroblastomas are relatively well differentiated variants with a comparatively favorable prognosis. She also found that such tumors usually occur with relatively young children, frequently under 2 years of age.

2.1.6.2 Cystic, Partially Differentiated Nephroblastoma

Cystic, partially differentiated nephroblastoma designates a distinctly uncommon lesion with considerable multilocular cystic changes and with minimal amounts of undifferentiated blastema [216]. The affected patients tend to be very young. Due to the high differentiation the prognosis is favorable, so that simple nephrectomy as a therapeutic measure may suffice. According to GONZALEZ-CRUSSI [144], there has not yet been a documented case of metastasizing cystic nephroblastoma.

2.1.6.3 Congenital Mesoblastic Nephroma

According to BOLANDE [45], congenital mesoblastic nephroma (fetal mesenchymal hamartoma) is not rarely observed among Wilms' tumor-related lesions in the newborn. However, STAMBOLIS [366] found only 142 cases in the literature.

The tumor consists predominantly of mesenchymal stromal elements and usually has a benign course. However, cases with a low grade of malignancy have been reported. Therefore, HARMS [168] considers the lesion a cytodifferentiated variant of Wilms' tumor with a low grade of malignancy.

Macroscopically, typical cases are not encapsulated. Fingerlike extensions of tumor parenchyma into the surrounding kidney tissue may be observed. The cut surface is markedly similar to that of leiomyoma of the uterus. The tumor tissue is firm and whitish. Necroses and hemorrhage are usually lacking. There are, however, cases in which the tumor tissue is relatively soft, and hemorrhage and necroses may also be found. If so, a more aggressive behavior must be suspected.

Microscopically (Fig. 35), one finds irregular bundles of spindle cells that contain cigarlike, oval-shaped nuclei. The fascicles are intermingled with collagenous fibers. There is a broad

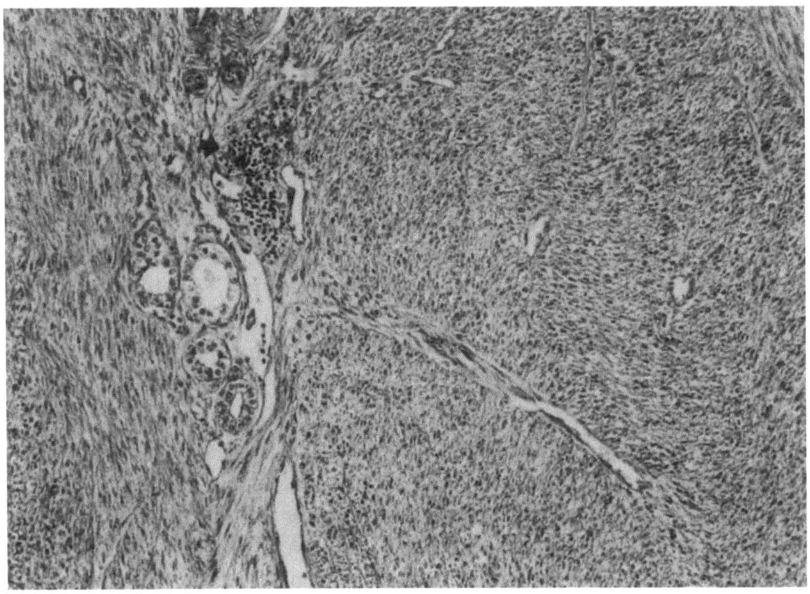

Fig. 35. Congenital mesoblastic nephroma with irregularly arranged bundles of spindle cells that entrap a group of four tubuli adjacent to a small nest of hematopoietic cells (*arrow*). H & E, ×140

spectrum of cellularity, and this is also true for the frequency of mitoses. Cases with a high frequency of mitoses no longer form tumor cell fascicles. Instead, diffuse masses of cells interrupted by necrotic zones may be found. A cystic component may be prominent. Since there is no well-developed capsule, there is no sharp delineation between the tumor and the renal parenchyma. At the boundary of the tumor, an angiomatous zone may be found. Sometimes one may find foci of hematopoiesis, especially around blood vessels. HARMS et al. [170] mentioned that these foci can be selectively demonstrated by the application of the chloroesterase method of LEDER [248]. Hyalin cartilage may also be formed by the tumor. Invasion of the perirenal fatty tissue may be observed especially with cell-rich variants. Entrapped dysplastic tubuli and glomeruli may be interspersed but are not considered components of the tumor itself.

Congenital mesoblastic nephroma is prognostically favorable if an operation is done early enough. In more advanced cases the tumor shows an aggressive behavior. Generally, cure can be achieved by total nephrectomy.

2.1.6.4 Fetal Rhabdomyomatous Nephroblastoma

The term fetal rhabdomyomatous nephroblastoma was proposed by WIGGER [422]. In this rare variant 30%–50% or more of the tumor tissue consist of rhabdomyomatous structures that correspond closely to fetal striated muscle. Characteristically, the muscle cells are intensely eosinophilic, elongated, very slender, and – in contrast to adult muscle cells – exhibit centrally placed nuclei arranged in single files. Identical cells are present in fetal rhabdomyomas of the soft tissue. The cells occur in fascicles that are separated by mature fibrous tissue (Fig. 36). In

a

b

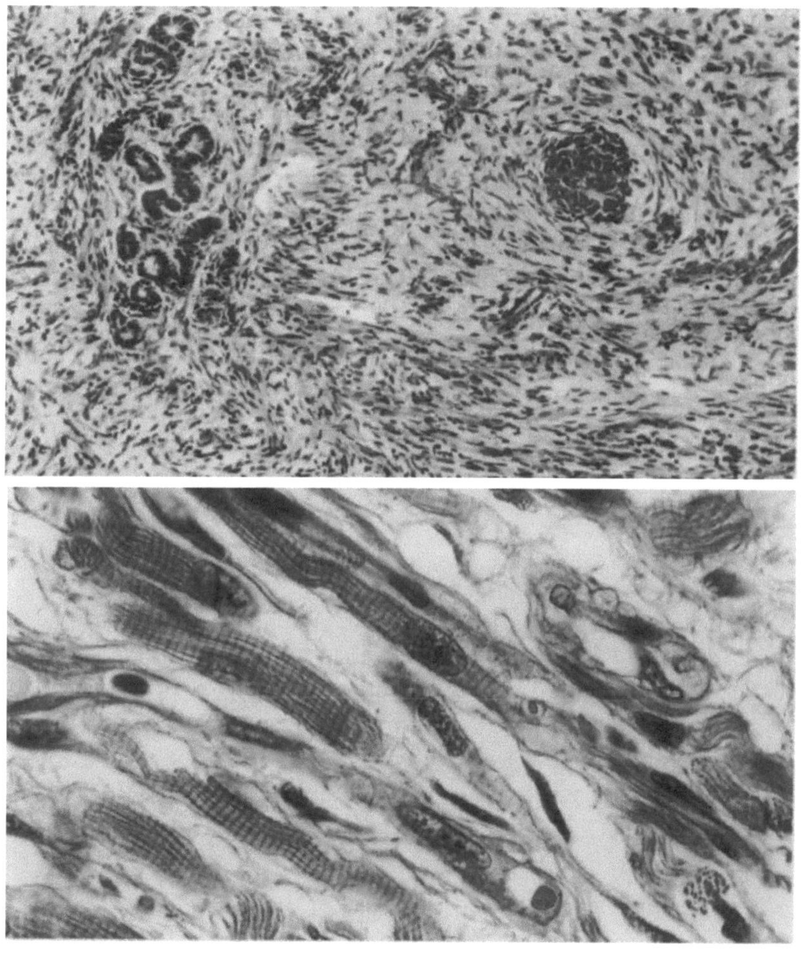

Fig. 36. (a) Fetal rhabdomyomatous nephroblastoma consisting mainly of fetal striated muscle with only minor amounts of embryonal tubules and blastomatous tissue H & E, × 140. Cross-striation and centrally placed nuclei are depicted in **(b)** at higher magnification (H & E, × 850)

addition, blastema cells may be present with evidence of epithelial differentiation. Sometimes the tumors are almost entirely made up of myogenous cells. Mitoses are not a prominent feature. The tumors do not usually metastasize, but unfortunately, the lesions frequently occur bilaterally [169]. The prognosis is relatively good [144].

2.1.6.5 Rhabdoid Sarcoma

Rhabdoid sarcoma [88, 157] is a highly aggressive lesion. The tumor is rare, comprising only 2% of all nephroblastomas. The neoplasia consists of medium-sized cells with round to oval nuclei that contain prominent nucleoli. The tumor shows numerous mitoses including atypical examples. Characteristically, the cells contain large eosinophilic cytoplasmic globoid inclusions that are weakly PAS positive. There is no cross-striation demonstrable. Blastomatous areas may rarely be formed [134, 348].

The nature of the rhabdoid tumor cells is unclear. From electron-microscope studies, no evidence of a rhabdomyoblastic differentiation could be detected [134, 348]. PALMER and SUTOW [312] discuss a neuroectodermal origin of the globule-containing cells.

The tumor occurs mainly in the first year of life, is prognostically unfavorable because of a high potential for metastases [312], and is frequently associated with brain metastases and second independent tumors of the posterior fossa. BECKWITH [25] reported over 80% mortality.

2.1.6.6 Clear Cell Sarcoma

A second very malignant renal neoplasia of children, the nature of which is as yet not quite clear, has been called bone metastasizing renal tumor of childhood (BMRTC) by MARSDEN and LAWLER [269]. This tumor is also known as clear cell sarcoma of the kidney [26]. The tumor affects girls and boys with approximately equal frequency. MARSDEN et al. [270] reported on 23 cases, and HAAS et al. [158] on 75 cases. Whereas metastases of typical Wilms' tumors often involve the liver and the lungs, clear cell sarcomas frequently produce metastases in the skeleton.

Microscopically (Fig. 37), the tumor is characterized by roundish, elongated, polygonal, or even spindle cells with medium-sized polymorphous nuclei that contain a finely dispersed chromatin and small inconspicuous nucleoli. The cytoplasm of the tumor cells is optically clear or difficult to stain, and mitoses occur with varying frequency. HAAS et al. [158] reported mitoses to be not very frequent. The presence of spaced fibrovascular septa coursing through the tumor is a diagnostically important feature. Sometimes osteochondrosarcomatous areas or hyalin deposits may be seen. Necroses may also be present. There is a rich vascular network but usually minimal collagen production. The nature of the clear cells remains uncertain.

Epithelial differentiation is not a feature of this variant. Sometimes tubular structures may be found that are interpreted by most authors

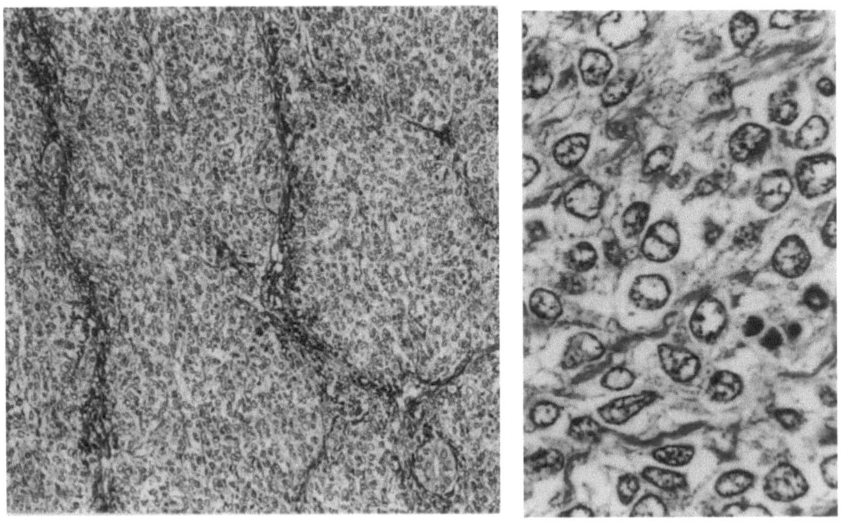

a b

Fig. 37 a, b. Clear cell sarcoma. **(a)** The low magnification discloses spaced fibrovascular septae and some entrapped tubuli (*bottom right*). H & E, ×140. **(b)** Polygonal tumor cells with clear or faintly stained cytoplasm and inconspicuous nucleoli. H & E, ×880 as entrapped normal tubules. However, SCHMIDT et al. [347] reported a case with unequivocal epithelial differentiation, from which finding a relationship to Wilms' tumor is deduced. The prognosis of this renal neoplasia is poor.

2.1.7 Grading

The grading system of LAWLER et al. [243, 244] considers the proportion of well-differentiated tubular structures as a main criterion. The authors could show that the grade of formation of tubules is a practicable, significant, and easily reproducible criterion for the histologic typing of Wilms' tumor. In short: the more tubules that are formed by a given nephroblastoma, the better the prognosis.

The grading procedure of BECKWITH and PALMER [26] is somewhat different. The authors speak of a favorable histology if a given nephroblastoma does not show anaplastic features and if a sarcomatous component is lacking. In contrast, an unfavorable histology is assumed if anaplastic changes and sarcomatous features are present. According to their data, approximately 50% of all fatalities from Wilms' tumor show either anaplastic or sarcomatous features.

HARMS [168] proposed a grading system of nephroblastomas that includes those variants with a high cytologic differentiation. According to his proposal, about 10% of cases are nephroblastomas of a low grade of malignancy, consisting of mesoblastic nephromas, fetal rhabdomyomatous nephroblastomas, cystic partially differentiated nephroblastomas, and monomorphic tubular nephroblastomas. The second group denotes cases of an intermediate grade of malignancy and comprises about 80% of all cases. This group includes the mixed type (triphasic) nephroblastoma, blastemic nephroblastoma, epithelial nephroblastoma, and stromal nephroblastoma without sarcomatous changes. The third group, of the remaining 10%, shows a high grade of malignancy. It includes nephroblastomas with focal or diffuse anaplasia, malignant rhabdoid tumor, clear cell sarcoma, and other sarcomatous nephroblastomas.

2.1.8 Staging

According to the recommendations of the "National Wilms' Tumor Study" [86], spread of nephroblastomas can be divided into five stages on the basis of pathologic findings at the time of diagnosis and nephrectomy.

Stage I comprises cases in which the tumor is confined to the kidney and can be completely removed. In these cases, the renal capsule should be intact, and no rupture of the tumor should have occurred during operation. It must also be verified that no recognizable rests of the tumor have been left at operation.

In stage II invasion of the capsule and/or continuing growth into the adjacent connective tissue have occurred. There are metastases within the regional lymph nodes. The renal veins may be infiltrated. Tumors of stage II should not show involvement of neighboring organs or abdominal metastases. Furthermore, they must be completely removable.

If the tumor has spread within the abdominal region, stage III is reached. One or several of the following findings may be present: direct involvement of neighboring organs, rupture of the tumor, metastases to the abdominal lymph nodes, tumor invasion of the inferior vena cava, and impossibility of total removal of the tumor.

Stage IV is characterized by the presence of hematogenous metastases in the lungs, liver, brain, bones, and other sites.

Stage V designates bilateral tumors. In such cases, both kidneys may each contain a primary nephroblastoma or there may be contralateral metastases from one kidney to the other.

2.1.9 Spread and Biologic Behavior

Interestingly enough, infiltration of the renal capsule and infiltrating growth into adjacent tissues are relatively rare and late events even with large tumors. In contrast, invasion of the intrarenal blood vessels and lymph channels can be frequently observed. Almost every fifth tumor shows invasion of the renal vein, and in 21% of cases the tumor attains the inferior vena cava [250]. In a review of the literature, HOLLAND [190] found that metastases were already present in about 20% of cases at the time of diagnosis.

Tumor metastases to the hilar and para-aortal lymph nodes are less frequent than 30% [271, 317] and JEREB et al. [209] found lymph node involvement in 15% of their cases. In 143 cases of nephroblastoma with distant metastases, the lungs were affected in 80%, the abdominal region in 33%, the liver in 19%, and the bones in 13% [250]. Rare sites of metastases include superficial lymph nodes, testes, spermatic cord, brain and intraspinal region, the contralateral kidney, and the adrenals [19].

2.2 Nodular Renal Blastema and Nephroblastomatosis

Nodular renal blastema and nephroblastomatosis consists of subcapsular collections of primitive metanephrogenic epithelial cells and are usually found bilaterally. Single lesions that can be found only microscopically are designated as nodular renal blastema. Their frequency is about 1% in children below the age of 4 months [31]. The lesions may involve the total of the outer renal cortex, so that the term nephroblastomatosis is appropriate.

There are intimate relationships between nodular renal blastema and Wilms' tumor, which shows that most nephroblastomas probably develop from such nodular renal blastemas [50, 367].

3 Tumors of the Renal Pelvis

3.1 General Remarks

Most epithelial tumors of the renal pelvis present the same histologic spectrum as those of the ureter and bladder since they all arise from urothelial cells. However, carcinomas of the kidney pelvis behave more aggressively than those of the bladder, which is probably due to anatomic factors.

3.2 Papilloma

Papillomas of the renal pelvis are derived from transitional cells. They are microscopically identical to papillomas of the urinary bladder and ureter and are relatively uncommon. However, they are of considerable interest because their biologic behavior cannot be predicted. Besides, they may be associated with carcinomas of the urinary tract. Of a series of patients with a renal pelvic papilloma, 25% subsequently developed carcinoma; in a series of patients with multiple papillomas as many as 50% developed carcinoma [146].

Morphologically, a papilloma consists of long processes that carry a fibrovascular core of the lamina propria. This core is covered by transitional epithelium. The epithelium is indistinguishable from normal transitional epithelium and the epithelial thickness must not exceed 5–10 cellular layers. Any marked deviation from the normal urothelial pattern must be regarded as indicative of carcinoma. In spite of this relatively clear definition of papilloma, there is no doubt that the transition point between benign papilloma and papillary carcinoma of the kidney pelvis is indefinite.

3.3 Inverted Papilloma

Occasionally, inverted papilloma may be found within the renal pelvis. Few cases have been described [394, 404, 242]. The tumors are considered benign but may undergo malignant transformation.

3.4 Fibroepithelial Polyp

Extremely rarely, a pelvic mass suspected to represent transitional cell carcinoma may turn out to be a fibroepithelial polyp. As of 1980, only seven cases had been reported [397]. Histologically, the lesion consists of a loosely structured edematous fibrous stroma covered by unremarkable transitional epithelium.

3.5 Carcinoma

3.5.1 Introduction

Carcinomas of the renal pelvis arise from urothelial cells, hence, most of them are transitional cell carcinomas. However, urothelial cells have the capacity to differentiate into squamous and glandular epithelium. Thus, approximately 10%–20% of the cases are either squamous cell carcinomas throughout or show squamous cell "metaplasia," and less than 1% are adenocarcinomas [146, 31].

It is important to distinguish between cases with squamous "metaplasia" and cases with epidermoid pattern throughout because according to PUGH'S experience with tumors of the bladder the biologic behavior of these two is different: transitional cell carcinomas metastasize earlier to the regional lymph nodes [325]. However, RAFLA [327] found that squamous cell carcinomas of the renal pelvis invade the peripelvic tissue more frequently than do transitional cell carcinomas.

Metaplasia is defined as a *benign* change of a particular type of differentiated tissue when it takes on the characteristics of another kind of differentiated tissue. If similar changes are observed in cancers, these probably reflect genetic instability of the neoplastic cells and, hence, express malignancy. Therefore, in the case of papillary carcinoma of the urinary tract, squamous epithelial changes must not be labelled "metaplasia" but "atypia" and are indicative of an increase of deviation from nonneoplastic.

The carcinomas may also develop tubular or glandular structures that are capable of mucus production. This may occur together with the development of squamous epithelial cell structures. Of transitional cell carcinomas, 24% may show this mixed pattern in the ureter [286], and it can also be found in the kidney pelvis. If in growths of the urinary tract no similarity to transitional, glandular, or squamous cells is recognizable, then the cancers are labelled "undifferentiated" [295].

In summary, carcinomas of the renal pelvis can be divided into the following groups: (1) papillary transitional cell carcinomas that may be pure, with squamous differentiation, with glandular differentiation, and with mixed squamous and glandular differentiation, (2) squamous cell carcinomas; (3) adenocarcinomas; and (4) undifferentiated carcinomas. Carcinosarcomas are extremely rare.

3.5.2 Causes

Transitional and squamous cell carcinomas of the renal pelvis can be experimentally produced by substances like dibenzanthracene, methylcholanthrene, benzpyrene, aflatoxin B, and lead salts. Possibly, RNA viruses play a causative role. Inflammation, calculus formation, metaplasia, and metabolites of certain chemical agents such as benzidine [321] have also been incriminated as causes of renal pelvis carcinoma. A history of retrograde pyelography with Thorotrast has been repeatedly reported in patients with carcinoma of the renal pelvis [10, 236, 104, 421, 213, 408, 129, 399, 311, 102]. Carcinoma of the kidney pelvis is approximately 40 times more common in persons who take large amounts of phenacetin as compared to other patients [28, 211]. Probably, phenacetin is metabolized to o-aminophenol, detoxified in the liver by conjugation with glucuronic acid, which may be split off again by β-glucuronidase within the urinary tract. The level of β-glucuronidase can be found elevated in the urine of patients with inflammatory diseases of the kidney. An association between tobacco use and the development of tumors of the renal pelvis is also discussed [31].

3.5.3 Epidemiology

Carcinoma of the renal pelvis is relatively rare. For example, 2340 cases of renal adenocarcinoma have been collected at the California Tumor Registry from 1942–1969. At the same time, however, only 775 cases of carcinoma of the kidney pelvis were registered [31]. Thus, kidney pelvis carcinomas occur at least three times less frequently than adenocarcinomas of the renal parenchyma. SAY and HORI [344] found 13 kidney pelvis carcinomas in 201 cases of renal malignancy, and in the series of WAGLE et al. [412] the corresponding figures were 12 of 334 cases. According to WAGLE et al. [412], 7%–8% of all renal tumors arise in the renal pelvis, and DEL REGATO and SPJUT [97] have reported that transitional cell carcinomas of the renal pelvis make up about 6%–12% of all malignant tumors of the kidney.

The majority of renal pelvis tumors are found in the elderly [240, 344], namely in the 6th to 8th decade. In most series, there is a preponderance of males [82] who are two to four times as commonly afflicted as females [215, 13]. There is no indication of heredity occurrence.

The simultaneous appearance of tumors in the pelvis, ureter, and bladder is not uncommon. This multicentricity very probably represents independent tumors rather than implantation metastases, since there are reports on bilat-

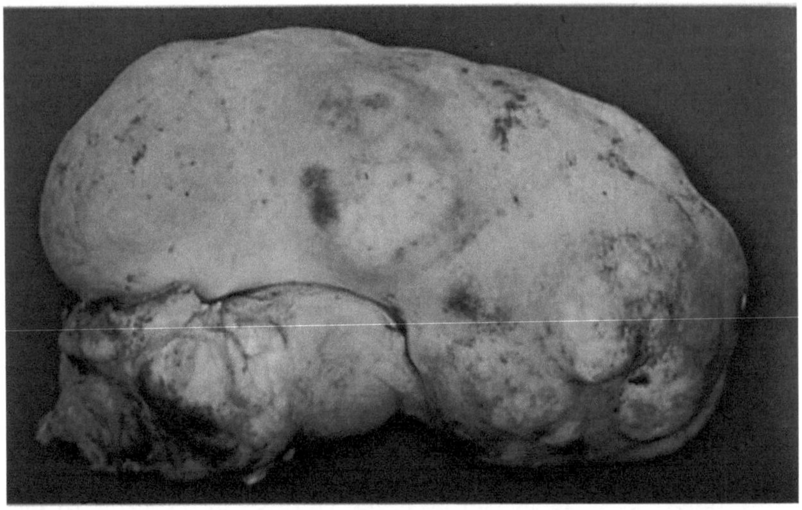

Fig. 38. Transitional cell carcinoma of the kidney pelvis. The tumor has infiltrated the ureter, renal vein, peripelvic tissue, and renal cortex

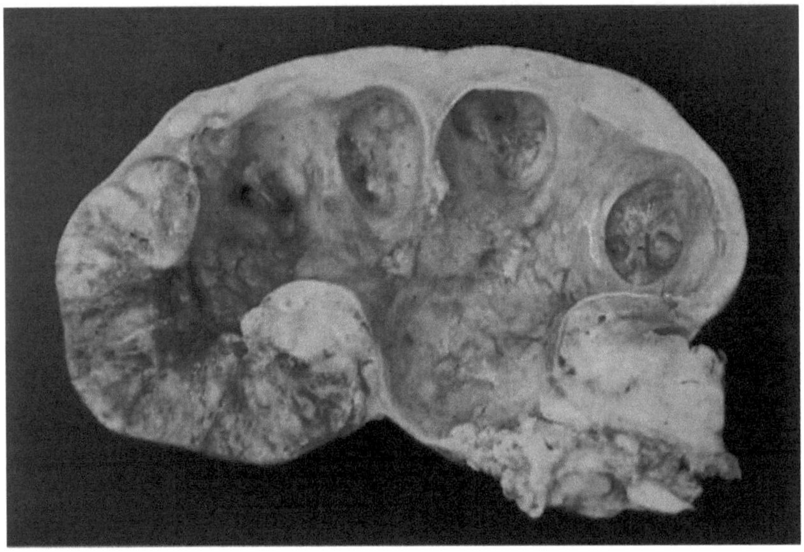

Fig. 39. Same case as Fig. 38. Obliteration of the ureter by tumor tissue with formation of hydronephrosis. Infiltration of the renal cortex (*left*) and of the peripelvic fatty tissue (*bottom right*)

eral carcinomas of the kidney, pelvis, and ureter [75, 146, 412]. Such "satellite" tumors may be present in 40%–50% of the cases of papillary renal tumors [384, 224, 276, 281, 336]. These attendant neoplasms may develop at the same time or subsequently. Therefore, surgical treatment of renal pelvis tumors should include ureterectomy [344, 381].

3.5.4 Transitional Cell Carcinoma

Macroscopically, there is a lobular surface that bulges into the renal pelvis. A papillary carcinoma has a much broader base and is bulkier and more friable than a transitional cell papilloma. It forms red or grey, soft, smooth, mamillated growths with a glistening surface. The neoplasm may arise anywhere in the renal pelvis. The larger the carcinoma, the more frequently one will find focal hemorrhages and secondary changes caused by obturation of the pelvis. This may result in hydronephrosis, depending on the localization of the tumor (Figs. 38 and 39).

Histologically, papillary carcinomas (Fig. 40) are made up of arborescent ramifying masses. The cores are covered by many layers of cells. These are more or less hyperchromatic and irregularly arranged, and invasion of the pelvic wall through the stalk may be seen. In comparison to papilloma, the villi are much thicker and

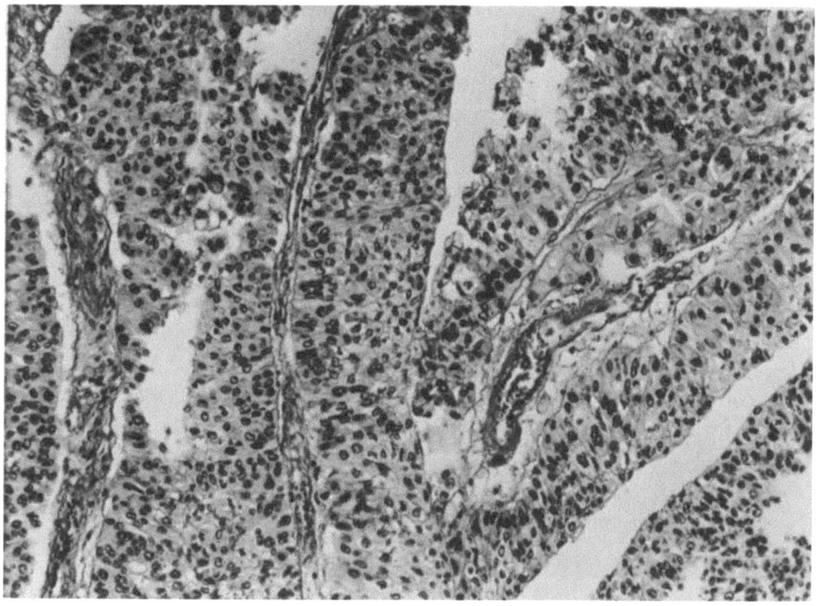

Fig. 40. Papillary transitional cell carcinoma. Same case as Fig. 38. There is marked anaplasia and disarrangement of the carcinomatous urothelial cells. H & E, ×140

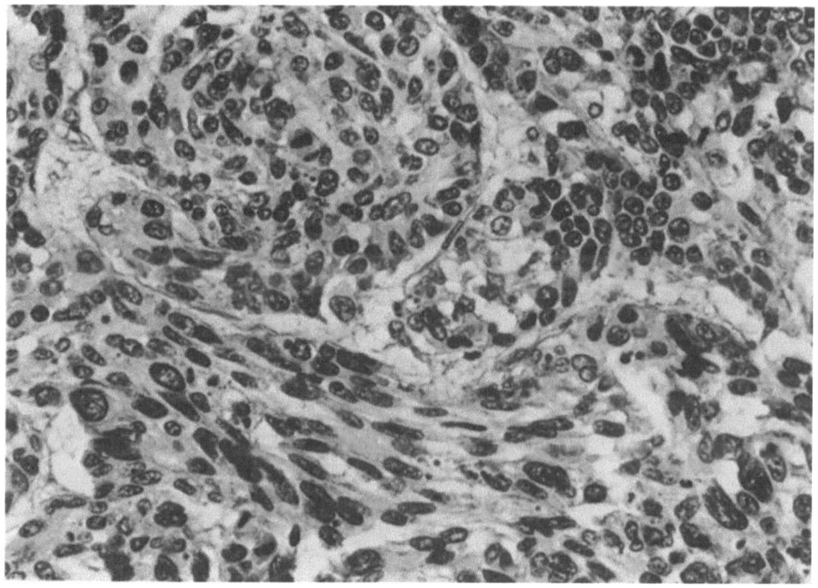

Fig. 41. Same case as Fig. 38. Areas of polymorphic and hyperchromatic spindle cells with several mitoses. H & E, ×350

have a much broader basis. There is no regular stratification, there is loss of polarity and maturation, and the epithelial thickness by far exceeds seven to ten layers. The number of mitoses differs from case to case and from area to area. Anaplasia may be marked. Occasionally, spindle cells are formed (Fig. 41), so the tumors may be confused with sarcomas or with sarcomatoid renal adenocarcinomas.

There are also flat, nonpapillary and noninfiltrating transitional cell carcinomas. These cases are usually markedly cellular with high grade atypicalities, hyperchromatism, and substantial numbers of mitoses.

Not rarely, cancer of the renal pelvis shows a so-called clear cell pattern. Cases with such a pattern together with those showing spindle cell development may be easily confused with adenocarcinoma of the renal parenchyma. If the tumor masses are very large and have destroyed large portions of the kidney, it may be impossible to decide whether there is adenocarcinoma of the renal parenchyma or carcinoma of the renal pelvis.

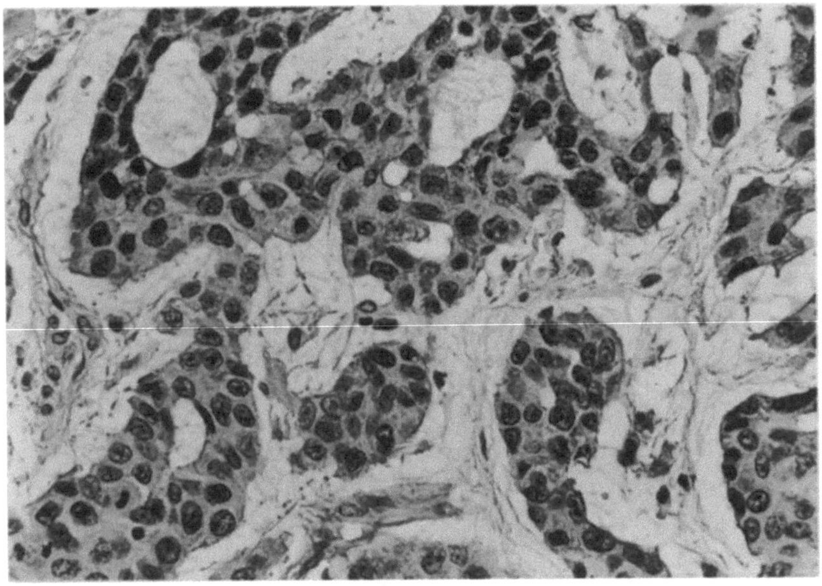

Fig. 42. Same case as Fig. 38. In the deeper infiltrates, a glandular pattern is elaborated by the tumor cells. H & E, ×350

Frequently, one finds submucosal inflammatory infiltrates composed of lymphocytes, macrophages, and plasma cells, sometimes together with germinal centers. Occasionally, these infiltrates may obscure the interface between epithelium and lamina propria so that a decision about a beginning infiltration cannot be made.

Foci of squamous and glandular changes, or both, may be seen in transitional cell carcinomas, particularly in the case of invasion (Fig. 42).

3.5.5 Squamous Epithelial Carcinoma

Pure squamous cell carcinoma of the renal pelvis is rare. In a series of 2166 renal neoplasias, Blacher et al. [40] found only 11 cases (0.5%). Patients with epidermoid carcinomas often have a long previous history of symptoms suggesting stones and infections with fever, tenderness and hematuria [97]. The course of epidermoid carcinoma is rapid because squamous carcinoma metastasizes early.

Macroscopically, these carcinomas are at most slightly papillary. One finds solid, flat, or slightly raised, friable growths. Most of these carcinomas tend to be extensive. Often they are ulcerated. The tumors are mostly firm and fixed due to the accompanying inflammation with concomitant fibrosis.

Histologically, the tumors are very cellular. They show unequivocal squamous epithelia with a variety of atypicalities. There are intercellular prickles and areas of keratinization. We have seen one case after pyelography with Thorotrast (Fig. 43).

If, histologically, mixtures of squamous and urothelial structures are observed, then transitional cell carcinoma should be diagnosed. Squamous cell carcinoma is often accompanied by or associated with chronic pyelonephritis, hydronephrosis, lithiasis, and leukoplakia [315, 58, 402].

3.5.6 Adenocarcinoma

Adenocarcinoma of the renal pelvis is very rare. Occasional instances have been reported [3, 329, 204, 222, 14, 326, 15, 99, 256]. From the study of the available literature, we estimate that fewer than 50–60 cases of pelvic adenocarcinoma have been published up to now. Kobayashi et al. [229] reviewed 47 cases and added 2 further examples.

Macroscopically, adenocarcinomas of the renal pelvis correspond largely to the gross appearance of colonic adenocarcinomas. There is a nodular mass of glistening, slimy, mucoid tumor tissue. Hydronephrosis and pyelonephritis may have developed.

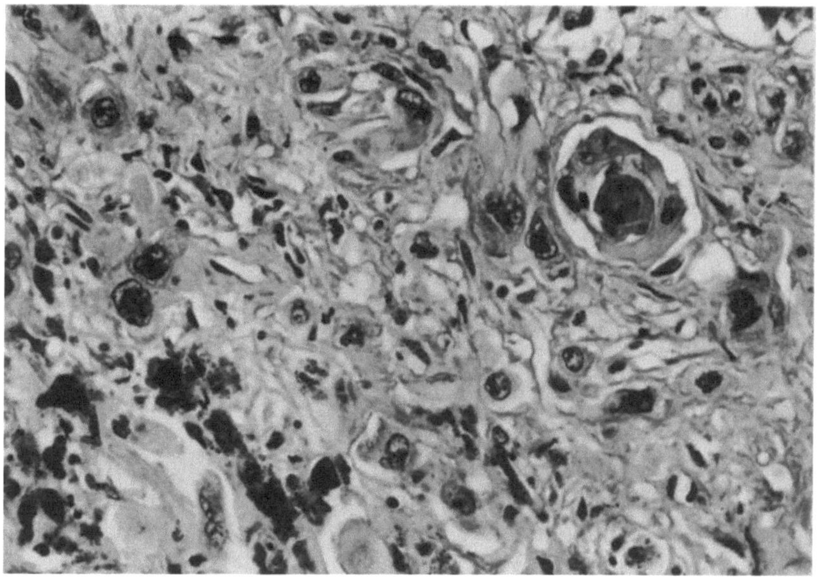

Fig. 43. Poorly differentiated squamous cell carcinoma of the kidney pelvis due to Thorotrast. To the *lower left* deposits of thorium-dioxide, to the *upper right* a horny pearl. H & E, ×350

Histologically, the tumors are mostly columnar cell adenocarcinomas. Sometimes the carcinomas form large masses of mucin.

3.5.7 Undifferentiated Carcinoma and Carcinosarcoma

These carcinomas do not show recognizable similarities to urothelial cells or glandular patterns. According to BENNINGTON and BECKWITH [31], they present histological patterns that differ from case to case. For instance, some cases strongly imitate small cell carcinoma of the lung. Others show so high a degree of anaplasia that classification is not at all possible.

Carcinosarcoma is rarely found to occur in the renal pelvis. Only a few cases have been documented in the literature [391, 69].

3.5.8 Grading

Grading is problematic. This can be shown by the fact that there are authors who use four grades and others who use up to seven. BENNINGTON and BECKWITH [31] feel that three grades are sufficient for routine purposes. These authors distinguish between slightly anaplastic tumors (grade I) and tumors that are markedly anaplastic (grade III). They apply the term grade II if the tumor lies somewhere in between grades I and III.

It is quite clear that the prognosis worsens from grade I to grade III. Such a differentiation of grades of malignancy can, of course, also be achieved by labels such as "slightly anaplastic," "moderately anaplastic," or "markedly anaplastic," with complementary comments if necessary. If such a description is used, the clinician is equally well informed and knows precisely the situation in a given individual case. Moreover, he understands much better that there are, in fact, many transitional cases between grades I and II, and also between grades II and III, which can only be grouped arbitrarily in such a grading system. The three numerals may suggest that there are no intermediate cases between grades I, II, and III, which is definitely not in keeping with biologic principles.

Therefore, we propose that grading of tumors as described above should be accompanied by well elaborated, descriptive diagnoses as has been done ever since. Thus, oversimplification by using numerals can be avoided. Pure grading expressed in Roman numerals is only justified for statistical purposes, here coding is necessary. We define grading as a kind of coding that must always be arbitrary, nonbiologic, and subjective. In statistics these disadvantages will be compensated for by the large number of cases, which is impossible in the individual case. In summary, we advise against grading as the only cytodiagnostic statement when individual cases are to be judged. Instead, grading should be used in the sense of complementary information in addition to traditional histopathology reports.

3.5.9 *Staging*

It is quite clear that the extent of invasion is important in predicting the prognosis. BENNINGTON and BECKWITH [31] propose the following stages:

Stage I	Papillary or planar carcinoma with no evidence of invasion
Stage II	Papillary or planar carcinoma, superficially invasive, but with invasion limited to the lamina propria
Stage III	Carcinoma extends to the level of the muscularis
Stage IV	Carcinoma extends to the adventitial surface involving adjacent structures, and metastases can be found.

3.5.10 *Spread*

Carcinoma of the renal pelvis first spreads locally. It may invade large parts of the renal cortex. In such cases, renal adenocarcinoma may be simulated, especially in cases of clear cell carcinoma. The lamina propria, muscularis, and adventitia of the renal pelvis may be involved and infiltrated by the tumor. Papillary carcinoma may extend into the renal vein and its tributaries and also into the perineural spaces in more than 45% of infiltrating cases [276]. Extension into the inferior vena cava is uncommon but has been described [174, 210]. Infiltration of the retroperitoneal space may occur. Distant metastases can be found in various organs, most often in the regional lymph nodes, liver, lungs, brain, and bones [240].

Solid tumors such as squamous cell carcinomas, in contrast to papillary growths, already have almost invariably infiltrating properties at the outset of their evolution [13]. Therefore, metastases in these cases may occur very early. Epidermoid carcinoma spreads directly into juxtarenal tissues via the lymphatics or the blood stream. Some tumors may invade the kidney parenchyma or extend to the ureter by direct continuity. Distant metastases of adenocarcinoma of the renal pelvis have been reported in the lungs, liver, pancreas, and gastrointestinal tract. We are not aware of a comprehensive statistical analysis of distant metastases from renal pelvis carcinoma, and the available data on this subject differ largely from author to author.

3.5.11 *Prognosis*

By and large, the prognosis of renal pelvis cancer is poor. The 15% of the growths that are keratinizing squamous cell carcinomas have a very poor outlook. According to RICHES [335], all patients with papillomas survived; 57% with low-grade papillary tumors survived 5 years, 38% with high-grade papillary cancers survived 5 years, but none of those with various solid infiltrating and highly malignant cancers survived more than 5 years. According to MCDONALD and PRIESTLEY [276], only one patient in six with papillary carcinomas and only one in fourteen with flat carcinomas survived for more than 5 years. However, as is the case with the distribution of distant metastases, no reliable prognostic data based on a large series of renal pelvis cancer are available as yet, due to the relative rareness of this kind of malignant neoplasia and its variants.

4 Tumors of the Adrenal

4.1 Introduction

The cortex and the medulla of the adrenal differ completely from each other with regard to their development, morphology, and function. The cortex originates from mesodermal coeloma epithelia in close vicinity to the gonadal anlage. Therefore, ectopic adrenal tissue including some respective neoplasms may sometimes be found within liver and perirenal tissues, along the spermatic cords, and in association with the female adnexa. The adrenal medulla develops from the neural crest and is of neuroectodermal origin: sympathogonia migrate to the mesodermal anlage of the cortex and develop there into the chromaffin cells of the adrenal medulla.

4.2 Tumors of the Adrenal Cortex

4.2.1 General Remarks

Although the adrenal cortex is of mesodermal origin, the respective neoplasms are designated as adenomas and carcinomas. Hormonally active and large cortical tumors are rare, but small, hormonally inactive adenomas can be found relatively often in autopsy material. The tumors occur at all ages. Some of them produce adrenocortical hormones, or their precursors, or both. Accordingly, they are divided into functioning (active) and nonfunctioning (inactive) neoplasms.

Active tumors evoke various clinical syndromes, depending not only on the kind of hormones produced but also on the age and sex of the patients. Thus, adrenogenital syndromes with feminization or virilization, precocious puberty, Cushing's syndrome, Conn's syndrome, or combinations of these may develop [255]. The following relationships between the various clinical syndromes and their respective underlying adrenocortical lesions are of considerable interest because they are indispensable for a properly pursued preoperative differential diagnosis.

An *adrenogenital syndrome* that follows a normal prepubertal development is much more often due to a cortical neoplasia than to a simple hyperplasia. The syndrome occurs much more often with females than with males, more than 50% of whom are children. In the case of a *congenital adreno-cortical syndrome,* a bilateral hyperplasia is usually found.

Cushing's syndrome (Fig. 44a) is caused by cortical tumors in 20%–30% of all cases, about half of which are carcinomas [350, 420]. Twenty per cent occur before puberty; two-thirds of these concern girls and are mostly due to carcinomas [155, 424].

a

b

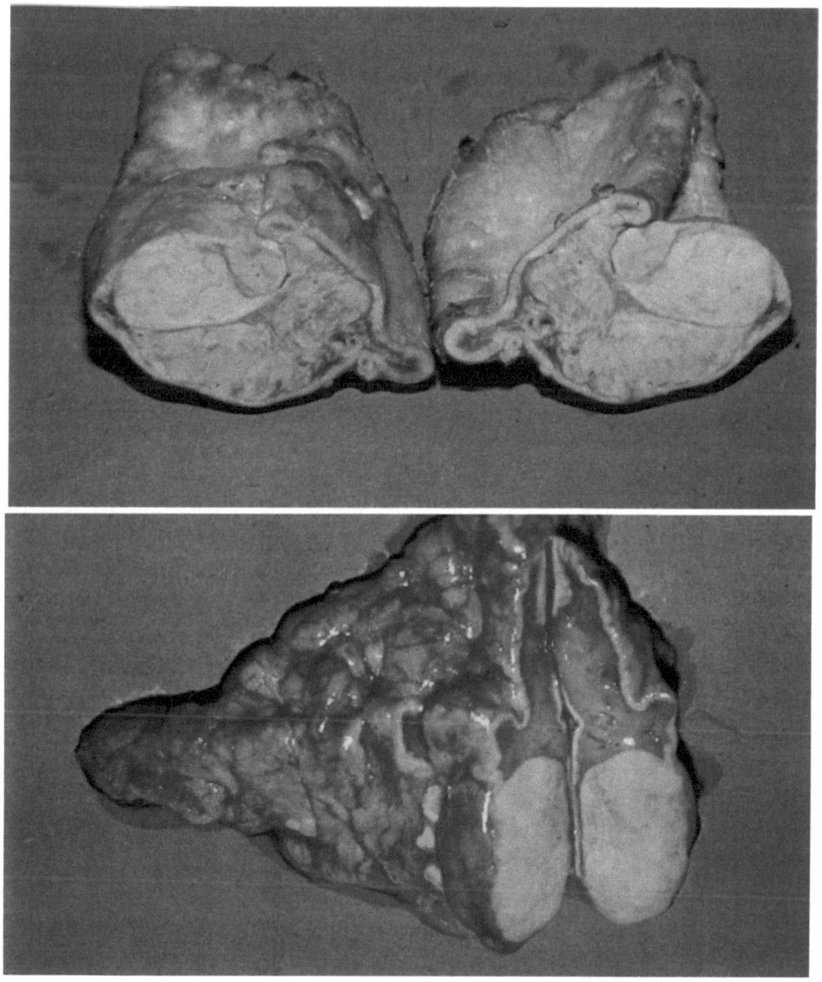

Fig. 44. (a) Nodular hyperplasia of the adrenal cortex with Cushing's syndrome. **(b)** Small adenoma of the adrenal cortex. This tumor had caused Conn's syndrome

Conn's syndrome is very rare and occurs usually in adults. Females predominate in the ratio of 2:1. The most frequent symptoms are hypertension, weakness of the skeletal muscle, nocturia, and polydipsia. The cause is most often an adenoma (aldosteronoma). According to NEVILLE and SYMINGTON [300], most aldosteronomas are small and weigh less than 10 g (Fig. 44b). In approximately 30% of the cases a cortical hyperplasia is present [91]. In very occasional cases a carcinoma may be the cause [300].

Feminizing syndromes due to adrenocortical lesions are very rare, and usually involve adult males. In most cases, metastasizing carcinomas can already be found at the first presentation [373]. GABRILOVE et al. [136] reviewed comprehensively 52 cases of feminizing adrenal tumors. Unilateral or bilateral gynecomastia is usually the presenting symptom.

Apart from this, the following general data can additionally be used for the preoperative differential diagnoses of adrenocortical growths. Most cortical neoplasias occurring in children are both endocrinologically active *and* malignant, and girls predominate. Interestingly, accompanying congenital malformations have been described [130] and a substantial array of secondary neoplasms, particularly of the brain, reported [289]. In contrast, hormonally inactive carcinomas concern predominantly elderly males, but are extremely rare [255, 201, 252, 383].

There are also certain differences between hyperplasiogeneous or adenoma-related syndromes and those due to carcinomas. The last often present as a mixture of symptoms that usually do not occur together and normally belong to two or more different syndromes. In comparison, hormonal disturbances evoked by hyperplasias or adenomas can be much more clearly defined. Therefore, a careful analysis of the clinical features may give important clues to the preoperative differential diagnosis [180, 178].

As a rule, no conclusions can be drawn from the histologic and cytologic picture as to the hormonal activity of a given tumor. There is, however, one exception: if aldosteronomas have been treated with spironolactone, they may reveal "spironolactone bodies" (see below) that indicate the production of aldosterone [206, 59, 6, 72]. AIBA et al. [5] found that adrenocortical tumors producing mineralocorticoids contain a substantial number of tissue mast cells, which differentiates them from those that produce cortisols. However, further studies are needed to confirm this finding.

Hormonally active tumors will usually be detected clinically in a relatively early stage [383]. Therefore, they are usually small at the time of diagnosis. In contrast, hormonally inactive tumors may attain large and rarely even gigantic proportions with weights of up to 5000 g [259]. However, in a clinicopathologic study of 49 adrenocortical carcinomas, KING and LACK [225] did not find a significant difference in size and weight between active and nonactive tumors.

Metastases usually produce the same hormonal substances as do the primary tumors. A few cases have been reported in which functioning tumors recurred as nonfunctioning growths or with a qualitative change of their function [331]. HALMI and LASCARI [163] described a carcinoma that converted from virilization to feminization with the advent of recurrence and metastases.

4.2.2 Adenomas

Inactive adenomas are often found incidentally at autopsy. However, with increasing usage of computerizised tomography they may probably be more frequently detected during life.

Macroscopically, adenomas are roundish, bulging, fairly well-circumscribed, noninfiltrating nodes (Fig. 44b). Usually, they do not grow larger than 5 cm, and their weight does not exceed 100 g. Cortical nodes exceeding 100 g and larger than 5 cm are suspected of carcinoma [350, 172, 252, 389]. The cut surface is yellow, sometimes with brownish patches due to lipofuscin. Calcification may be seen. Necroses and hemorrhages are rare, occurring more often in large adenomas (Fig. 45) than in small varieties. However, *pronounced* regressive changes should always raise the suspicion of a carcinoma [406].

Adenomas that cause Cushing's syndrome are accompanied by a bilateral atrophy of the normal cortical tissue, whereas aldosteronomas will produce hypertrophy rather than atrophy. However, there are cases of hormonally active

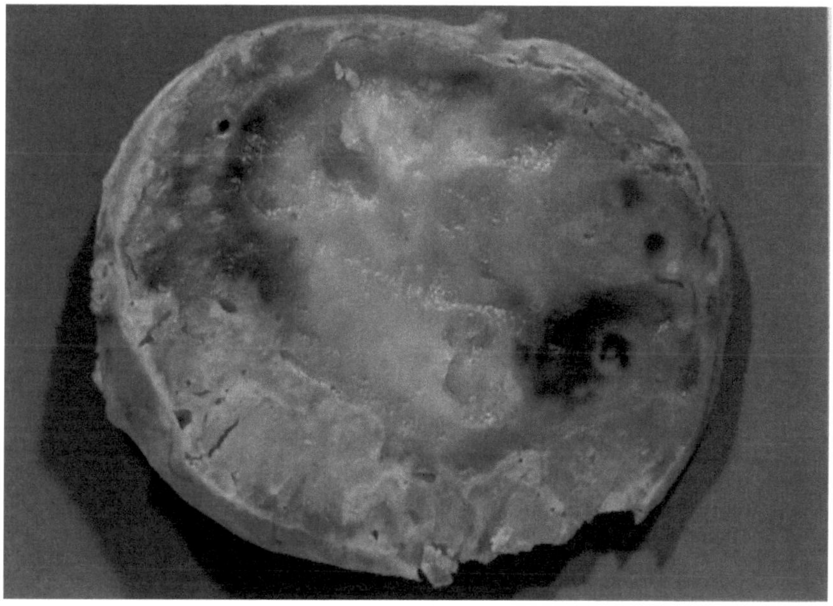

Fig. 45. Large adenoma of the adrenal with pronounced regressive changes and hemorrhages that are not normally observed with adenomas but rather with carcinomas

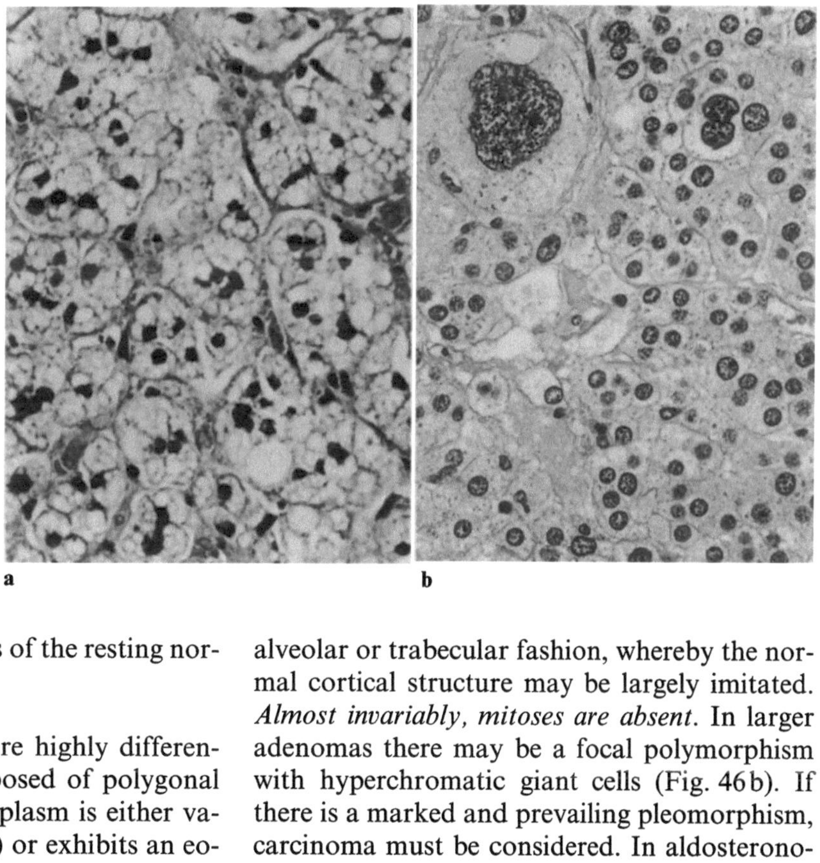

Fig. 46 a, b. Adenoma of the renal cortex. **(a)** Vacuolated "clear" cells with small, dark, slightly polymorphous nuclei. **(b)** "Compact cells" with granulated cytoplasm and pronounced nuclear polymorphism. H & E, ×350

adenomas without alterations of the resting normal parenchyma.

Microscopically, adenomas are highly differentiated lesions (Fig. 46) composed of polygonal medium-sized cells. The cytoplasm is either vacuolized (so-called clear cells) or exhibits an eosinophilic granulation ("compact cells"). Compact cells may be arranged in small groups forming "microadenomas." Intermediate cells with features both of clear cells and compact cells may occur. The cells are arranged in an alveolar or trabecular fashion, whereby the normal cortical structure may be largely imitated. *Almost invariably, mitoses are absent.* In larger adenomas there may be a focal polymorphism with hyperchromatic giant cells (Fig. 46b). If there is a marked and prevailing pleomorphism, carcinoma must be considered. In aldosteronomas, spironolactone bodies may be found. These are eosinophilic, round, laminated cytoplasmic inclusions surrounded by clear halos [206, 6]. Adenomas usually possess a delicate vascular stroma. Larger examples may

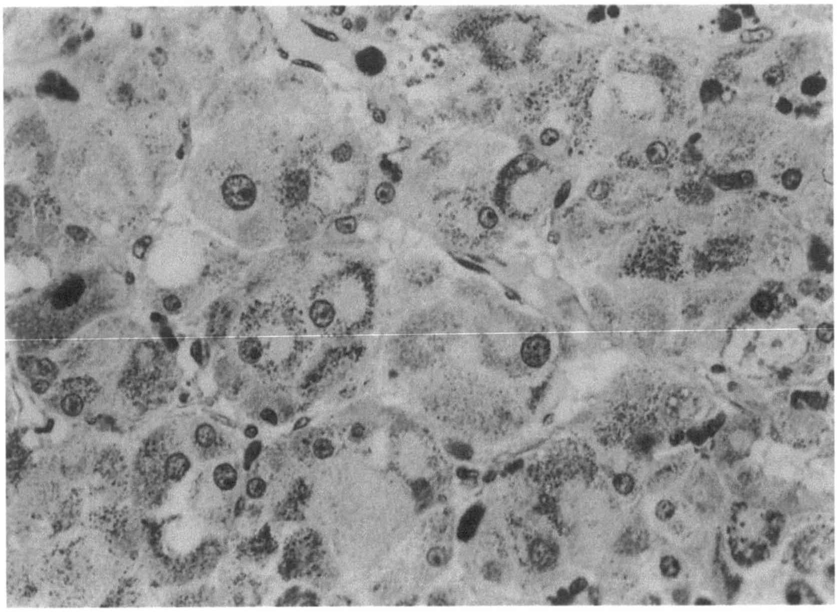

Fig. 47. "Black adenoma" of the adrenal cortex. Note the deposits of finely granular lipofuscin that are concentrated particularly at the cytoplasmic margins of the adenoma cells. H & E, ×350

show pronounced stromal sclerosis. Not rarely, small aggregates of lymphocytes may be admixed.

A very rare variant is the so-called "black" adenoma of the adrenal cortex (Fig. 47). This peculiar tumor stands out by its dark brown color caused by large amounts of lipofuscin within the tumor cells [258, 261]. Since lipofuscin is regularly observed within the cells of the normal zona reticularis, black adenomas may derive from this zone [341]. The lesion can cause endocrine disturbances, for instance Cushing's syndrome [411, 233].

The *differential diagnosis* includes nodular hyperplasia (Fig. 44a). Adenomas are usually unilateral, whereas nodular hyperplasia concerns both adrenals. Hyperplastic nodules do not exceed 2 cm in diameter. The histology of adenomas and hyperplasia does not principally differ. For the differential diagnosis between adenoma and carcinoma see below.

4.2.3 Primary Carcinoma

This carcinoma is rare and accounts for only 0.2% of all cancer deaths in the USA [200]. Most cases occur in the fourth or fifth decade. Two-thirds of the patients are females. Functioning and nonfunctioning varieties show a different age distribution [177, 201]. Active carcinomas occur mainly in the first 4 decades and predominantly in females [177], whereas inactive carcinomas affect predominantly the elderly. Two-thirds of the patients with inactive carcinomas are males [255]. The left adrenal is affected twice as often as the right [177, 201, 225].

Macroscopically, carcinomas are much larger than adenomas and may weigh more than 1000 g (Fig. 48). They tend to exhibit a pronounced nodularity and are incompletely encapsulated and often intimately adherent to the neighboring organs such as kidney, pancreas, or liver. Their consistency is soft and friable. The cut surface is greyish-red or yellowish-white and mottled. Large areas of hemorrhage and necrosis are frequent. Calcification is rare.

Microscopically, there is a broad range of possible pictures, depending on the differentiation of a given tumor. The average one presents polygonal cells with an eosinophilic or vacuolated cytoplasm. They are arranged in trabecules or in an alveolar fashion but in many cases there is no characteristic arrangement. Highly atypical cells with giant nuclei and multinucleation, as well as typical and atypical mitoses can be found with varying frequency (Figs. 49 and 50).

In some examples the tumor cells are fairly monomorphous although unequivocally atypical (Fig. 49). In highly differentiated cases the morphology may be very similar to that of ad-

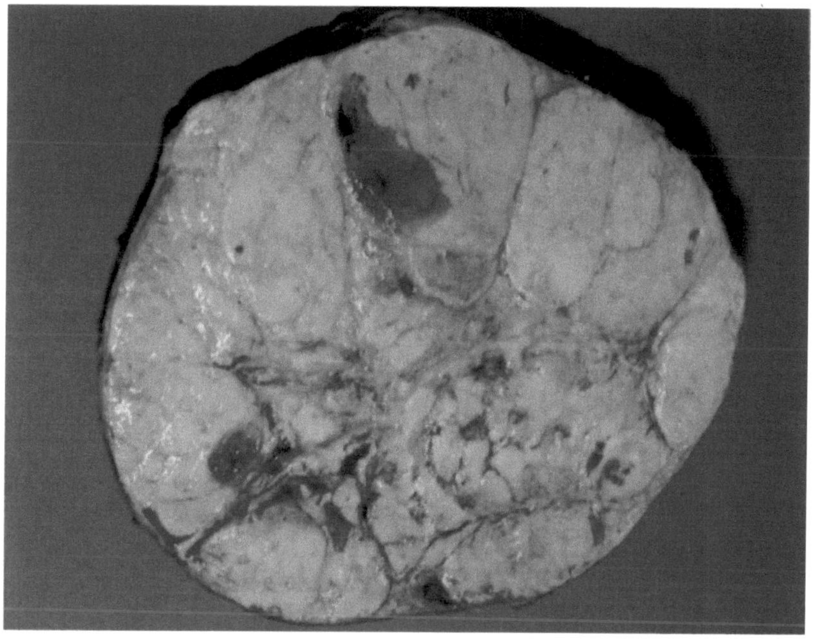

Fig. 48. This carcinoma of the adrenal cortex measured 17 cm in diameter with a weight of 1800 g. Note the pronounced nodularity, hemorrhages, and yellowish areas of necrosis near the center of the growth. These macroscopic features virtually exclude adenoma

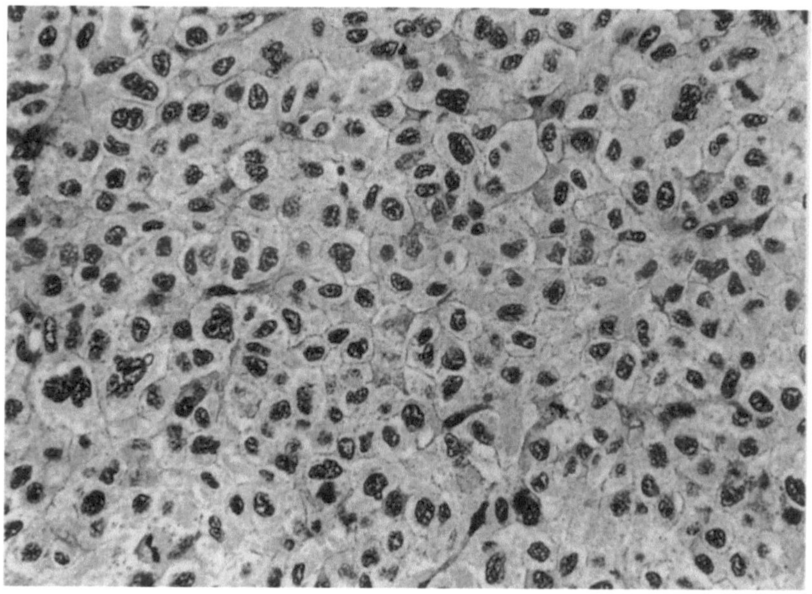

Fig. 49. Carcinoma of the adrenal cortex. Relatively monomorphous nuclei. There are some mitotic figures. H & E, ×350

enomas so that the distinction from large adenomas can be very difficult if histological criteria alone are used. In such cases a thorough evaluation of other criteria such as age, sex, and functionality may help in establishing the correct diagnosis.

4.2.3.1 Grading

Grading of adrenocortical carcinomas is not commonly applied. LEWINSKY et al. [252] graded 20 cases of "nonhormonal" carcinomas with respect to cellular and nuclear pleomorphism, nuclear vesicularity, and mitotic activity. According to their data, patients with highly malignant variants died within the first 7 months, those with a moderate grade of malignancy within 6 years, while those with a low grade of malignancy survived for up to 18 years postoperatively. HOGAN et al. [189] graded 21 cases and distinguished differentiated from anaplastic forms. A case was labeled anaplastic

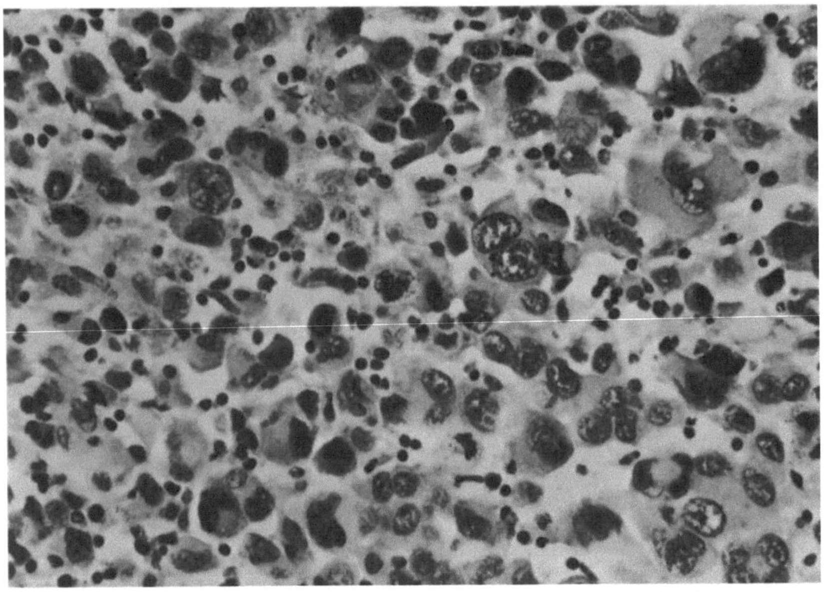

Fig. 50. Carcinoma of the adrenal cortex. Pronounced atypia of the cells with formation of small giant cells. For comparison, note the small lymphocytes that intermingle with the tumor cells. H & E, ×350

if 50% or more of the cells were large and pleomorphic. The median survival time of patients with anaplastic carcinomas was only 5 months, while those with differentiated carcinomas survived for 40 months. Thus, grading of adrenocortical carcinomas seems to be feasible, but its informational value is clearly not superior to that provided by the general criteria of malignancy.

4.2.3.2 Staging

Staging of adrenocortical carcinomas is rarely performed although the stage is an important prognostic factor. SULLIVAN et al. [383] modified the original proposal of MACFARLANE [262] as follows: in stage I the tumor is smaller than 5 cm in diameter; in stage II the tumor exceeds 5 cm. In both stages there should be no local invasion and no metastases. In stage III regional lymph node metastases or local invasion or both are present. Stage IV is defined by the presence of distant metastases.

4.2.3.3 Spread

Spread of adrenocortical carcinomas may take three main routes, namely, directly, lymphogenous, and hematogenous. Direct spread affects the soft tissue bed of the adrenals and adjacent organs, particularly the kidneys. Local spread was observed in 65% of 127 cases by HUTTER and KAYHOE [200]. Spread to the regional lymph nodes is reported to be present in 10%–31% of the cases at operation. Distant lymph node involvement may affect the hilar, supraclavicular, cervical, and axillary nodes. Hematogenous metastases are most often found in the liver, lungs, and bones. At autopsy, KING and LACK [225] reported the following distribution in 29 patients: liver 93%, lungs 79%, bone 24%, pancreas 17%, kidney and brain 10%. Cutaneous metastases have been reported to be particularly frequent with cases of anaplastic carcinomas [189].

4.2.3.4 Differential Diagnosis

The differential diagnosis of adrenocortical carcinoma includes secondary carcinoma, pheochromocytoma, and adrenocortical adenoma. Only the distinction between carcinoma and adenoma will be considered here; with respect to the remaining two differential diagnoses, see Sects. 4.2.4 and 4.4.4.

Clinical symptoms that favour the diagnosis of a carcinoma over that of an adenoma are weight loss [192], a palpable abdominal mass [225], and an endocrinopathia with "mixed" features. For example, mixed syndromes in adult females exhibiting features both of adrenogenital *and* Cushing's syndrome are almost always caused by a carcinoma.

Macroscopically, large tumor weight (more than 100 g) and size (more than 5 cm) together with significant degenerative changes are considered relatively reliable criteria of malignancy by many authors [225, 389, 406].

Microscopically, a high proliferative activity, atypical mitoses, capsule invasion, and vascular invasion all indicate carcinoma [180, 350, 192, 225, 406, 418]. If all these criteria are carefully analysed, the differential diagnosis between adenoma and carcinoma can generally be made with accuracy [389].

4.2.3.5 Prognosis

The prognosis is poor. The five-year mortality ranges between 75% and 90% [225] due to the fact that most of these cancers are nonfunctioning, undifferentiated, and rapidly growing. TANG and GRAY [389] and VAN SLOOTEN et al. [406] observed a rather favourable outcome for virilizing cancers after radical surgery since functioning carcinomas are highly differentiated. Accordingly, they enlarge slowly and are still small at the first presentation.

4.2.4 Secondary Carcinoma

Metastases to the adrenals occur very frequently secondary to many different neoplasms. In particular many carcinomas metastasize to the adrenals, e.g., lung cancer. Furthermore, carcinoma of the breast, carcinoma of the stomach, and also adenocarcinoma of the kidney may lead to metastases in the adrenals. The lesions are usually manifestations of a second generation of metastases except for carcinoma of the lung. Adrenal metastases of malignant melanoma are also relatively frequent. Metastases to the adrenals hardly evoke clinical symptoms and are usually incidental findings at autopsy.

4.3 Tumors of the Adrenal Medulla

4.3.1 General Remarks

The cells of the adrenal medulla derive from the neural crest and migrate to the adrenal. The migrating cells may give rise to (1) neuroblasts, sympathogonia, sympathicoblasts, and ganglion cells as well as to (2) pheochromoblasts and pheochromocytes. Accordingly, two different groups of tumors may be found within the adrenal medulla: (1) neuroblastomas, ganglioneuroblastomas, and ganglioneuromas and (2) pheochromocytomas. Thus, adrenal medullary tumors comprise neoplasias of the chromaffin tissue as well as neurogenic neoplasias. Both groups of tumors may produce catecholamines and/or their metabolites which may be detected in the urine. This unique property not only aids in diagnosis but is a useful means of assessing the response to therapy or detection of recurrence.

4.3.2 Neuroblastoma and Ganglioneuroblastoma

Neuroblastoma is one of the most frequent neoplasias of childhood. More than 90% occur in children below 10 years of age, 43% in the first 2 years of life [290]. Furthermore, it is not so rare to find these tumors in fetuses or in newborns [112]. Rarely, neuroblastomas develop in adolescents and very rarely in adults. The male–female ratio is 3:2 [142]. Familial occurrence has been described [65, 150, 48].

In some cases, malformations like spina bifida, aortal coarctation, hydrocephalus, polydactylia, and visceral malformations accompany the tumor [385]. Neuroblastoma may also be combined with dominantly hereditary neurofibromatosis [428].

According to GRONCY and FINKLESTEIN [152], the most common sites are the adrenals (43.6%), followed by the abdominal ganglia (23.6%), and the dorsal mediastinum (15.8%). Some authors [154, 247] described multiple neuroblastomas with various grades of maturation. However, whether such cases are neuroblastomas with different grades of maturation of their metastases rather than multiple primaries independent from each other remains to be cleared.

Neuroblastomas are poorly differentiated neoplasms. Ganglioneuroblastomas are partly differentiated neuroblastomas containing undifferentiated neuroblasts side by side with well-developed ganglion cells. Two subtypes of ganglioneuroblastoma are distinguished, namely,

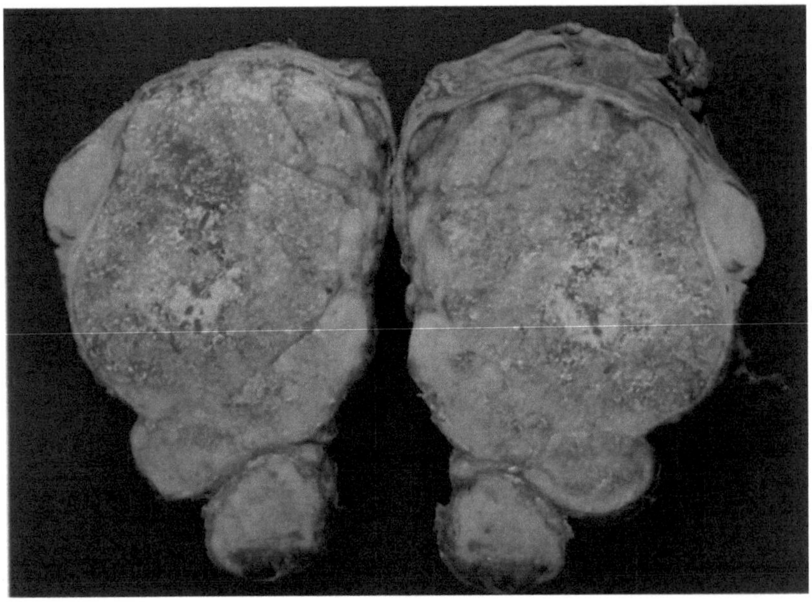

Fig. 51. Neuroblastoma of the adrenal. The cut surface exhibits finely stippled yellowish deposits of calcification. This feature is almost pathognomonic

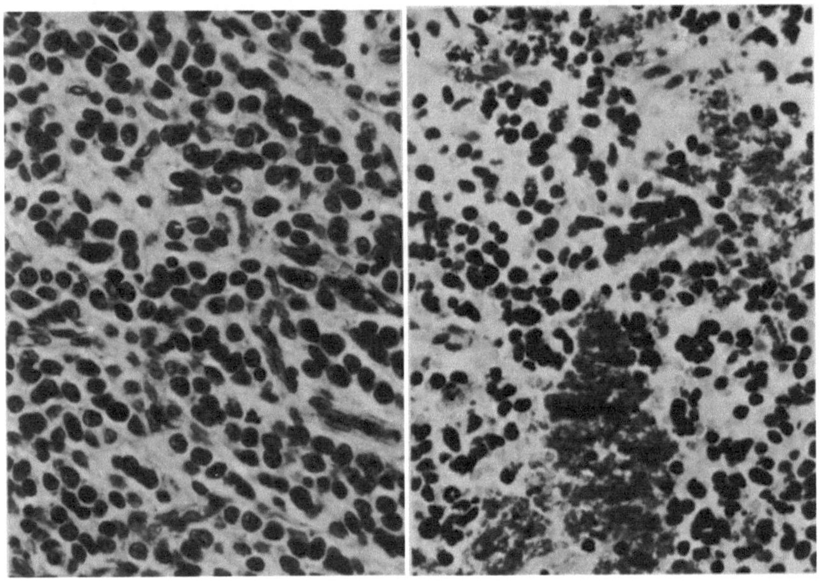

a b

Fig. 52 a, b. Neuroblastoma. **(a)** Uniformly shaped cells mimicking sympathicogonias. Dense but finely stippled chromatin. **(b)** Small blocklike or granular microcalcifications. H & E, ×350

(1) a diffuse type and (2) a composite type, of which the latter is prognostically unfavourable [4, 375].

Macroscopically, neuroblastomas are large, roundish or lobated tumors that are relatively well delineated, mostly, however, without a true capsule. The tumors are soft and friable, and the cut surfaces reveal solid medullary greyish-white tumor tissue. Hemorrhages, necroses, cystic changes, and calcification that can be demonstrated roentgenologically can all be observed (Fig. 51). The most undifferentiated forms very often show a marked local invasion, whereas the more differentiated tumors tend to be better delineated.

Microscopically, undifferentiated neuroblastomas consist of densely packed, uniformly shaped cells (Fig. 52), closely imitating sympathogonias. The cells are small with round or oval nuclei. The chromatin is finely structured, evenly distributed, and delicately stippled, which distinguishes them clearly from lympho-

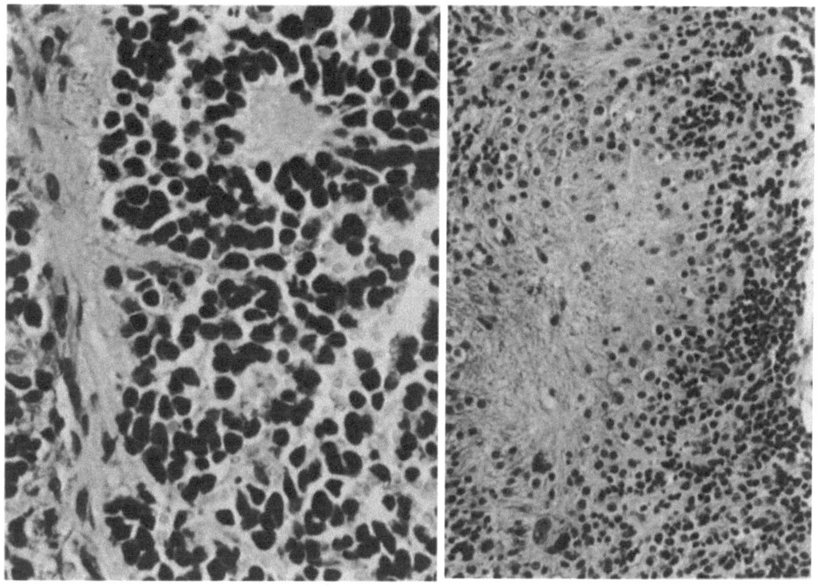

a b

Fig. 53 a, b. Neuroblastoma. **(a)** A typical rosette can be seen at the *top*. H & E, × 350. **(b)** Cell-free fibrillar area resembling glial tissue. At the *bottom* some larger cells similar to ganglion cells. H & E, × 140

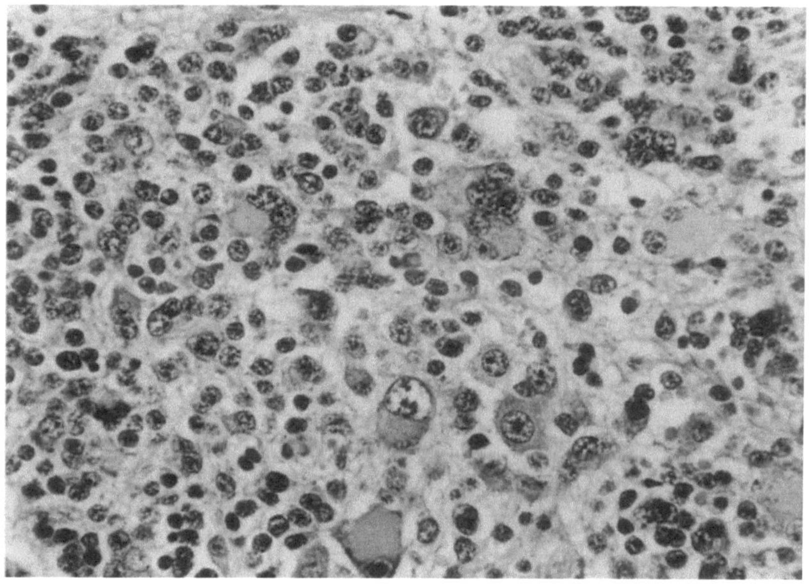

Fig. 54. Ganglioneuroblastoma, diffuse type. Note the admixture of large differentiated ganglion cell-like elements. H & E, × 350

cytes provided thoroughly prepared paraffin sections are used. The cytoplasmic rim is very small, so that the nuclei often appear naked. There are very often granular or blocklike microcalcifications that are highly characteristic.

The tumor cells tend to be arranged in groups of small dense morulalike structures. In one-third of cases, rosettes can be demonstrated. These diagnostic structures consist of groups of cells that surround a central network of very delicate fibrils (Fig. 53). Furthermore, cell-free fibrillar areas that strongly resemble glial tissue may be observed with varying frequency.

If the cases show larger tumor cells with vesicularly structured nuclei and a well-defined eosinophilic cytoplasm, many authors will diagnose a more advanced differentiated form of neuroblastoma as compared with the form described above [264].

If well-developed ganglion cells occur, one speaks of ganglioneuroblastoma. An irregular mixture of mature ganglion cells defines the so-called diffuse ganglioneuroblastoma (Fig. 54). If there are one or more nodules consisting of pure neuroblastoma tissue, then the diagnosis of a composite ganglioneuroblastoma must be made [4, 375].

4.3.2.1 Grading

Hughes et al. [195] have proposed three grades of malignancy for neuroblastoma including ganglioneuroblastoma. Grade I is identical with the diagnosis of ganglioneuroblastoma, showing a mixture of immature cells with mature ganglion cells. It is said that diffuse ganglioneuroblastomas have a better prognosis than composite ganglioneuroblastomas [358]. Grade II is applied if a mixture of undifferentiated cells with moderately differentiated neuroblastoma cells can be found. Grade III labels cases that consist exclusively of undifferentiated cells without any recognizable tendency for differentiation.

4.3.2.2 Staging

Staging of neuroblastoma is important because it helps in assessing prognostic predictions. Evans et al. [109] have proposed four stages. In stage I the tumor is confined to the organ or structure of origin. Stage II comprises tumors extending in continuity beyond the organ but not crossing the midline, and homolateral regional lymph nodes may be involved. In stage III the tumor extends beyond the midline and there is bilateral involvement of lymph nodes. In stage IV distant metastases have developed. The authors further discriminate a special stage, which they call IV-S. This stage takes into consideration the extraordinary peculiarity that a localized primary tumor with distant metastases in liver, skin, or bone marrow, and any combination of these without roentgenologically recognizable skeletal metastases shows a markedly better prognosis than is to be expected in the case of other malignancies with corresponding spread [87, 110].

4.3.2.3 Spread

Neuroblastomas and ganglioneuroblastomas may show macroscopically a more or less sharp delineation. However, microscopically one always finds infiltration. Metastases within the regional para-aortal lymph nodes are frequent. From here, spread to the mediastinal and supraclavicular lymph nodes may occur. Hematogenous metastases will be found frequently in the liver and bones.

According to the literature, there are varying data about distant metastases in neuroblastoma. Stowens [378] studied autopsy cases and found metastases in various organs in the following frequency: liver 65%, regional lymph nodes 60%, lungs 60%, skeleton 50%, gastrointestinal tract 43%, bone marrow 23%, skull 23%, kidney 19%, orbit 17%.

Typically, distant metastases of neuroblastoma occur very early. The bone marrow is relatively often involved even with small occult primary neuroblastomas. Of all patients 70% already have distant metastases at first diagnosis [154].

4.3.2.4 Differential Diagnosis

As a rule, the diagnosis can readily be made if a given tumor shows typical behavior concerning localization, age, morphology, and metabolism: catecholamines and their metabolites are produced in approximately 95% of cases [142]. Ganglioneuroblastomas are diagnosable by morphology alone. If the first symptoms are produced by early involvement of long bones, Ewings' sarcoma may be imitated. However, a meticulous search will detect rosettes in a neuroblastoma, and the PAS-reaction will usually be negative. In Ewings' sarcoma no true rosettes and no differentiation into ganglion cells can be found, and the PAS-reaction in most cases is strongly positive [345].

In more than 50% of cases, neuroblastoma cells can be found in bone marrow smears and may be misinterpreted as undifferentiated cells of leukemia. Here again, a meticulous analysis of the cytology together with appliance of cytochemical reactions should enable one to make the correct diagnosis.

Other malignant tumors that have to be separated from neuroblastomas are embryonal rhabdomyosarcomas, seminomas, and dysgerminomas. These last three will all give a more or less intensely positive reaction with the PAS-method, whereas neuroblastoma cells are negative. Moreover, rhabdomyosarcomas may show myxoid areas, which is not found with neuroblastomas, and rhabdomyosarcomas may contain cells that are cross-striated. Seminomas and dysgerminomas present a very typical stromal reaction, namely, a delicate framework of connective tissue that is infiltrated by lymphocytes, macrophages, epithelioid cells, and even foreign body giant cells. Such structures will never be found within neuroblastomas. Finally, seminoma cells and dysgerminoma cells are very large and usually show broad clear cytoplasms. This, too, is not the case with neuroblastoma cells.

4.3.2.5 Prognosis

With exceptions, neuroblastomas behave very aggressively and are highly malignant. Irrespective of treatment, there is a fatal outcome within a very short period of time. However, in certain distinct, particular cases, spontaneous regression or differentiation resulting in cure have been reported (see below). Apart from these exceptions, prognosis is influenced by at least four factors: age, localization, differentiation, and spread. By and large, the following rule of thumb can be given: the younger the patient, the better the prognosis [154]. The most favourable outcomes are seen in the first 12 months of life [378]. In reviewing a total of 246 patients, BRESLOW and MCCANN [54] found 2-year survival in 74% at age 0 to 11 months, in 26% at age 12 to 23 months, and in 12% for children older than 24 months. KINNIER WILSON and DRAPER [226] in a series of 487 cases reported similar experiences.

The localization of a neuroblastoma is also a well recognized prognostic factor. In fact, an intrathoracic localization correlates positively with better survival data [154, 96, 109, 121]. According to DE LORIMIER et al. [96], the survival rate for mediastinal cases was 48.5%, whereas retroperitoneal cases showed only a 20% survival. This better prognosis for patients with mediastinal neuroblastoma was due to a 100% survival rate in the infant group.

That grade of differentiation of a neuroblastoma is an important prognostic factor is reflected by the division of the tumors into neuroblastomas which are very undifferentiated, those that are moderately differentiated, and ganglioneuroblastomas that are partly differentiated, while the most advanced differentiation is reached by ganglioneuromas which are benign.

As is the case with all other malignant neoplasias, spread is very important in assessing the prognosis. The farther advanced a given neuroblastoma, the worse the prognosis: survival drops progressively from 90% in stage I to 2.4% in stage IV [230]. However, very exceptional courses are observed with patients in stage IV-S, i.e., localized, small primaries accompanied by extensive distant metastases in liver, skin, or bone marrow (without bone destruction), or any combination of these. Such cases show a markedly better prognosis than would be expected if the general criteria of malignancy were applied [87, 110]. These cases concern children younger than one year. The underlying process is spontaneous regression with the possible result of even complete disappearance of the disease [111], the mechanism of which is not yet fully understood. For this group of patients, HASSENBUSCH et al. [176] stated that death is more likely to result from vigorous treatment than from the disease itself. Therefore, careful consideration should be given before selecting treatment for young infants with stage IV-S [87, 351].

A second exception from the rule comprises those cases that show maturation into typical benign ganglioneuromas [83, 150, 279]. The mechanism of such a maturation remains highly speculative, and it is debatable whether or not these cases in fact represent truly malignant neoplasias. The prognostic meaning or not of lymphocytic infiltration of neuroblastoma tissue has also not been resolved [241, 195]. The number of mitoses does not play a significant role in the prognosis. This seems to be generally true for all cancers in infancy and childhood [298]; however, atypical mitoses may mean anaplasia. Finally, it should be mentioned that the prognosis for girls is said to be better than that for boys [226].

4.3.3 Ganglioneuroma

Ganglioneuroma of the adrenal is rare, the most common site being the mediastinum [378]. It is defined as a relatively mature benign tumor of the sympathetic system of neck, mediastinum, pelvis, and adrenal medulla. Ganglioneuromas are found in young patients below 20 years of age. Most of the tumors occur in the first decade. Girls may slightly outnumber boys.

Macroscopically, the tumor is well demarcated and well encapsulated. Its consistency is firm and solid. The tumors may attain considerable sizes. The cut surface is greyish-white with opaque patches. Often there are whorls or plexiform structures with myxomatous slimy areas. Hyalinization and calcification may occur.

Histologically, the tumor consists of more or less regularly layered bundles of nerve fibers. These may be accompanied by Schwann's cells. Ganglion cells of different sizes and in varying numbers can be found scattered in the tissue. These may contain lipofuscin. Sometimes there are large groups of ganglion cells. Occasionally, even satellite cells can be observed. There are practically no mitoses. In spite of this, the tumors may grow larger by and by, for instance, through increase of nerval fibers, connective tissue, and edematous fluid within the tissue.

The diagnosis usually does not present any difficulties. It is very important to investigate many sections from many regions in this kind of tumor to exclude immature tumor tissue. If immature structures can be detected, ganglioneuroblastoma must be diagnosed. It should be emphasized that lymphocytes that can be often found within ganglioneuromas must not be confused with immature neuroblastoma cells.

4.3.4 Pheochromocytoma

In most cases, pheochromocytoma is an adrenal tumor, although extra-adrenal development such as from the organs of Zuckerkandl and the paraganglionic system does occur [283]. Most of these growths appear between the 25th and 55th year of life. In adults there is no sex preponderance, but in childhood the incidence was found to be twice as frequent in boys than in girls [364]. The right gland is more often affected than the left. Remine et al. [334] have reported that of 124 intra-adrenal tumors, 56.5% were located in the right gland and 38.7% in the left.

In the adult, more than 90% of the pheochromocytomas involve the adrenal, while in childhood about 25% of these tumors originate from extra-adrenal chromaffin structures. Extra-adrenal tumors most commonly involve the organs of Zuckerkandl. Multiple pheochromocytomas are much more common in children (about 30%) than in adults. Approximately 25% of those tumors that occur in children are bilateral [199]. It is important to know that a second pheochromocytoma may appear many years after the removal of an earlier one.

Of the infantile pheochromocytomas 10% are associated with identical tumors in other members of the family. These familial pheochromocytomas may be combined with C-cell (medullary) carcinoma of the thyroid [360, 426] and are often bilateral (Sipple's syndrome). In addition, there are many examples of pheochromocytomas occurring in association with multiple neurofibromatosis [179, 62].

Familial syndromes of multiple endocrine neoplasias (MEN) have been described. If a pheochromocytoma occurs together with medullary thyroid carcinoma and parathyroid hyperplasia, the syndrome is called "MEN II" [371]. If a pheochromocytoma is combined with mucosal neuroma and medullary thyroid carcinoma the term "MEN III" is applied [223]. However, it has been discussed whether or not such pheochromocytomas might only be adrenal medullary hyperplasias [410, 63, 95].

Of all pheochromocytomas in the adult 10% arise from chromaffin tissue outside the adrenal medulla. Such extra-adrenal chromaffin tissue is widely distributed in the fetus, especially in association with the sympathetic nervous system. It disappears during childhood but may persist and give rise to extra-adrenal pheochromocytomas. These are located retroperitoneally in the vicinity of the renal capsule, within the scrotum, in the wall of urinary bladder [133], neck, thorax, and intracranial sites [357].

The designation of adrenal medullary tumors as "pheochromocytomas" expresses the ability of the tumor tissue to react with dichromate salts or chromic acid to form dark-brown pigments that represent oxidation products of adrenaline and noradrenaline. This chromaffin reaction (Fig. 55) was first described by Henle [182] and is of great importance in the diagnosis of pheochromocytoma.

Macroscopically, pheochromocytomas (Fig. 56) can be very small and not larger than 1–2 cm

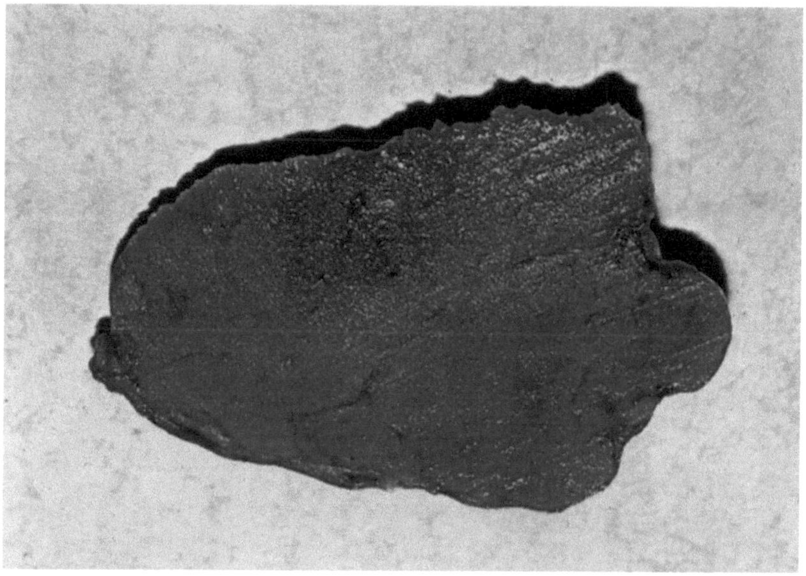

Fig. 55. Pheochromocytoma tissue subjected to Henle's chromoreaction. The tissue has taken on a brownish color

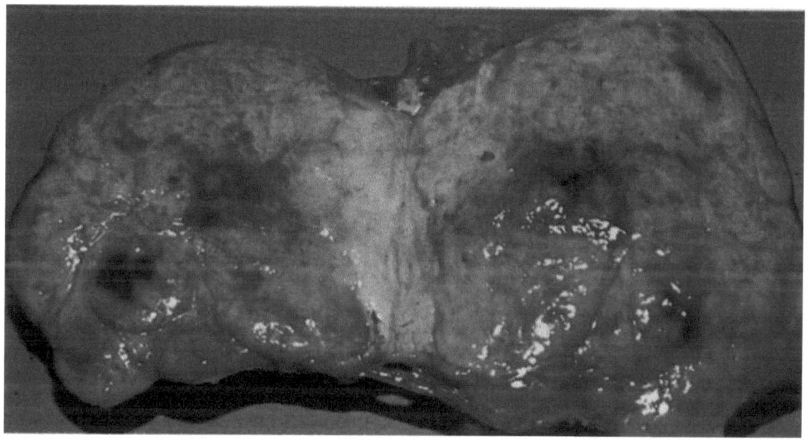

Fig. 56. Pheochromocytoma measuring 10 × 7 cm. The cut surface exhibits a greyish-red color. There are several hemorrhages

in diameter but may reach 25 cm. They may weigh more than 2000 g. Symptoms and signs do not correlate with their size, localization, or histopathology.

On the cut surface the tumors exhibit a grey or greyish-red to dusky red color together with a more or less pronounced lobulation. Larger tumors often reveal extensive hemorrhage, necrosis, and cystic changes. The tumors are generally rounded and enveloped by a compressed residual rim of cortical tissue.

Very characteristic and helpful in the diagnosis is the tendency of the tumor tissue to take on a yellowish to brown color if exposed to air or formalin solution, and the solution is also colored brown. As has already been mentioned, this reflects oxidation of catecholamines into brownish pigments.

Microscopically, pheochromocytomas reveal a very variegated appearance (Figs. 57 and 58). The stroma contains many thin-walled sinusoids together with smaller and larger, sometimes thick-walled vessels. In some cases, the grade of vascularization may be exceedingly high, so that a vascular tumor may be mimicked [359]. Polygonal cells of differing sizes are located in between this well-vascularized stroma. The cells are often arranged in a mosaiclike or in an alveolarlike fashion.

According to the cytology, three types are distinguished [334]: 55% show an epithelial differ-

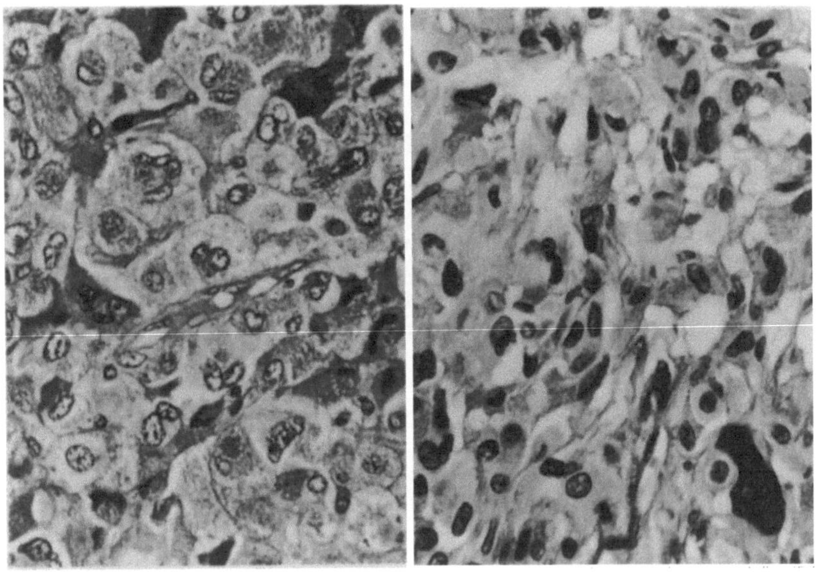

a b

Fig. 57 a, b. Pheochromocytoma. **(a)** Typical mosaic-like pattern. **(b)** Polymorphous pattern. H & E, ×350

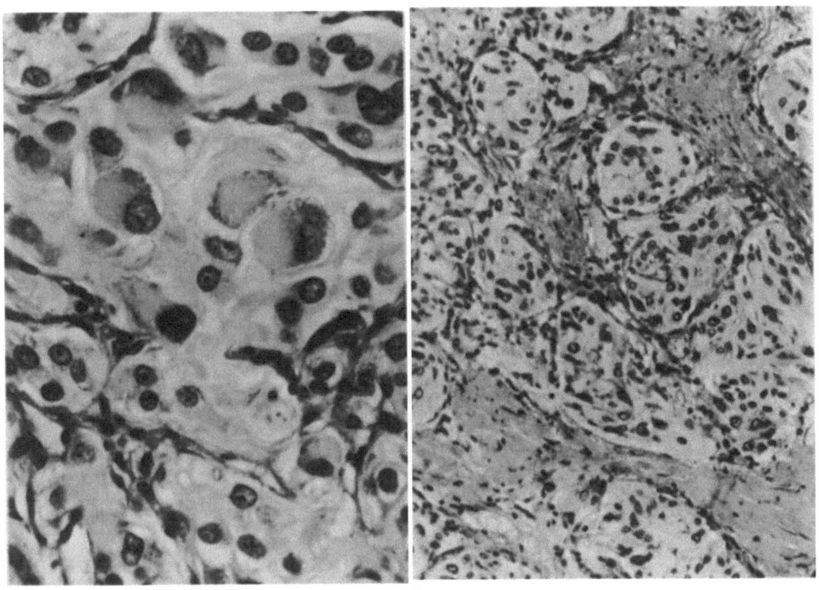

a b

Fig. 58 a, b. Pheochromocytoma. **(a)** Ganglion cell-like pattern. H & E, ×350. **(b)** Alveolar pattern. H & E, ×56

entiation, 43% are pleomorphic, and 2% consist of spindle cells. The tumor cells are usually larger than the cells of the normal medulla and possess a broad, foamy or granular cytoplasm that may be eosinophilic, amphophilic, or basophilic. The cell borders are not always distinctively recognizable. Some cases contain cells with a prominent vacuolization of the cytoplasm.

The nuclei may be vesicular or compact. They tend to take on an eccentric position. A marked pleomorphism of the nuclei is very characteristic, as are nuclear inclusions of cytoplasm. Multinucleation and bizarre nuclei can often be found. Mitotic figures are rare; hyperchromatic degenerating nuclei are frequent and must not be confused with mitoses. Some occasional cells may exhibit features of ganglion cells, occur in small clusters, and be sometimes accompanied by neurofibrils and Schwann's cells.

Not rarely, strongly PAS-positive hyaline corpuscles can be found singly or in small groups within the tumor cells. They are known to occur also in cells of the normal medulla. Histochemical studies have indicated a proteinaceous nature of these globules [173]. According to

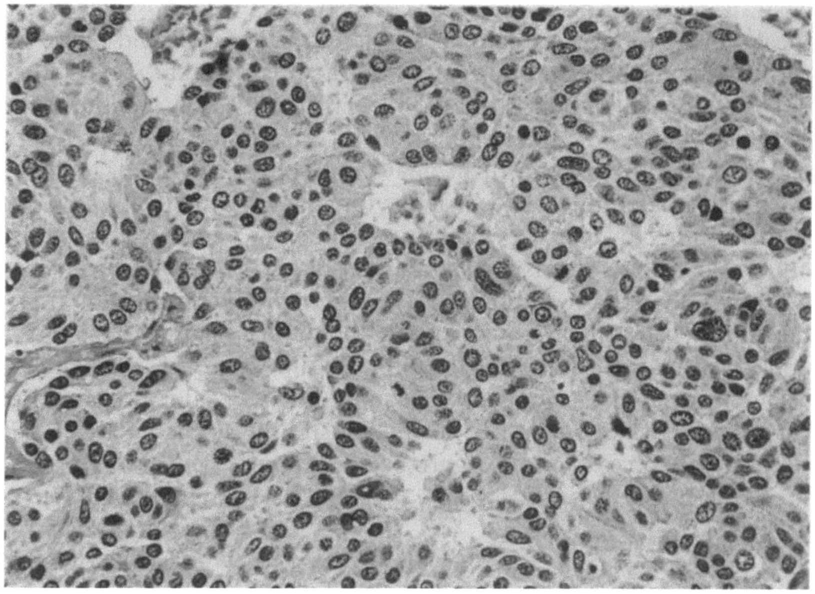

Fig. 59. Malignant pheochromocytoma. Note the relatively small and uniform tumor cells. There are some mitoses. Patient died two years later with widespread disease. H & E, ×350

DECKER and OEHRLE [93], these bodies are possibly products of lipid peroxidation. The association of fetal fat cells with pheochromocytomas has been noticed by GRAHAM [148] and has been well documented by MELICOW [282].

The biologic behavior of pheochromocytoma is extremely difficult to assess. The only certain criterion of malignancy is the presence of secondary tumor deposits *in sites where chromaffin tissue is not normally found* [386]. This restriction is important to know, in order to avoid confusion of multiple pheochromocytomas with distant metastases of a single solitary pheochromocytoma.

Common characteristics of malignancy such as cellular and nuclear pleomorphism cannot be applied to pheochromocytomas. Even infiltration of the capsule or of blood vessels is not a reliable criteria of malignancy. The same is true for the presence of spindle cells. However, frequent and atypical mitoses as well as a relatively monotonous cytologic pattern are highly suggestive of malignancy (Fig. 59).

Many widely differing opinions about the frequency of benign and malignant pheochromocytomas can be found in the literature. LEWIS [253] thinks approximately 10% and REMINE et al. [334] 13.1% to be malignant. However, HUME [199] estimates only 2.8% of all pheochromocytomas to be cancers. This corresponds well to the data of SYMINGTON and GOODALL [386] who suggest that 2.5% would be a reasonable figure. At least malignant pheochromocytomas are extremely rare.

Spread of malignant pheochromocytoma first of all involves the tumor capsule, adjacent tissue, and regional lymph nodes. Involvement of the renal vein and its tributaries and spread into the inferior vena cava have been observed, though not necessarily associated with the occurrence of distant metastases. If distant metastases do occur, then these involve liver, lungs, and bone. There may be a peculiar tendency towards isolated vertebral involvement. Therefore, a preoperative bone scan is recommended in all patients with pheochromocytoma. Metastases are generally functional. With their advent, symptoms reappear and hypertension becomes difficult to manage.

Usually, pheochromocytoma is clinically diagnosed by the fact that the patient develops high blood pressure. This is caused by the noradrenaline and adrenaline that are produced by the tumor cells. The amount of the hormones daily produced can be assessed by investigation of catecholamines within the urine. A main problem for the clinicians is – particularly with small tumors – finding the exact preoperative locality of the tumor.

Differential diagnosis should consider polymorphous carcinomas of the adrenal cortex. If the cells of an adrenocortical carcinoma possess a broad granulated eosinophilic cytoplasm, discrimination may be difficult. However, the demonstration of fat-positive, honeycombed cells speaks in favor of a carcinoma of the adrenal cortex. Heavy pigmentation is more characteristic of a cortical tumor than of pheochromocytoma, whereas the development of brownish pigment after fixation in dichromate salt solutions clearly identifies pheochromocytoma.

According to SHERWIN [357] the following morphologic characteristics should be sought: (1) tumor–medulla continuity, (2) tumor and medullary cell similarity, including the uninvolved adrenal medulla, (3) the typical tumor cell mosaic pattern, (4) pseudoacinar formation, (5) droplet formation that is not diagnostic by itself, (6) absence of mitotic figures, and (7) fetal fat in the tumor periphery.

4.4 Myelolipoma and Cysts

4.4.1 Myelolipoma

This lesion does not represent a true neoplasia but is probably a metaplasia that originates within the adrenal cortex. According to OLSSON et al. [307] the autopsy incidence ranges from 0.08%–0.4%.

Macroscopically, the appearance of the cut surface resembles fatty tissue. However, unlike lipoma, some patchy, dark red areas may be conspicuous.

Microscopically, the lesion is composed of fat cells and blood-forming cells that comprise megakaryocytes, the myeloid, and the erythroid series, together with reticulum cells, some plasma cells, and some occasional lymphocytes (Fig. 60).

Myelolipoma is completely benign and in most cases is an incidental finding at autopsy. However, there are very rare cases that produce clinical symptoms due to the bulk of the tumor, hemorrhage, or necrosis [16]. Single lesions may reach a weight of up to 1590 g [29]. Thus, clinically a retroperitoneal malignant neoplasm may be simulated [118]. The lesions do not occur before puberty [319]. Rarely, endocrine derangements have been described in association with myelolipomas [107].

Up to now, the pathogenesis of myelolipoma is not known. According to OLSSON et al. [307] and AYYAT et al. [16], tissue necrosis may be the major stimulus for the pathogenesis of myelolipoma.

4.4.2 Cysts

Cysts develop rarely in the adrenals. FOSTER [128] collected 220 cases from the literature. They have been reported at all ages. Generally, they evoke only slight symptoms such as dull pain, gastrointestinal symptoms, and a palpable mass. In rare cases, hypertension may be present [140]. Morphologically, pseudocysts due to

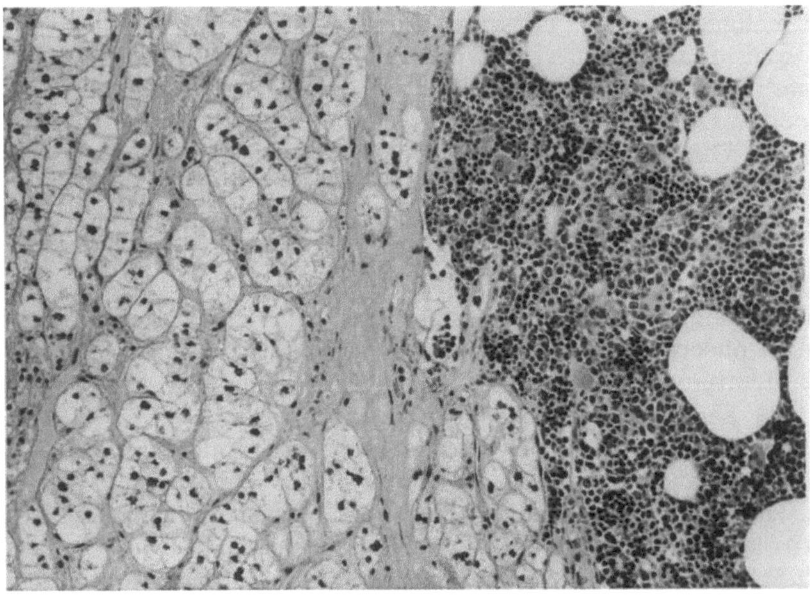

Fig. 60. Myelolipoma and cortical adenoma of the adrenal. Myelolipoma tissue to the *right*, adenoma tissue to the *left*. H & E, ×140

hemorrhages must be separated from true cysts. These latter can be divided into congenital epithelial retention cysts, cystic adenomata, and angiomatous pseudocysts. Occasionally, echinococcal cysts may be found [2]. Some cases may attain gigantic dimensions [128]. No malignancies associated with adrenal cysts have been reported so far.

References

1. Abeshouse BS, Abeshouse G (1960) Endometriosis of the urinary tract: a review of the literature and a report of four cases of vesical endometriosis. J Int Coll Surg 34:43–63
2. Abeshouse GA, Goldstein RB, Abeshouse BS (1959) Adrenal cysts: review of the literature and report of three cases. J Urol 81:711–719
3. Ackerman LV (1946) Mucinous adenocarcinoma of the pelvis of the kidney. J Urol 55:36–45
4. Adam A, Hochholzer L (1981) Ganglioneuroblastoma of the posterior mediastinum. A clinicopathologic review of 80 cases. Cancer 47:373–381
5. Aiba M, Iri H, Suzuki H, Kageyama K, Kawai P, Abe O, Murai M, Pazaki H, Saruta P (1985) Numerous mast cells in an 11-deoxycorticosterone-producing adrenocortical tumor. Histologic evaluation of benignancy and comparison with mast cell distribution in adrenal glands and neoplastic counterparts of 67 surgical specimens. Arch Pathol Lab Med 109:357–360
6. Aiba M, Suzuki H, Kageyama K, Murai M, Tazaki H, Abe O, Saruta P (1981) Spironolactone bodies in aldosteronomas and in the attached adrenals. Am J Pathol 103:404–410
7. Akhtar M, Kott E (1979) Oncocytoma of kidney. Urology 14:397–400
8. Akhtar M, Kott E, Brooks B (1977) Extrarenal Wilms' tumor. Report of a case and review of the litarature. Cancer 40:3087–3091
9. Allred CD, Cathey WJ, McDivitt RW (1981) Primary renal angiosarcoma: a case report. Hum Pathol 12:665–668
10. Alken CE, Roucayrol JC, Oberhausen E, Taupitz A, Überberg H (1960) Zur Frage der Carcinom-Entstehung nach Pyelographie mit Thorotrast. Urol Int 10:137–156
11. Amtrup F, Bech Hansen J, Thybo E (1974) Prognosis in renal carcinoma evaluated from histological criteria. Scand J Urol Nephrol 8:198–202
12. Apitz K (1944) Die Geschwülste und Gewebsmißbildungen der Nierenrinde. Virchows Arch 311:285–327
13. Ashley DJB (1978) Evans' histological appearances of tumors. Livingstone, Edinburgh
14. Ashley DJB, Hickey BB (1964) Adenocarcinoma of the renal pelvis. Br J Urol 36:309–312
15. Aufderheide AC, Streitz JM (1974) Mucinous adenocarcinoma of the renal pelvis. Cancer 33:167–173
16. Ayyat F, Fosslin E, Kent R, Hudson HC (1980) Myelolipoma of the adrenal. Urology 16:415–418
17. Babaian RJ, Skinner DG, Waisman J (1980) Wilms' tumor in the adult patient: diagnosis, management, and review of the world medical literature. Cancer 45:1713–1719
18. Balsaver AM, Gibley CW Jr, Tessmer CF (1968) Ultrastructural studies in Wilms' tumor. Cancer 22:417–427
19. Bannayan GA, Huvos AG, D'Angio GJ (1971) Effect of irradiation on the maturation of Wilms' tumor. Cancer 27:812–818
20. Barajas L (1966) The development and ultrastructure of the juxtaglomerular cell granule. J Ultrastruct Res 15:400–413
21. Bartone NF, Grieco RV (1968) Renal hemangioma. JAMA 205:118–120
22. Baruch D, Corvol P, Alhenc-Gelas F, Dufloux MA, Guyenne TT, Gaux JC, Raynaud A, Brisset JM, Duclos JM, Menard J (1984) Diagnosis and treatment of renin-secreting tumors. Report of three cases. Hypertension 6:760–766
23. Bazaz-Malik G, Gupta DN (1966) Leiomyosarcoma of kidney: report of a case and review of the literature. J Urol 95:754–758
24. Bazaz-Malik G, Saraf V, Rana BS (1980) Endometrioma of the kidney: case report. J Urol 123:422–423
25. Beckwith JB (1981) Histologic classification of nephroblastoma and other renal tumors of childhood. Am J Surg Pathol 5:194
26. Beckwith JB, Palmer NF (1978) Histopathology and prognosis of Wilms' tumor. Results from the first national Wilms' tumor study. Cancer 41:1937–1948
27. Bell ET (1952) Renal diseases. Lea and Febiger, Philadelphia
28. Bengtsson U, Angervall L, Ekman H, Lehmann L (1968) Transitional cell tumors of the renal pelvis in analgesic abusers. Scand J Urol Nephrol 2:145–150
29. Bennett BD, McKenna PJ, Hough AJ, Dean R, Page DL (1980) Adrenal myelolipoma associated with Cushing's disease. Am J Clin Pathol 73:443–447
30. Bennington JL (1973) Cancer of the kidney – etiology, epidemiology, and pathology. Cancer 32:1017–1029
31. Bennington JL, Beckwith JB (1975) Tumors of the kidney, renal pelvis and ureter. Atlas of tumor pathology, second series, fascicle 12. Armed Forces Institute of Pathology, Washington DC
32. Bennington JL, Kradjian RM (1967) Renal carcinoma. Saunders, Philadelphia
33. Bennington JL, Laubscher FA (1968) Epidemiologic studies on carcinoma of the kidney. I. Association of renal adenocarcinoma with smoking. Cancer 21:1069–1071
34. Berger L, Sinkoff MW (1957) Systemic manifestations of hypernephroma. A review of 273 cases. Am J Med 22:791–796
35. Biava CG, West M (1966) Fine structure of normal juxtaglomerular cells. II. Specific and non-specific cytoplasmic granules. Am J Pathol 49:955–979
36. Biggers R, Stewart J (1979) Primary renal osteosarcoma. Urology 13:674–676
37. Bigler JA, Killingsworth WP (1949) Cartilage in the kidney. Arch Pathol 47:487–493
38. Bittencourt AL, Britto JF, Fonseca LE (1981) Wilms' tumor of the uterus. First report of the literature. Cancer 47:2496–2499
39. Bjelke E (1964) Malignant neoplasms of the kidney in children. Cancer 17:318–321
40. Blacher EJ, Johnson DE, Abdul-Karim FW, Ayala AG (1985) Squamous cell carcinoma of renal pelvis. Urology 25:124–126
41. Bloom DA, Scardino PT, Ehrlich RM, Waisman J

(1982) The significance of lymph nodal involvement in renal angiomyolipoma. J Urol 128:1292–1295
42. Boczko S, Fromowitz FB, Bard RH (1979) Papillary adenocarcinoma of kidney: a new perspective. Urology 14:491–495
43. Böttiger LE, Ivemark BI (1959) The structure of renal carcinoma correlated to its clinical behaviour. J Urol 81:512–514
44. Bogaert R, deLoecker W, Tverdy G (1966) Amyloidosis secondary to renal carcinoma. Clinical study of 3 cases. Acta Chir Belg 15:81–95
45. Bolande RP (1973) Congenital mesoblastic nephroma of infancy. Perspect Pediatr Pathol 1:227–250
46. Bolande RP (1977) Childhood tumors and their relationship to birth defects. In: Mulvihill JJ, Miller RW, Fraumeni JF Jr (eds) Genetics of human cancer. Raven, New York, pp 43–75
47. Bond JV (1975) Bilateral Wilms' tumour. Age at diagnosis, associated congenital anomalies, and possible pattern of inheritance. Lancet II:482–484
48. Bond JV (1976) Familial neuroblastoma and ganglioneuroblastoma. JAMA 236:561–562
49. Borski AA, Kimbrough JC (1954) Bilateral carcinoma in polycystic renal disease – an unique case. J Urol 71:677–681
50. Bove KE, McAdams AJ (1976) The nephroblastomatosis complex and its relationship to Wilms' tumor: a clinicopathologic treatise. Perspect Pediatr Pathol 3:185–223
51. Bracken RB, Chica G, Johnson DE, Luna M (1979) Secondary renal neoplasms: an autopsy study. South Med J 72:806–807
52. Brantley RE, Mashni JW, Bethards RE, Chernys AE, Chung WM (1985) Computerized tomographic demonstration of inferior vena caval tumor thrombus from renal angiomyolipoma. J Urol 133:836–837
53. Brauman A, Gur H, Leibovitz A, Kopolovic J, Gilboa Y, Eliakim M (1985) Primary fibroxanthosarcoma of the kidney presenting as fever of unknown origin. Eur Urol 11:134–135
54. Breslow N, McCann B (1971) Statistical estimation of prognosis for children with neuroblastoma. Cancer Res 31:2098–2103
55. Brown WT, Puranik SR, Altman DH, Hardin HC Jr (1972) Wilms' tumor in three successive generations. Surgery 72:756–761
56. Budin RE, McDonnell PJ (1984) Renal cell neoplasms. Their relationship to arteriolonephrosclerosis. Arch Pathol Lab Med 108:138–140
57. Busch FM, Bark CJ, Clyde HR (1976) Benign renal angiomyolipoma with regional lymph node involvement. J Urol 116:715–717
58. Cabot H, Allen RB (1933) Epithelioma primary in the renal pelvis. Report of 45 cases. Lancet II:1301–1306
59. Cain DR, van de Velde RL, Shapiro StJ (1974) Spironolactone inclusions in an aldosteronoma. Am J Clin Pathol 61:412–416
60. Cajfinger H, Bothier F, Lafon H, Boulud B (1973) A propos d'un nouveau cas de métastase d'hypernéphrome en ORL: une métastase amygdalienne. J Fr Otorhinolaryngol 22:69–71
61. Campbell EW, Brantley R, Harrold M, Simson LR (1974) Angiomyolipoma presenting as fever of unknown origin. Am J Med 57:843–846
62. Carman CT, Brashear RE (1960) Pheochromocytoma as an inherited abnormality. N Engl J Med 263:419–423
63. Carney JA, Sizemore GV, Sheps SG (1976) Adrenal medullary disease in multiple endocrine neoplasia, type 2. Pheochromocytoma and its precursors. Am J Clin Pathol 66:279–290
64. Chatten J (1976) Epithelial differentiation in Wilms' tumor: a clinicopathologic appraisal. Perspect. Pediatr. Pathol. 3:225–254
65. Chatten J, Voorhess ML (1967) Familial neuroblastoma. N Engl J Med 277:1230–1236
66. Chatterjee D, Powell A (1982) Renal hemangioendothelioma. Int Surg 67:373–375
67. Chen KT (1983) Multifocal renal oncocytoma. J Urol 130:546–547
68. Chen KT (1984) Malignant fibrous histiocytoma of the kidney. J Surg Oncol 27:248–250
69. Chen KT, Workman RD, Flam MS, DeKlotz RJ (1983) Carcinosarcoma of renal pelvis. Urology 22:429–431
70. Choi H, Almagro UA, McManus JT, Norback DH, Jacobs SC (1983) Renal oncocytoma. A clinicopathologic study. Cancer 51:1887–1896
71. Churg J, Gordon AJ (1942) Multiple myeloma with unusual visceral involvement. Arch Pathol 34:546–556
72. Cohn D, Jackson RV, Gordon RD (1983) Factors affecting the frequency of occurrence of spironolactone bodies in aldosteronomas and non-tumorous cortex. Pathology 15:273–277
73. Cohnheim J (1878) Vorlesungen über allgemeine Pathologie. Ein Handbuch für Ärzte und Studierende. Hirschwald, Berlin
74. Cole AT, Gill WB (1973) Dual renal cell carcinomas in an unilateral polycystic kidney. J Urol 109:182–185
75. Colston JAC, Arcadi JA (1955) Bilateral renal papillomas: transpelvic electro resection with preservation of kidney. Contralateral nephrectomy; 4 years survival. J Urol 73:460–467
76. Colvin SH (1942) Certain capsular and subcapsular mixed tumors of the kidney herein called "capsuloma". J Urol 48:585–600
77. Cooper PH, Waisman J (1973) Tubular differentiation and basement membrane production in a renal adenoma: ultrastructural features. J Pathol 109:113–121
78. Cristol DS, McDonald JR, Emmett JL (1976) Renal adenomas in hypernephromatous kidneys: A study of their incidence, nature and relationship. J Urol 55:18–27
79. Critchley M, Earl CJC (1932) Tuberous sclerosis and allied conditions. Brain 55:311–346
80. Cromie WJ, Davis CJ, DeTure FA (1979) Atypical carcinoma of kidney: possibly originating from collecting duct epithelium. Urology 13:315–317
81. Csapo Z, Bartok I, Kahan IL, Ormos J (1973) Malakoplakia of the kidney. A light microscopic, fine structural and chromatographic study. Beitr Pathol 148:407–415
82. Cummings KB, Correa RJ Jr, Gibbons RP, Stoll HM, Wheelis RF, Tate Mason J (1975) Renal pelvic tumors. J Urol 113:158–162
83. Cushing H, Wolbach SB (1927) The transformation of a malignant paravertebral sympathicoblastoma into a benign ganglioneuroma. Am J Pathol 3:203–215
84. Dahlin DC (1970) Bone tumors. Thomas, Springfield
85. Damon A, Holub DA, Melicow MM, Uson AC (1958)

Polycythemia and renal carcinoma. Report of ten new cases, two with long hematologic remission following nephrectomy. Am J Med 25:182–197
86. D'Angio GJ (1972) Management of children with Wilms' tumor. Cancer 30:1528–1533
87. D'Angio GJ, Evans AE, Koop CE (1971) Special pattern of widespread neuroblastoma with a favourable prognosis. Lancet I:1046–1049
88. D'Angio GJ, Beckwith JB, Breslow NE, Bishop HC, Evans AE, Farewll V, Fernbach D, Goodwin WE, Jones B, Leape LL, Palmer NF, Tefft M, Wolff JA (1980) Wilms' tumor: an update. Cancer 45:1791–1798
89. Dao AH, Pinto AC, Kirchner FK, Halter SA (1984) Massive nodal involvement in a case of renal angiomyolipoma. Arch Pathol Lab Med 108:612–613
90. Davidson JK, Clark DC (1974) Renin secreting juxtaglomerular cell tumor. Br J Radiol 47:594–597
91. Davis WW, Newsome HH, Wright LD, Hammond WG, Easta J, Bartter FC (1967) Bilateral adrenal hyperplasia as a cause of primary aldosteronism with hypertension, hypokalaemia and suppressed renin activity. Am J Med 42:642–647
92. Dehner LP, Leestma JE, Price EB (1970) Renal cell carcinoma in children. A clinicopathologic study of 15 cases and review of the literature. J Pediatr 76:358–368
93. Dekker A, Oehrle JS (1971) Hyaline globules of the adrenal medulla of man. Arch Pathol 91:353–363
94. Del Carmen BV, Korbitz BC (1970) Oral metastasis from hypernephroma. J Am Geriat Soc 18:743–746
95. DeLellis RA, Wolfe HJ, Gagel RF, Feldman LP, Miller HH, Gang DL, Reichlin S (1976) Adrenal medullary hyperplasia. A morphometric analysis in patients with familial medullary thyroid carcinoma. Am J Pathol 83:177–190
96. De Lorimier AA, Bragg KU, Linden G (1969) Neuroblastoma in childhood. Am J Dis Child 118:441–450
97. Del Regato JA, Spjut HJ (1977) Cancer. Diagnosis, treatment and prognosis. Mosby, St Louis
98. Deyhle P (1970) Zur Frage paraneoplastischer Amyloidose bei hypernephroidem Nierencarcinom. Zentralbl Allg Pathol 113:10–15
99. Diamond SM, Russo JF (1974) Primary adenocarcinoma of the renal pelvis: case report. Milit Med 139:859–961
100. Dineen MK, Venable DD, Misra RP (1984) Pure intrarenal lipoma – report of a case and review of the literature. J Urol 132:104–107
101. Dolin S, Dewar JP (1956) Extramedullary plasmocytoma. Am J Pathol 32:83–103
102. Donhuijsen K, Heidemann HJ (1979) Thorotrastose und Thorotrastkarzinom der Niere. Schweiz Med Wochenschr 109:1230–1234
103. Drivsholm A (1960) Hypernephroma and polycythaemia. Br Med J II:1063–1065
104. Dunant JH, Rutishauser G (1966) Thorotrast-Tumoren der Niere. Drei weitere Fälle. Schweiz Med Wochenschr 96:1156–1160
105. Eble JN, Hull MT (1984) Morphologic features of renal oncocytoma: a light and electron microscopic study. Hum Pathol 15:1054–1061
106. Enzinger FM, Weiss SW (1983) Soft tissue tumors. Mosby, St Louis
107. Escuin F, Gomez P, Martinez I, Perez-Fontan M, Selgas R, Sanchez-Sicilia L (1985) Myelolipoma associated with bilateral adrenocortical hyperplasia and hpertension. J Urol 133:655–657
108. Essex WB (1966) Renal angiomyolipomata. J Pathol Bacteriol 91:81–84
109. Evans AE, D'Angio GJ, Randolph J (1971) A proposal staging for children with neuroblastoma. Cancer 27:374–378
110. Evans AE, Chatten J, D'Angio GJ, Gerson JM, Robinson J, Schnaufer L (1980) A review of 17 IV-S neuroblastoma patients at the Children's Hospital of Philadelphia. Cancer 45:833–839
111. Evans AE, Gerson J, Schnaufer L (1976) Spontaneous regression of neuroblastoma. Natl Cancer Inst Monogr 44:49–54
112. Evans AR (1965) Congenital neuroblastoma. J Clin Pathol 18:54–62
113. Evans JA, Halpern M, Finby N (1961) Diagnosis of kidney cancer. An analysis of 100 consecutive cases. JAMA 175:201–203
114. Evans RW (1968) Histologic appearances of tumors. Livingstone, Edinburgh
115. Faarup P (1971) Morphological aspects of the renin-angiotensin system. Acta Pathol Microbiol Scand [Suppl] 222:1–96
116. Farrow GM, Harrison EG, Utz DC, Jones DR (1968) Renal angiomyolipoma. A clinico-pathologic study of 32 cases. Cancer 22:564–570
117. Farrow GM, Harrison EG, Utz DC, Remine WH (1968) Sarcomas and sarcomatoid and mixed malignant tumors of the kidneys in adults – part I. Cancer 22:545–550
118. Fernandez-Sanz J, Galera H, Garcia-Donas A, Gonzalez-Campona R, Llamas R, Matilla A (1981) Adrenal myelolipoma simulating a retroperitoneal malignant neoplasm. J Urol 126:780–782
119. Ferrer-Roda J, Sanjuan C, Vilar J, Villanueva A, Baeza R (1983) Hemangioma of the kidney. Eur Urol 9:189–190
120. Fetissof F, Benatre A, Dubois MP, Lanson Y, Arbeille-Brassart B, Jobard P (1984) Carcinoid tumor occurring in a teratoid malformation of the kidney. An immunohistochemical study. Cancer 54:2305–2308
121. Filler RM, Traggis DG, Jaffe N, Vawter GF (1972) Favourable outlook for children with mediastinal neuroblastoma. J Pediatr Surg 7:136–143
122. Fischer W (1911) Die Nierentumoren bei der tuberösen Hirnsklerose. Beitr Pathol 50:235–282
123. Fisher ER, Horvat B (1972) Comparative ultrastructural study of so-called renal adenoma and carcinoma. J Urol 108:382–386
124. Fite GL (1945) Classifications of tumors of the kidney. Arch Pathol 39:37–41
125. Flocks RH, Kadesky MC (1958) Malignant neoplasms of the kidney: an analysis of 353 patients followed five years or more. J Urol 79:196–201
126. Foot NC, Humpreys GA (1948) The importance of accurate pathologic classification in the prognosis of renal tumors. Surgery 23:369–376
127. Foot NC, Papanicolaow GN, Holmquist NC, Seybolt JF (1958) Exfoliative cytology of urinary sediments. A review of 2829 cases. Cancer 11:127–137
128. Foster DG (1966) Adrenal cysts. Review of literature and report of case. Arch Surg 92:131–143
129. Fransen G, Bultinck J, van Camp K (1975) Un cas de cancer rénal après pyélographie au Thorotrast. Acta Urol Belg 43:268–281

130. Fraumeni JF, Miller RW (1967) Adrenocortical neoplasms with hemihypertrophy, brain tumors, and other disorders. Med Prog 70:129–138
131. Frey WG (1958) Polycythemia and hypernephroma. Review and report of a case with apparent surgical cure. N Engl J Med 258:842–844
132. Friedmann PS, Solis-Cohen L (1948) Hemangioma of the kidney; its roentgen diagnosis. AJF 60:408–410
133. Fries JG, Chamberlin JA (1968) Extra-adrenal pheochromocytoma: literature review and report of a cervical pheochromocytoma. Surgery 63:268–279
134. Fung CH, Gonzalez-Crussi F, Yonan TN, Martinez N (1981) "Rhabdoid" Wilms' tumor: an ultrastructural study. Arch Pathol Lab Med 105:521–523
135. Futter NG, Collins WE (1974) Renal angiomyolipoma causing hypertension: a case report. Br J Urol 46:485–487
136. Gabrilove JL, Sharma DC, Wotiz HH, Dorfman RI (1965) Feminizing adrenocortical tumors in the male. A review of 52 cases including a case report. Medicine 44:37–79
137. Gaulin EJ (1951) Simultaneous Wilms' tumors in identical twins. J Urol 66:547–550
138. Geschickter CF, Widenhorn H (1934) Nephrogenic tumors. Am J Cancer 22:620–658
139. Gherardi GJ, Arya S, Hickler RB (1974) Juxtaglomerular body tumor: a rare occult but curable cause of lethal hypertension. Hum Pathol 5:236–240
140. Gigax JH, Bucy JG, Proxler G, Chunn SP (1972) Cystic hamartoma of the adrenal gland associated with hypertension. J Urol 107:161–163
141. Giger K (1967) Sekundäre Polyglobulie bei Nierentumoren. Schweiz Med Wochenschr 97:1067–1070
142. Gitlow StE, Dziedzig LB, Stouss L, Greenwood StM, Dziedzig StV (1973) Biochemical and histologic determinants in the prognosis of neuroblastoma. Cancer 32:898–905
143. Goldberg MF, Tashjian AH, Order SR, Dammin GJ (1964) Renal adenocarcinoma containing a parathyroid hormone-like substance and associated with marked hypercalcemia. Am J Med 36:805–814
144. Gonzalez-Crussi F (1984) Variants and miscellaneous. In: Gonzalez-Crussi F (ed) Wilms' tumor (nephroblastoma) and related renal neoplasms of childhood. CRC, Boca Raton, pp 77
145. Gonzalez-Crussi F, Hsueh W (1984) Epidemiology. In: Gonzalez-Crussi F (ed) Wilms' tumor (nephroblastoma) and related renal neoplasms of childhood. CRC, Boca Raton, pp 39
146. Grabstald H, Whitmore WF, Melamed MR (1971) Renal pelvic tumors. JAMA 218:845–854
147. Graham AP (1947) Malignancy of the kidney, survey of 195 cases. J Urol 58:10–21
148. Graham JB (1951) Pheochromocytoma and hypertension; analysis of 207 cases. Int Abstr Surg 92:105–121
149. Grawitz PA (1883) Die sogenannten Lipome der Niere. Virchows Arch 93:39–63
150. Griffin ME, Bolande RP (1969) Familial neuroblastoma with regression and maturation to ganglioneurofibroma. Pediatrics 43:377–382
151. Griffiths IH, Thackray AC (1949) Parenchymal carcinoma of the kidney. Br J Urol 21:128–151
152. Groncy P, Finklestein JZ (1978) Neuroblastoma. Pediatr Ann 7:548–559
153. Gross H (1955) Hypernephrom und Polyglobulie. Med Welt 1:706–708
154. Gross RE, Farber S, Martin LW (1959) Neuroblastoma sympathicum: a study and report of 217 cases. Pediatrics 23:1179–1191
155. Guin GH, Gilbert EF (1956) Cushing's syndrome in children associated with adrenal cortical carcinoma. A case report with review of the literature. Am J Dis Child 92:297–307
156. Gupta OP, Dube MK (1971) Rare primary renal sarcoma. Br J Urol 43:546–571
157. Haas JE, Palmer NF, Weinberg AG, Beckwith JB (1981) Ultrastructure of malignant rhabdoid tumor of the kidney – a distinctive renal tumor of children. Hum Pathol 12:646–657
158. Haas JE, Bonadio JF, Beckwith JB (1984) Clear cell sarcoma of the kidney with emphasis on ultrastructural studies. Cancer 54:2978–2987
159. Hai MA, Diaz-Perez R (1982) Atypical carcinoma of kidney originating from collecting duct epithelium. Urology 19:89–92
160. Haining RB, Poole FE (1936) Osteoblastoma of the kidney, histologically identical with osteogenic sarcoma. Arch Pathol 21:44–54
161. Hajdu SI, Foote FW (1969) Angiomyolipoma of the kidney: report of 27 cases and review of the literature. J Urol 102:396–401
162. Hallahan JD (1959) Spontaneous remission of metastatic renal cell adenocarcinoma: a case report. J Urol 81:522–525
163. Halmi KA, Lascari AD (1971) Conversion of virilization to feminization in a young girl with adrenal cortical carcinoma. Cancer 27:931–935
164. Hamer HG, Wishard WN (1948) Osteogenic sarcoma involving the right kidney. J Urol 60:10–17
165. Hamilton WJ, Mossman HW (1972) Human embryology, 4th edn. Williams and Wilkins, Baltimore
166. Hanna W, Tepperman B, Logan AG, Robinette MA, Colapinto R, Phillips MJ (1979) Juxtaglomerular cell tumour (reninoma) with paroxysmal hypertension. Can Med Assoc J 120:957–959
167. Harding ML (1972) Renal carcinoma or sweat gland tumour? Br J Clin Pract 26:391–393
168. Harms D (1984) Tumoren des Kindesalters. In: Remmele W (ed) Pathologie, vol 3. Springer, Berlin Heidelberg New York Tokyo
169. Harms D, Gutjahr P, Hohenfellner R, Willke E (1980) Fetal rhabdomyomatous nephroblastoma. Pathologic histology and special clinical and biologic features. Eur J Pediatr 133:167–172
170. Harms D, Leder L-D, Rossius H, Albani M, Tillmann W (1975) Congenital mesoblastic nephroma of infancy. Beitr Pathol 154:83–87
171. Harms D, Löhr J (1978) Inguinaler Wilms-Tumor. Klin Padiatr 190:54–56
172. Harrison JH, Mahoney EM, Bennett AH (1973) Tumors of the adrenal cortex. Cancer 32:1227–1235
173. Hart MN, Cyrus A (1968) Hyaline globules of the adrenal medulla. Am J Clin Pathol 19:387–391
174. Hartman DS, Pyatt RS, Dailey E (1983) Transitional cell carcinoma of the kidney with invasion into the renal vein. Urol Radiol 5:83–87
175. Hartveit F, Halleraker B (1960) A report of three angiomyolipomata and one angiomyoliposarcoma. Acta Pathol Microbiol Scand 49:329–336
176. Hassenbusch S, Kaizer H, White JJ (1976) Prognostic factors in neuroblastic tumours. J Pediatr Surg 11:287–297

177. Haupt R (1964) Über Besonderheiten der Nebennierenrindencarcinome. Frankf Z Pathol 73:602–610
178. Hayles AB, Hahn HB Jr, Sprague RG, Bahn RC, Priestley JP (1966) Hormone-secreting tumors of the adrenal cortex in children. Pediatrics 37:19–25
179. Healey FH Jr, Mekelatos CJ (1958) Pheochromocytoma and neurofibromatosis. N Engl J Med 258:540–543
180. Heinbecker P, O'Neal LV, Ackerman LV (1957) Functioning and nonfunctioning adrenal cortical tumors. Surg Gynecol Obstet 105:21–33
181. Helmbrecht LJ, Cosgrove MD (1974) Triple therapy for leiomyosarcoma of kidney. J Urol 112:581–584
182. Henle J (1865) Über das Gewebe der Nebenniere und der Hypophyse. Z Rat Med 24:143–152
183. Herbeuval R, Cuny G, Larcan A (1957) Maladie des Vaquez et hypernéphrome. Presse Med 65:132–134
184. Hermanek P, Sigel A, Chlepas S (1976) Histological grading of renal cell carcinoma. Eur Urol 2:189–191
185. Herzog H (1939) Nierengeschwülste mit quergestreifter Muskulatur. Z Krebsforsch 48:424–446
186. Hickey BB, Evans CJ, Sharp ME, Ashley DJB (1962) Renal and pulmonary tuberose sclerosis: the relationship of the renal lesion to haemangiopericytoma. Br J Surg 49:396–400
187. Higgins TT, Williams DI, Nash DFE (1951) The urology of childhood. Mosby, Butterworth, London
188. Ho J, Ma L, Wong KC (1981) An extrarenal Wilms' tumor arising from an undescended testis. Pathology 13:619
189. Hogan PF, Gilchrist KV, Westring DW, Citrin DL (1980) A clinical and pathologic study of adrenocortical carcinoma. Therapeutic implications. Cancer 45:2880–2883
190. Holland P (1976) Clinical and biochemical manifestations of Wilms' tumor. In: Pochedly C, Miller DR (eds) Wilms' tumor. Wiley, New York
191. Hou LT, Willis RA (1963) Renal carcino-sarcoma, true and false. J Pathol Bacteriol 85:139–144
192. Hough AJ, Hollifield JV, Page DL, Hartmann WH (1979) Prognostic factors in adrenal cortical tumors. A mathematical analysis of clinical and morphologic data. Am J Clin Pathol 72:390–399
193. Howard RM, Young JD (1969) Two malignant tumors in a polycystic kidney. J Urol 102:162–164
194. Hudson HC (1956) Osteogenic sarcoma involving the left kidney. J Urol 75:21–24
195. Hughes M, Marsden HB, Plamer MK (1974) Histologic patterns of neuroblastoma related to prognosis and clinical staging. Cancer 34:1706–1711
196. Hughson MD, Hennigar GR, McManus JFA (1980) Atypical cysts, acquired renal cystic disease, and renal cell tumors in endstage dialysis kidneys. Lab Invest 42:475–480
197. Hulbert JC, Graf R (1983) Involvement of the spleen by renal angiomyolipoma: metastasis or multicentricity? J Urol 130:328–329
198. Hulse CA, Palik EE (1951) Renal hamartoma. J Urol 66:506–515
199. Hume DM (1960) Pheochromocytoma in the adult and in the child. Am J Surg 99:458–496
200. Hutter AM, Kayhoe DE (1966) Adrenal cortical carcinoma. Clinical features of 138 patients. Am J Med 41:572–580
201. Huvos AG, Hajdu SI, Brasfield RD, Foote FV Jr (1970) Adrenal cortical carcinoma. Clinicopathologic study of 34 cases. Cancer 25:354–361
202. Innis MD (1973) Nephroblastoma: index cancer of childhood. Med J Aust 2:322–323
203. Ito J, Johnson WW (1969) Ultrastructure of Wilms' tumor. I. Epithelial cell. JNCI 42:77–99
204. Jacob NH, Mau WJ (1951) Metaplasia of ureteral epithelium resulting in intestinal mucosa and adenocarcinomatous transformation. Report of two cases. J Urol 65:20–24
205. Jacobi GH, Philipp TH (1975) Stauffer's syndrome. Diagnostic help in hypernephroma. Clin Nephrol 4:113–115
206. Janigan DP (1963) Cytoplasmic bodies in the adrenal cortex of patients treated with spirolactone. Lancet I:850–852
207. Jenkins GD (1959) Regression of pulmonary metastasis following nephrectomy for hypernephroma: eight-year follow-up. J Urol 82:37–40
208. Jensen OA (1970) Metastatic tumors of the eye and orbit. A histopathological analysis of a Danish series. Acta Pathol Microbiol Scand [Suppl] 212:201–214
209. Jereb B, Tournade MF, Lemerle J, Voûte PA, Delemarre JF, Ashtrom L, Flamant R, Gérard-Marchant R, Sandstedt B (1980) Lymph node invasion and prognosis in nephroblastoma. Cancer 45:1632–1636
210. Jitsukawa S, Nakamura K, Nakayama M, Osawa A, Matsui K (1985) Transitional cell carcinoma of kidney extending into renal vein and inferior vena cava. Urology 25:310–312
211. Johansson S, Angervall L, Bengtsson W, Wahlqvist L (1974) Uroepithelial tumors of the renal pelvis associated with abuse of phenacetin-containing analgesics. Cancer 33:743–753
212. Johnson LA, Ancona VC, Johnson T, Pineda NB (1970) Primary osteogenic sarcoma of the kidney. J Urol 104:528–531
213. Jonas D, Bigalke KH (1973) Nierenbeckencarcinom nach retrograder Thorotrastpyelographie. Z Urol 66:353–357
214. Jonas D, Thoma B, Beckert H, Weber W (1985) The value of morphological prognostic criteria in the assessment of renal cell carcinoma. Urol Int 40:148–154
215. Jones DB (1977) Kidneys. In: Anderson WAD, Kissane JM (eds) Pathology. Mosby St Louis
216. Joshi VV (1979) Cystic partially differentiated nephroblastoma: an entity in the spectrum of infantile renal neoplasia. Perspect Pediatr Pathol 5:217–235
217. Kandel LB, Harrison LH, Woodruff RD, Williams CD, Ahl ET Jr (1984) Renal plasmacytoma: a case report and summary of reported cases. J Urol 132:1167–1169
218. Kaufman JJ (1968) Reasons for nephrectomy. Palliative and curative. JAMA 204:607–608
219. Kaufman JJ, Mims MM (1966) Current problems in surgery. Tumors of the kidney. Year Book Medical, Chicago
220. Kazal LA, Erslev AJ (1975) Erythropoietin production in renal tumors. Ann Clin Lab Sci 5:98–109
221. Kempson RL, Kyriakos M (1972) Fibroxanthosarcoma of the soft tissues. A type of malignant fibrous histiocytoma. Cancer 29:961–976
222. Kennedy JS, Fidler HK (1958) Primary adenocarcinoma of the renal pelvis. J Urol 80:208–213
223. Khairi MRA, Dexter RN, Burzynski NJ, Johnston CC (1975) Mucosal neuroma, pheochromocytoma and

medullary thyroid carcinoma: multiple endocrine neoplasia type 3. Medicine 54:89–112
224. Kimball FN, Ferris HW (1934) Papillomatous tumors of pelvis associated with similar tumors of ureter and bladder; review of literature and report of two cases. J Urol 31:257–304
225. King DR, Lack EE (1979) Adrenal cortical carcinoma. A clinical and pathologic study of 49 cases. Cancer 44:239–244
226. Kinnier Wilson LM, Draper GJ (1974) Neuroblastoma, its natural history and prognosis: a study of 487 cases. Br Med J 3:301–307
227. Klapproth HJ (1959) Wilms' tumor. A report of 45 cases and an analysis of 1351 cases reported in the world literature from 1940 to 1958. J Urol 81:633–648
228. Klein MJ, Valensi QJ (1976) Proximal tubular adenomas of kidney with so-called oncocytic features. A clinico-pathologic study of 13 cases of a rarely reported neoplasm. Cancer 38:906–914
229. Kobayashi S, Ohmori M, Akaeda T, Ohmori H, Miyaji Y (1983) Primary adenocarcinoma of the renal pelvis. Report of two cases and brief review of literature. Acta Pathol Jpn 33:589–597
230. Koop CE, Schnaufer L (1975) The management of abdominal neuroblastoma. Cancer 35:905–909
231. Korst DR, Whalley BE, Bethell FA, Arbor A (1959) Erythropoietic activity of plasma in polycythemia. J Lab Clin Med 54:916
232. Koss LG (1979) Diagnostic cytology and its histopathologic bases, 3nd edn. Lippincott, Philadelphia
233. Kovacs K, Horvath E, Feldman PS (1976) Pigmented adenomas of adrenal cortex associated with Cushing's syndrome. Light and electron microscopic study. Urology 7:641–645
234. Kradjian RM, Bennington JI (1965) Renal carcinoma recurrent 31 years after nephrectomy. Arch Surg 90:192–195
235. Kragel PJ, Toker C (1985) Infiltrating recurrent renal angiomyolipoma with fatal outcome. J Urol 133:90–91
236. Krückemeyer K, Lessmann HD, Pudwitz KR (1960) Nierencarcinom als Thorotrastschaden. Fortschr Roentgenstr 93:313–321
237. Lambird PA, Yardley JH (1970) Urinary tract malakoplakia: report of a fatal case with ultrastructural observations of Michaelis-Gutmann-bodies. Johns Hopkins Med J 126:1–14
238. Largiader F (1958) Morphologie, Histogenese und Klassifikation der Nierentumoren. Urol Int 6:273–367
239. Lassen UV, Sagild W (1960) Salt-losing syndrome due to unilateral renal disease (hypernephroma). Acta Med Scand 168:65–70
240. Latham HS, Kay S (1974) Malignant tumors of the renal pelvis. Surg Gynecol Obstet 138:613–622
241. Lauder I, Aherne W (1972) The significance of lymphocytic infiltration in neuroblastoma. Cancer 26:321–328
242. Lausten GS, Anagnostaki L, Thomsen OF (1984) Inverted papilloma of the upper urinary tract. Eur Urol 10:67–70
243. Lawler W, Marsden HB, Palmer MK (1975) Wilms' tumor – histologic variation and prognosis. Cancer 36:1122–1126
244. Lawler W, Marsden HB, Palmer MK (1977) Histopathological study of the first medical research council nephroblastoma trial. Cancer 40:1519–1525
245. Lawrence JJ, Donald WG (1959) Polycythemia and hydronephrosis or renal tumor. Ann Intern Med 50:959–969
246. Lawson RS (1970) Hypernephroma presenting with hypertension. Br Med J I:301
247. Leape LL, Lowman JP, Loveland GC (1978) Multifocal nondisseminated neuroblastoma. Report of two cases in siblings. J Pediatr 92:75–77
248. Leder L-D (1964) Über die selektive fermentcytochemische Darstellung neutrophiler myeloischer Zellen und Gewebsmastzellen im Paraffinschnitt. Klin Wochenschr 42:553
249. Ledlie EM, Mynors LS, Draper GJ, Gorbach PD (1970) Natural history and treatment of Wilms' tumour: an analysis of 335 cases occurring in England and Wales, 1962–1966. Br Med J 4:195–200
250. Lemerle J, Tournade M-F, Gerard-Marchant R, Flamant R, Sarrazin D, Flamant F, Lemerle M, Jundt S, Zucker J-M, Schweisguth O (1976) Wilms' tumor: natural history and prognostic factors. A retrospective study of 248 cases treated at the Institut Gustave-Roussy 1952–1967. Cancer 37:2557–2566
251. Lerman RJ, Pitcock JA, Stephenson P, Muirhead EE (1972) Renomedullary interstitial cell tumor (formerly fibroma of renal medulla). Hum Pathol 3:559–568
252. Lewinsky BS, Kenneth MG, Symington T, Neville AM (1974) The clinical and pathological features of "non-hormonal" adrenocortical tumors. Cancer 33:778–790
253. Lewis PD (1971) A cytophotometric study of benign and malignant phaeochromocytomas. Virchows Arch 9:371–376
254. Lindop GB, Stewart JA, Downie TT (1983) The immunocytochemical demonstration of renin in a juxtaglomerular cell tumour by light and electron microscopy. Histopathology 7:421–431
255. Lipsett MB, Hertz R, Ross GP (1963) Clinical and pathophysiologic aspects of adrenocortical carcinoma. Am J Med 35:374–383
256. Liwnicz BH, Lepow H, Schutte H, Fernandez R, Caberwal D (1975) Mucinous adenocarcinoma of the renal pelvis: discussion of possible pathogenesis. J Urol 114:306–310
257. Loomis RC (1972) Primary leiomyosarcoma of the kidney: report of a case and review of the literature. J Urol 107:557–560
258. Lüders CJ (1953) Zur Frage der pigmentierten Nebennierenrindenadenome. Virchows Arch 324:123–135
259. Lumb G (1950) Adrenal cortical tumours of unusually large size. Br Med J I:582–584
260. Ma MKG, Chan KW (1974) Renal angiomyolipoma. Report of 5 cases. Br J Urol 46:481–484
261. Macadam RF (1971) Black adenoma of the human adrenal cortex. Cancer 27:116–119
262. Macfarlane DA (1958) Cancer of the adrenal cortex. The natural history, prognosis, and treatment in a study of fifty-five cases. Ann R Coll Surg Engl 23:155–156
263. Mackenzie DH (1970) The differential diagnosis of fibroblastic disorders. Blackwell Scientific, Oxford
264. Mäkinen J (1972) Microscopic patterns as a guide to prognosis of neuroblastoma in childhood. Cancer 29:1637–1646
265. Malhotra CM, Doolittle CH, Rodil JV, Vezeridis MP (1984) Mesenchymal chondrosarcoma of the kidney. Cancer 54:2495–2499
266. Manabe T, Tasaka Y, Amano M, Okunobo T (1984)

Regional lymph node involvement in benign renal angiomyolipoma. Acta Pathol Jpn 34:889–893
267. Mancilla-Jimenez R, Stanley RJ, Blath RA (1976) Papillary renal cell carcinoma. A clinical, radiologic and pathologic study of 34 cases. Cancer 38:2469–2480
268. Marsden HB, Steward (1968) Wilms' Tumors. In: Marsden HB, Steward JK (eds) Tumors in Children. Springer, Berlin Heidelberg New York
269. Marsden HB, Lawler W (1980) Bone metastasizing renal tumour of childhood. Histopathological and clinical review of 38 cases. Virchows Arch 387:341–351
270. Marsden HB, Lennox EL, Lawler W, Kinnier-Wilson LM (1980) Bone metastases in childhood renal tumours. Br J Cancer 41:875–879
271. Martin LW, Reyes PM Jr (1969) An evaluation of 10 years' experience with retroperitoneal lymph node dissection for Wilms' tumor. J Pediatr Surg 4:683–687
272. Martinez-Maldonado M, Ramirez De Arrelano GA (1966) Renal involvement in malignant lymphomas: a survey of 49 cases. J Urol 95:485–488
273. Mathias DB (1971) A case of spontaneous regression of pulmonary metastases arising from hypernephroma following nephrectomy. Br J Urol 43:65–68
274. McCrea LE (1951) Hemangioma of the kidney, review of the literature. Urol Cutan Rev 55:670–680
275. McDonald JR, Priestley JT (1943) Malignant tumors of the kidney; surgical and prognostic significance of tumor thrombosis of the renal vein. Surg Gynecol Obstet 77:295–306
276. McDonald JR, Priestley JT (1944) Carcinomas of the renal pelvis. Histopathologic study of 75 cases with special reference to prognosis. J Urol 51:245–258
277. McDonald EC, Mukai K, Burke BA, Sibley RK (1983) Primary carcinoid tumor of the kidney: a light and electron microscopic and immunohistochemical study. J Urol 130:333–335
278. McFarland WL, Wallace S, Johnson DE (1972) Renal carcinoma and polycystic disease. J Urol 107:530–532
279. McLaughlin JE, Ulrich H (1977) Maturing neuroblastoma and ganglioneuroblastoma: a study of four cases with long survival. J Pathol 121:19–26
280. Meadows AT, Lichtenfeld JL, Koop CE (1974) Wilms' tumor in three children of a woman with congenital hemihypertrophy. N Engl J Med 291:23–24
281. Melicow MM (1945) Tumors of the urinary drainage tract: urothelial tumors. J Urol 54:186–193
282. Melicow MM (1957) Hibernating fat and pheochromocytoma. Am Med Assoc Arch Pathol 63:367–372
283. Melicow MM (1977) One hundred cases of pheochromocytoma (107 tumors) at the Columbia-Presbyterian Medical Center (1926–1976). Cancer 40:1987–2004
284. Merino MJ, Livolsi VA (1982) Oncocytomas of the kidney. Cancer 50:1852–1856
285. Messinger WJ, Jarman WD (1937) Rhabdomyosarcoma of the kidney: case report with autopsy findings. Surgery 2:26–32
286. Meyer PC (1969) The histological grading of primary epithelial neoplasms of the ureter. J Urol 102:30–36
287. Micolonghi TS, Liang D, Schwartz S (1984) Primary osteogenic sarcoma of the kidney. J Urol 131:1164–1166
288. Miller RW (1974) Childhood cancer epidemiology: two international activities. Natl Cancer Inst Monogr 40:71–74
289. Miller RW (1978) Peculiarities in the occurrence of adrenal cortical carcinoma. Am J Dis Child 132:235–236
290. Miller RW, Fraumeni JF Jr, Hill JA (1968) Neuroblastoma: epidemiologic approach to its origin. Am J Dis Child 115:253–261
291. Moertel CG, Dockerty MB, Baggenstoss AH (1961) Multiple primary malignant neoplasms. III. Tumors of multicentric origin. Cancer 14:238–248
292. Mondal A, Choudhury S, Mukherjee PK (1983) Primary malignant haemangiopericytoma of kidney (a case report). J Postgrad Med 29:120–122
293. More IAR, Jackson AM, Macsween RNM (1974) Renin secreting tumor associated with hypertension. Cancer 34:2093–2102
294. Mostofi FK (1967) Pathology and spread of renal cell carcinoma. In: King JS (ed) Renal neoplasia. Little, Brown, Boston
295. Mostofi FK (1968) Pathological aspects and spread of carcinoma of the bladder. JAMA 206:1764–1769
296. Mulcahy JJ, Furlow WL (1970) Vaginal metastasis from renal cell carcinoma: radiographic evidence of possible route of spread. J Urol 104:50–52
297. Murphy GP, Mostofi FK (1970) Histologic assessment and clinical prognosis of renal adenoma. J Urol 103:31–36
298. Murphy ML (1968) Curability of cancer in children. Cancer 22:779–784
299. Nativ O, Horowitz A, Lindner A, Many M (1985) Primary chondrosarcoma of the kidney. J Urol 134:120–121
300. Neville AM, Symington T (1966) Pathology of primary aldosteronism. Cancer 19:1854–1868
301. Newman HR, Schulman ML (1969) Renal cortical tumors: a 40-year statistical study. Urol Survey 19:2–12
302. Nourse MH, Yurdin DH (1959) Renal cell carcinoma in children. J Urol 82:21–25
303. Oberling C (1935) Retroperitoneal xanthogranuloma. Am J Cancer 23:477–489
304. Oberling C, Riviere M, Hagueneau F (1960) Ultrastructure of the clear cells in renal carcinomas and its importance for the demonstration of their renal origin. Nature 186:402–403
305. O'Grady AS, Morse LJ, Lee JB (1965) Parathyroid hormone-secreting renal carcinoma associated with hypercalcemia and metabolic alkalosis. Ann Intern Med 63:858–868
306. Ojeda LM, Johnson DE, Ames FC, Raymond AK, Ayala AG (1984) Primary renal malignant fibrous histiocytoma. Urology 24:491–494
307. Olsson CA, Krane RJ, Klugo RC, Selikowitz SM (1973) Adrenal myelolipoma. Surgery 73:665–670
308. Olsson PJ, Fierer JA, Kelly CE, Wright RW, Blaise D, Anderson KB, Peterson JC, Alexander RW (1985) Renal carcinoma and dialysis in end-stage renal disease. South Med J 78:507–512
309. Omland G (1959) Polycythemia in renal carcinoma. Acta Med Scand 164:451–454
310. Orlowski JP, Levin HS, Dyment PG (1980) Intrascrotal Wilms' tumor developing in a heterotopic anlage of probable mesonephric origin. J Pediatr Surg 15:679
311. Oser W, Fladerer H (1976) Angiographischer Nachweis eines thorotrastbedingten Nierenbeckencarcinomes. Röntgenblätter 29:115–118
312. Palmer NF, Sutow W (1983) Clinical aspects of the rhabdoid tumor of the kidney: a report of the National Wilms' Tumor Study Group. Med Pediatr Oncol 11:242–245

313. Palma LD, Kenny GM, Murphy GP (1970) Childhood renal carcinoma. Cancer 26:1321–1324
314. Pasmantier MW, Azar HA (1969) Extraskeletal spread in multiple plasma cell myeloma. A review of 57 autopsied cases. Cancer 23:167–174
315. Patch FS (1929) The association between leukoplakia and squamous cell carcinoma in the upper urinary tract. N Engl J Med 200:423–436
316. Penman HG, Thomson KJ (1972) Amyloidosis and renal adenocarcinoma. A post-mortem study. J Pathol 107:45–47
317. Perez CA, Kaiman HA, Keith J, Mill WB, Vietti TJ, Powers WE (1973) Treatment of Wilms' tumor and factors affecting prognosis. Cancer 32:609–617
318. Petkovic SD (1959) An anatomical classification of renal tumors in the adult as a basis for prognosis. J Urol 81:618–623
319. Plaut A (1958) Myelolipoma in the adrenal cortex (myeloadipose structures). Am J Pathol 34:487–502
320. Plimpton GH, Gellhorn A (1956) Hypercalcemia in malignant disease without evidence of bone destruction. Am J Med 21:750–759
321. Poole-Wilson DS (1969) Occupational tumours of the renal pelvis and ureter arising in the dye-making industry. Proc R Soc Med 62:93–94
322. Pratt-Thomas HR, Spicer SS, Upshur JK, Greene WB (1973) Carcinoma of the kidney in a 15 year old boy. Unusual histological features with formation of microvilli. Cancer 31:719–725
323. Price EB, Mostofi FK (1965) Symptomatic angiomyolipoma of the kidney. Cancer 18:761–774
324. Prince CL (1942) Primary angioendothelioma of the kidney: report of a case and brief review. J Urol 47:787–792
325. Pugh RCB (1959) The pathology of bladder tumours. In: Wallace DM (ed) Monographs on neoplastic disease at various sites, vol II. Tumors of the bladder. Livingstone, Edinburgh
326. Quattlebaum RB, Shirley SW (1968) Adenocarcinoma of the renal pelvis. J Urol 99:384–386
327. Rafla S (1975) Tumors of the upper urothelium. AJR 123:540–551
328. Raghavaiah NV, Mayer RF, Hagitt R, Soloway MS (1980) Malignant fibrous histiocytoma of the kidney. J Urol 123:951–953
329. Ragins AB, Rolnick HC (1950) Mucus producing adenocarcinoma of the renal pelvis. J Urol 63:66–73
330. Raney RB Jr, Palmer N, Sutow WW, Baum E, Ayala A (1983) Renal cell carcinoma in children. Med Paediatr Oncol 11:91–98
331. Rapaport E, Goldberg MB, Gorman GS, Hinman F (1952) Mortality in surgically treated adrenocortical tumours. Review of cases reported for the 20-year period 1930–1949 inclusive. Postgrad Med J 11:325–353
332. Rawlins MD, Luff RH, Cranston WI (1970) Pyrexia in renal carcinoma. Lancet I:1371–1373
333. Reese AJM, Winstanley DP (1958) The small tumorlike lesions of the kidney. Br J Cancer 12:507–516
334. Remine WH, Chong GC, van Heerden JA, Sheps SG, Harrison EG Jr (1974) Current management of pheochromocytoma. Ann Surg 179:740–748
335. Riches EW (1964) Monographs on neoplastic disease at various sites, vol V. Tumours of the kidney and ureter. Williams and Wilkins, Baltimore
336. Riches EW, Griffiths IH, Thackray AC (1951) New growths of the kidney and ureter. Br J Urol 23:297–356
337. Richmond J, Sherman RS, Diamond HD, Craver LF (1962) Renal lesions associated with malignant lymphomas. Am J Med 32:184–207
338. Risdon RA (1971) Renal dysplasia, part I. A clinicopathological study of 76 cases. J Clin Pathol 24:57–71
339. Roberts PF (1973) Bilateral renal carcinoma associated with polycystic kidneys. Br Med J III:273–274
340. Robertson PW, Klidjian A, Harding LK, Walters G, Lee MR, Robb-Smith ATH (1967) Hypertension due to a renin-secreting renal tumor. Am J Med 43:963–976
341. Robinson MJ, Pardo V, Rywlin AM (1972) Pigmented nodules (black adenomas) of the adrenal. Hum Pathol 3:317–325
342. Robson CJ, Churchill BM, Anderson W (1969) The results of radical nephrectomy for renal cell carcinoma. J Urol 101:297–301
343. Rousseau MF, Nabarra B (1974) Tumeurs embryonnaires du rein. Virchows Arch 363:149–162
344. Say CC, Hori JM (1974) Transitional cell carcinoma of the renal pelvis: experience from 1940–1972 and literature review. J Urol 112:438–442
345. Schajowicz F, Ackerman LV, Sissons HA, Sobin LH, Torloni H (1972) Histological typing of bone tumours. WHO, Geneva
346. Schambelan M, Howes EL, Stockigt JR, Noakes CA, Biglieri EG (1973) Role of renin and aldosterone in hypertension due to a reninsecreting tumor. Am J Med 55:86–92
347. Schmidt D, Harms D, Evers KG, Bliesener JA, Beckwith JB (1985) Bone metastasizing renal tumor (clear cell sarcoma) of childhood with epithelioid elements. Cancer 56:609–613
348. Schmidt D, Harms D, Zieger G (1982) Malignant rhabdoid tumor of the kidney. Histopathology, ultrastructure and comments on differential diagnosis. Virchows Arch 398:101–108
349. Schmidt U, Donhuijsen K (1983) Nierenzystenkarzinom oder zystisches Nierenkarzinom? Med Welt 34:763–764
350. Schteingart DE, Oberman HA, Friedman BH, Conn JW (1968) Adrenal cortical neoplasms producing Cushing's syndrome. A clinicopathologic study. Cancer 22:1005–1013
351. Schwartz AD, Dadash-Ladeh M, Lee H, Swaney JJ (1974) Spontaneous regression of disseminated neuroblastoma. J Pediatr 85:760–763
352. Scotti DW (1939) Malignancies in infancy and childhood; clinical and pathological survey of 64 consecutive cases. NY State J Med 39:1188–1208
353. Scriven RR, Thrasher TV, Smith DC, Stewart SC (1984) Primary renal malignant fibrous histiocytoma: a case report and literature review. J Urol 131:948–949
354. Seabury JC (1967) Renal rhabdomyosarcoma. JAMA 201:1043–1044
355. Seljelid R (1966) An electron microscopic study of the formation of cytosomes in a rat kidney adenoma. J Ultrastruc Res 16:569–583
356. Seljelid R, Ericsson JLE (1965) Electron microscopic observations on specializations of the cell surface in renal clear cell carcinoma. Lab Invest 14:435–447
357. Sherwin RP (1959) Histopathology of pheochromocytoma. Cancer 12:861–877
358. Shimada H, Chatten J, Newton VA, Sachs N, Hamoudi AB, Chiba P, Marsden HB, Misugi K (1984) Histopathologic prognostic factors in neuroblastic tumors: definition of subtypes of ganglioneuroblastoma

and an age-linked classification of neuroblastomas. J Natl Cancer Soc 73:405–416
359. Shin W-Y, Groman GS, Berkman JI (1977) Pheochromocytoma with angiomatous features. A case report and ultrastructural study. Cancer 40:275–283
360. Sipple JH (1961) The association of pheochromocytoma with carcinoma of the thyroid gland. Am J Med 31:163–166
361. Squires JP, Ulbright TM, DeSchryver-Kecskemeti K, Engleman W (1984) Juxtaglomerular cell tumor of the kidney. Cancer 53:516–523
362. Skinner DG, Colvin RB, Vermillien CD, Pfister RC, Leadbetter WF (1971) Diagnosis and management of renal cell carcinoma. Cancer 28:1165–1177
363. Soto PJ, Radler ES, Martin JM, Gregowicz A (1965) Osteogenic sarcoma of the kidney: report of a case. J Urol 94:532–535
364. Stackpole RH, Melicow MM, Uson AC (1963) Pheochromocytoma in children. Report of 9 cases and review of the first 100 published cases with follow-up studies. Med Progr 63:315–330
365. Stahl RE, Sidhu GS (1979) Primary carcinoid of the kidney: light and electron microscopic study. Cancer 44:1345–1349
366. Stambolis C (1984) Benigne und potentielle maligne metanephrogene Neoplasmen. Thieme, Stuttgart
367. Stambolis Chr (1978) Zur Natur und Bedeutung des nodulären renalen Blastems. Zentralbl Allg Pathol 123:3–8 (1979)
368. Stanley RJ, Cubillo E, Mancilla-Jimenez R, Geisse G, Melson GL (1975) Cavernous hemangioma of the kidney. AJR 125:682–687
369. Stauffer MH (1961) Nephrogenic hepatosplenomegaly. Gastroenterology 40:694
370. Steiner PE (1954) Sources, materials, racial composition, age, sex, methods, comments and comparisons with sedentes. In: Steiner PE (ed) Cancer: race and geography. Williams and Wilkins, Baltimore
371. Steiner AL, Goodman AD, Powers SR (1968) Study of a kindred with pheochromocytoma, medullary thyroid carcinoma, hyperparathyroidism and Cushing's disease: multiple endocrine neoplasia, type 2. Medicine 47:371–409
372. Sternby NH (1955) Studies in enlargement of leukemic kidneys. Acta Hematol 14:354–362
373. Stewart WK, Fleming LV,Wotiz HH (1964) The feminizing syndrome in male subjects with adrenocortical neoplasms. Am J Med 37:455–472
374. Störkel S, Thoenes W, Rumpelt H-J, Becht E, Düber C (1985) Zur Morphologie und Klinik des Onkozytoms der Niere. Verh Dtsch Ges Pathol 69:615
375. Stout AP (1947) Ganglioneuroma of the sympathetic system. Surg Gynecol Obstet 84:101–110
376. Stout AP (1953) Atlas of tumor pathology. Tumors of soft tissues, fascicle 5. Armed Forces Institute of Pathology, Washington
377. Stout AP, Murray MR (1942) Hemangiopericytoma. A vascular tumor featuring Zimmermann's pericytes. Ann Surg 116:26–33
378. Stowens D (1957) Neuroblastoma and related tumors. Arch Pathol 63:451–459
379. Strauss FH, Scanlon EF (1956) Five year survival after hepatic lobectomy for metastatic hypernephroma. Arch Surg 72:328–331
380. Strauss MB, Welt LG (1963) Diseases of the kidney. Little, Brown, Boston
381. Strong DW, Pearse HD (1976) Recurrent urothelial tumors following surgery for transitional cell carcinoma of the upper urinary tract. Cancer 38:2178–2183
382. Sudeck P (1893) Zwei Fälle von Adenosarkom der Nieren. Virchows Arch 133:558–562
383. Sullivan M, Boilean M, Hodges CV (1978) Adrenal cortical carcinoma. J Urol 120:660–665
384. Swift-Joly J (1933) Tumours of the renal pelvis and ureter. Br J Urol 5:327–329
385. Sy WM, Edmonson JH (1968) The developmental defects associated with neuroblastoma – etiologic implications. Cancer 22:234–238
386. Symington P, Goodall AL (1953) Studies in phaeochromocytoma; pathological aspects. Glasgow Med J 34:75–96
387. Takats LJ, Czapo Z (1966) Death from renal carcinoma 37 years after its original recognition. Cancer 19:1172–1176
388. Takeuchi T, Tanaka T, Tokuyama H, Kuriyama M, Nishiura T (1984) Multilocular cystic renal adenocarcinoma: a case report and review of the literature. J Surg Oncol 25:136–140
389. Tang CP, Gray GF (1975) Adrenocortical neoplasms. Prognosis and morphology. Urology 5:691–695
390. Tannenbaum M (1971) Ultrastructural pathology of human renal cell tumors. Pathol Ann 6:249–277
391. Tarry WF, Morabito RA, Belis JA (1982) Carcinosarcoma of the renal pelvis with extension into the renal vein and inferior vena cava. J Urol 128:582–585
392. Taylor CR (1978) Immunoperoxidase techniques. Arch Pathol Lab Med 102:113–121
393. Taylor WF, Myers M, Taylor WR (1980) Extrarenal Wilms' tumor in an infant exposed to intrauterine phenytoin. Lancet 2:481
394. Theoret G, Paquin F, Schick E, Martel A (1980) Inverted papilloma of urinary tract. Urology 16:149–151
395. Thomson WHF, Karat ABA (1966) Hypercalcemia associated with adenocarcinoma of kidney without demonstrable bone lesions. Br Med J II:745–746
396. Tomera KM, Farrow GM, Lieber MM (1983) Sarcomatoid renal carcinoma. J Urol 130:657–659
397. Toppercer A (1980) Fibroepithelial tumour of the renal pelvis. Can J Surg 23:269–270
398. Tremblay M (1971) Ultrastructure of a Wilms' tumour and myogenesis. J Pathol 105:269–277
399. Tschubel K, Helpap B, Boldt I, Bastian P (1975) Metastasierendes Nierenbeckencarcinom nach Thorotrastpyelographie. Fortschr Röntgenstr 122:103–106
400. Tuttle RJ, Salama S, Matthews WR (1985) Primary osteosarcoma of kidney with liposarcomatous elements. J Can Assoc Radiol 36:76–78
401. Umiker W (1964) Accuracy of cytologic diagnosis of cancer of the urinary tract. Acta Cytol 8:186–193
402. Utz DC, McDonald JR (1957) Squamous cell carcinoma of the kidney. J Urol 78:540–552
403. Utz DC, Warren HW, Gregg JA, Ludwig J, Kelalis PP (1970) Reversable hepatic dysfunction associated with hypernephroma. Mayo Clin Proc 45:161–169
404. Uyama T, Moriwaka S (1981) Inverted papilloma with malignant change of renal pelvis. Urology 17:200–201
405. van der Walt JD, Reid HA, Risdon RA, Shaw JH (1983) Renal oncocytoma. A review of the literature and report of an unusual multicentric case. Virchows Arch 398:291–304

406. Van Slooten H, Schaberg A, Smenk D, Moolenaar AJ (1985) Morphologic characteristics of benign and malignant adrenocortical tumors. Cancer 55:766–773
407. Varkarakis MJ, Bhanalaph T, Moore RH, Murphy GP (1974) Prognostic criteria of renal cell carcinoma. J Surg Oncol 6:97–107
408. Verhaak RLOM, Harmsen AE, von Unni AJM (1974) On the frequency of tumor induction in a thorotrast kidney. Cancer 34:2061–2068
409. Vilits P, Fladerer H (1975) Angiomyolipome beider Nieren mit spontaner Massenblutung. Z Urol Nephrol 68:125–128
410. Visser JW, Axt R (1975) Bilateral adrenal medullary hyperplasia: a clinico-pathological entity. J Clin Pathol 28:298–304
411. Visser JV, Boeijinga JK, Meer CvD (1974) A functioning black adenoma of the adrenal cortex: a clinicopathological entity. J. Clin Pathol 27:955–959
412. Wagle DG, Moore RH, Murphy GP (1974) Primary carcinoma of the renal pelvis. Cancer 33:1642–1648
413. Wagle DG, Moore RH, Murphy GP (1975) Secondary carcinomas of the kidney. J Urol 114:30–32
414. Wallace AC, Nairn RC (1972) Renal tubular antigens in kidney tumors. Cancer 29:977–981
415. Walter P, Vetter JM (1976) Epithelioma rénal à cellules claires chez l'enfant. Etude de deux observations et revue de la literature. Semin Hôp Paris 52:541–550
416. Wapnick S, Lazarovici I, Baratz M, Solowiejczyk M (1975) Spontaneous rupture of an angiomyolipoma of the kidney. Int Surg 60:485–487
417. Weigensberg IJ (1972) Metastatic renal carcinoma: unusual and deceptive presenting features. South Med J 65:611–616
418. Weiss LM (1984) Comparative histologic study of 43 metastasizing and nonmetastasizing adrenocortical tumors. Am J Surg Pathol 8:163–169
419. Weiss JP, Pollack HM, McCormick JF, Malloy TM, Hanno PM, Carpiniello VL (1984) Renal hemangiopericytoma: surgical, radiological and pathological implications. J Urol 132:337–339
420. Welbourn RB, Montgomery DAD, Kennedy TL (1971) The natural history of treated Cushing's syndrome. Br J Surg 58:1–16
421. Westin J, Lanner L-O, Weinfeld A, Zettergren L (1973) Renal pelvic carcinoma after thorotrast pyelography. Acta Med Scand 194:141–143
422. Wigger HJ (1976) Fetal rhabdomyomatous nephroblastoma – a variant of Wilms' tumor. Hum Pathol 7:613–623
423. Wigger HJ (1976) Histopathology of Wilms' tumor and related lesions. In: Pochedly C, Miller D (eds) Wilms' tumor. Wiley, New York, pp 103–131
424 Wilkins L (1957) The diagnosis and treatment of endocrine disorders in childhood and adolescence. Thomas, Springfield
425. Williams DI (1964) Nephroblastoma: clinical picture and diagnosis. In: Riches EW (ed) Monographs on neoplastic disease at various sites, vol V. Tumours of the kidney and ureter. William and Wilkins, Baltimore
426. Williams ED (1965) A review of 17 cases of carcinoma of the thyroid and phaeochromocytoma. J Clin Pathol 18:288–292
427. Williams JP, Savage PS (1958) Liposarcoma of the kidney. Br J Surg 46:225–231
428. Witzleben CL, Landy RA (1974) Disseminated neuroblastoma in a child with von Recklinghausen's disease. Cancer 34:786–790
429. Xippel JM (1971) The incidence of benign renal nodules (a clinicopathological study). J Urol 106:503–506
430. Young JL, Miller RW (1975) Incidence of malignant tumors in US children. J Pediatr 86:254–258
431. Yu GSM, Rendler S, Herskowitz A, Molnar JJ (1980) Renal oncocytoma. Report of five cases and review of the literature. Cancer 45:1010–1018
432. Yum M, Ganguly A, Donohue JP (1984) Juxtaglomerular cells in renal angiomyolipoma. Ultrastructural observation. Urology 24:283–286
433. Zak FG, Jindrak K, Capozzi F (1983) Carcinoidal tumor of the kidney. Ultrastruct Pathol 4:51–59
434. Zangemeister W (1936) Untersuchungen über Altersverteilung, Häufigkeit und Morphologie der Nierenfibrome unter Mitberücksichtigung der übrigen ausgereiften Tumoren. Beitr Pathol 97:142–183
435. Zhang G, Monda L, Wasserman NF, Fraley EE (1985) Bilateral renal oncocytoma: report of 2 cases and literature review. J Urol 133:84–86
436. Zippel L (1942) Zur Kenntnis der Onkozyten. Virchows Arch 308:360–382

Ultrasound Diagnosis of Renal and Pararenal Tumors

R. HECKEMANN

1 Introduction

The introduction of sonography and computerized tomography (CT) resulted in drastic changes in the strategy of diagnosing renal masses. The excretory urogram combined with conventional tomography and angiography represented the classical equipment of imaging renal tumors. Sonography and CT not only complement these and thus extend the possibility of detecting renal masses, but additionally they lead to a reorientation in the diagnostic decision.

In the following chapter the possibilities and limitations of ultrasound in the diagnosis of various renal masses are to be evaluated.

2 Method

2.1 Apparatus

Real-time scanning is preferred to compound scanning since it permits a stepless and immediate evaluation of the kidney and the perirenal compartments. The combined employment of a linear and a sector array in the same machine seems to be optimal for abdominal ultrasound.

2.2 Technique of Examination

Anterior sagittal, transverse, and subcostal sections, and lateral longitudinal and cross sections are carried out in a supine and lateral decubitus. More rarely the patient is examined in the prone position. It is important to assess dynamic processes such as the mobility of the kidney during deep inspiration, pulsations of the vessels, peristalsis of the intestine in the differentiation of retroperitoneal tumors, and the contraction of the psoas muscle which can be mistaken as a solid mass.

The mobility of the kidney is disclosed in lying and standing or sitting position.

Always the whole abdomen (pansonography) including the base of the lungs (pleural effusions) should be examined routinely.

3 The Abnormal Kidney

3.1 Cysts

3.1.1 Simple Cysts

Simple cysts occur singly and multiply, arising in the renal cortex. They are uncommon before 40 years of age although they have been described in children [11]. They contain clear, yellowish, or watery fluid [16]. The sonographic criteria for a renal cyst have been well documented in early publications [7, 23, 25, 26]. The following signs are characteristic (Fig. 1):

1. The typical cyst should be free of structural echoes. However echoes may be observed in small cysts due to reverberations and the effect of beam width [20]. A cyst is resistant to artifactual signals when it lies in the focal zone of the transducer. This can be achieved by changing the position of the patient. Echoes originating from within a mass do not change and are more persistent than artifacts.
2. Distal sonic enhancement.
3. Round shape which is due to the uniform internal pressure within the cyst [25].
4. The wall of a cyst is thin, smooth, and sharply outlined.
5. The compression of the cyst may excavate the renal parenchyma and the adjacent organs and structures.

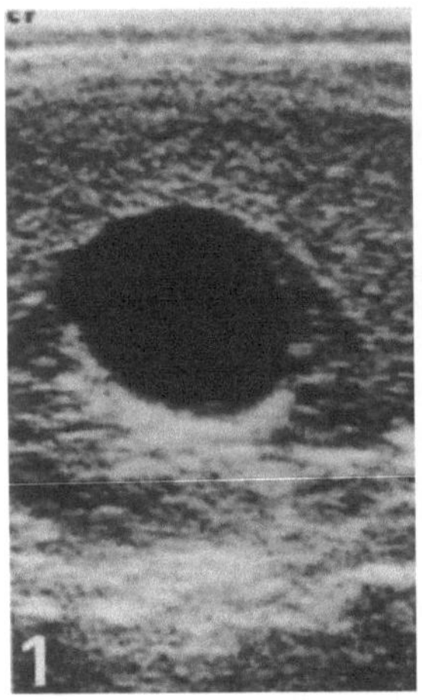

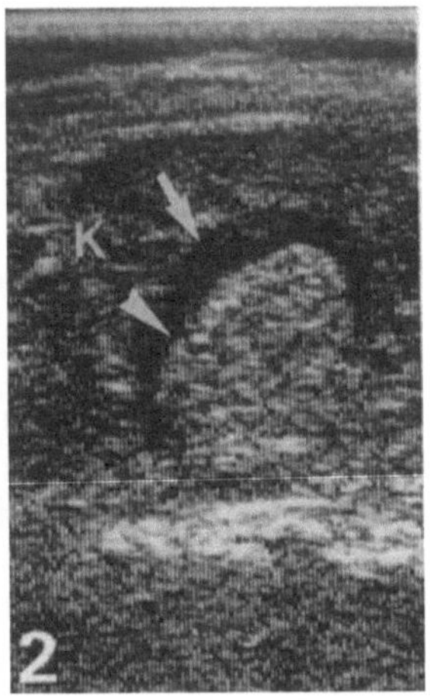

Fig. 1. Typical cyst: echofree, spherical, thin-walled, distal enhancement. **Fig. 2.** Hemorrhagic cyst. Echogenic clots are due to trauma from cyst puncture. *Arrow*, cyst wall; *arrowhead*, clot; *K* kidney

3.1.2 Atypical Cysts

Space-occupying lesions that do not fulfil the above criteria 1–4 may be considered malignant tumors unless proven otherwise. Such lesions are called atypical cysts and require a thorough evaluation. Atypical cysts are caused by:

1. Hemorrhage, which is observed in 6% of simple cysts [19]. These cysts are characterized by echogenic contents caused by blood clots (Fig. 2). The hemorrhage is due to trauma, bleeding diathesis, marginal tumor growth, varicosis of the cyst wall, necrotized pseudocystic carcinomas, cystic benign tumors (cystadenoma, cystic hamartoma), and liquified hematomas.
2. Infected cysts or infected hydronephroses in a duplicated kidney. The purulent fluid may be accompanied by a low echogenicity and a thick wall; however, densely echogenic and echofree abscesses are known [16].
3. Septated renal cysts show clearly defined highly echogenic septations and normal renal tissue in the rest of the kidney (Fig. 3). These multilocular cysts involve a part of the kidney and are well encapsulated, consisting of multiple noncommunicating cysts, sharply separated from the surrounding normal tissue [12]. This rare lesion behaves generally like a benign tumor. About half occur in young children and half in adults.
4. Multicystic dysplasia is a common abdominal mass in the newborn. Septa separate the cysts and are seen throughout the whole kidney (Fig. 4). Generally, the multicystic dysplasia is unilateral. Compared with unilateral hydronephrosis the cystic spaces are not confluent with each other. Multiple oval or round cysts do not communicate, there is an absence of an identifiable renal sinus, and an absence of parenchymal tissue [34]. Although the morphology of multicystic renal dysplasia usually differs substantially from that of hy-

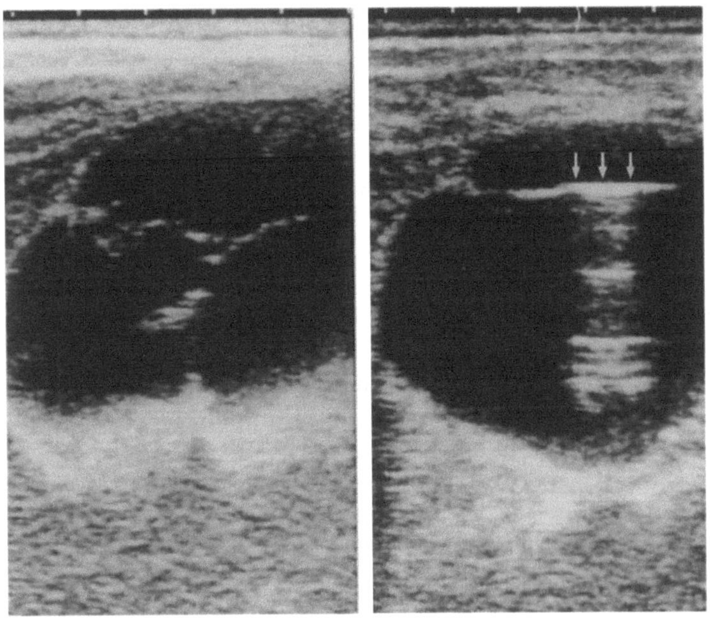

Fig. 3. Septated renal cyst. Highly echogenic septations. Reverberations caused by a septum (*arrows*)

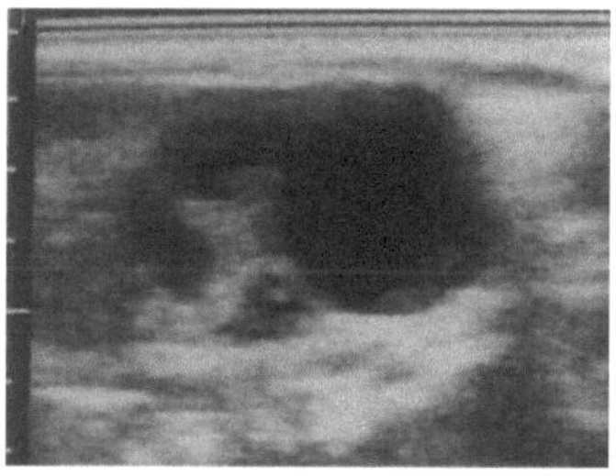

Fig. 4. Multicystic dysplasia of a newborn. Cysts throughout the whole kidney

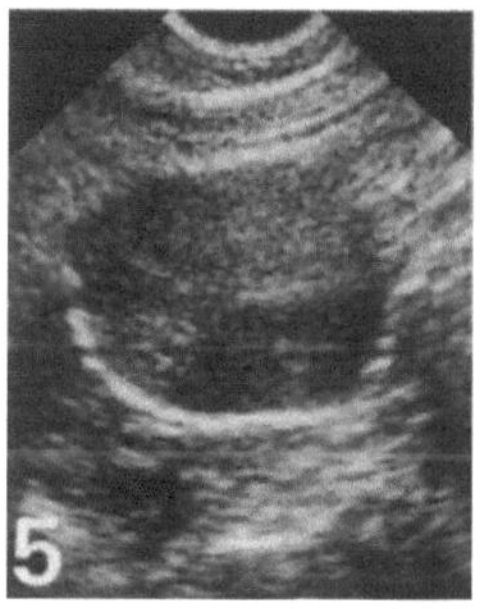

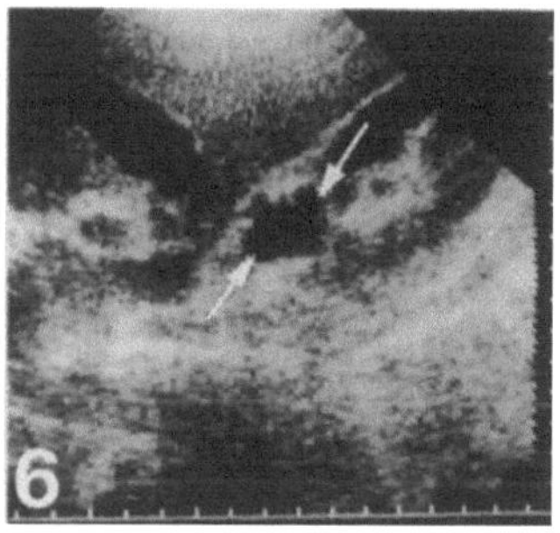

Fig. 5. Calcified cyst with a solid pattern. The thin layer of calcifications shows an echogenic rim. **Fig. 6.** Renal artery aneurysm. An anechoic, oval-shaped mass with irregular wall and low sonic enhancement is located in the upper half of the right kidney (*arrows*)

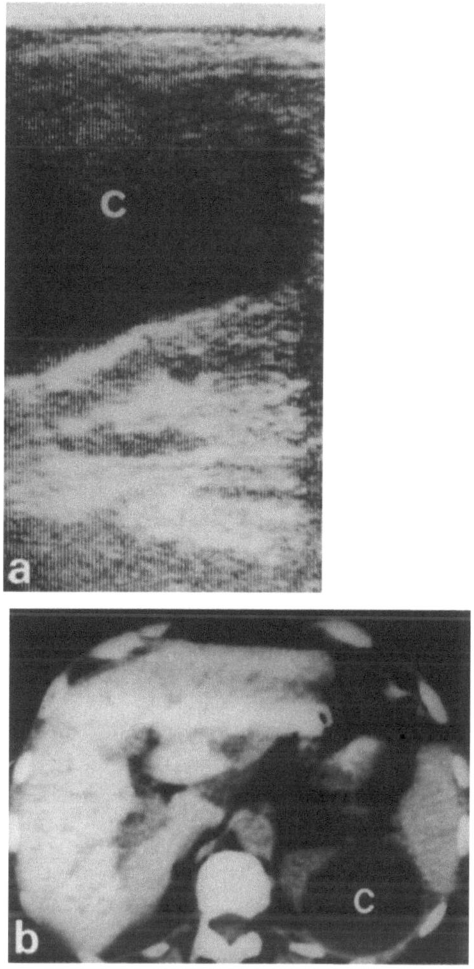

Fig. 7 a, b. A pancreatic pseudocyst has entered the renal capsule laterally mimicking a renal cortex cyst. There are no criteria for differentiating by ultrasound (**a**) or CT (**b**). *C* cyst

dronephrosis, occasionally the hydronephrotic type of multicystic kidney [10] may be indistinguishable from hydronephrosis. Radionuclide scanning is the most effective means of identifying the blood flow in hydronephrosis; if there is no perfusion, multicystic kidney is the more likely diagnosis [34].

5. Calcified cysts may be difficult to image by ultrasound since the thin layer of calcification in the cyst wall produces a solid pattern of the lesion (Fig. 5), although a cystic pattern will be seen in the calcium-free portions.
6. Renal artery aneurysms may mimic a renal cyst (Fig. 6). In our observation an anechoic, oval-shaped mass was seen with irregular borders and a low sonic enhancement. A giant renal artery aneurysm was reported by HANTMAN et al. [13] meeting all the criteria for a simple cyst. Parapelvic anechoic masses may not always be simple cysts, and a vascular etiology must be considered as well, especially in a young patient suffering from hypertension and hematuria. Contrast CT will confirm the diagnosis.
7. Pancreatic pseudocysts may enter the renal capsule and mimic a cyst (Fig. 7) [35]. In our case a fine needle puncture was performed and the high level of amylase lead to the definite diagnosis. The liquid consistency of hyperdense cysts in CT can be proven by sonography (Fig. 8).

3.1.3 Parapelvic Cysts

Cysts located in the renal hilum are referred to as parapelvic cysts. They do not communicate with the collecting systems and their pathogenesis is uncertain. Frequently a lymphatic origin and development from embryologic rests are discussed [18]. The parapelvic cyst is an anechoic mass with a well demarcated wall and

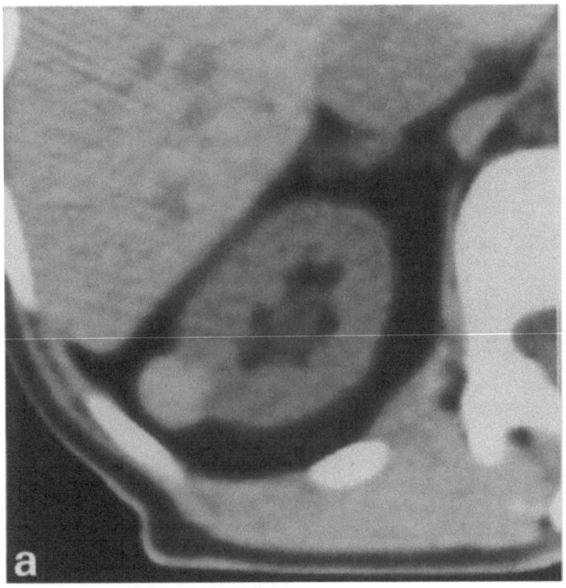

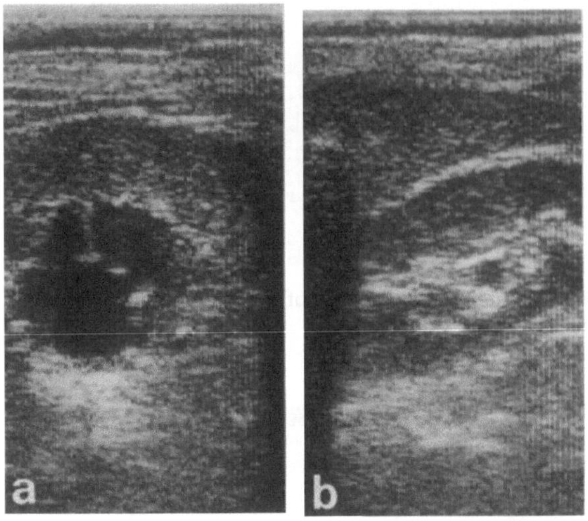

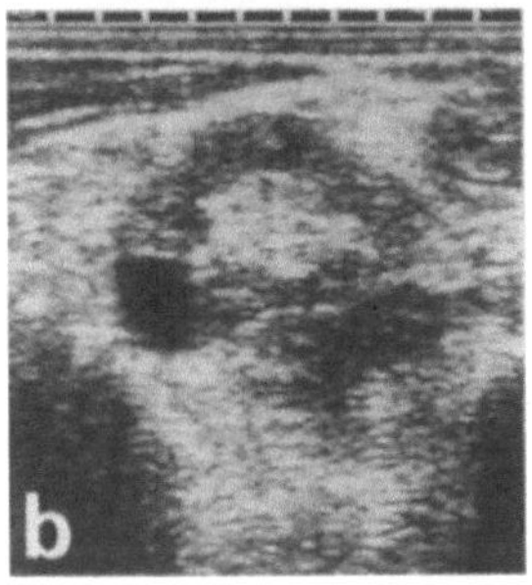

Fig. 8 a, b. Hyperdense cyst detected by CT (**a**). Sonography (**b**) reveals a typical liquid content

sonic enhancement, but when multiple they seem to compress each other in the narrow space of the renal sinus (Fig. 9). In some cases it may be difficult to differentiate parapelvic cysts from hydronephrosis or renal sinus lipomatosis by means of sonography alone. A CT examination with contrast administration will disclose the problem. If CT is not available an intravenous urogram is necessary in order to conclusively exclude hydronephrosis.

Abnormal urine collections within a portion of the kidney as a diverticulum of a calyx (Fig. 10) cannot be differentiated from renal cysts by ultrasound alone, but together with an intravenous urogram the correct diagnosis can be made.

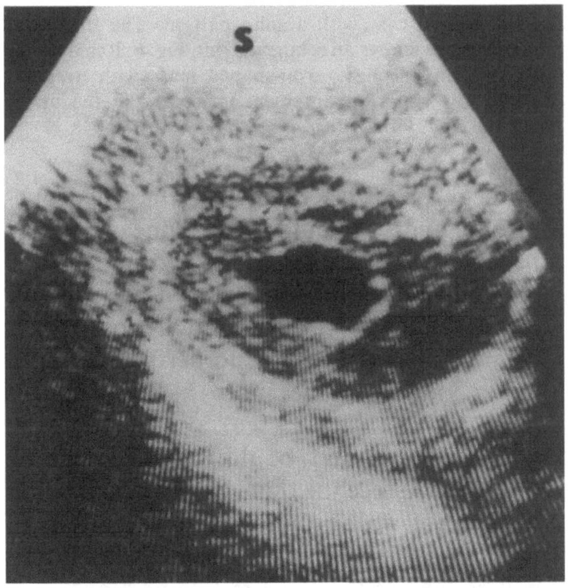

Fig. 10. Diverticulum of a calyx. It cannot be differentiated from renal cysts by ultrasound alone

3.1.4 Adult Polycystic Disease

This autosomal dominant hereditary disease is characterized by increased bilateral renal size, nodular cortical surface, and multiple cysts of various shapes and sizes replacing the normal parenchyma (Fig. 11) and the renal sinus completely. They may take up a large part of the whole abdomen and present a honeycomb echo pattern. The value of making early diagnoses by examining all the members of an affected family was pointed out by WEITZEL et al. [36]. The interface of multiple microcysts gives rise to numerous echoes, and on occasion to a misleading echotexture of solid type [35]. Asso-

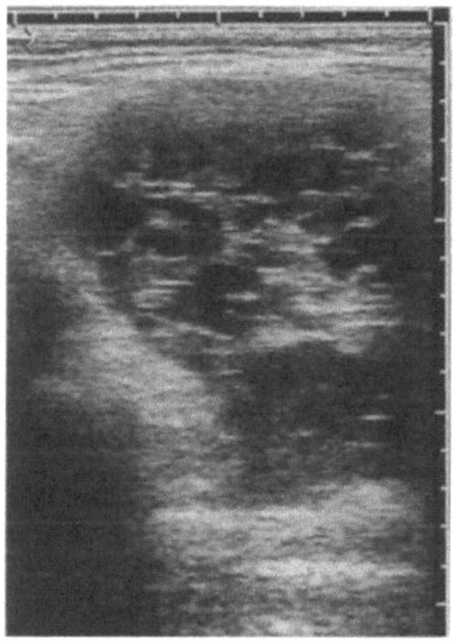

Fig. 11. Adult polycystic disease. Multiple cysts of various shapes and sizes replace the normal parenchyma and renal sinus and take up a large part of the whole abdomen

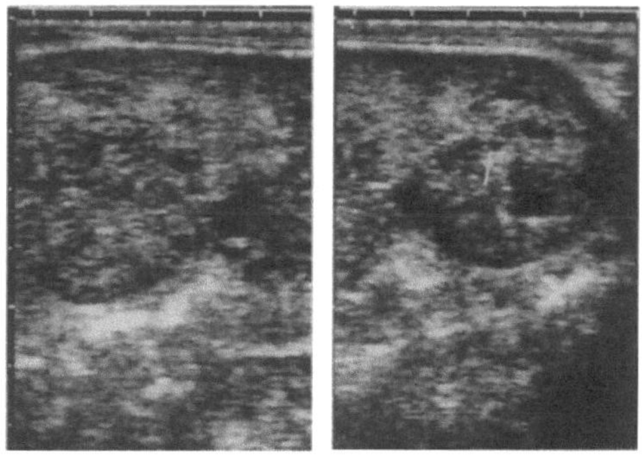

Fig. 12. Infantile polycystic disease, "pepper and salt" pattern. The improved resolution of newer scanners shows cysts down to 2 mm in diameter (*arrow*)

ciated hepatic and pancreatic cysts can be clearly detected by ultrasound. In most cases the diagnosis of polycystic disease can be confirmed by sonography alone; however, an acute hemorrhage or associated lithiasis causing violent pain will require complementary CT. Sonography is an appropriate method with which to follow this chronic progressive disease.

3.1.5 Infantile and Juvenile Polycystic Disease

Clinically, infants present with renal failure, hypertension, or portal hypertension with esophageal varices.

Polycystic disease of the kidney is divided into two major categories: child and adult polycystic disease. Polycystic disease of the young encompasses a spectrum of disease from the newborn type at one end to the childhood type at the other end. It is a two organ disease involving both the kidneys and the liver. Multiple epithelial hepatic cysts, dilated bile ducts, and periportal fibrosis are invariably present. In younger children the kidneys are more severely involved, while in older children it is the liver. Both types are genetically inherited as an autosomal recessive disease. Sonograms show increased bilateral renal size. There is an increased echogenicity of the cortex and the medulla [30]. Analyses with newer real-time scanners of improved resolution reveal a specific pattern called "pepper and salt" and a striped pattern (Fig. 12). Even minute cysts down to 2 mm in diameter ("pepper") can be detected [37]. In association with bilaterally enlarged kidneys and poor definition among the renal sinuses, this pattern suggests the final diagnosis, but it does not offer any correlation with the clinical course or state of renal function.

3.2 Solid Tumors

3.2.1 Renal Cell Carcinoma

Renal cell carcinomas are by far the most common primary malignancy of the kidney in the adult with 75% of the total [8], but they are still relatively rare, accounting for approximately 2% of all malignancies [9]. When a solid mass is diagnosed in all probability it will be renal cell carcinoma, due to its frequency. However this finding can never represent a definite diagnosis. The same signs can be seen in sarcomas of the kidney, metastases, lymphomas, oncocytomas, and advanced transitional cell carcinomas of the kidney. The following sonographic criteria are characteristic:

1. A superficial bulge breaks the kidney's even contours, the tumor-bearing part of the kidney is distended and deformed (Fig. 13). The contours of small masses are sharply delineated. Once the tumor has extended beyond Gerota's fascia the boundaries will become irregular and difficult to delineate.
2. The echo pattern of renal cell carcinomas differs widely. The most frequent patterns displayed are: (a) a weakly echogenic pattern which may contain a few reflective nodules (89%) [35] (Fig. 13), (b) a strongly and densely echogenic structure (2%) (Fig. 14),

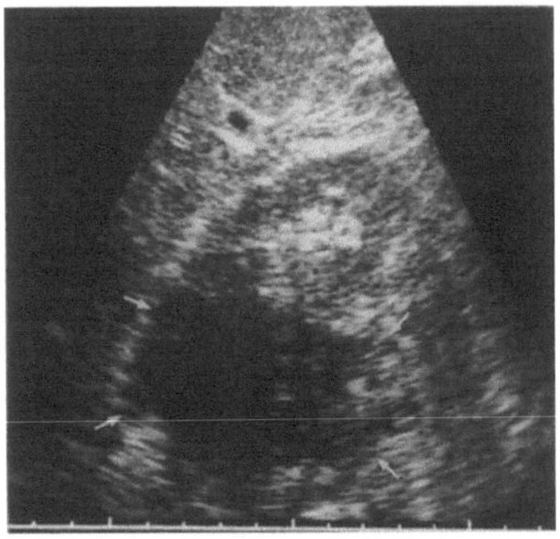

Fig. 13. Renal cell carcinoma. Weakly echogenic tumor, superficial bulge, and irregular margins (*arrows*)

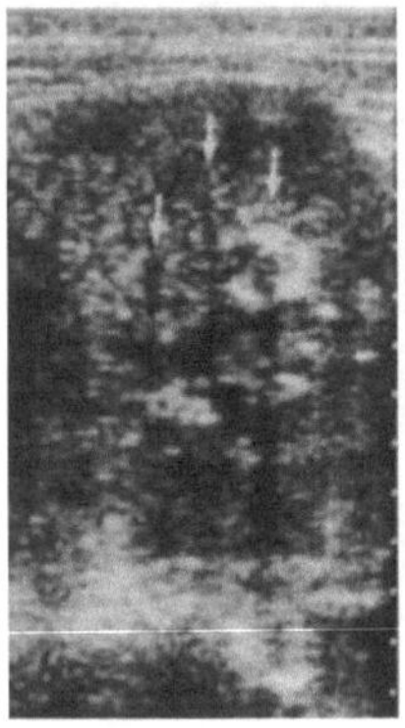

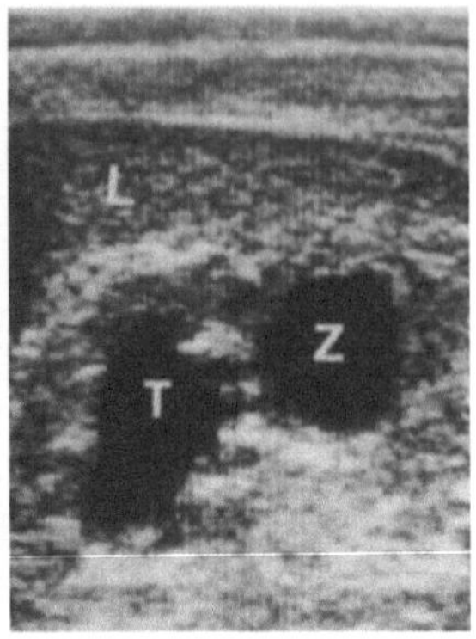

Fig. 15. (*left*)

Fig. 16.

Fig. 15. (*left*) Renal cell carcinoma. Mixed pattern of strongly reflective and decreased echogenicity, shadowing calcifications (*arrows*). **Fig. 16.** Tumor (*T*) and cyst (*Z*) in one kidney. The tumor (renal adenocarcinoma) is strongly liquid, necrotized, and shows an irregular wall. *L*, liver

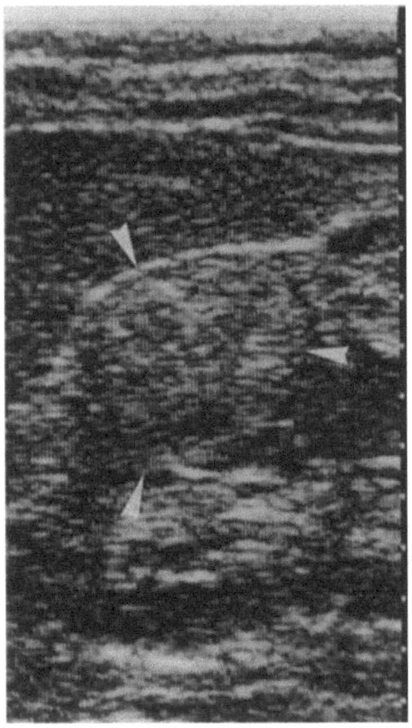

Fig. 14. Renal cell carcinoma. Strongly and densely echogenic pattern (*arrowheads*)

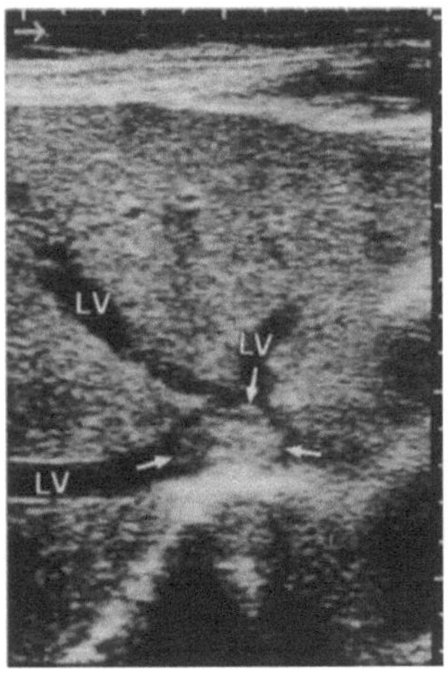

Fig. 17. (*left*)

Fig. 18.

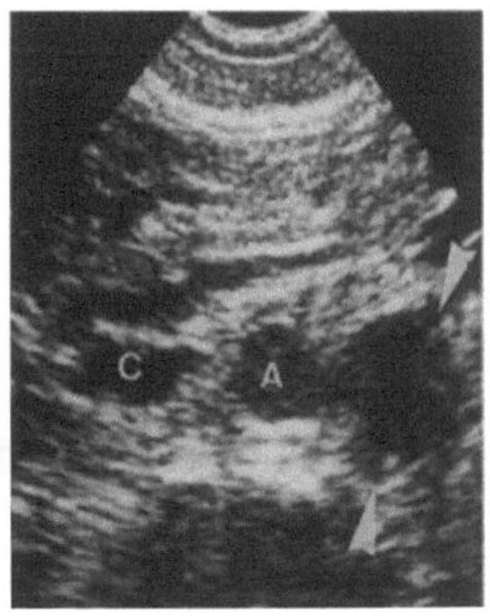

Fig. 17. (*left*) Tumor invasion (*arrows*) into the cranial part of the inferior caval vein. *LV*, liver vein. **Fig. 18.** Para-aortal lymph node involvement (*arrowhead*). *A*, aorta; *C* inferior caval vein

(c) a mixed pattern of strongly reflective and decreased echogenicity, which can be combined with shadowing calcifications (4.5%) (Fig. 15), and (d) a cystic echo pattern in strongly necrotizing tumors (4.5%). In contrast to a benign cyst, the cyst wall is several millimeters thick and irregular (Fig. 16).

3. The renal sinus may be deformed or amputated (Fig. 13).
4. The mobility of the kidney during inspiration is reduced or suspended.
5. The involvement of the renal vein can be seen. Intracaval tumor growth (Fig. 17) is documented in up to 90% of cases [27, 33].
6. Lymphatic spread to the para-aortal nodes is readily displayed. A correct delineation was reported in 74% [27]. Limitations include the volume and flatulence of the patient. The use of sector scanning improves the accuracy of detecting lymph nodes in our own practice (Fig. 18).
7. Ascites can be recognized early and is of importance in the follow-up of postnephrectomy patients. It is evidence of a poor prognosis in the adult [15]. However, in Wilms' tumor, ascites is detectable during the primary examination (Fig. 19).
8. Pleural effusions should be displayed by ul-

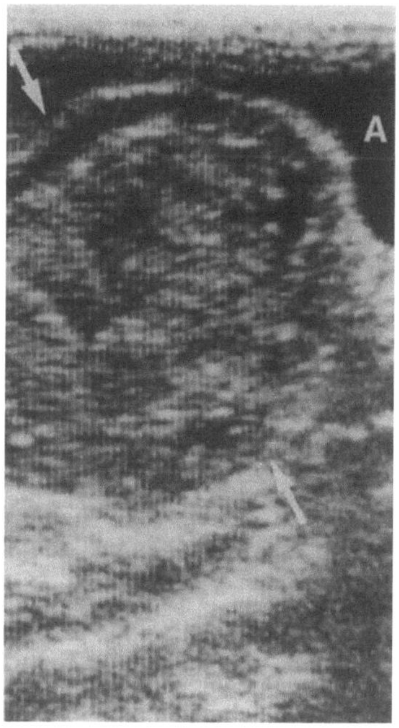

Fig. 19. Wilms' tumor. Ascites (*A*) is detected during primary examination

trasound especially with Wilms' tumors and large adult renal masses. Encouraging results about the sonographic visualization of mediastinal lymph nodes by a suprajugular port were reported by K. WERNECKE (personal communication).

9. Metastases of the liver smaller than 1 cm in diameter are successfully diagnosed.

3.2.1.1 Diagnostic Problems

Statements about the accuracy of a method always demonstrate that results of various investigators cannot be compared due to differences between patients, technical equipment, experience of the investigators, and the parameters of the examination. Nevertheless the following data [27] will give an insight into the efficiency of sonography and CT in detecting renal masses (Table 1).

Table 1. Diagnostic accuracy

Sonography of malignant tumors	x=85% (52–100%)
cysts	x=87% (64–98%)
CT of malignant tumors	x=96% (84–100%)
cysts	x=87% (64–98%)

Diagnostic problems in solid renal masses include the various morphological changes of the kidneys' shape with isoechogenic pattern, especially cortical humps in the middle portion and the central dividing parenchyma in a dichotomous renal pelvis. It is difficult to detect small tumors (1–3 cm in diameter) without differences in impedance. Regeneration nodules are observed as pseudotumors encountered in chronic pyelonephritis; they are usually accompanied by chronic atrophy with local indentations [35]. Frequently inflammatory processes such as carbuncles are poorly visualized.

3.2.2 "Adenomas" and Oncocytomas

Epithelial neoplasms of the renal cortex smaller than 3 cm in diameter usually behave benign although rare metastasizing examples are known. If a node is larger than 3 cm its biologic behavior is more likely to be malignant. The malignant potential increases with size, but large examples without metastases have also been reported. In short: There is no sharp borderline between adenomas and carcinomas, so that all renal cortical nodes should be removed. The sonographic pattern of small nodes is readily derived: small homogeneous tumors of low echogenicity located in the renal cortex. There are no necrotic or hemorrhagic areas influencing the echotexture. A "papillary adenoma" of low echogenicity is shown in Fig. 20. Renal oncocytomas have no malignant potential [24]. However, there are no urographic, scintigraphic, angiographic, sonographic, and com-

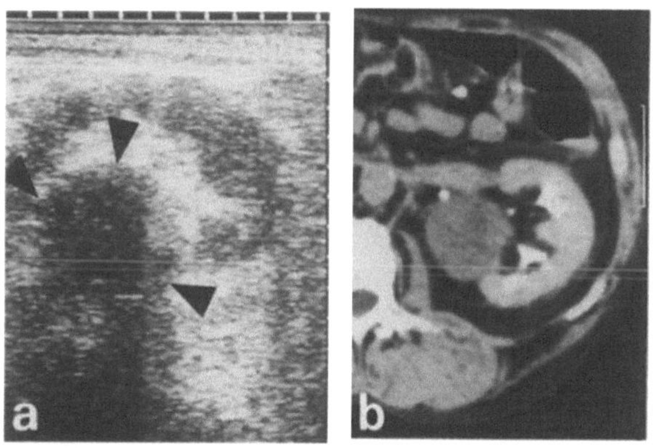

Fig. 20a, b. "Papillary adenoma". (a) Low homogeneous echogenicity and a pronounced shadowing by absorption. (b) CT shows a hypodense, centrally located tumor puted tomographic criteria to differentiate oncocytoma from adenocarcinoma of the kidney [5].

3.2.3 Angiomyolipoma

Angiomyolipoma, or hamartoma, is the most common benign solid mass of the kidney. Frequently the tumor is associated with tuberous sclerosis. In 42% of cases tuberous sclerosis is combined with angiomyolipoma of the kidney [21]. However angiomyolipomas also occur without evidence of tuberous sclerosis. These tumors tend to have unilateral site, to be larger in size, and to be symptomatic. Pathologically angiomyolipomas are composed of widely varying quantities of fat, vascular tissue, and musculature, resulting in different echopatterns. When the fatty component predominates, sonographically a strongly and densely echogenic area is recognized (Fig. 21). However there are reports of angiomyolipomas with low echogenicity [14]. In the presence of a strong reflection pattern a benign tumor must be considered, in all probability an angiomyolipoma. However, the same reflective displays are known in renal adenocarcinoma, hemangioma, angiosarcoma, and metastases [28]. The definite confirmation of an angiomyolipoma is available with density evaluation on CT.

3.2.4 Metastases

The frequency of metastases in the kidney of tumor patients is reported in one pathologic anatomic study as 12.6%, in another as 45% [1, 6]. Though the kidney is frequently a site of metastases, these are seldom clinically noted because of the microscopical size [2, 29]. The most frequent primary tumor is bronchogenic carcinoma and melanoma, but gastrointestinal carcinomas, squamous cell carcinoma of the sublingual salivary gland and buccal mucosa, and seminoma of the testis are also mentioned. We have seen in addition the following: thymic carcinoma, breast carcinoma, and liposarcoma of the thigh. It is noteworthy that metastases of the kidney were accompanied by metastases in other sites and that the kidneys were in preference invaded bilaterally. We agree with Bhatt et al. [2] that metastases of the kidneys show a homogenous structure; Nishitani et al. [29] however observed three necroses in five cases.

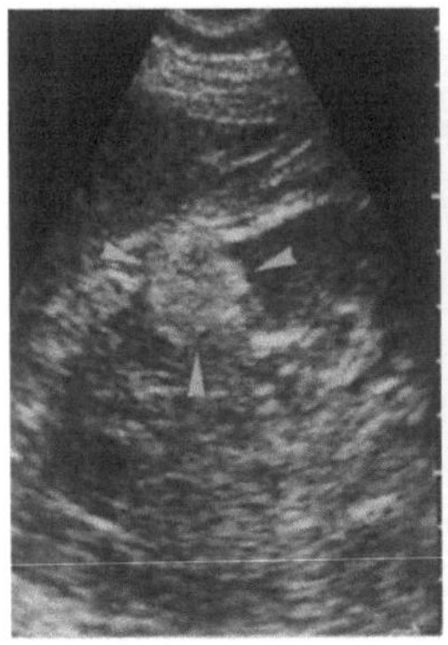
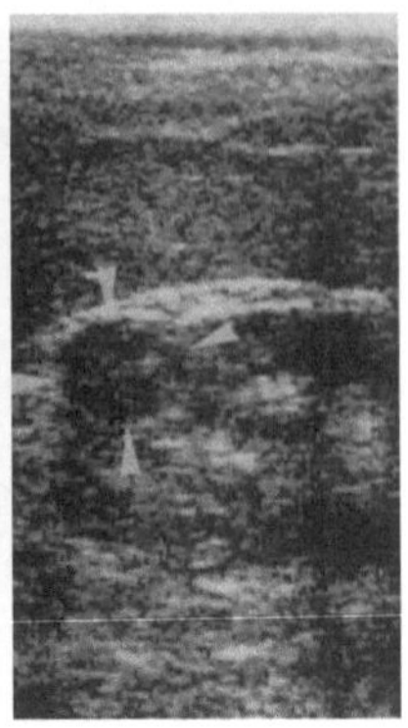

Fig. 21. (*left*)

Fig. 22.

Fig. 21. Angiomyolipoma. A roundish shaped tumor of strongly and densely homogeneous echogenicity, 2 cm in diameter. **Fig. 22.** Metastasis of the kidney. The primary tumor was a bronchogenic carcinoma. Low homogeneous echogenicity and bulging contour evident

Sonographically, all the metastases we observed were of low homogeneous echogenicity, were located in the renal cortex, and showed bulging contours (Fig. 22). Metastases of lymphomas are more frequently found. In most cases, renal lymphoma is a manifestation of long-standing disease [4]. Lesions of the kidney are rarely due to primary lymphoma but rather to local extension from adjacent perinephric nodal masses or distant hematogenous metastases [22]. Metastases of lymphomas may show such low level echogenicity due to their uniform cellularity that they may be mistaken for cysts. The appearance of lymphomas may be various: multiple large and small nodules, single large masses (Fig. 23), diffuse infiltration, and lesions of the renal hilum [31].

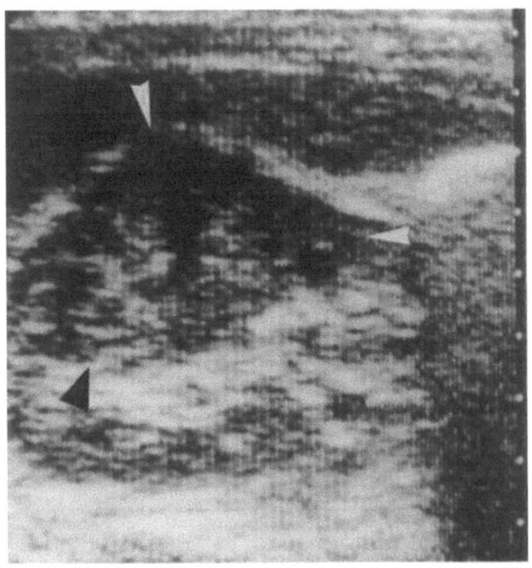

Fig. 23. Renal metastasis in Hodgkins' disease. Large mass of low echogenicity (*arrow*). This tumor cannot be differentiated from a renal adenocarcinoma

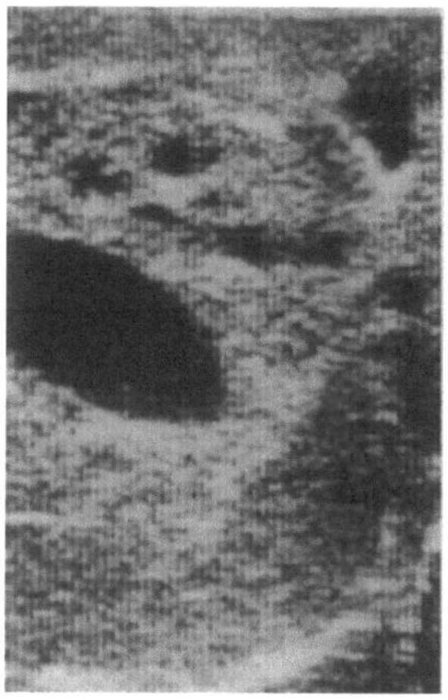

Fig. 24. Wilms' tumor. Bulky mass extending within one-half of the abdomen. The echogenicity imitates that of liver. Echofree areas are due to hemorrhage and necrosis

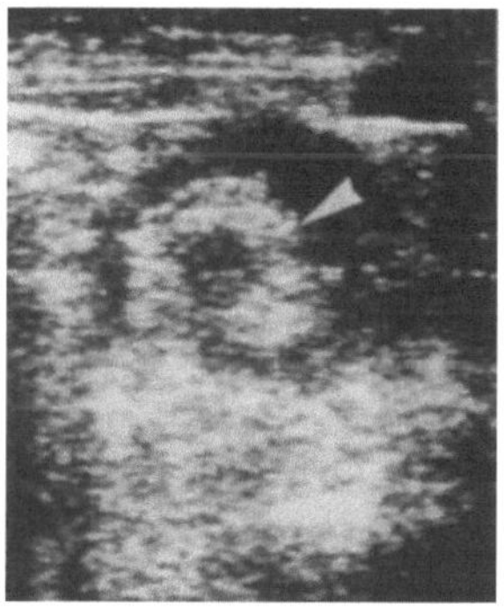

Fig. 25. Transitional carcinoma. A solid central mass divides the renal sinus (*arrow*)

When there are no other manifestations of metastases in a known primary, we use fine needle puncture for cytological confirmation when therapeutic decisions are required.

3.2.5 Wilms' Tumor

Wilms' tumor is the most common malignancy in childhood, particularly between 2 and 5 years of age. Bilateral tumors have an incidence of about 5%–10%. Clinically, an asymptomatic abdominal mass is the most frequent finding. Typically, the sonogram shows a bulky mass expanding within one-half of the abdomen. Frequently it is difficult to identify the invaded kidney. The mass is solid, and echogenicity can imitate that of the liver. There are characteristic echofree areas due to necrosis and hemorrhage (Fig. 24). In contrast to renal cell carcinoma of the adult, ascites is frequently demonstrated during primary examination. Further findings are the same as those described for other solid renal masses.

3.2.6 Transitional Cell Carcinoma of the Kidney

Transitional carcinomas constitute approximately 10% of all renal carcinomas. They are four times more common in men than in women and appear to be 40% multicentric. The intravenous urogram including a conventional tomogram and a retrograde pyelogram dominates as the diagnostic procedure of choice. Sometimes transitional tumors are recognized by sonography (Fig. 25). Small tumors are difficult or impossible to visualize by means of ultrasound. But larger tumors can also be missed when the pattern is highly reflective and a delineation against the echogenic renal sinus is obscured. Nevertheless there are some remarkable characteristics of renal transitional cell carcinomas: there is no bulging of the kidney's contour even in advanced tumors and calcifications are unusual. Frequently an early loss of function is found.

3.3 Perirenal Lesions

Perinephric fluid collections are caused by hematomas, abscesses, seromas, lymphoceles, urinomas, and pancreatic pseudocysts [32].

3.3.1 Hematomas

The sonographic appearance of hematomas spans a wide range. In the early phase (some hours) they are of dense echogenicity (see also Fig. 2); later there is a low echogenic or cystic pattern (Fig. 26). Hematomas surrounding the kidney can be responsible for hypertension.

3.3.2 Abscesses

The sonographic pattern of abscesses varies widely [16]: cystic, low echogenic, isoechoic, highly echogenic, and shadowing if the abscess contains gas. Abscesses tend to disrupt the fascial boundaries and move along the psoas muscle. Clinical features such as pain, leucocytosis, and fever are essential for the definite diagnosis.

3.3.3 *Lymphoceles*

Lymphoceles are a common complication in renal transplants. However urinomas and seromas have the same appearance. Sonographically, these lesions are echofree and cystic (Fig. 27a). Lymphoceles may appear septated (Fig. 27b).

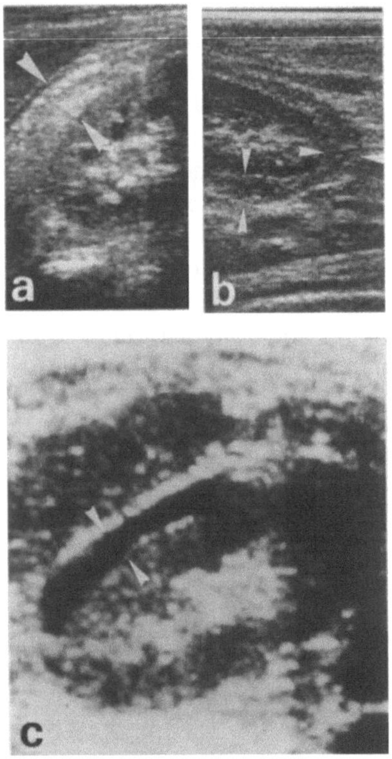

Fig. 26 a–c. Perirenal hematomas. (**a**) Perirenal hematoma of high echogenicity in a slim, 18-year-old man 1 h after a moped accident. (**b**) Perirenal hematoma of low echogenicity 24 h after renal biopsy. (**c**) Subcapsular hematoma of liquid and echofree appearance following renal trauma

3.3.4 *Pancreatic Pseudocysts*

Perirenal invasion of a pancreatic cyst is mentioned under atypical cysts (Fig. 7).

4 Extrarenal Lesions

Splenic and retroperitoneal tumors can mimic a renal mass, especially adrenal lesions (Fig. 28). Despite this Fig. 29 shows a patient in whom a primary retroperitoneal tumor was diagnosed by ultrasound and CT. Operation revealed a peduncled renal adenocarcinoma.

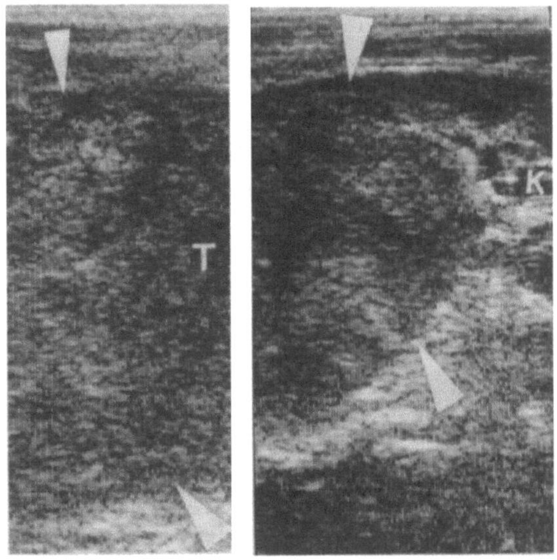

Fig. 28. Metastases of the left adrenal in a patient with bronchogenic carcinoma. A huge mass (*T*) is poorly delimited (*arrows*) from the upper pole of the kidney (*K*)

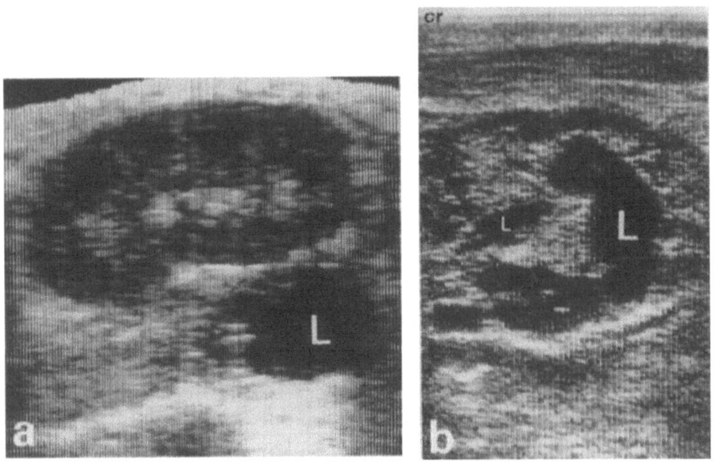

Fig. 27 a, b. Lymphoceles in a renal transplant (*L*). (**a**) Cystic appearance with sonic enhancement and a diameter of 3 cm. (**b**) Irregular, septated, and "polycystic" appearance

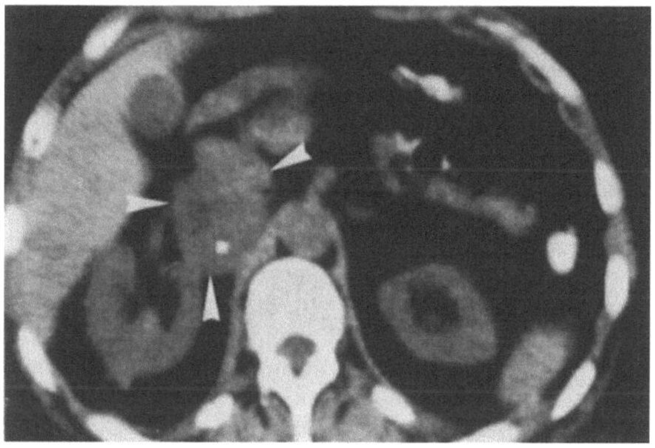

Fig. 29. Peduncled renal adenocarcinoma mimicking a retroperitoneal lymph node tumor (*arrwos*)

5 Diagnostic Procedure in Renal Tumors

The diagnostic procedure is summarized in a decision tree (Fig. 30). The first steps in demonstrating a solid renal mass are taking a urogram and a sonogram and vice versa, of which one complements the other. The advantage of ultrasound is the detection of peripheral lesions localized in the renal cortex, whereas the urogram is especially suitable for delineating central masses by indicating subtle changes of the central collecting system. The possibility of determining the consistency of a tumor is the benefit of employing sonography. Ultrasound examination is independent of renal function and thus application of contrast medium is not required. This advantage, however, is reduced by the poor visualization of the ureter. Frequently, parapelvic cysts cannot be distinguished from hydronephrosis by only using ultrasound. In such cases, an additional urogram may be essential for a definite diagnosis, although a CT scan is unnecessary. When a renal mass is discovered, both a urogram and a sonogram should be performed except for small-sized cortical cysts which can be proved sonographically. When the renal sinus is altered, a urogram should be performed as a basic examination, especially when a follow-up is planned. We only recommend surgery when a cyst is symptomatic(pain) or induces hydronephrosis. In the typical cyst – anechoic, spherical, sharply outlined, distal enhancement – sonography is sufficient and further studies are redundant. When classical sonographic characteristics are not portrayed, the cyst must be considered atypical, requiring a CT evaluation. If the CT scan provides equivocal results as well, a sonographically guided fine needle puncture should be performed. Should hemorrhagic aspirate be obtained, surgery is indicated in our opinion, provided that the hemorrhage is not caused iatrogenically.

In cases where both ultrasound and CT suggest an atypical cyst, there are several possible reasons: hemorrhagic cysts, inflammatory cysts, cystadenomas, necrotized tumors, lymphomas tumor and cyst lying next to each other in one kidney, and, finally and very rarely, malignancy of the cyst wall.

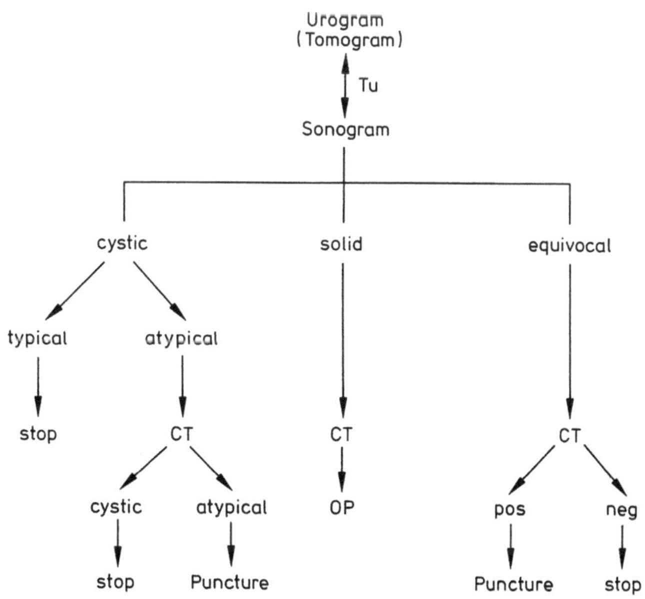

Fig. 30. Decision tree of diagnostic procedures in renal tumours

When a solid mass is diagnosed, a CT scan should preferably be performed before surgery because of its superiority in staging the tumor and because it is able to provide a specific diagnosis in an angiomyolipoma. Angiography has lost its diagnostic value and is applied only in organ-preserving surgery and for tumor embolization.

The diagnosis of renal masses is based on sonography, excretory urography, and CT. Though CT continues to be superior to ultrasound in the detection of renal masses, sonography is the method of choice with regard to expense and capacity.

References

1. Abrams HL, Spiro R, Goldstein N (1950) Metastases in carcinoma, analysis of 1000 autopsied cases. Cancer 3:74
2. Bhatt GM, Bernardino ME, Graham SD Jr (1983) CT diagnosis of renal metastases. J CAT 7:1032
3. Chan JCM, Kodroff MB (1980) Hypertension and hematuria secondary to parapelvic cyst. Pediatrics 65:821–822
4. Coleman BG, Arger PH (1984) Renal neoplasm. In: Resnick MJ, Sandes RC (eds) Ultrasound in urology. Williams and Wilkins, Baltimore
5. Cohan R, Dumnick NR, Degesys GE (1984) Computed tomography of renal oncozytoma. J CAT 8:284–287
6. Das Gupta T, Brasfield R (1964) Metastatic melanoma. A clinicopathological study. Cancer 17:1323–1339
7. Doust VL, Doust BD, Redman H (1973) Evaluation of ultrasonic B-mode scanning in the diagnosis of renal masses. Radiology I:112–119
8. Emmet JL, Levine SR, Woolner LB (1963) Coexistence of renal cyst and tumor: incidence in 1007 cases. Br J Urol 35:403–410
9. Evans RW (1968) Histologic appearances of tumors. Livingstone, Edinburgh
10. Felson B, Cussen LJ (1975) The hydronephrotic type of unilateral congenital multicystic disease of the kidney. Semin Roentgenol 10:113–123
11. Gordon RL, Pollack HM, Popky GL, Duckett JW Jr (1979) Simple serous cysts of the kidney in children. Radiology 131:357–361
12. Grossman H, Rosenberg ER, Bowie DJ, Ram P, Merten DF (1983) Sonographic diagnosis of renal cystic disease. AJR 140:81–85
13. St Hantman S, Barie JJ, Glendening TB, Eisenberg MN, Rapoport KD (1982) Giant renal artery aneurysm mimicking a simple cyst on ultrasound. J Clin Ultrasound 10:136–139
14. Hartman DS, Goldman SM, Friedman AC, Davis ChJ, Madewell JE, Sherman JL (1981) Angiomyolipoma. Ultrasonic-pathologic correlation. Radiology 139:451
15. Heckemann R, Heimann H, Holfeld H (1980) Die Sonographie in Therapie und Nachsorge von malignen Nierentumoren. In: Hinselmann H, Anliker M, Meudt R (eds) Ultraschalldiagnostik in der Medizin. Thieme, Stuttgart
16. Heckemann R, Krüger K, Wernecke K (1982) Echomorphologie und Punktionsdiagnostik von intraabdominellen Abszessen. Fortschr Roentgenstr 137 [5]:517–522
17. Heckemann R, Heimann H, Meyer-Schwickerath M, Paar D, Eickenberg H-U (1982) Ultraschallgeführte Nierenzystenpunktion. Fortschr Roentgenstr 137:1
18. Hidalgo H, Dumnick NR, Rosenberg ER, Ram CP, Korobkin M (1982) Parapelvic cysts: appearance on CT and sonography. AJR 138:667–671
19. Jackman RJ, Stevens GM (1974) Benign hemorrhagic renal cyst. Nephrotomography, renal arteriography and cyst puncture. Radiology 110:7–13
20. Jaffe CC, Rosenfield AT, Sommer G, Taylor KJW (1980) Technical factors influencing the imaging of small anechoic cysts by B-scan ultrasound. Radiology 135:429–433
21. Jardin A, Richard F, Le Duc A, Chatelain A, Le Gulliou M, Fourcade R, Camey M, Küss R (1980) Diagnosis and treatment of renal angiomyolipoma. Eur Urol 6:69
22. Kaude JV, Lacy GD (1978) Ultrasonography in renal lymphoma. J Clin Ultrasound 6:321
23. King DL (1972) Renal ultrasonography. An aid in the clinical evaluation of renal masses. Radiology 105:633–640
24. Klein MJ, Valensi QJ (1976) Proximal tubular adenomas of kidney with so-called oncocytic features: a clinicopathologic study of 13 cases of a rarely reported neoplasm. Cancer 38:906–914
25. Kosoff G, Garret WJ, Carpenter DA, Jellins J (1976) Principles and classification of soft tissues by grey scale echography. Ultrasound Med Biol 2:89–105
26. Kristensen JK, Gammelgard PA, Holm HH, Rasmussen SN (1972) Ultrasound in the demonstration of renal masses. Br J Urol 44:517–527
27. Lackner K, Koischwitz D, Molitor B, Vogel J, Schmidt S (1984) Treffsicherheit in der Diagnostik renaler Raumforderungen. Fortschr Roentgenstr 140(4):363–372
28. Lingard DA, Lawson TL (1979) Accuracy of ultrasound in predicting the nature of renal masses. J Urol 122:724
29. Nishitani H, Onitsuka H, Kawahira K et al. (1984) Computed tomography of renal metastasis. J CAT 8:727–730
30. Rosenfield AT, Curtis AM, Putman CE, Taylor KJW, Allen WE, Siegel NJ, Hsia YE (1977) Gray scale ultrasonography, computerized tomography, and nephrotomography in evaluation of polycystic kidney and liver disease. Urology 9:436–438
31. Rubin BE (1979) Computed tomography in the evaluation of renal lymphoma. J Comput Assist Tomogr 3:759–764
32. Sanders RC (1984) Retroperitoneal pathology. In: Resnick MI, Sanders RC (eds) Ultrasound in urology, 2nd edn. Williams and Wilkins, Baltimore
33. Schwerk WB, Schwerk WN, Drews H, Rodeck G (1984) Ultraschalldiagnostik venöser Tumorthromben bei Nierenkarzinomen. Urologe 23:214
34. Stuck KJ, Koff A St, Silver TM (1982) Ultrasonic feature of multicystic dysplastic kidney: expanded diagnostic criteria. Radiology 143:217–221
35. Weill FS, Rohmer P, Zeltner F (1981) Renal sonography. Springer, Berlin Heidelberg New York
36. Weitzel D, Bahlmann J, Otto P (1974) Die Wertigkeit der Sonographie für die Diagnostik von Zystennieren. Dtsch Med Wochenschr 99:1587
37. Wernecke K, Heckemann R, Bachmann H, Peters PE (1985) Sonography of infantile polycystic kidney disease. Urol Radiol 7:138–145

Computed-Body-Tomography of Renal Carcinoma and Perirenal Masses

E. LÖHR, P.E. BILLIMORIA, and M. SERDAREVIC

1 Introduction

In the last 10 years the concept of detection of renal tumors has been completely renovated. Before then i.v. urography, and renal angiography developed by SELDINGER, OLSSON, and BOIJSEN were the main diagnostic tools. The introduction of ultrasound and CT has entirely changed all diagnostic procedures and devices. In addition magnetic resonance imaging (MR) enriches the spectrum of diagnostic possibilities. For this reason a special chapter is dedicated to the diagnosis of the kidney and adrenals by magnetic resonance (MR).

Today the primary diagnosis is mostly incidental during a check-up by ultrasound in apparently healthy patients. In 1 year we treated ten patients with renal cell carcinoma by tumor embolization after the tumor had been detected accidentally as it was without any clinical signs. It can perhaps be assumed thus that the survival rate of these patients will increase in contrast to other groups in former times.

Before ultrasound and CT the primary diagnosis to localise a supposed malignant renal tumor started with an i.v. urogram when there were clinical urgent symptoms such as fever, flank pain, macrohematuria, and anemia. When detected by this means and by angiography, tumor spread had already taken place in many cases. With our patients it occurred in more than 40% according to a follow-up study of 15 years which ended by 1979 (LÖHR). Nowadays if urography is used it should come after the first detection of the neoplasm by ultrasound, followed by CT.

Angiography should only be done as a "second-look" examination if embolization therapy is being discussed (LANG 1983) or, if the urologic surgeon wants a survey of the extra- and intrarenal vasculature in the preoperative phase. There are rare cases when angiography is necessary for the primary diagnosis of a malignant renal tumor. This may only happen in cases of so-called poorly vascularized neoplasms with tumorous vessels and a cystic wall (LÖHR and MELLIN 1971).

2 Anatomy

Knowledge of the normal CT appearance of the kidney is important for evaluating and differentiating between normal and pathological findings. The kidneys are part of the extraperitoneum. They have a harmonious shape with round contours of the cortex. With a good scanner differentiation between the cortical zone and the medullar region is possible.

Towards the center the calices and the pelvis can be visualized, and towards the hilum the large vessels, i.e., the renal artery and the renal vein situated before it, can be observed. It can easily be noticed too that the left renal vein communicates with the right renal vein, draining into the inferior vena cava. This becomes obvious after enhancement with contrast medium (see below).

In his monography *Dynamic Radiology of the Abdomen* M.A. MEYERS (1976, 1979) clearly describes the anatomical relationships of the kidneys and the adrenals; they are embedded in the extraperitoneal space which is defined by the surrounding anatomical structures, especially by the different fascia.

Following the example of MEYERS, the retroperitoneal space (RPS) is demarcated by its distinctly defined fascia into different components:

1. The anterior pararenal space extending from the posterior parietal peritoneum to the anterior renal fascia (Gerota's fascia)
2. The perirenal space encompassing the kidney and its surrounding fat

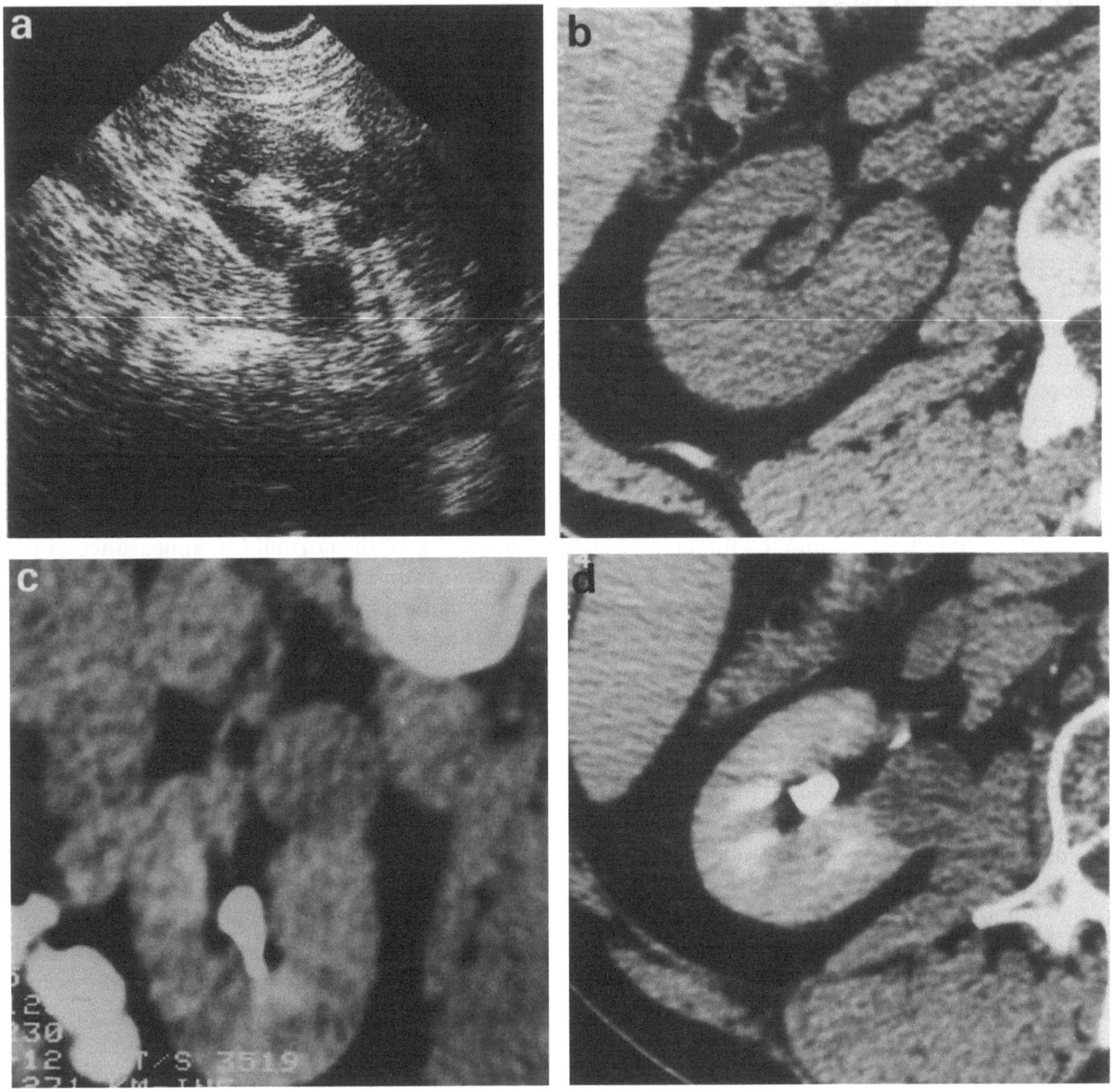

Fig. 1. **a** Ultrasonogram, pre- and post-contrast, CT scan of a solid lesion centrally located between the kidney and the psoas muscle. This lesion can be delineated very well in the ultrasonogram as a solid mass. In the precontrast CT scan the lesion seems to be adherent to the cortex (**b**); after contrast (**c**), however, the invasion of the lesion towards the normal kidney tissue can be seen. The lesion proved to be a renal cell carcinoma stage I–II, not invading the psoas muscle (**d**)

3. The posterior pararenal space extending from the posterior renal fascia to the transversalis fascia.

According to McLennan (1983) Gerota's fascia may be detected in some normal individuals, particularly on sections at the level of the renal hilum where this fascia is perpendicular to the scanning plain. Vertical sections in coronal projection (Blümm 1981) give additional information of topographical relation. In cases of inflammatory diseases originating from the kidneys or the pancreas, this fascia is supposed to be thickened, and similarly in cases of neoplastic processes in the retroperitoneum.

The delineation of these anatomical structures is useful for the staging of tumorous growth and defining tumorous spread to the adjoining organs, especially the lymph nodes (Hata et al. 1983; Clausen 1984; Richie et al. 1983).

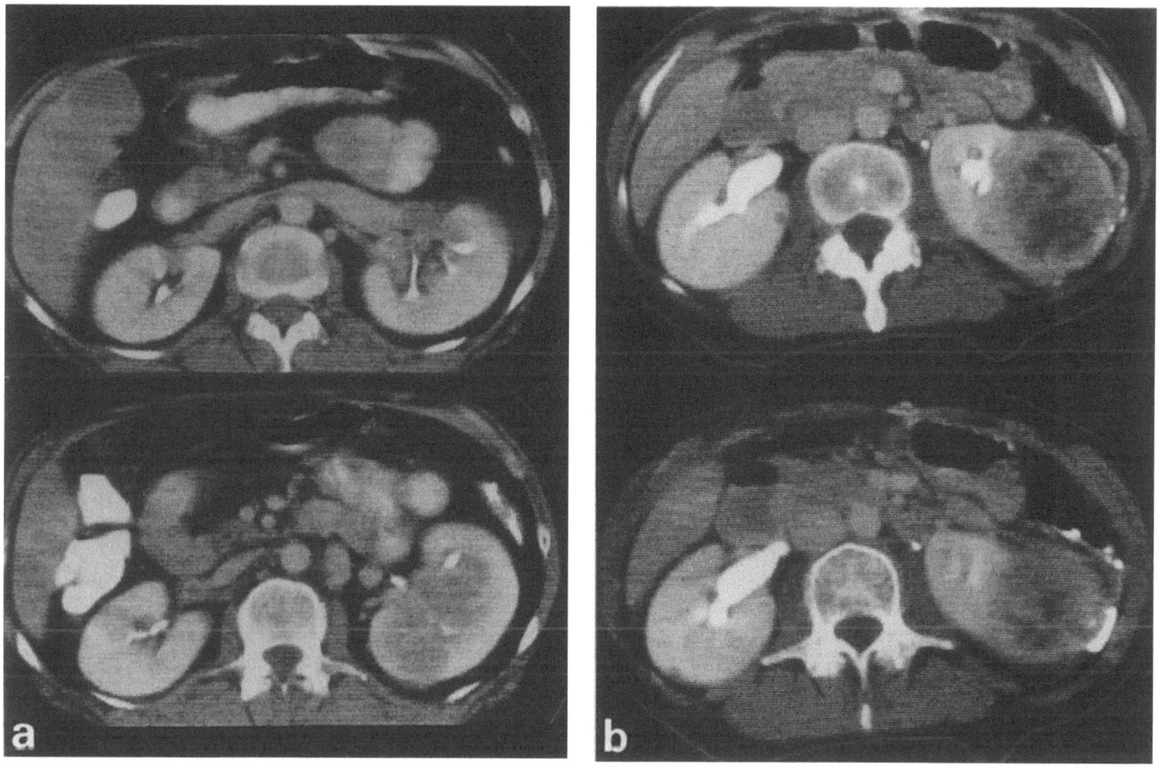

Fig. 2 a, b. Dynamic CT of a space-occupying parenchymal lesion of the left kidney which surpasses the renal capsule. It becomes obvious that this lesion consists of solid tissue with an irregularly shaped hypodense area, corresponding to a necrosis. The normal tissue, especially the collecting system in the postcontrast scan, is compressed. There is no invasion of the renal vein by tumorous growth. The tumor adheres to the muscular wall, but has not invaded it (renal cell carcinoma stage II)

3 Methods

3.1 General Considerations

A CT scanner is an instrument which is by far more sensitive than X-ray examination; the space resolution is high, the possibility of manipulating and maneuvering it is impressive, and it can measure structures by their densities. For these reasons we should like to present a catalogue of criteria which should be followed to delineate and localize a malignant mass lesion of the kidneys:

1. A lesion must be defined regarding its size, localization, and density
2. The lesion must be demarcated from its surroundings
3. Renal abnormalities must be estimated
4. A lesion must be characterized by its typical signs.

The aim of the examination must be to obtain reliable diagnostic data that can be used for the assessment of surgical and nonsurgical therapy and for prognosis of the illness as well. As to methods of examination we must consider that techniques will change with the progress in technology. Several factors influence technique:

1. the slice thickness
2. the use of i.v. contrast
3. the method of viewing, e.g., hard copy, imaging of the structures in windows.

3.2 Positioning of the Patient

For CT scanning of the kidneys and adrenals the patient lies horizontally on the examination table in the ordinary way, with the gantry positioned vertically. It is more convenient to incline the gantry from 6–10°. Normally the kidneys

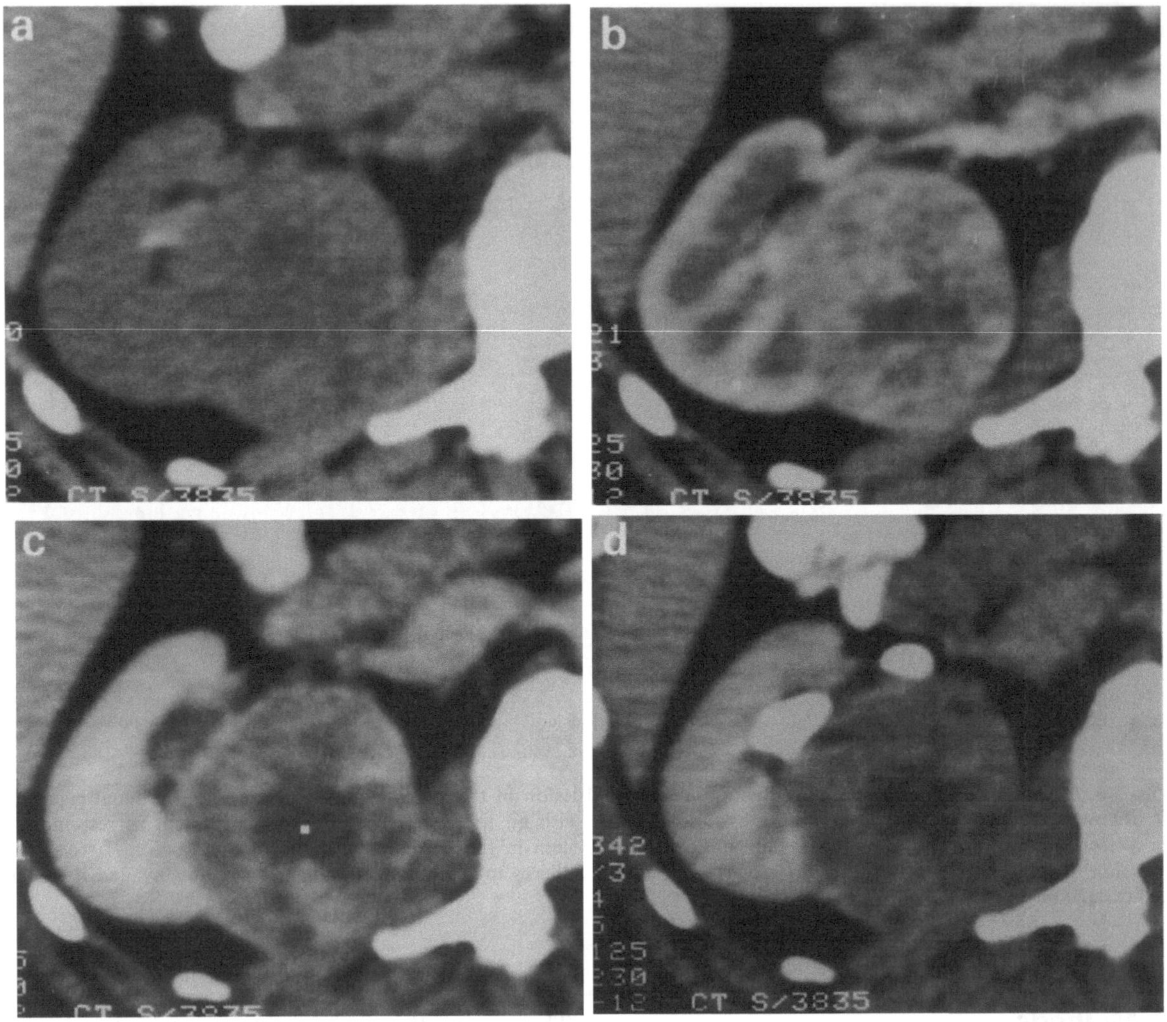

Fig. 3 a–d. Dynamic CT of a 44-year-old patient with renal cell carcinoma, involving the psoas muscle. In the first stages of the CT the tumorous lesion, extending the normal shapes of the kidney, is almost isodense with the renal tissue. After enhancement with contrast medium there is a steady attenuation of the tumorous lesion and the kidney as well. In the first slices there is a very good enhancement of the cortical zone and the columns of Bertini. A central hypodense area (beginning necrosis) is demarcated 20 s and 120 s post injection. Later on the collecting system is filled. At the end of the examination there is a strong opacification of the normal tissue and less attenuation of the tumorous area, which shows central necrosis. The tumor has passed through the renal capsule and has invaded the psoas muscle

are scanned without contrast medium (native scan), and each section is in a sequence of every 2–4 mm.

3.3 Contrast

In all cases a precontrast scan must be done; it is useful in localizing the lesion and getting an idea of its size. Areas of calcification can only be differentiated correctly and distinguished from contrast medium in the collecting system if a precontrast scan is done. After finishing the noncontrast scan, the examination is continued by means of bolus injection of contrast medium.

After contrast injection there is enhancement of the renal parenchyma and a good differentiation of the corticomedullary zone, which takes place in about 20 s. The parenchyma becomes homogeneous after about 45 s, and the collecting system can be distinguished in 1 min. This time sequence is related to the amount of iodine

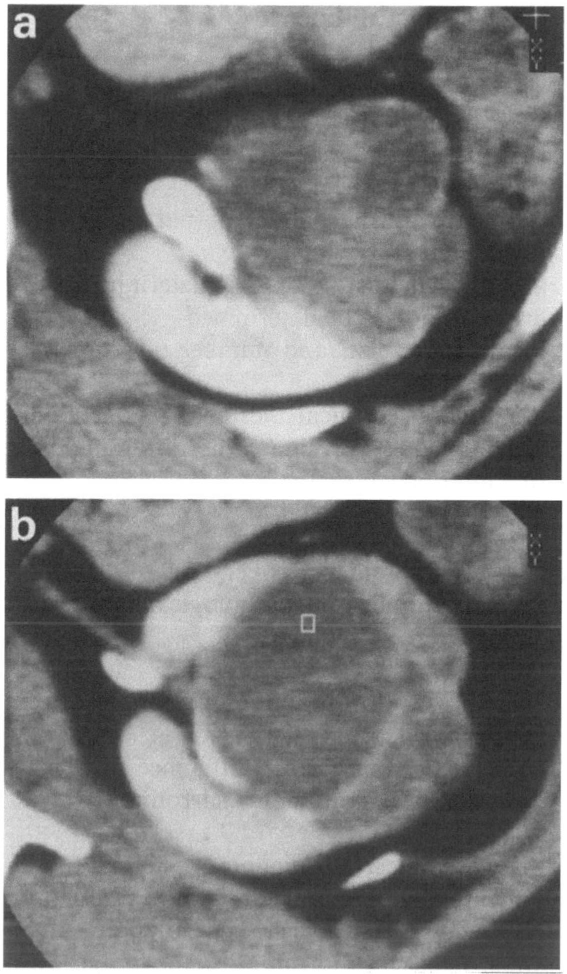

Fig. 4 a, b. Presentation of a large renal mass of the left kidney with different zones of attenuation. There is obviously a thickened wall, demarcating the normal tissue from the tumorous area (**b**). The tumor itself is nonhomogeneous. The collecting system is compressed by its growth. Histology indicated a poorly vascularized renal cell carcinoma with necrosis

injected, the rapidity of injection, the cardiac status, and, most of all, the arterial perfusion of the kidney. Within seconds the venous compartments and the renal veins are being contrasted with a simultaneous visualization of the inferior vena cava. Within some minutes the pelvic structures and the proximal ureter are enhanced according to the further progress of the excretion phase. The normal attenuation of the kidney increases from 40 HU for the noncontrast scan to 100 HU for the postcontrast scan.

In cases of difficult discrimination of renal structures a fast sequential scan (dynamic scan) after application of contrast medium should be carried out. With modern CT equipment six images/min can be taken. Minimal differences of enhancement of the cortex can be observed and measured, which is useful in the detection of adenomas, small renal tumors, vascular lesions, and complicated cysts (Krahe 1985; Freitag et al. 1983).

On the other hand, in order to decide whether a tumorous lesion has surpassed the fascia and invaded the fatty tissue or even in the psoas muscle a *second look scan*, i.e., involving turning the patient into an oblique or lateral position, will be helpful. Additionally the possibilities of direct coronal scanning (Blümm 1983) are useful to obtain better information about the topographic situation of the retroperitoneum. Of course, MR possesses better technical devices to achieve these coronal sections and they normally are not necessary for a definite diagnosis.

3.4 CT Enhancement Values

According to our experience with the Somatom D 2 and the Somatom DR 3 Scanner there are quite definite enhancement values for the different types of tissue in the native scan and also with the application of contrast medium (Table 1). The CT absorption lies between 30–40 HU with Siemens SOMATOM D 2 and DR 3 or 20 HU for the G.E.-Scanner 9090, respectively.

Table 1. CT enhancement values

Noncontrast scan	
Parenchyma	30–40 HU
Renal pelvis	±0 HU
Fatty tissue	−20/−100 HU
Abscess	about 30 HU
Cysts	5 HU ± 5 to 15 HU <15 HU if from hemorrhage or infection
Postcontrast scan	
Parenchyma	100 HU (infusion)
Cortex and columns of Bertin	12 s (i.p. injection)
Medulla	60 s (injection)
Renal carcinoma	Mostly hypodense against normal tissue

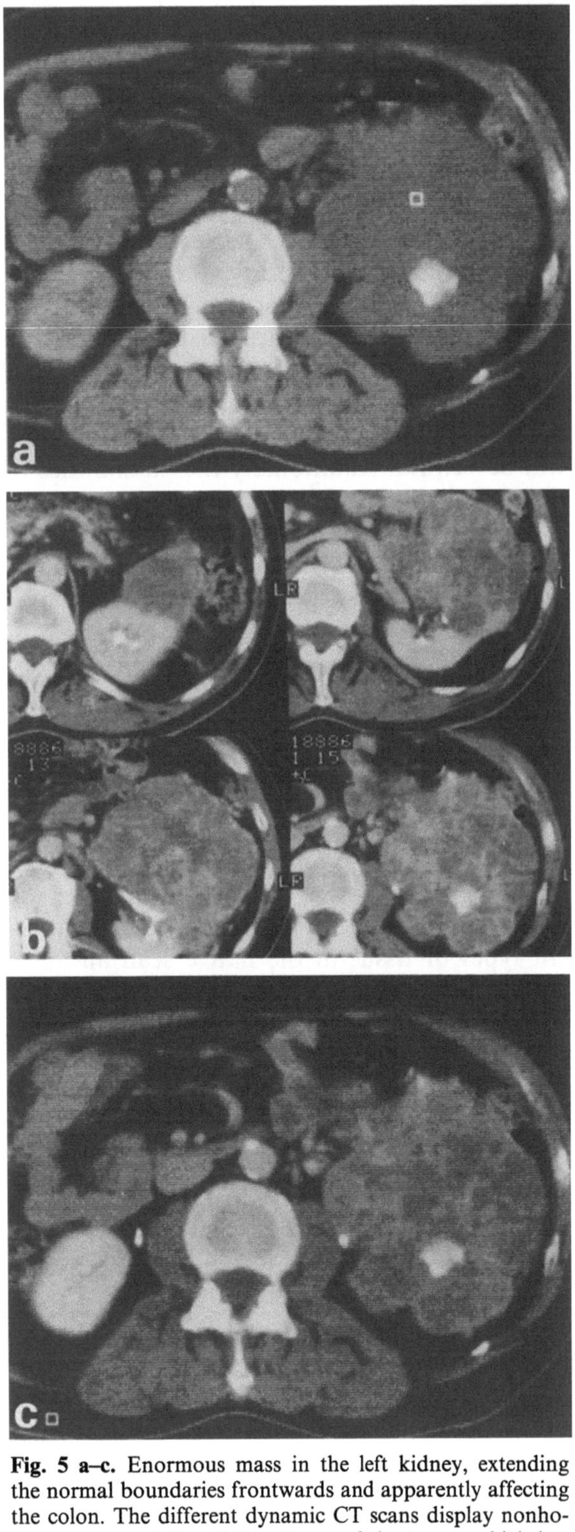

Fig. 5 a–c. Enormous mass in the left kidney, extending the normal boundaries frontwards and apparently affecting the colon. The different dynamic CT scans display nonhomogeneous and "cystic" patterns of the tumor which has invaded large parts of the kidney. The collecting system is compressed, the inferior part of the calyces is obstructed, and congestion can be seen. There is obviously not yet an obstruction of the renal vein. During operation it became clear that the tumor tissue had not invaded the transverse colon

3.5 Levels of Confidence

There is a high degree of confidence, if:

1. there is a totally normal renal parenchyma (following enhancement)
2. it is an obviously benign cyst (particularly following enhancement)
3. areas of calcification can be determined
4. areas of fat can be determined
5. localization, size, and number of lesions ascertainable
6. identifying "surgical" lesions; it is generally not efficient to evaluate the different kinds of "internal" disease.

The level of confidence is very low in determining abnormalities and pathological findings of the kidney, if:

1. there is no formation of a border or the border is distorted
2. there is no appreciable difference of density between the lesion and its surroundings

In cases of uncertain diagnosis one has to discuss many differential diagnostic modalities such as complicated cyst, e.g., adenoma, lymphoma, degenerating tumor, hemorrhage without tumor abscess, and inflammatory mass.

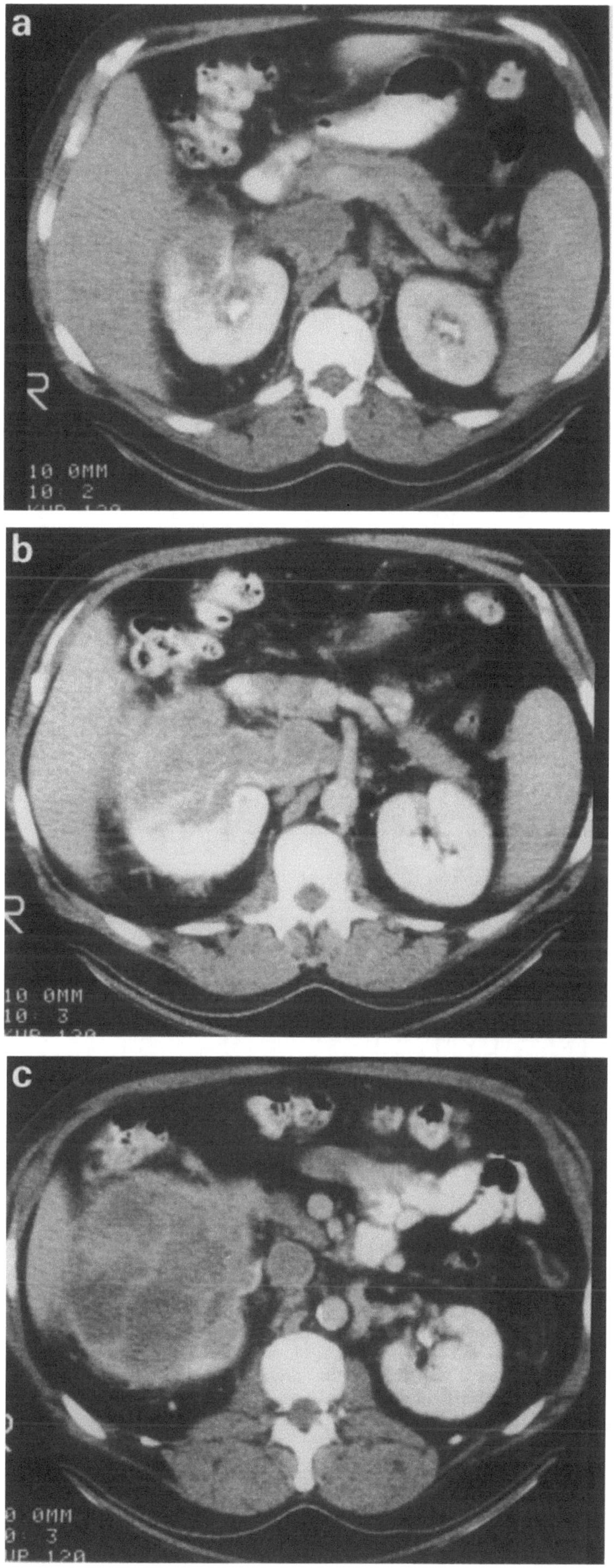

Fig. 6 a–c. Renal cell carcinoma stage III–IV of the right kidney with obstruction of the renal vein and the vena cava inferior. The different CT scans demonstrate the extension of a large tumor with irregular intratumorous patterns. The tumor has invaded the renal vein, as shown by the irregular hypodense shape of the vessel's contours. The shape of the vena cava is irregular. There is a small rim of enhancement, corresponding to the demarcation between the tumorous thrombus and the wall of the vessel (**c**)

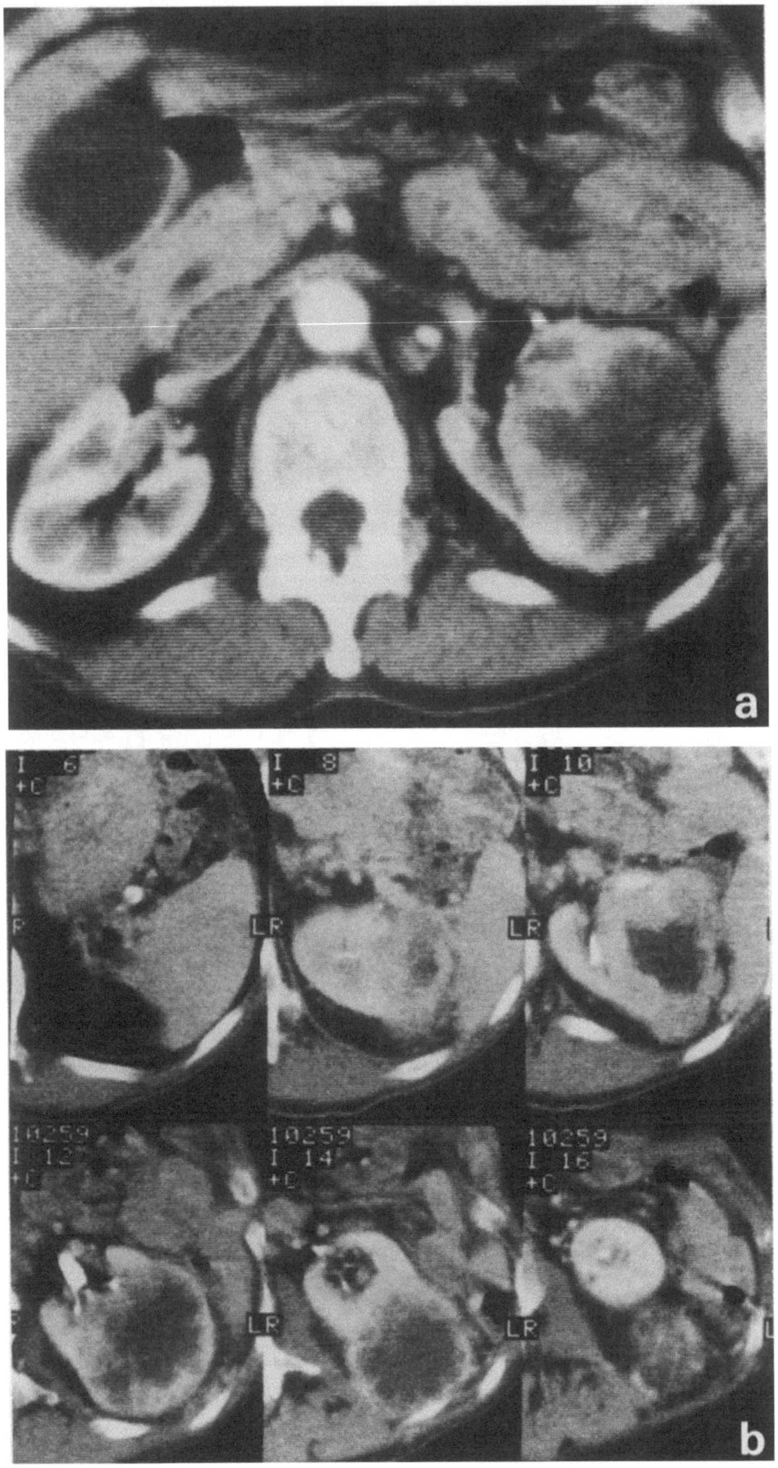

Fig. 7 a, b. Renal carcinoma stage III of the left kidney with thrombotic obstruction of the left renal vein and the vena cava. The left kidney is enlarged, and the boundaries are irregular, especially backwards. The tumor reaches to the retroperitoneal wall and encloses the area up to the spleen. After contrast, it becomes obvious that the renal vein is obstructed either by thrombus or tumor tissue, as is the vena cava, which is demarcated by peripheral contrast enhancement

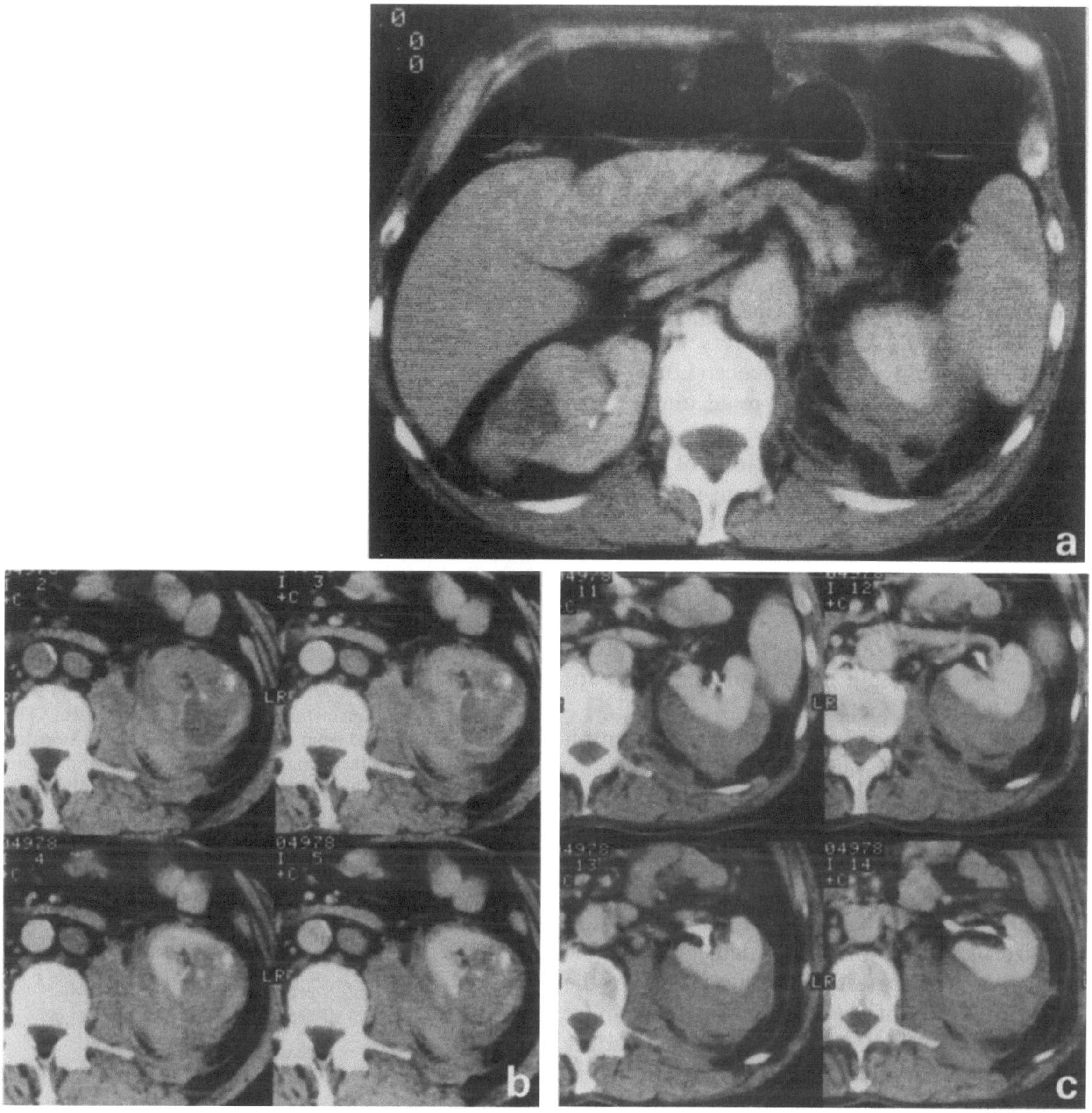

Fig. 8 a–c. Representation of one mass lesion in either kidney. *Left kidney* has sarcoma-mesenchymoma with perinephric blood assembly, while the *right kidney* has a carcinoma (**a**). The tumor of the left kidney has surpassed the renal capsula and has spread into the contiguous tissue (psoas muscle and fascia of Gerota). After enhancement there is a relatively good demarcation between the normal kidney and tumorous tissue, whilst in the more proximal slices there is a progressive destruction of the parenchyma and invasion of the collecting system. Hypodense areas can be distinguished and are due to focal necrosis (**b, c**). The mass tumor of the right kidney develops towards the liver, but can be distinguished from it. The dorsal fascia has been invaded at the point of junction with the anterior fascia. As far as can be seen there is no invasion by tumorous masses into the renal vein

4 Renal Carcinoma

4.1 Staging

The most frequent renal tumors in adults are renal cell carcinomas (so-called hypernephroma). These tumors are mostly vascularized and they possess "tumorous vessels" with arteriovenous shunts. Therefore, before the introduction of ultrasound and especially CT, renal mass lesions could be detected very well by angiography. In our own experience (Löhr 1979) the rate for the detection of renal tumors was about 96%.

We follow the classification of Robson (1968), who devised four different stages of tumor growth:

Stage I, the tumor is situated within the fibrous capsule
Stage II, the tumor has surpassed the fibrous capsule but has not invaded the capsule of Gerota
Stage III, the tumor has spread into the lymph nodes or vena cava
Stage IV, the tumor has spread into the surrounding organs and/or has distant metastases

The prognosis of renal neoplasms depends on the size of the tumors being detected, i.e., the stage and the progress of the neoplasm. In the follow-up study of Jaschke et al. (1982), more than 90% of the detected tumors were invading neighbouring organic structures. According to C. Ney and M. Friedenberg (1972) the prognosis of survival is defined for these stages (Table 2).

It becomes clear by this that there exists a close relationship between size and staging of renal tumors. Also age, sex histological grading, cytoplasmic content, extent of tumor spread into the renal vein or vena cava (i.e., the local extension), and especially the extent of invasion of the lymph nodes are important factors which are responsible for the future of the patient and the prognosis (Probst et al. 1982; Handel et al. 1983; McLennan and Lee 1983).

Ultrasound and CT are most excellent radiological instruments for the detection of renal tumors and their staging (Cronan et al. 1982; Pamilo et al. 1983; Heckemann et al. 1985). Therefore the possibility exists that renal neoplasms will generally be examined at an earlier stage than previously.

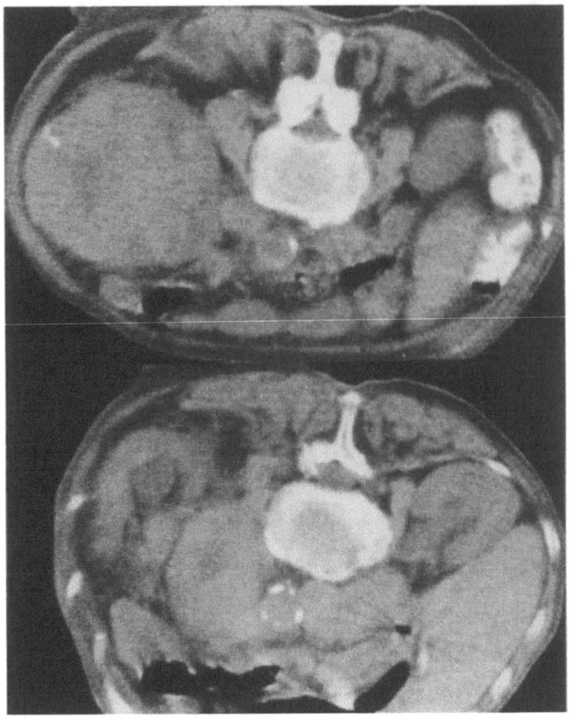

Fig. 9. Large mass of a renal carcinoma (*left kidney*) with focal lymph node metastases bilaterally to the aorta. The kidney is compressed from its medial contour and dislocated laterally. In the precontrast scan some calcifications can be distinguished. The vena cava is involved and obviously obstructed

Table 2. Prognosis of survival by stages

	Follow-up	%
Stage I	5-year	65
	10-year	56
Stage II	5-year	47
	10-year	20
Stage III	5-year	51
	10-year	37
Stage IV	5-year	8
	10-year	7

4.2 CT Findings

The detection of intrarenal tumors is sometimes difficult. Often the irregular shape of the con-

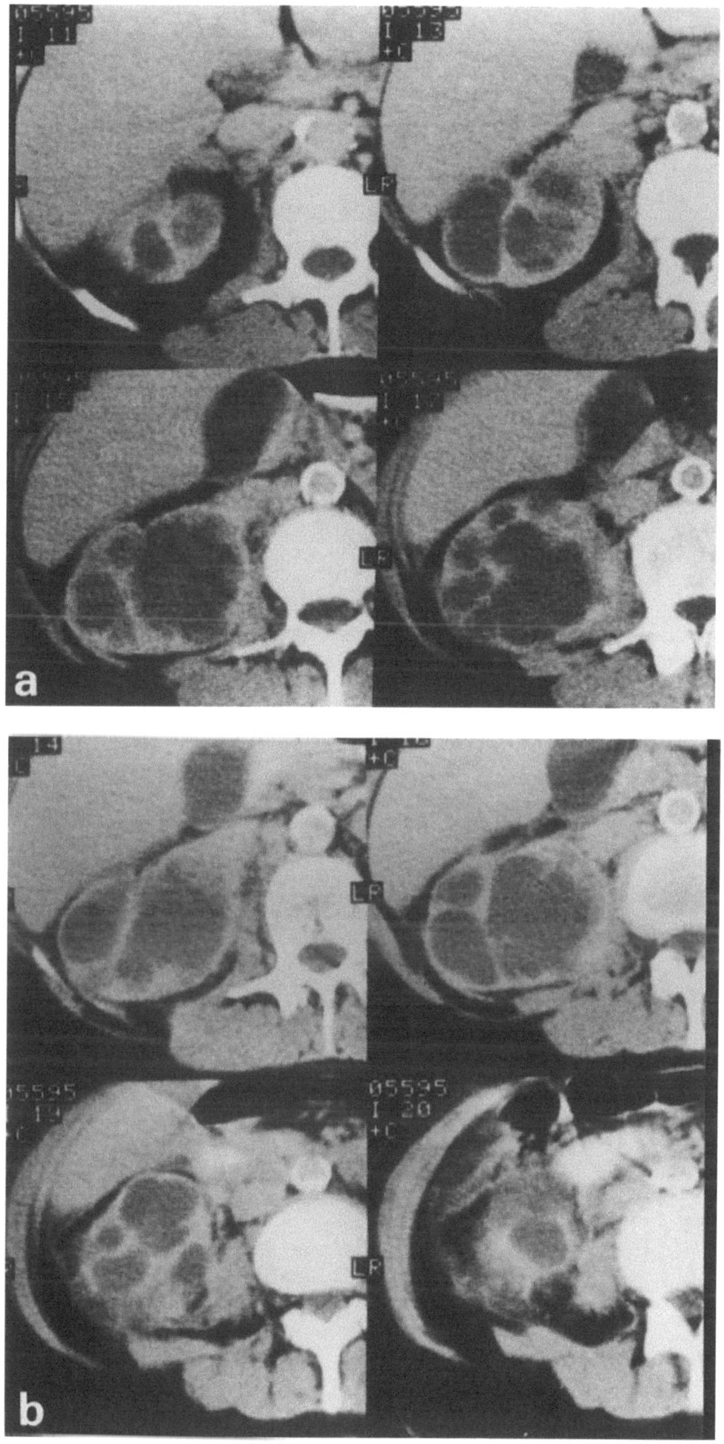

Fig. 10 a, b. Dynamic scans of a mass lesion of the right kidney with several confluent hypodense areas. The mass lesion has surpassed the posterior renal fascia and invaded the soft tissue. From the patient's history there were flank pain, chills, and fever, suggesting a pyonephrosis. After nephrectomy a renal carcinoma was found

ture is the first reliable sign of tumor growth. Sometimes there are central necroses or calcifications; both signs are of great value for further identification. The attenuation of the tumor is mostly isodense to the surrounding tissue (BAERT 1979). The values of the normal tissue will increase steadily with contrast enhancement, while the tumorous lesion remains hypodense. On the other hand a tumorous lesion may primarily have an increased enhancement towards the surrounding tissue, owing to hemorrhage into tumorous tissue.

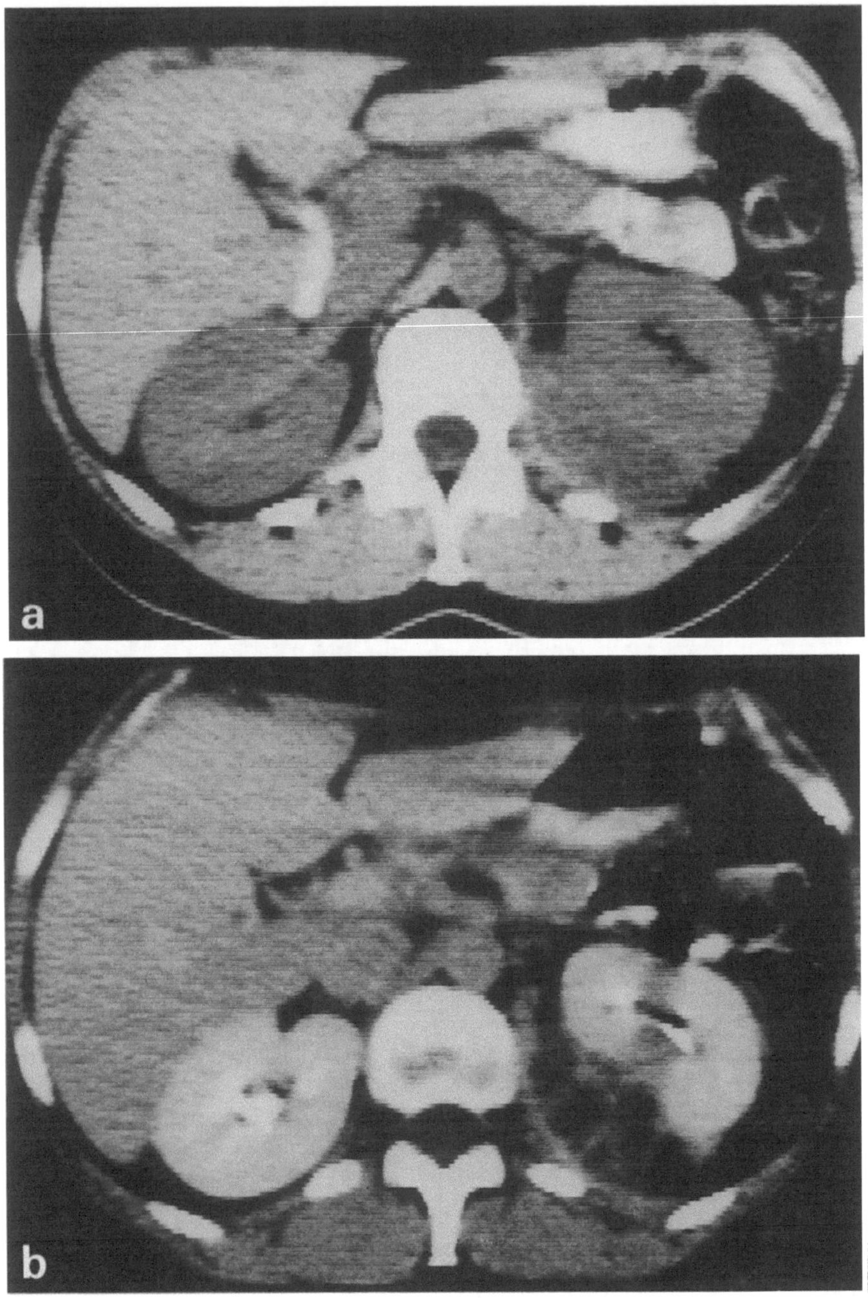

Fig. 11 a, b. Representation of the so-called cystic, poorly vascularized renal carcinoma (*left kidney*). The sections of CT scan reveal an indistinct delineation of the cortical region and a broad line of the invasion of the psoas muscle. After contrast application a scarce enhancement of this cystic lesion appears. The collecting system is compressed by the hypodense infiltrating tumor, which proved to be a cystic renal carcinoma (**b**)

After bolus injection this tumorous area will become isodense to the neighboring tissue. By this, it is obvious that in any case a CT examination has to be carried out before and after application of contrast medium. Calcification can occur with cysts and neoplasms as well (KIM et al. 1981). They are in any case suspicious. Renal calculi must be excluded. According to CANNON and ZANON (1976) and LARGIADER (1958) poorly vascularized tumors tend to calcification even if they primarily begin as "cysts". In such cases correlations between sonography and CT must be done. The "cyst" may be punctured, followed by a chemical and cytologic analysis of the punctate. If there are contraindications to puncture, a preoperative selective angiography in combination with electronical harmonization and magnification (LÖHR and MELLIN

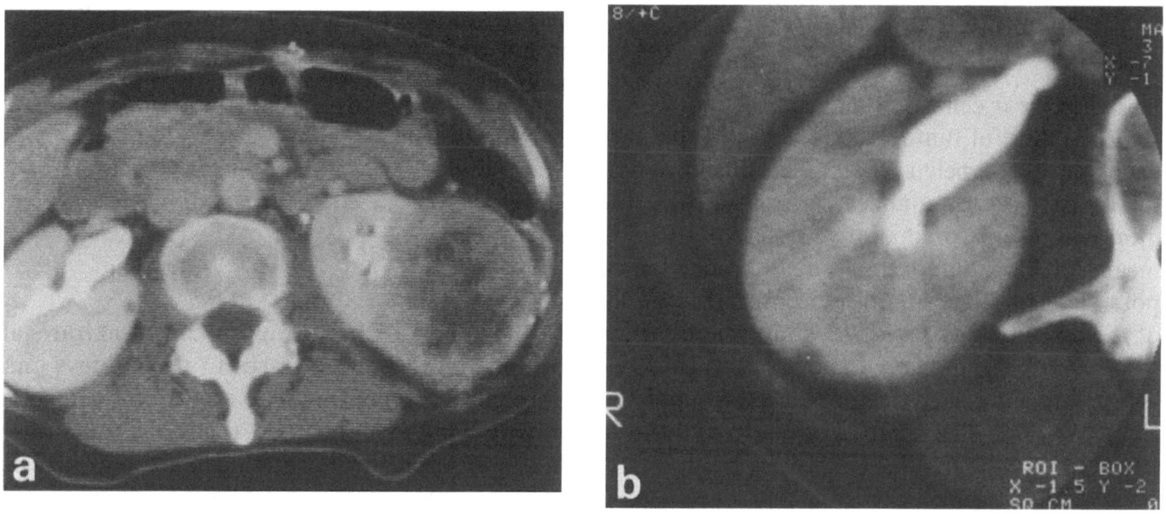

Fig. 12 a, b. Hypodense mass lesion with necrotic areas of the left kidney. The kidney is totally enlarged, while the border-lines are seemingly intact with the exception of the posterior portion. After enhancement there are irregular densities at the center and relatively good demarcation towards the normal tissue with signs of compression of the collecting system. In the right kidney there is another small "cystic" lesion at the cortex. Both lesions proved to be metastases of a vaginal tumor

1971, 1979) can lead to further progress in diagnosis. In certain cases renal angiography will be performed even if the tumor has already been diagnosed, for preoperative visualization of the renal vessels or for embolization therapy (LÖHR and ROSS 1985; LANG, this volume).

4.3 Tumor Spread

A mass lesion surpassing the borders of the normal kidney is easily detected on a CT scan. If i.v. urography is to be administered (and to examine the function of the contralateral kidney), we combine it with subtraction angiography (DSA). Thus, one bolus injection additional information can be obtained. At this state of tumorous growth further questions must be answered, e.g., spread to neighboring structures, blockade of large vessels, or dislocation.

4.4 Tumor Invading Vena Cava

Measuring tumor spread and metastatic growth into the renal vein and the inferior vena cava is of practical importance regarding operability. Tumorous cones can be distinguished by means of CT. At the level of the hilum the shape of the wall of the vena cava disappears; this is a reliable sign for intraluminal tumorous growth (HANDEL et al. 1983; PROBST et al. 1982). Today the operative aim is to perform an en bloc resection of the kidney with the middle segment of the vena cava.

To confirm the diagnosis of obstruction, cavography is preferred. This can be performed with intravenous DSA, applying the contrast medium by injection into the femoral vein. If the possibility exists to prolong the series, the arterial structures can also be visualized in the same examination (aorta, renal vessels).

5 Clear Cell Carcinoma

So-called clear cell carcinomas of the kidney are a special kind of tumor development of the parenchyma of the pelvis (see LEDER, this volume). In comparison to renal cell carcinoma these tumors are rare. A preoperative differentiation by means of CT and contrast enhancement is not possible. The same situation occurs with tumors of the collecting system, which are usually transitional cell carcinomas. In some cases they develop into so-called clear cell carcinomas; the differentiation between a transitional cell carcinoma and a clear cell carcinoma cannot be achieved neither by CT or ultrasound.

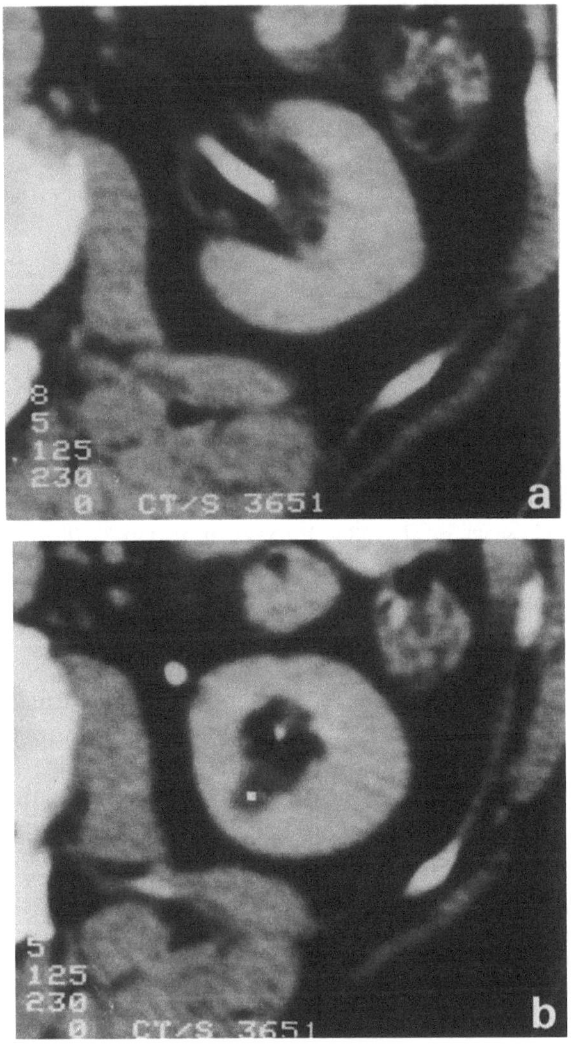

Fig. 13 a, b. Postcontrast scan of the left kidney, demonstrating a hypodense mass lesion of the corticomedullary zone, which reaches to the pelvis. At the border of the pelvis there are irregular structures. The collecting system is partly compressed. At operation a clear cell carcinoma of the left kidney was revealed

6 Metastases Simulating Primary Renal Carcinoma

In the course of tumorous spread of extrarenal primary tumors, metastases in the kidneys and adrenals are common. The metastatic spread is mostly hematogenous and therefore sometimes bilateral; multifocal growth can also occur. The most common metastases derive from small cellular bronchial carcinomas. The invasion of tumorous tissue from paravertebral tumors or metastases can be observed, and it is not so unusual for metastatic growth from the lymph nodes to surpass anatomical borders and invade the kidney. On the other hand tumors of the pancreas invade the kidneys very seldom.

The clinical symptoms are dependent on the localization, local irritation, and velocity of metastatic growth. So all clinical signs may be quite variable and are not specific. Like primary renal tumors the detection of metastases may be incidental or deduced because of their clinical symptoms (MITNICK et al. 1985; PAGANI 1983).

Ultrasound examinations and CT images of metastases may be similar to those of renal cell carcinoma. If the primary tumor is highly vascularized, metastases of it will show similar hypervascularized patterns.

7 Malignant Tumors of Different Histologic Pattern

The renal and adrenal perinatal tumors are being discussed in other chapters. The detection of those malignant processes follows identical procedures. Most of these primary tumors are sarcomatous such as *angiopericytomas* and *leiomyosarcomas*. *Angiopericytomas* develop from the vessel's wall and therefore they are very often highly vascularized. Their detection is easily accomplished by angiography. With CT examination the enhancement is remarkable. But preoperative detection may not lead to a more precise diagnosis as "malignant tumor". This can only be correctly done by histological examination. *Leiomyosarcomas* may develop at any site of organic structures containing smooth musculature. Therefore the localisation of those tumors does not follow a specific pattern.

The tumorous structures of an *oncocytoma* are rather dense; they possess a central scar. Differentiation between oncocytoma and renal cell carcinoma is not possible by means of CT (Cohan et al. 1984; Levine et al. 1983).

The development and intrarenal localization of an extramedullary *plasmocytoma* are very rare. The clinically unsuspected renal mass of a patient who 18 months previously had presented with a solitary plasmocytoma of the bone was diagnosed by CT (Twomey and Katz 1983).

8 Benign Tumors

Benign tumors of the kidney and pelvis are very rare. They comprise *cysts, lipomas, angiomyolipomas,* and angiomas. These benign tumors must be separated from so-called pseudotumors (see below) which are mostly inflammatory mass lesions and anatomical variants.

Most frequently *cysts*, as solitary lesions, can be found in all anatomical structures of the cortex. Single cysts develop during life, whilst polycystic degeneration depends on hereditary defects. Multicystic degeneration will always be found bilaterally with cystic lesions of various diameters.

A cystic lesion can be diagnosed during i.v. urography if the local mass is augmented by a stretching, dislocation, or compression of the calices or pelvic structures. We know from experience that by i.v. urography alone the differentiation between cyst and tumor is impossible. Instead, ultrasound possesses a better validity which only will be surpassed by CT. The diagnostic procedures typical for ultrasound are discussed in a previous chapter (Heckemann, this volume).

The CT characteristics for cysts are well defined: hypodense areas contrasted with normal tissue of higher density. The mean values for cystic lesions lie between 5 and 20 HU. After contrast the neighboring tissue enhances, while cysts show an additional enhancement that is very low, sometimes completely lacking. This finding commonly concerns peripheral cysts. The diagnosis "cyst" becomes more difficult if some are found with a higher enhancement, even after contrast. Such "complicated cysts" have to undergo further investigation.

Hemorrhages into normal cysts may occur at any time (Dunnick et al. 1984), transforming it into a "complicated cystic mass lesion." The CT values then may attain 40 HU or more. Further CT examinations, and especially ultrasonography in combination with puncture, are necessary for histological differentiation and improvement.

The cystic puncture and evaluation of the cyst will give clear evidence whether it is a hypodense and hypovascular cystic tumorous lesion.

A local infarction with subsequent necrosis must be considered, as it presents similar images. Here ultrasonography may be helpful and also angiography, if ultrasonography and CT alone do not lead to a convincing diagnosis.

8.1 Lipomas

The best procedure for detecting lipomas and angiolipomas is done sequentially by ultrasound and CT. Urography is here of not so great value, it will only demonstrate a possible mass dislocation. The criteria for ultrasound are listed in Chapt. 2. Lipomas may be examined by low levels of enhancement, commonly lying about 40 HU. After contrast no considerable change is obvious.

8.2 Angiomyolipomas

This is a hereditary disease belonging to the phakomatoses. Angiomyolipomas are rare. Klumair found 3 in 8500 CT examinations. Angiomyolipomas grow slowly and steadily. The mass lesion can be observed very often in i.v. urography by the central displacement of the pelvis and calices. Just like fat, the angiomatous portion after contrast influences the enhancement by increasing density values (Hantelmann 1981; Hochhauser et al. 1983). Distinction is possible with angiography by which hypervascularized areas can be noted. Also angiomyolipomas can occur bilaterally.

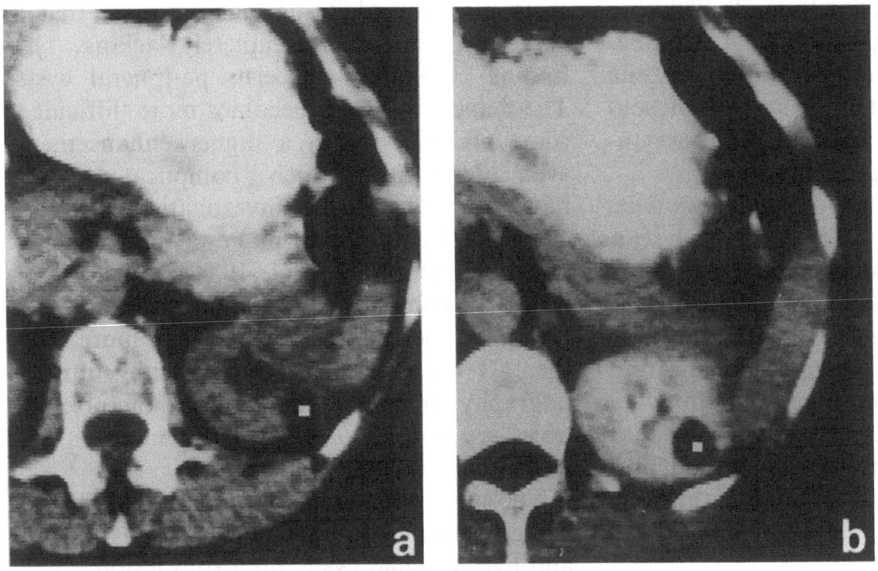

Fig. 14 a, b. Pre- and post-contrast scan of a "cystic" mass lesion of the left kidney with a low density ranging to −100 HU. After contrast there is a relatively sharp demarcation with the normal kidney. This lesion proved to be a lipoma

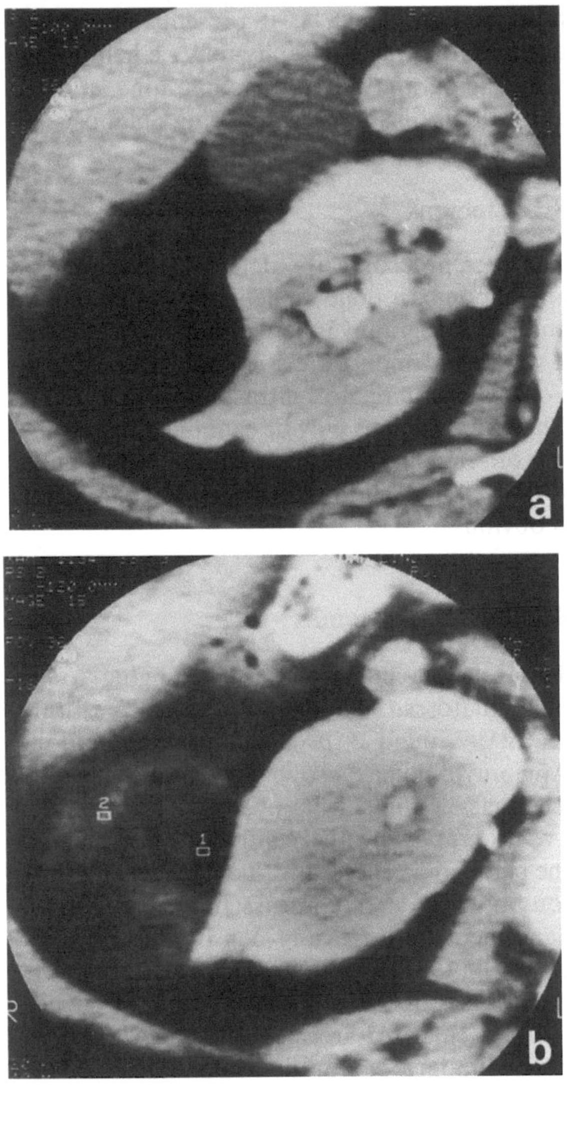

Fig. 15 a, b. Postcontrast scan of the right kidney of a 47-year-old female. A mass lesion is represented, which has relatively sharp boundaries with the well-enhanced kidney. Within this lesion there are different areas with different amounts of attenuation (see ROI)
At operation an angiomyolipoma was found. This finding is typical because this benign tumor contains both fatty and vascular compartments (**a**). In addition there is hyperplasia of the right adrenal without any clinical symptoms (**b**)

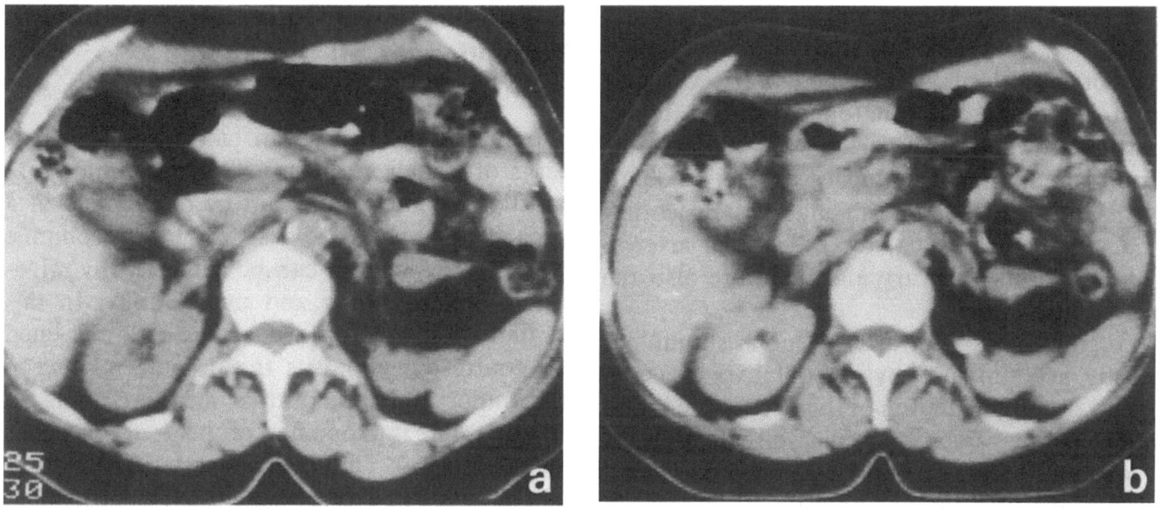

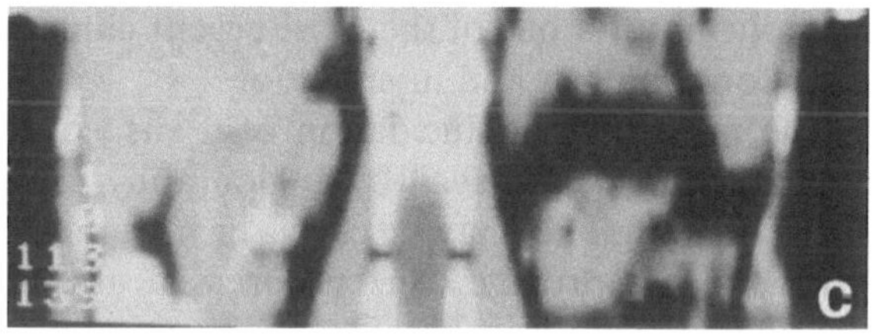

Fig. 16 a–c. Representation of a large hypodense mass lesion, separating the left kidney into two parts. After contrast enhancement the two parts of the kidney appear almost completely divided by a beltlike lesion which contains fat. This situation is demonstrated in the coronal scan. At operation an angiomyolipoma was found

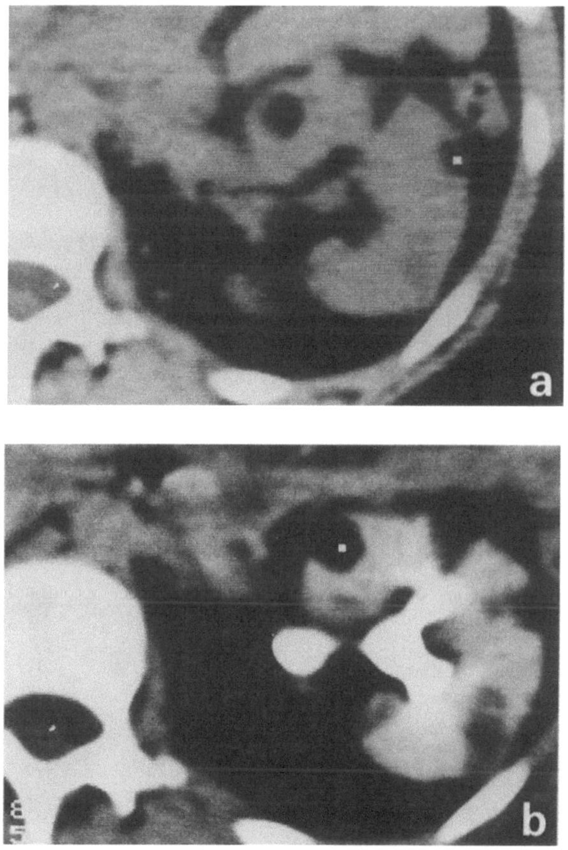

Fig. 17 a, b. Diffuse angiomyolipoma of the left kidney of a 35-year-old female. The several, mostly circular, partly cut lesions of the left kidney have a density of more than −40 HU on the pre- and postcontrast scan. This finding is a typical demonstration of multilocular, mostly bilateral angiomyolipoma

8.3 Angiomas, Aneurysms

Angiomas belong to the hereditary vascular malformations. The anatomical substrate, in particular whether the arterial or venous portion is predominant, influences various the patterns of torqued and irregular vessels (LÖHR et al. 1976). The proportion of vascular arteriovenous shunts will vary and therefore also the visualisation.

Angiomatosis with arteriovenous shunts are mostly accompanied by arterial hypertension, due to the augmentation of the circulating blood value. As in cerebral vascular disease there is a constant threat of hemorrhage from these malformations into the neighboring structures. In the kidneys the proximity of the tubuli makes macrohematuria one of the most urgent clinical signs for diagnosis and intervention.

The most certain elucidation of a suspected angioma can be achieved by angiography. The site of the angioma may be extra- or intrarenal. With CT hemorrhage can be observed as can the dilated renal vein because of the arteriovenous shunt.

In certain cases it will be possible to occlude an arteriovenous shunt by embolization.

9 Tumors of the Collecting System, Transitional Cell Carcinoma

Tumors of the pelvis can cause different patterns of visualization in CT. These tumors are mostly hypodense and can be overlooked in a precontrast scan. The best and most economic way of visualization can be achievied by retrograde ureterography and pyelography. In this examination the tumorous masses are framed by contrast medium as the boundary between the tumor and the contrast medium forms an irregular line in the lumen of the ureter or pelvis (KRIEDEMANN). The same characteristic features can be found in CT. After contrast enhancement the tumor's growth, centralized towards the pelvis and the upper ureter, will be become obvious in subsequent and overlapping CT scans. Here also the borderline between the contrasted ureter and tumor is irregular; the structures of the wall conceal the exact site where the tumor invades the centrally localised pelvis. In contrast to ureterography and sonography, CT possesses the ability to visualize the neighboring structures and artline the spread of the tumor.

According to BARON et al. (1982), GATEWOOD (1982), FUND et al. (1983), and BREATNACH et al. (1984) CT can be used for preoperative staging. One can distinguish between a focal intraluminal mass, ureteral wall thickening with

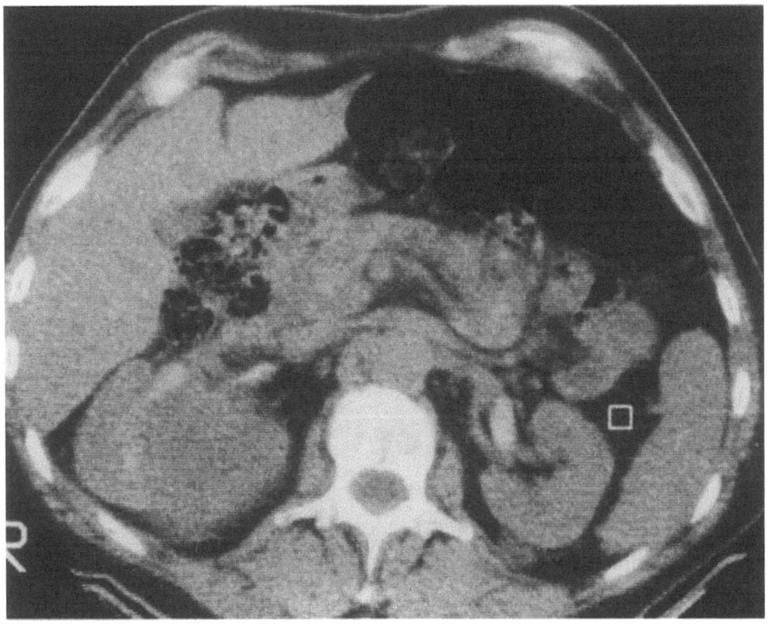

Fig. 18. Demonstration of a space-occupying complicated cyst with compression of the collecting system. In the postcontrast scan the density of the mass lesion was low. There is a surpassing of the posterior fascia and the delineation of the renal hilum is indistinct. At operation a renal cell carcinoma was revealed

Fig. 19 a–e. Ultrasonography (**a**), sequential CT scan (**b**), and selective renal angiography (**c–e**) of a 65-year-old patient with a "cystic" lesion of the right kidney, which had been known for 4 years. There were multiple pulmonary metastases which had led to a search for the primary tumor. In CT after contrast there is an increasing attenuation of the cystic lesion. Sonography shows the echo of a solid mass. In the angiograms the vessels are distorted and curved, but no "tumor vessels" are present. In the late parenchymal phase the round lesion can be distinguished emerging from the cortex. After operation the histologic examination revealed an oncocytoma. This tumor would not be responsible for the multiple pulmonary metastases

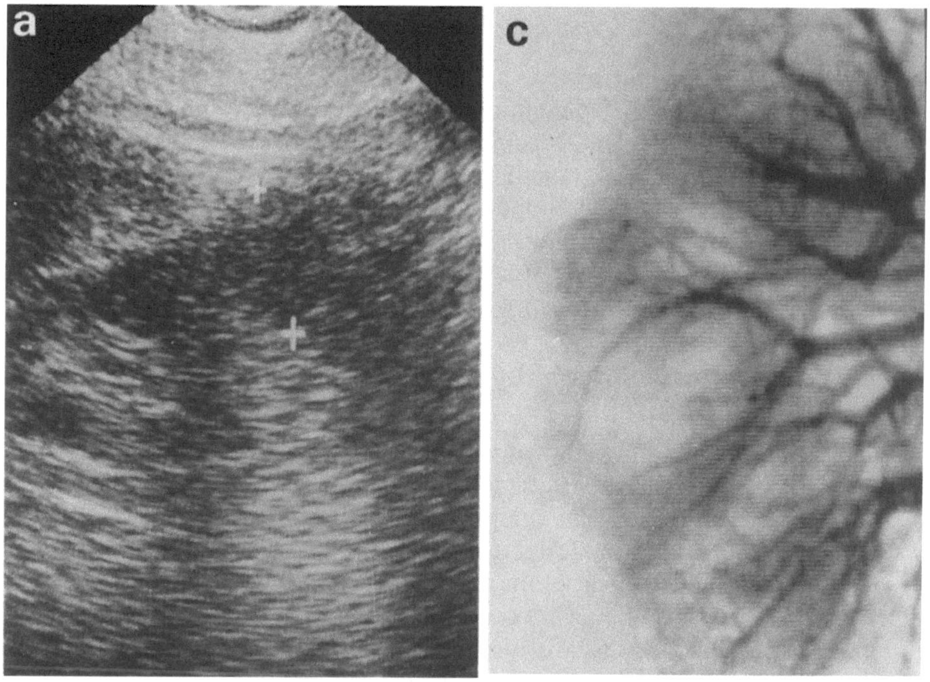

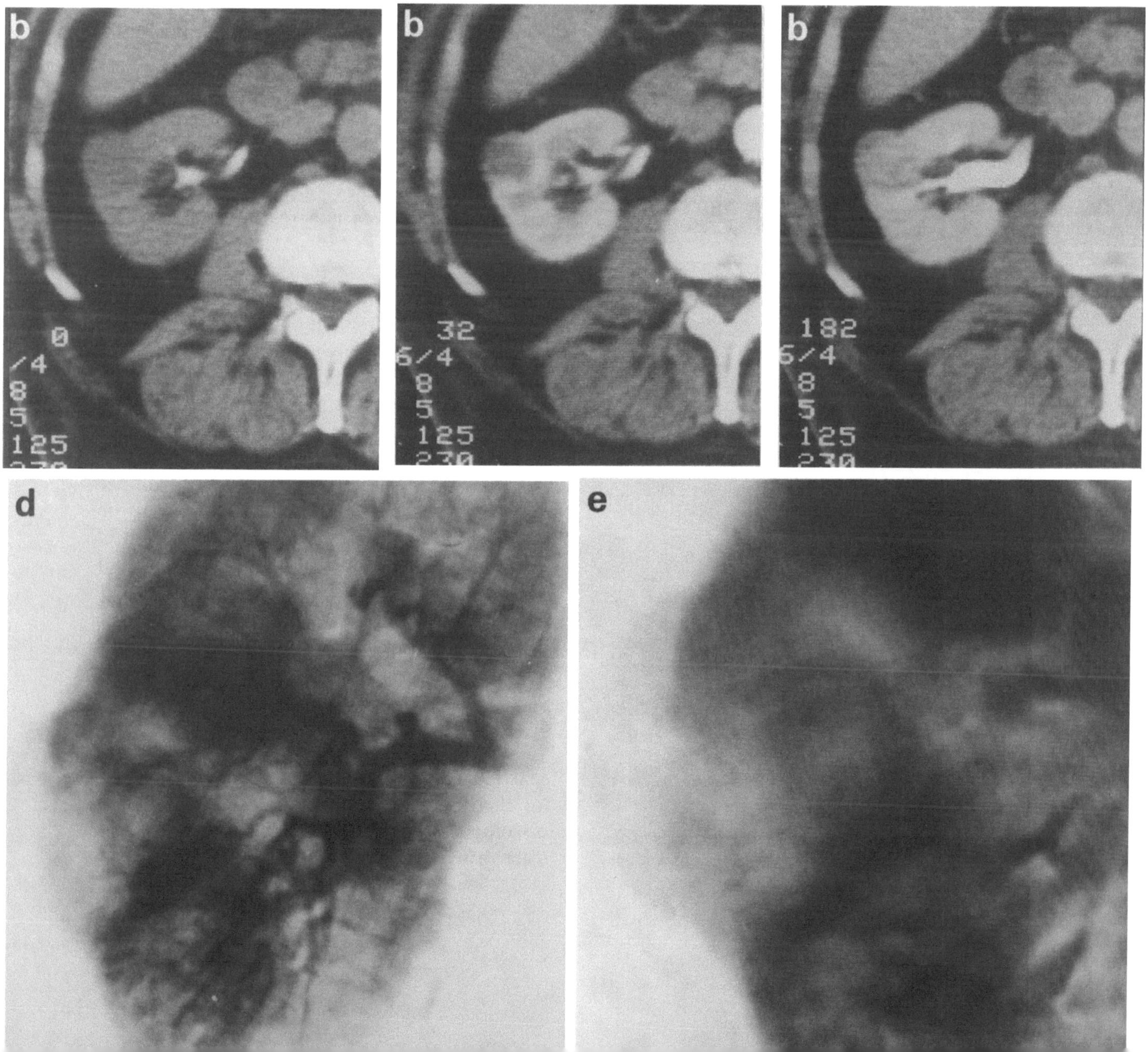

intraluminal narrowing, and infiltrating mass. In most cases the attenuation was similar to that of soft tissue. Of 21 tumors 1 was calcified. KRIEDEMANN et al. (1984) point out that in the detection and differentiation of pelvic tumors CT is superior to i.v. urography and angiography.

10 Retroperitoneal Lymphomas

Lymphomas of the retroperitoneal space came from quite different origins. In the course of primary illness of the lymphatic system (Hodgkin's disease, non-Hodgkin's disease, and leukemia) the assessment of the kidney is rare (KLOSE 1983; HORI 1983; CHILCOTE 1983; MCMILLIN et al. 1985). Metastatic lymphatic growth in the retroperitoneal space is mostly caused by tumors of the ovary and the testis (MITNICK et al. 1985).

With normal CT the paraaortal and paralumbar lymph nodes can hardly be observed. The normal size does not exceed a diameter of 1 cm. The visualization of large lymph nodes can be achieved by sonography and CT; CT communicates a better impression of tumorous and metastatic growth of the paraaortal lymph nodes, which can completely strangulate the vena cava and the aorta.

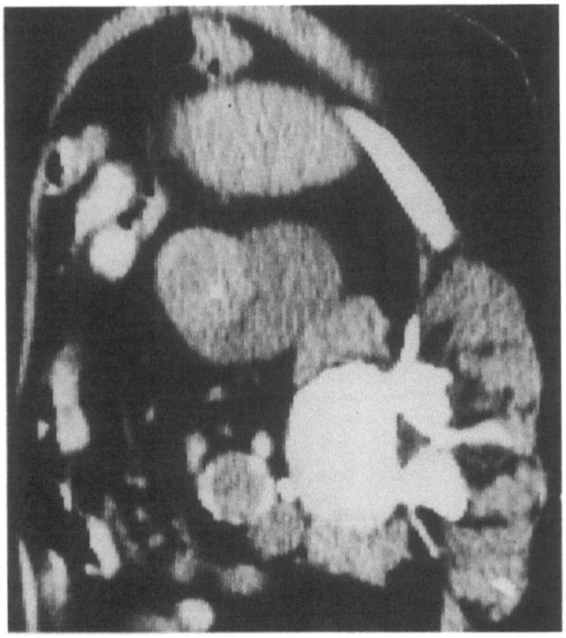

Fig. 20. Indefinite mass lesion of the left kidney with hypodensity in a precontrast scan. This lesion with a density of about 48 HU proved to be a lymphoma of the kidney

To obtain better details of the character of the lymphatic assessment additional lymphography is necessary. With CT it often becomes obvious that only parts of the lymph nodes are being opacified by the oily contrast medium during lymphography. Therefore sonography and especially CT are more certain to detect exclusion of retroperitoneal growth. This also includes metastatic disease from a renal tumor (see above).

11 Neuroblastoma and Nephroblastoma

Neuroblastoma is the commonest malignant tumor in children under the age of 4 years; more than half originate in the abdomen with two-thirds of those arising from the adrenal glands (SIEGEL 1983). When detected by CT (or at first by ultrasound), these lesions are generally large, dislocating the kidney back- and downwards. Almost always there is a relationship with the vertebral column (PERETZ et al. 1985).

The density of these tumors is low; calcifications are found in about 80% (KUHN and BERGER 1980). After enhancement the density remains low, and only a ring appearance will be found very often. An invasion of the stomach and liver is one of the main complications and is usually incurable. The nephroblastoma (Wilms' tumor) originates from the kidney. It possesses a reduced attenuation which will persist in the postcontrast scan. Calcifications occur, as do necrotic areas which are more central. The tumor, emerging from the kidney, will always compress the collecting system. The interface with the normally enhanced parenchyma of the kidney is indistinct. Very often a tumorous spread towards the liver and an occlusion of the vena cava will be observed (COUANET et al. 1982; FISHMAN et al. 1983).

Although a nephroblastoma is rather radiosensible, recurrences are observed. In our hospital there was a patient with a recurrence of a histologically proven nephroblastoma 25 years after primary treatment.

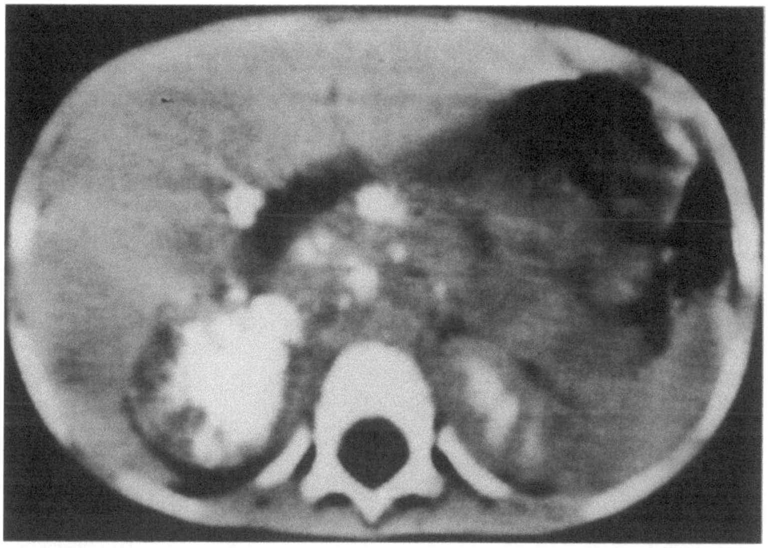

Fig. 21. CT scan of an extended neuroblastoma of a young child with multiple calcifications at the originating site, the portal, and the prevertebral region. The tumor extends to the pancreas. The aorta and vena cava are completely seized by the tumor. The kidney is dislocated backwards and compressed; a small rim of the cortex can be observed

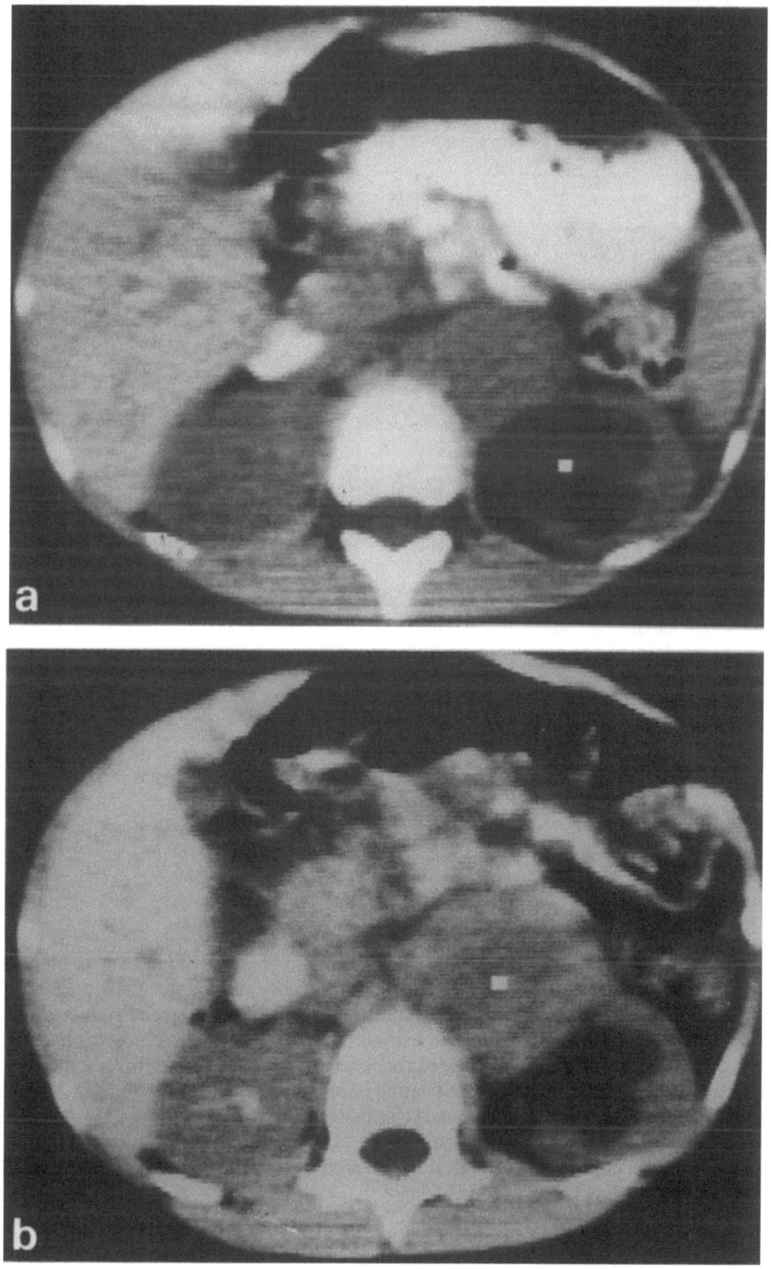

Fig. 22 a, b. Pre- and postcontrast scan of a neuroblastoma situated in the left paravertebral side. The primary isodense mass enhances after contrast application, whilst the left kidney remains hypodense. By tumorous compression the blood supply has been strangulated and a hydronephrosis is originating (**b**)

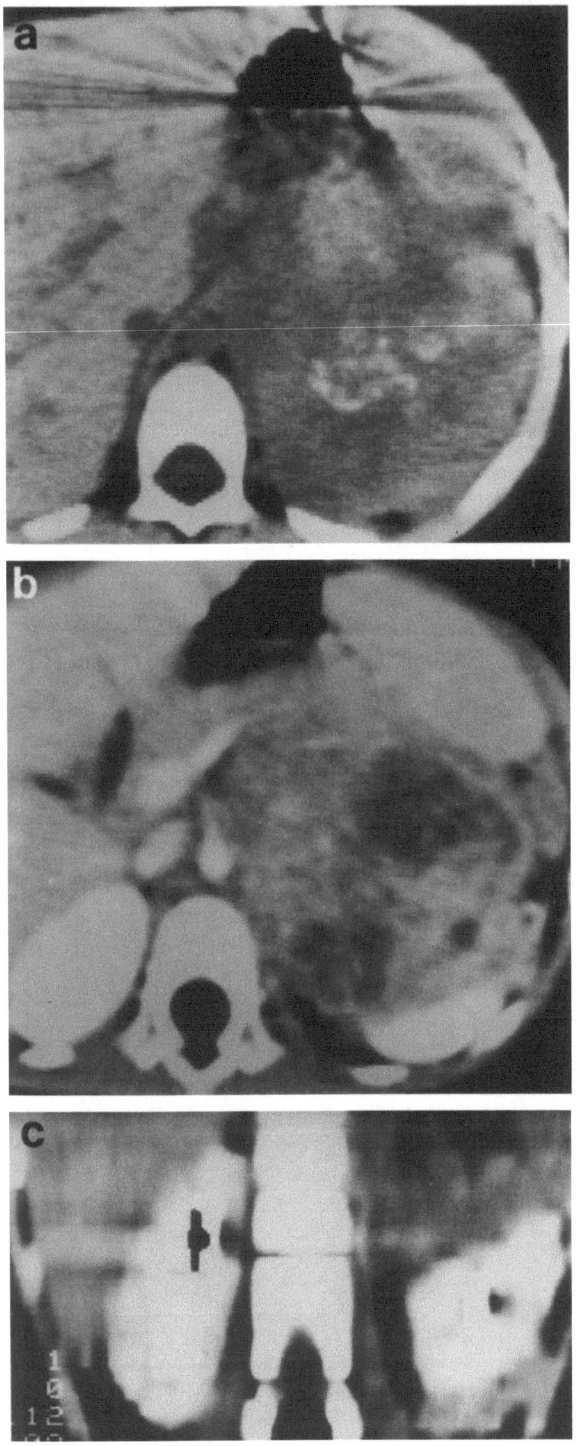

Fig. 23 a–c. Neuroblastoma of a 7-year-old child (pre- and postcontrast CT scan). The neurogenic tumor performs typically in the paravertebral region assessment (**a**). The left kidney is compressed and dislocated backwards (**b**) and downwards (**c**). Disseminated calcifications were found in three locations (**c**). In the postcontrast scan (**b**) a central, hypodense, irregularly defined area can be differentiated against a more enhanced cortical zone. It seems that the fascia of Gerota has been invaded

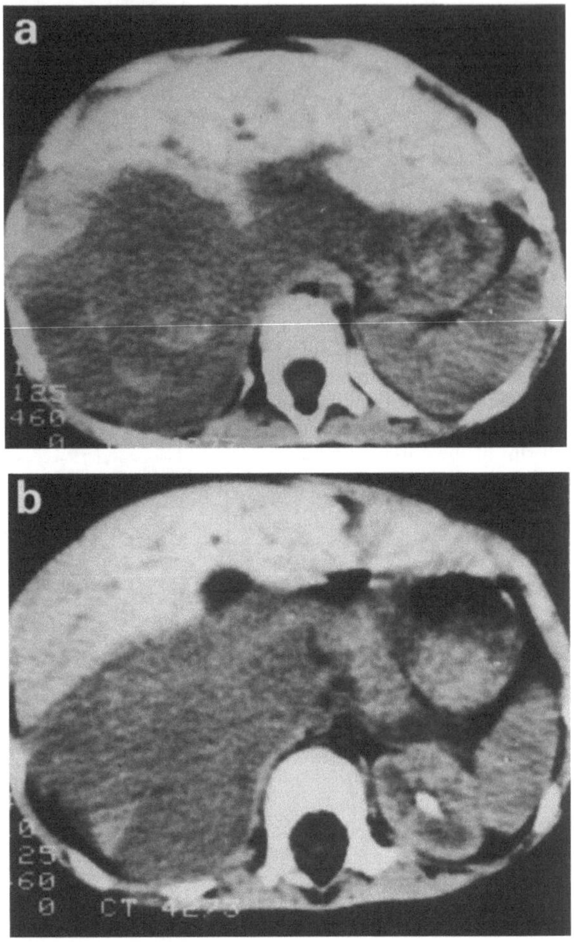

Fig. 24 a, b. Postcontrast scan of a large neuroblastoma, originating from the right paravertebral ganglia and invading the right lobe of the liver. By tumorous spread the aorta and the vena cava are being compressed; the structures of the pancreas cannot be delineated (**b**). In the precontrast scan calcifications can be observed inside the tumor (**a**)

Fig. 25 a–c. Nephroblastoma or Wilms' tumor of a 4-year-old girl. In the i.v. urogram there is presentation of an enlarged right kidney, whose borders cannot be defined. There is congestion of the collecting system and a distortion of the lower caliceal group; the proximal ureter is compressed also too (**a**). The CT examinations (**b, c**) represent a large tumorous mass emerging from the retroperitoneum towards the liver and compressing the right lobe. Parts of the collecting system can be observed (**c**); after contrast irregular "cystic" structures with calcifications become obvious ▶

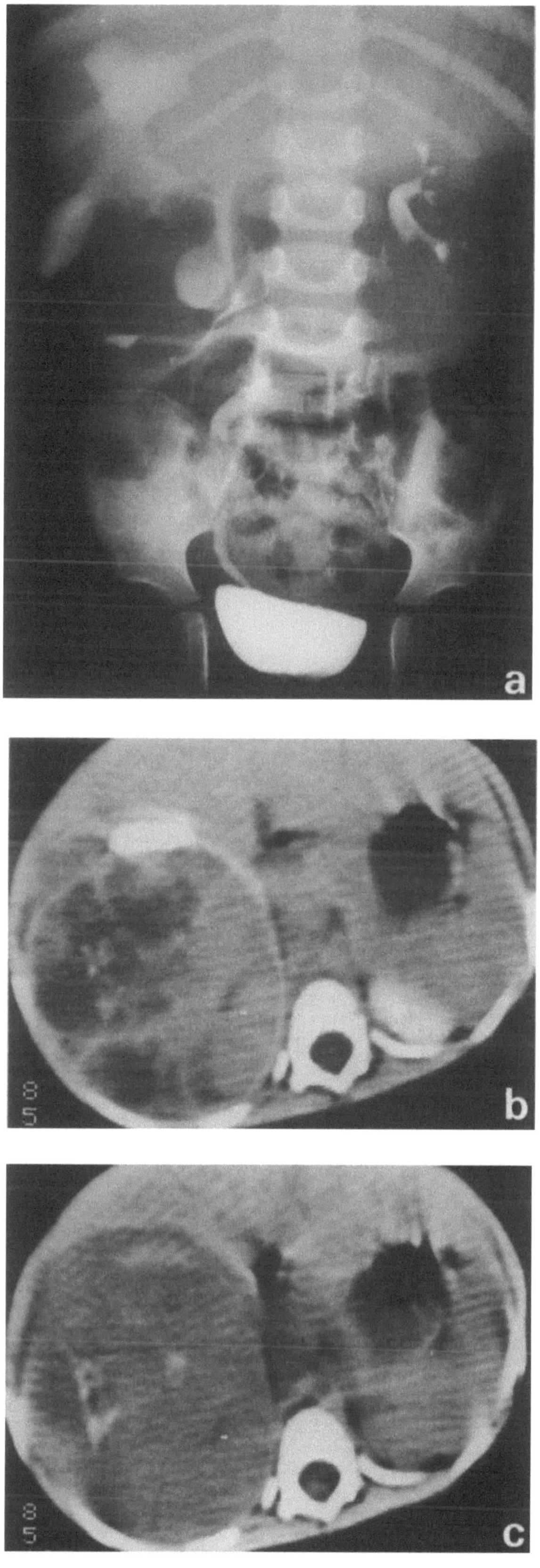

12 Differential Diagnostic Considerations: Pseudotumorous Mass Lesions vs Renal Tumor

In the detection of renal mass lesions spontaneous hemorrhage may pour into tumorous tissue, camouflaging any tumor growth. Comparative and sequential CT scans and also angiograms are necessary to ascertain the existence of tumorous growth or to exclude it. Vascular lesions (see above), recent infarction, and inflammatory disease (nephritis, carbuncle) must be excluded also.

12.1 Peri- and Paranephritic Abscesses

An acute *abscess* can be detected as a hypodense area in a noncontrast-enhanced CT scan. The kidney is enlarged by edema. After intravenous application of contrast medium a thickened wall around the mass lesion can be seen, contrasting with the normal enhanced tissue of the kidney which has compressed calices.

The inflammatory region may be restricted to the kidney or it can invade the surrounding areas. With abscess we will find necrosis and so-called air pockets in the capsula and paranephritic region, which are typical.

12.2 Xanthogranulomatous Nephritis

The clinical signs of xanthogranulomatous pyelonephritis (XGPN) are similar to those of acute bacterial nephritis or abscess with chills, flank pain, fever, and sometimes macrohematuria. Because of its frequent co-occurrence with diabetes, XGPN is often found bilaterally. Sections of sonography indicate poorly defined solid masses. On CT indeterminate masses are found with a swollen kidney and a frequent paranephritic extension. There are areas of high and low attenuation (McClennan and Lee 1983). Angiography indicates extended segmental vessels, but so-called pathological lacunae are missing. The correct diagnosis can be gained from clinical symptoms and bilateral assessment. Finally the diagnosis must be confirmed by operative exploration.

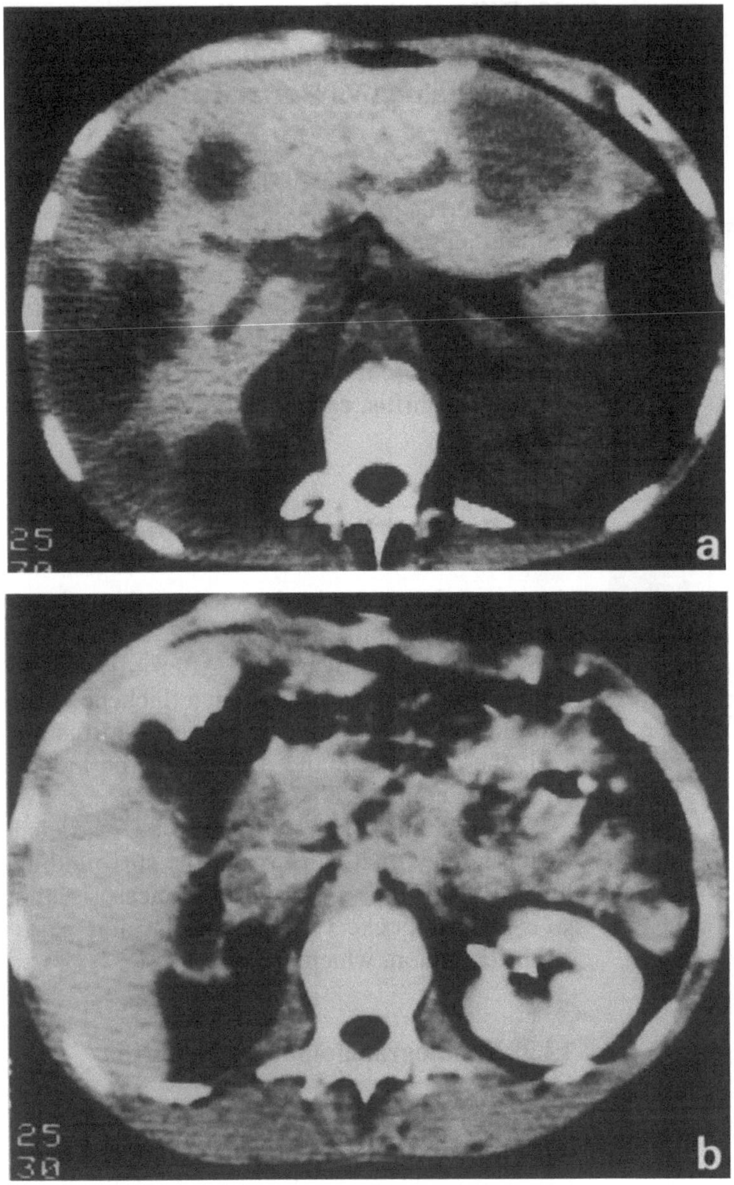

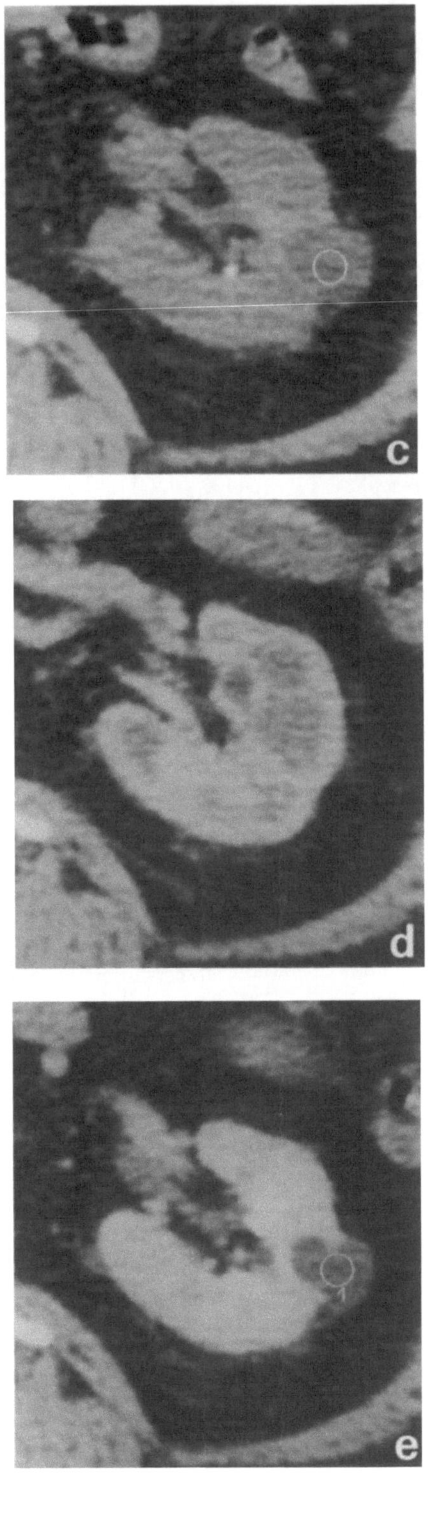

Fig. 26 a–e. Pre- (**a**) and post-contrast scans (**b**) of a 25-year-old patient with a recurrence of Wilms' tumor. Nephrectomy of the right kidney had been carried out in childhood. Now multiple metastases in the right and left lobe of the liver are delineated, whilst the left secondary kidney is obviously intact. Also the paravertebral and para-aortal lymph nodes seem to be unaffected

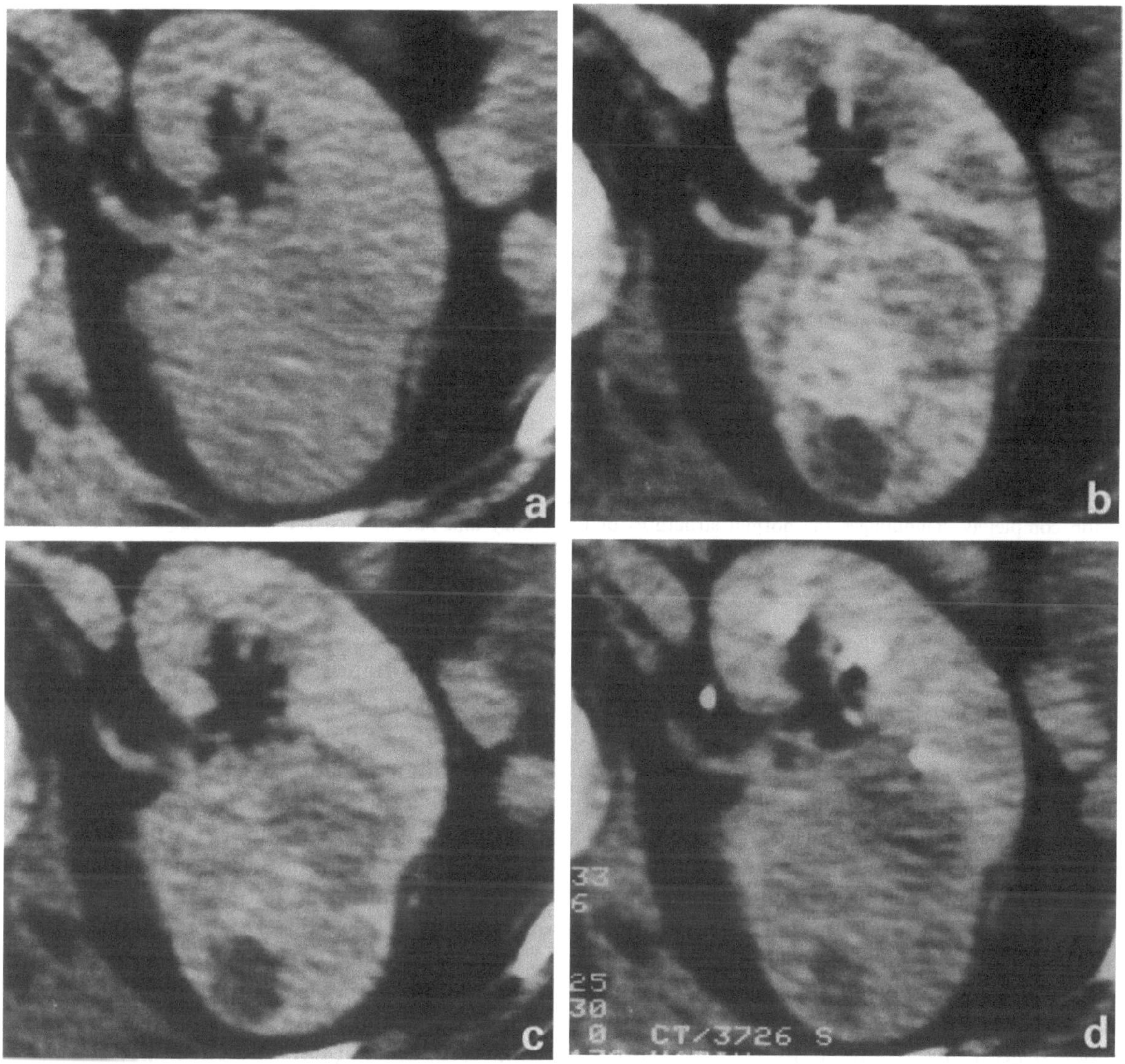

Fig. 27 a–d. Dynamic scan of a 59-year-old patient was sent to the hospital with the clinical symptoms of urosepsis (flank pain, chills, and fever). The first scans with and without low contrast (**a**, **b**) demonstrate a scarcely delineated hypodense mass lesion of the left kidney. The kidney is enlarged, but the posterior fascia is not actually surpassed. After contrast there is a steady increase of attenuation of the left kidney and an indistinct delineation to the lesion, which shows areas of different enhancement. At the dorsal portion an irregular cystic formation can be seen. The patient was operated on. The tumor proved to be a large carcinoma of the kidney with multiple necrosis

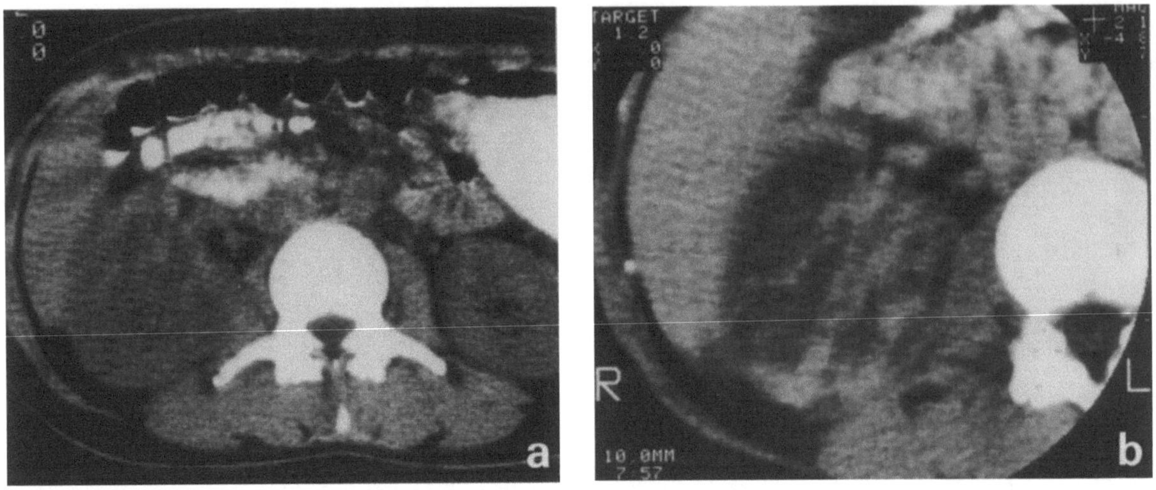

Fig. 28 a, b. Hypodense mass lesion of the right kidney, completely distorting the normal shape of the kidney. This lesion completely camouflages the normal structures of the kidney and has invaded the surroundings (liver, fascia of Gerota, and psoas muscle). After contrast (**b**) there are different zones of attenuation, partly with "cystic character." The lesion proved to be a septic renal abscess in a case of bacterial endocarditis

12.3 Hyperdense Cysts

One common, but sometimes very difficult, differentiation is that between the common cystic lesion and cystic hypernephroma. It must be stated that for the diagnosis of "cystic lesion" a noncontrast scan has to precede an examination with contrast enhancement, which should be carried out as a dynamic CT. If there is an attenuation of more than 40 HU every step must be taken to exclude malignant growth. A normal cyst can present higher attenuation when it contains an unusually large amount of protein due to a previous hemorrhage into it. Hyperdense cysts, even with an increasing enhancement after contrast, are therefore suspected suspicious of tumorous growth (Dunnick 1984).

12.4 Pseudotumors of Different Origin

Similar CT scan characteristics to those of renal mass lesions are found with patients under *treatment with anticoagulants*. In contrast to renal tumors the record of illness, particularly flank pain and fever, is commonly short. The patient's history with anticoagulation therapy must be recognized.

In cases of doubt still remaining after CT (pre- and postcontrast scan), renal angiography is necessary, and also for therapeutic embolisation. With one patient who developed macrohematuria in the course of anticoagulant therapy we successfully occluded the main renal vessel, and so the bleeding could be stopped. The primary CT diagnosis was doubtful.

In some cases a hypertrophied tail of the pancreas overlapping the left kidney imposes like a renal tumor (Moss et al. 1983). In order to perform a better differentiation ultrasonographic studies are required as well and CT sections in an oblique diameter (Marchal and Baert 1979).

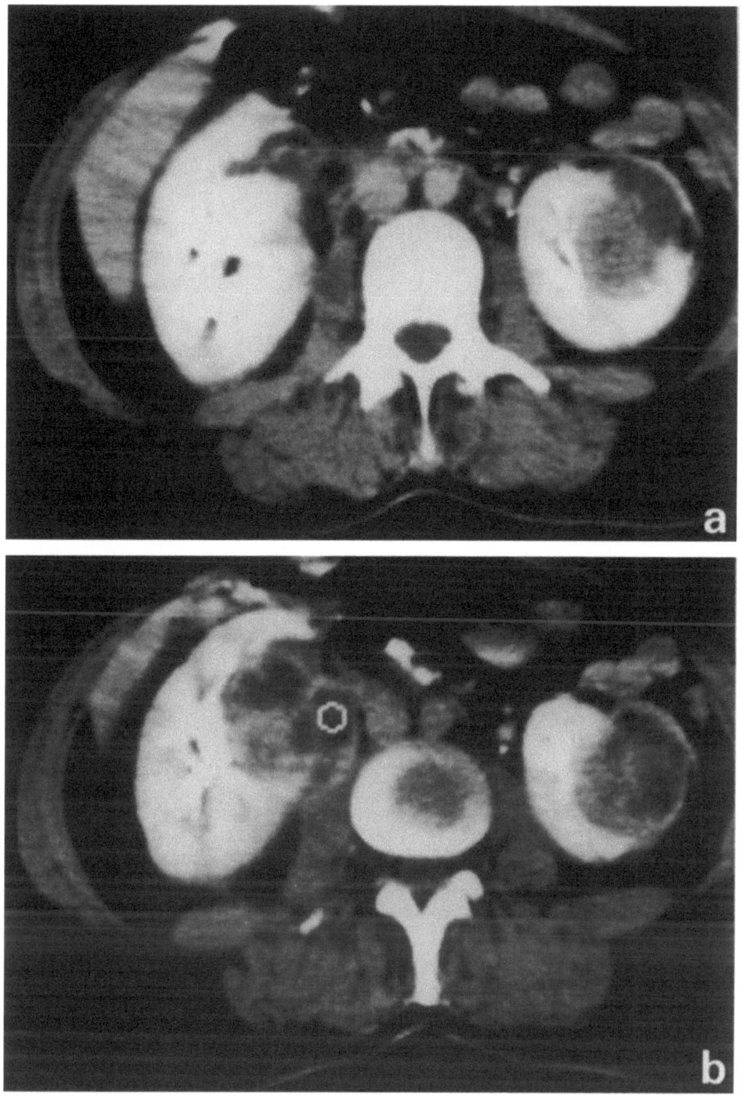

Fig. 29 a, b. Presentation of a bilateral, nonhomogeneous, partly cystic mass lesion in the kidneys of a 45-year-old patient. After application of contrast medium there is a good opacification of the intact renal parenchyma and a partly indefinite demarcation, especially in the right kidney. The normal structures are being invaded and surpassed, and the psoas muscle is partly infiltrated (**a, b**)

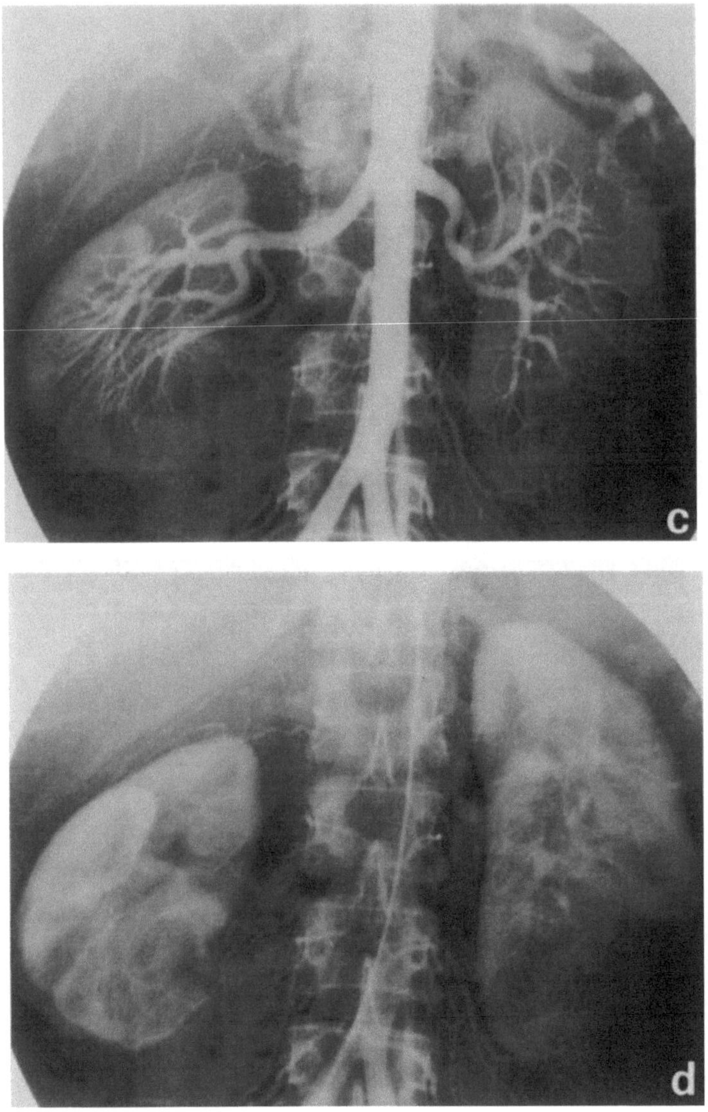

Fig. 29 c, d. A renal angiogram showed a distortion of the vessels, but no so-called pathological vessels (**c**, **d**) are present. At operation a perinephritic abscess on the background of a xanthogranulomatous nephritis was found. This finding is typical for this illness, which is usually bilateral and often found in patients with diabetes. (Fig. 29c, d by courtesy Professor Günther, University of Aachen)

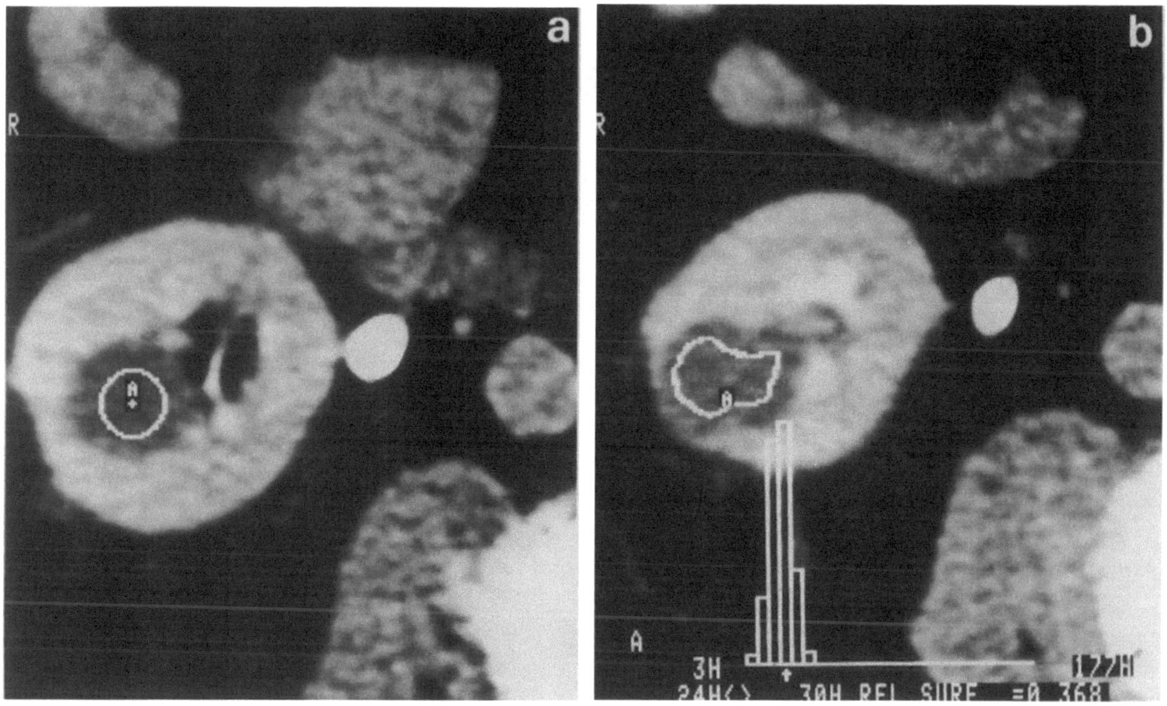

Fig. 30 a, b. Representation of a (mistakenly) supposed renal carcinoma of the right kidney. The patient had been examined only in this postcontrast scan and the examiner urgently expressed the diagnosis of a cystic tumor. The enhancement after contrast ranged up to 40 HU. The patient was operated on and nephrectomized. The histological diagnosis was a protein-containing cyst without any hints of neoplastic tissue (external examination)

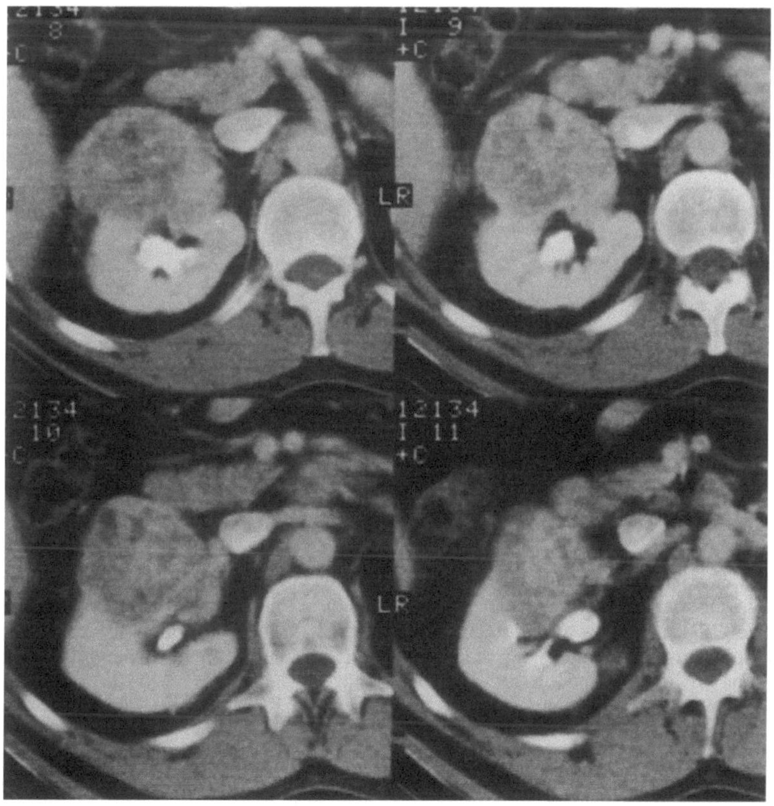

Fig. 31. Demonstration of a large intrarenal hemorrhage with blood enclosures and a relatively good delineation of the renal tissue. There are no actual signs of invasion of the neighboring tissue, although the kidney is being enlarged.
These particular items help to strengthen the diagnosis of a hemorrhage

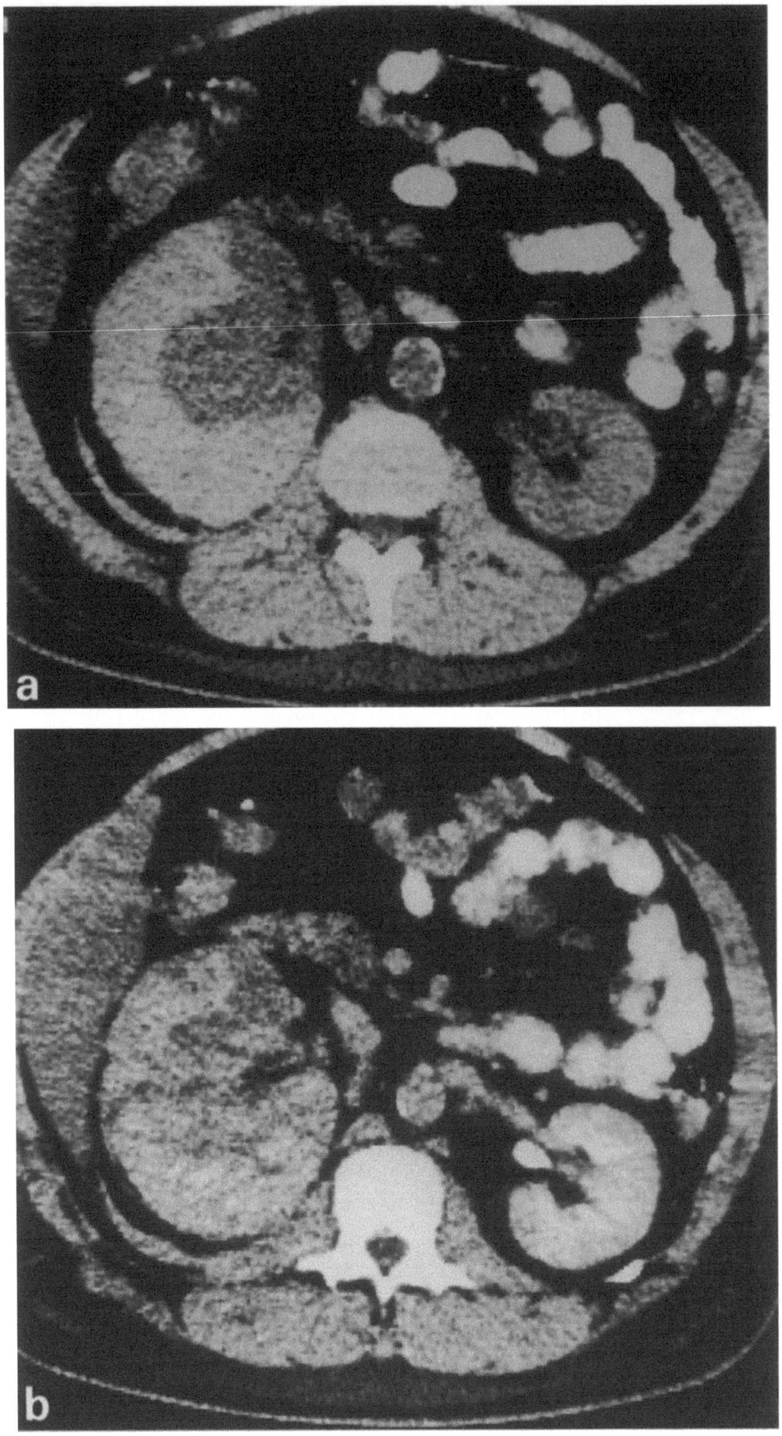

Fig. 32 a, b. Acute hemorrhage of the right kidney of a 54-year-old patient with mitral valve and coronary disease. Clinical symptoms were recurrent macrohematuria and flank pain. The patient was receiving anticoagulant therapy. The CT scan shows an enlargement of the right kidney, although the capsular boundaries are not being surpassed (**a**). After contrast enhancement there is a good differentiation of the hypodense coagulated blood and the normal renal tissue (**b**)

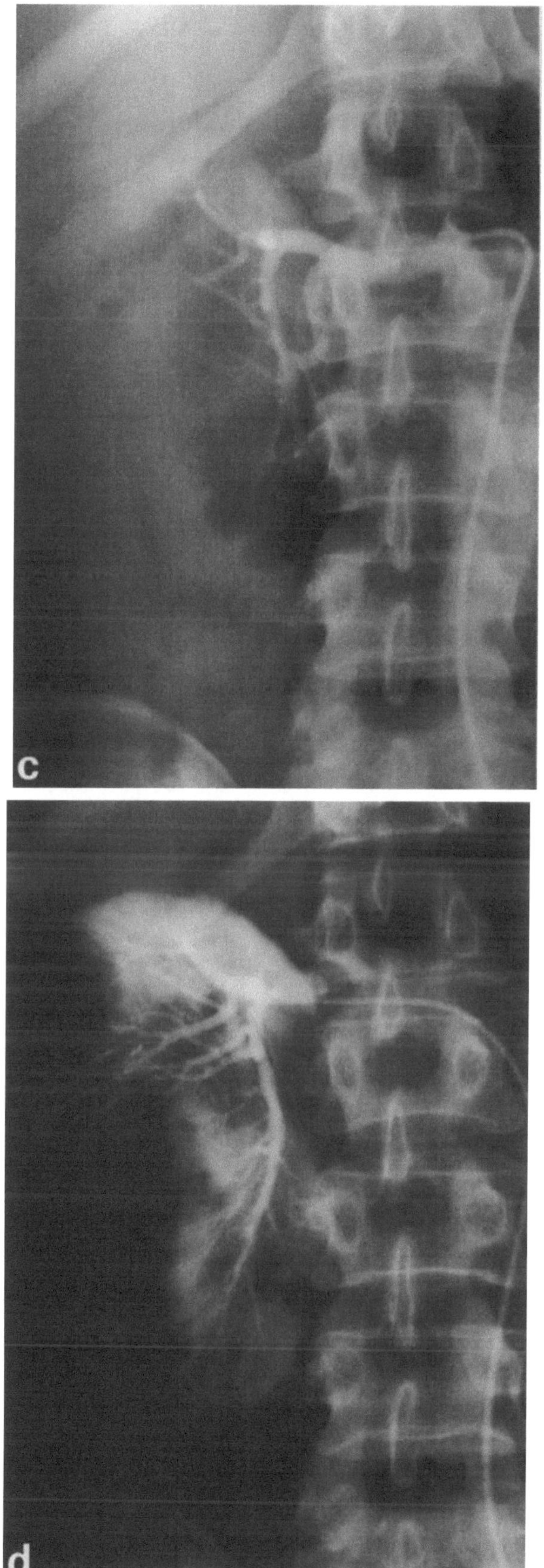

Fig. 32 c, d. A selective angiogram of the right kidney shows destruction of the intrarenal vessel and a large avascular zone reaching from the upper poleto the center of the kidney (**c**). This finding appears like an intrarenal hematoma. Occlusion of the right renal artery by means of Ethibloc applied via a balloon catheter stopped the bleeding (**d**)

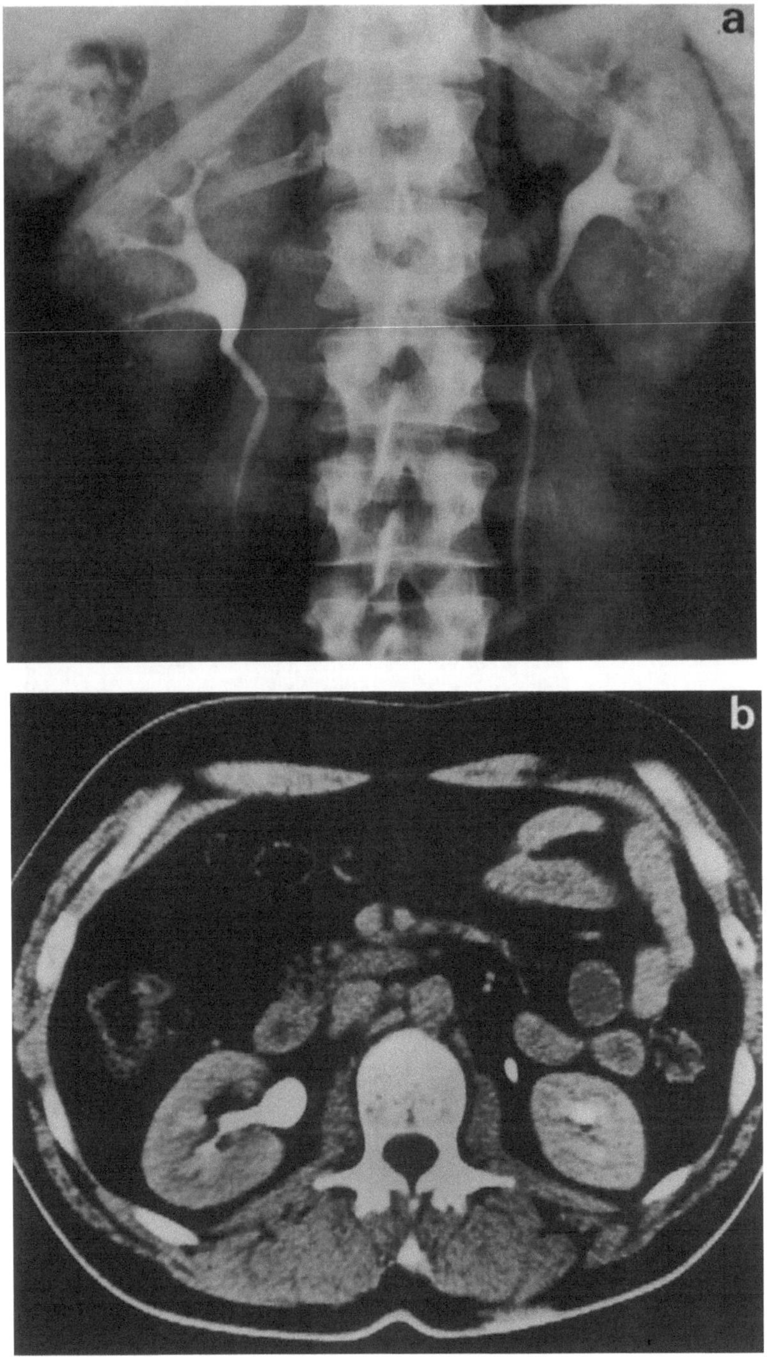

Fig. 33 a–c. Space-occupying lesion of the left kidney in a patient suffering from recurrent macrohematuria without flank pain and chills. In the i.v. urograph there is a distortion of the upper and medial caliceal group of the left kidney. There is an oval, well-delineated, hyperdense area which is partly compressing the upper caliceal group (**a**). The contrast CT reveals a distinct, localized, increased enhancement in the medullary zone, which reaches to the pelvic structures. The borders of the pelvis and of the parenchyma are not disrupted. The reason of the hemorrhage could be nephritis or a ruptured vessel (angioma?)

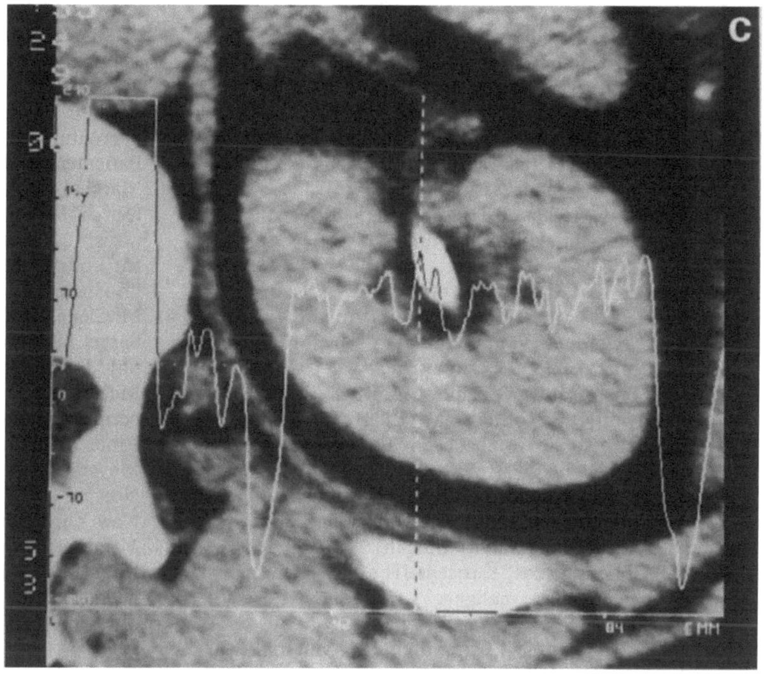

Fig. 33c

References

1. Baert A (1982) Computed Tomography and Digital Subtraction Angiography in the detection of renal tumors. Paper presented at the meeting of Deutsche Röntgengesellschaft Köln, Dec 2
2. Baron RL, McClennan BL, Lee JK, Lawson TL (1982) Computed tomography of transitional-cell carcinoma of the renal pelvis and ureter. Radiology 144(1):125–130
3. Blümm RG (1983) Direct intracranial sagittal and coronal CT scanning: anatomy and pathology. Amer J Neuroradiol 4:484
4. Brasch RC, Randel SB, Gould RG (1981) Follow-up of Wilms' tumor: comparison of CT with other imaging procedures. Amer J Radiol 137(5):1005–1009
5. Breatnach E, Stanley RJ, Carpenter JT Jr (1985) Intrarenal chloroma causing obstructive nephropathy: CT characteristics. J Comput Assist Tomogr 9(4):822–824
6. Breatnach, ES, Stanley RJ, Lloyd K (1984) Focal obstructive nephrogram: an unusual CT appearance of a transitional cell carcinoma. J Comput Assist Tomogr 8(5):1019–1022
7. Canon, Zanon, ref. by Löhr E, Mellin P, Göbbeler Th (1968) Über die Grenzen der angiographischen Diagnostik parenchymatöser Nierentumoren. Fortschr Röntgenstr 109:695–701
8. Chilcote WA, Borkowski GP (1983) Computed tomography in renal lymphoma. J Comput Assist Tomogr 7(3):439–443
9. Claussen C, Ludwigsen B, Knipper H, Weiss T, Fiegler W (1984) Computertomographische Stadieneinteilung des hypernephroiden Karzinoms. (Computed tomographic staging of hypernephroid carcinoma) Fortschr Röntgenstr 141(4):390–394
10. Cohan RH, Dunnick NR, Degesys GE, Korobkin M (1984) Computed tomography of renal oncocytoma. J Comput Assist Tomogr 8(2):284–287
11. Cohen MD, Weber T, Grosfeld J (1984) Preoperative evaluation of pediatric abdominal tumor volumes by computerized tomography. J Pediatr Surg 19(3):273
12. Coleman BG, Arger PH, Mintz MC, Pollack HM, Danner MP (1984) Hyperdense renal masses: a computed tomographic dilemma. Amer J Roentgenol 143(2):291–294
13. Cronan JJ, Zeman RK, Rosenfield AT (1982) Comparison of computerized tomography, ultrasound and angiography in staging renal cell carcinoma. J Urol 127(4):712–714
14. Couanet D, Geoffray A, Le Bras F, Piekarski JD, Vanel D, Masselot J (1982) Computerized tomography and nephroblastomas. Proc Clin Biol Res 100:67–70
15. Dunnick NR, Korobkin M, Clark WM (1984) CT demonstration of hyperdense renal carcinoma. J Comput Assist Tomogr 8(5):1023–1024
16. Fishman EK, Hartman DS, Goldman SM, Siegelman SS (1983) The CT appearance of Wilms' tumor. J Comput Assist Tomogr 7(4):659–665
17. Freitag J, Mueller GW, Freitag G, Theuring F, Blume P, Rabe F (1983) Korrelation computertomographischer und histologischer Untersuchungsergebnisse bei soliden Tumoren der Nieren. Z Urol Nephrol 76(11):689–697
18. Fund G, Fischedick AR, Mueller RP, Langenbruch K, Mueller-Rensing R (1983) Die Bedeutung der Computertomographie in der Stufendiagnostik von Nierenbekkentumoren. (Significance of computed tomography in the staging of renal pelvic tumors). Fortschr Röntgenstr 138(4):473–476
19. Gatewood OM, Goldman SM, Marshall FF, Siegelman SS (1982) Computerized tomography in the diagnosis of transitional cell carcinoma of the kidney. J Urol 127(5):876–887
20. Handel DB, Heaston DK, Korobkin M, Silverman PM, Dunnick NR (1983) Circumaortic left renal vein with tumor thrombus: CT diagnosis with angiographic and pathologic correlation. Amer J Roentgenol 141(1): 97–98

21. Hantelmann W, Rost A, Wegener OH, Loy L (1981) Diagnostik des Angiomyolipoms mit besonderer Hinsicht auf die Computertomographie. (Diagnosis of angiomyolipomas with special attention of computer tomography). Helv Chir Acta 48(3–4):359–364
22. Hata Y, Tada S, Kato Y, Onishi T, Masuda F, Machida T (1983) Staging of renal cell carcinoma by computed tomography. J Comput Assist Tomogr 7(5):828–832
23. Heckemann, R, Heimann H, Löhr E (1985) Renale Tumordiagnostik mit Ultraschall und CT. Urologe (A), 24(5):243–252
24. Hochhauser L, Grosman H, Gray RR, St Louis EL, Rankin JT, Gosevitz B (1983) Renales Angiomyolipom in der Computer-Tomographie. Urologe (A), 22(2):100–102
25. Horii SC, Bosniak MA, Megibow AJ, Raghavendra BN, Subramanyam BR, Rothberg M (1983) Correlation of CT and Ultrasound in the evaluation of renal lymphoma. Urol Radiol 5(2):69–76
26. Jaschke W, van Kaick G, Peter S, Palmtag H (1982) Accuracy of computed tomography in staging of kidney tumors. Acta Radiol (Diagn) (Stockh) 23(6):593–598
27. Klose, KC, Schwartz R, Karstens JH (1983) Computertomographie renaler maligner Lymphome. Fortschr Röntgenstr 139(5):515–520
28. Kim WS, Goldman SM, Gatewood OM, Marshall FF, Siegelman SS (1981) Computed tomography in calcified renal masses. J Comput Assist Tomogr 5(6):855–860
29. Klumair J, Walcher G (1985) Sonographische und computertomographische Differentialdiagnose des Angiomyolipoms. Digitale Bilddiagn. 5(2):76–79
30. Krahe T, Harder T, Lackner K (1985) Seriencomputertomographie. Wertigkeit densitometrischer Messungen in der Diagnostik benigner und maligner Laesionen von Leber, Pankreas und Niere. Fortschr Röntgenstr 143(1):28–35
31. Kriedemann E, Rotte KH, Marciniak H, Wehry B (1984) Tumoren des Nierenbeckens – Diagnostische Moeglichkeiten mit CT. Z Urol Nephrol 77(5):257–267
32. Largiader F (1938) Morphologie, Histogenese und Klassifikation von Nierentumoren. Urol Int 6:273–367
33. Lang EK (1984) Comparison of dynamic and conventional computed tomography, angiography, and ultrasonography in the staging of renal cell carcinoma. Cancer 54(10):2205–2214
34. Lang EK (1984) Angio-computed tomography and dynamic tomography in staging or renal cell carcinoma. Radiology 151(1):149–155
35. Levine E, Huntrakoon M (1983) Computed tomography of renal oncocytoma. Amer J Roentgenol 141(4): 741–746
36. Löhr E, Mellin P, Rodeck G, Rohen JW (1976) Atlas der Urologischen Röntgendiagnostik. 2nd Edition. Schattauer, Stuttgart New York
37. Löhr E (1979) Angiographic diagnosis of poorly vascularized renal tumors with emphasis on electronic harmonisation and magnification in: Löhr E (Edit) Renal and Adrenal Tumors. Springer, Berlin Heidelberg New York, pp 143–154
38. Löhr E, Mellin P (1971) Angiographische Diagnose von gefäßarmen Nierentumoren unter besonderer Berücksichtigung des elektronischen Subtraktions- und Harmonisierungsverfahrens. Electromedica 4:121–124
39. Löhr E, Ross S (1985) Embolisations-Therapie von Nierentumoren-Erfahrung an einem Krankengut von 60 Patienten. Radiologe 25:354–358
40. Marchal G, Baert A, Wilms G (1979) Value of computerized Tomography and Ultrasonography in the Diagnosis of Renal and Adrenal Space Occupying Lesions. In: Löhr E: Renal and Adrenal Tumors. Springer, Berlin Heidelberg New York, pp 98–118
41. McClennan BL, Lee JKT (1983) Kidney. In: Lee JKTE, Sargel SS, Stanley RJ (eds) Computed Body Tomography. Raven Press, New York, pp 341–378
42. McMillin KI, Gross BH (1985) CT demonstration of peripelvic and periureteral non-Hodgkin lymphoma. Amer J Roentgenol 144(5):945–946
43. Meyers MA (1979) Dynamic Radiology of the Abdomen Normal and Pathologic Anatomy (2nd Ed). Springer, New York Heidelberg Berlin
44. Mitnick JS, Bosniak MA, Rothberg M, Megibow AJ, Raghavendra BN, Subramanyam BR (1985) Metastasic neoplasm to the kidney studied by computed tomography and sonography. J Comput Assist Tomogr 9(1):43–49
45. Moss GD, Malvar TC (1983) CT demonstration of an ectopic pancreatic tail causing a renal pseudotumor. J Comput Assist Tomogr 7(4):724–726
46. Pagani JJ (1983) Solid renal mass in the cancer patient: second primary renal cell carcinoma versus renal metastasis. J Comput Assist Tomogr 7(3):444–448
47. Pamilo M, Suramo I, Paeivaensalo M (1983) Characteristics of hypernephromas as seen with ultrasound and computed tomography. JCU 11(5):245–249
48. Parvey LS, Warner RM, Callihan TR, Magill HL (1981) CT demonstration of fat tissue in malignant renal neoplasms: atypical Wilms' tumors. J Comput Assist Tomogr 5(5):851–854
49. Peretz GS, Lam AH (1985) Distinguishing neuroblastoma from Wilms' tumor by computed tomography. J Comput Assist Tomogr 9(5):889–893
50. Probst P, Kruker T, Hoogewoud HM (1982) Cavographie und Computertomographie zum Nachweis der Tumorinfiltration in die Vena cava bei malignen Nierentumoren. Radiologe 22(6):272–278
51. Richie JP, Garnick MB, Seltzer S, Bettmann MA (1983) Computerized tomography scan for diagnosis and staging of renal cell carcinoma. J Urol 129(6):1114–1116
52. Robson CJ, Churchill MB, Anderson W (1968) The results of radical nephrectomy for renal cell carcinoma. Trans Am Ass Genitourin. Surg 60:122–131
53. Siegel MJ (1983) Pediatric Applications in Computed Body Tomography. Lee JKT, St Sargel S, Stanley RS (Edit.) Raven Press, New York, pp 517–557
54. Twomey BP, Katz D (1983) Computed tomography in the diagnosis of extramedullary plasmacytoma. J Comput Tomogr 7(4):407–408

Magnetic Resonance Imaging of Renal Mass Lesions

J.V. KAUDE and R.E. KINARD

1 Introduction

In recent years the development of technology has added another imaging modality to the armamentarium of radiologists which can be used in the investigation of renal disease – magnetic resonance imaging (MRI). The accumulated experience with MRI in renal mass lesions – both experimental and clinical – was rather limited just a year or two ago. It included descriptions of only a few cases of malignant or benign renal tumors, cysts, inflammatory and posttraumatic mass lesions of the kidney [1, 2, 3, 4, 5]. However, the clinical importance and usefulness of MRI in the diagnosis and differential diagnosis of renal mass lesions have been rapidly recognized. HRICAK and coworkers recently reported a 96% success rate in staging 31 renal and perirenal neoplasms with MRI [6]. In this chapter we will discuss our experiences in the diagnosis of renal mass lesions with a 0.15 Tesla resistive magnet scanner.

2 Equipment

The high costs purchasing and operating a MRI-scanner have been, are, and will continue to be of concern for health care providers, insurers, and patients. In the investigation of renal mass lesions, it can be questioned whether the high cost of MRI is justified in exchange for diagnostic information that is already available from computed tomography or from other noninvasive diagnostic procedures such as ultrasound.

Since January 1984, we have operated a 0.15 Tesla resistive magnet unit (Teslacon, Technicare, Cleveland, Ohio). The acquisition and operation costs of this unit are comparable with those of a CT-scanner. For body imaging the scanner is equipped with software-C and a high performance half-saddle coil. Lately, we have used an ovoid surface coil for renal imaging which has further improved the image quality, allowing excellent analysis of renal parenchyma.

3 Technique of Examination

For the examination of kidneys, first a rapid, 1 or 2 min axial scan (SE 250/30) is performed. The scan is "noisy," but it permits adequate kidney localization. Patients with renal disease are then examined with three scanning sequences. In axial projection the scans are obtained with spin echo images (SE) for T1 information, using repetition time (TR) of 500 ms and echo delay time (TE) of 30 ms (SE 500/30). Multislice-multiecho technique is used for T2 weighted images (TE 30, 60, 90, 120 ms; TR 2000 or 2500 ms). In coronal projection T1 weighted scans are obtained. The scans are usually contiguous, but in the presence of larger kidneys we leave a 3 mm wide gap between the sections. The section thickness most often used is 10 mm, although sections as thin as 4.5 mm can be obtained. The data acquisition time for each of three sequences is about 8–10 min and the total time of a complete kidney examination including positioning the patient is approximately 45 min.

In the presence of larger renal malignancies or large masses in which the organ of origin is uncertain, we supplement the three standard projections with sagittal scans which are helpful in assessing adjacent organ or soft tissue involvement by renal masses.

The cases presented herein are renal mass lesions found in a total study of some 400 patients who had MRI examination for known or suspected kidney disease, while searching for a primary tumor in patients with metastatic disease of unknown origin, or after renal lesions were detected incidentally during investigation for other abdominal disorders.

3.1 Normal Kidney

Analysis of normal renal anatomy is best accomplished on spin echo T1 weighted images (SE 500/30) (Figs. 1 and 3) [1, 3, 7, 8]. Inversion recovery (IR) scans with good T1 weighting show the corticomedullary demarcation equally well but are not used routinely because of the decreased signal to noise ratio and increased examination time [7, 8, 9]. There is good demarcation between the cortex and the medulla which has a lower signal intensity relative to the cortex (Figs. 1 and 3). These signal differences may vary somewhat depending upon the state of hydration [3]. The sinus fat has the highest signal intensity, equal to that of perirenal fatty tissue. Urine in the renal pelvis has the lowest signal intensity and the renal vessels are well defined because of the absence of the signal from flowing blood (Figs. 2, 12, 19a, 20b, 28). The perinephric fascia is not routinely seen using body coils but is easily demonstrated using surface coils or when there is thickening. The renal capsule is not imaged. A low image intensity artifact is sometimes noted at the periphery of the kidney at the interface with the perinephric fat and should not be mistaken for the renal capsule. The exact cause of this artifact (Fig. 6a) is not known but may be secondary to chemical shift or edge enhancement [8, 10].

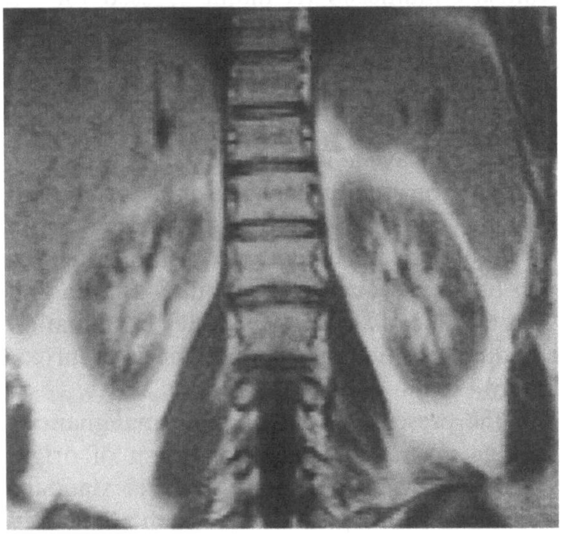

Fig. 1. Normal kidneys, MRI, coronal T1 weighted scan (SE 500/30). There is good demarcation between the cortex (higher signal intensity) and the medulla (lower signal intensity). Renal sinus fat has the highest signal intensity (equal to retroperitoneal fat). Intrarenal vessels (flowing blood) and urine in the collecting system have the lowest signal intensity

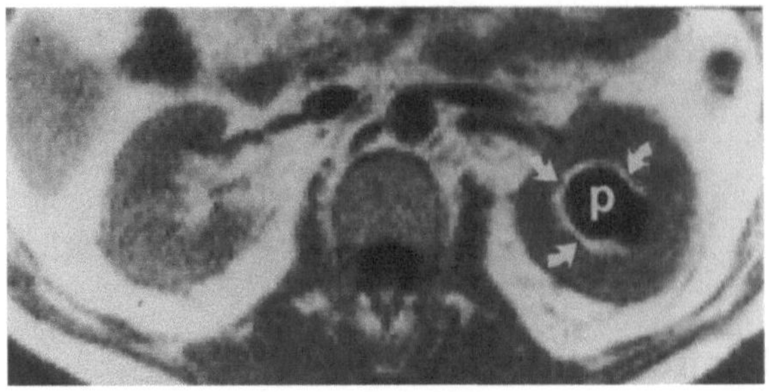

Fig. 2. Hydronephrosis, T1 weighted axial MRI scan (SE 500/30). The left kidney is enlarged, the kidney pelvis (*P*) is dilated. The sinus fat (of high signal intensity, *arrows*) is compressed by the dilated kidney pelvis. There is also a loss of the corticomedullary demarcation

4 Benign Lesions

4.1 Renal Edema

In kidney enlargement associated with edema, MRI demonstrates loss of corticomedullary demarcation (Figs. 2, 5a, 10a) as the differences in signal intensity between the cortex and medulla have been eliminated. This appearance is not specific for any renal disease but is found in conditions such as acute glomerulonephritis, renal artery stenosis, renal vein thrombosis, chronic hydronephrosis [9, 11], renal trauma associated with extracorporeal shock wave lithotripsy [12], and renal abscess [13]. In renal transplants the demarcation between the cortex and medulla is frequently lost in the presence of immunologic rejection [14, 15]. The reasons for the loss of corticomedullary demarcation are not well understood. It has been speculated that in chronic ureteral obstruction the water content in the cortex is increased resulting in longer T1 relaxation times and lower signal [9]. This appears to be true also in other conditions which produce circulatory disturbances and edema in the kidney.

4.2 Hydronephrosis

A dilated collecting system due to ureteral obstruction, with or without enlargement of the kidney, or a large extrarenal kidney pelvis is easily recognized by its low intensity signal (Fig. 2).

4.3 Cysts

For differentiation of cysts from solid mass lesions, we generally use ultrasound which is more cost-effective than CT or MRI. Only when differential diagnostic problems after ultrasound still exist do we proceed further with these more sophisticated imaging modalities. Most of the renal cysts we have examined with MRI have been incidental findings in patients who have had scans for other reasons. Some scans were obtained for comparison with cysts already diagnosed by computed tomography or ultrasound.

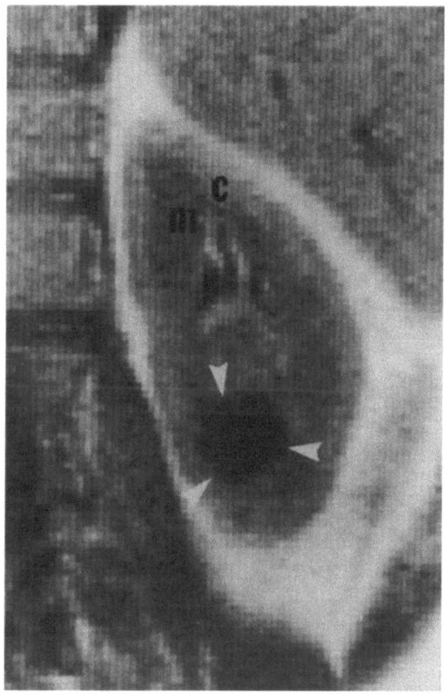

Fig. 3. Simple renal cyst. T1 weighted coronal MRI scan (SE 500/30). The cyst (*arrowheads*) is well-defined and of very low signal intensity (fluid). The kidney is otherwise normal. Note the high signal intensity of the cortex (*c*) relative to the medulla (*m*)

Simple cysts (Figs. 3 and 6) present on MRI scans as well-defined, smoothly outlined mass lesions with homogenously low signal intensity on T1 weighted images (long T1) [8, 10, 16]. On T2 weighted images the signal intensity increases and becomes markedly more intense than that of renal parenchyma. With more delayed echo sequences signal intensity of the fluid in a simple cyst becomes almost identical with or even greater than that of fat (long T2) (Figs. 6b, 8b, 11b). The use of late (90 and 120 ms) echoes is not universal, but we feel it is helpful because potentially misleading information may be gained when only using two relatively short echoes (i.e., 30 and 60 ms).

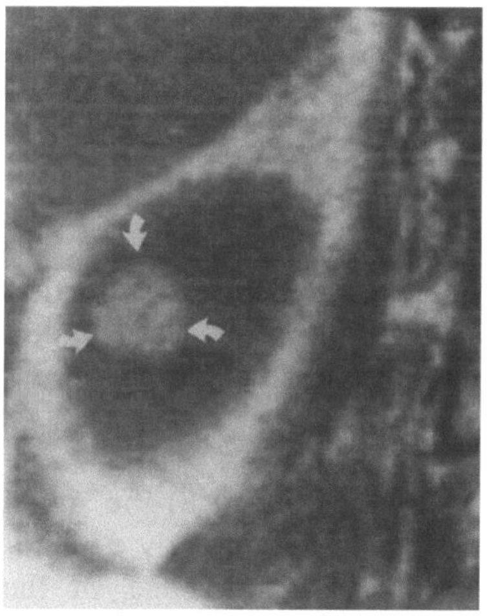

Fig. 4. Hemorrhagic cyst. Well-defined mass lesion of high intensity signal (*arrows*) on coronal T1 weighted MRI scan (SE 500/30). The hemorrhage is probably older (compare the high intensity signal from a 6-week-old subcapsular hemorrhage in Fig. 10b)

Hemorrhagic cysts (Figs. 4 and 5) can be differentiated from simple cysts by their appearance on T1 weighted images. Contrary to simple cysts, blood shortens the T1 relaxation time and increases the signal intensity. The signal intensity of hemorrhagic cysts may vary with the concentration of blood and the length of time elapsed since the bleeding accurred [3, 7, 8, 16]. In acute bleeding (Fig. 5) the signal intensity may be approximately the same as that of renal parenchyma or even higher [7, 9].

"Milk of calcium" in a cyst can be recognized by MRI because of the lack of signal in the

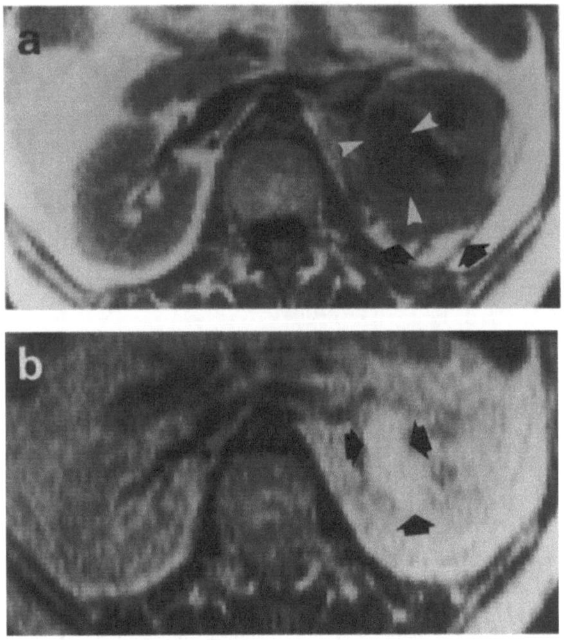

Fig. 5 a, b. Hemorrhage into a renal cyst, 24 h post extracorporeal lithotripsy. **a** T1 weighted axial MRI scan (SE 500/30). The left kidney is enlarged, there is loss of the corticomedullary demarcation (compared with the normal right kidney). There is also fluid dissecting into the retroperitoneal fat (*black arrows*). The signal intensity of this fresh hemorrhage into an earlier diagnosed parapelvic cyst (*white arrowheads*) is slightly lower than that of renal parenchyma, but higher than that of a simple cyst. From [12]. **b** On T2 weighted scan (SE 2500/60) the cyst is better identified by high intensity signal (*arrows*)

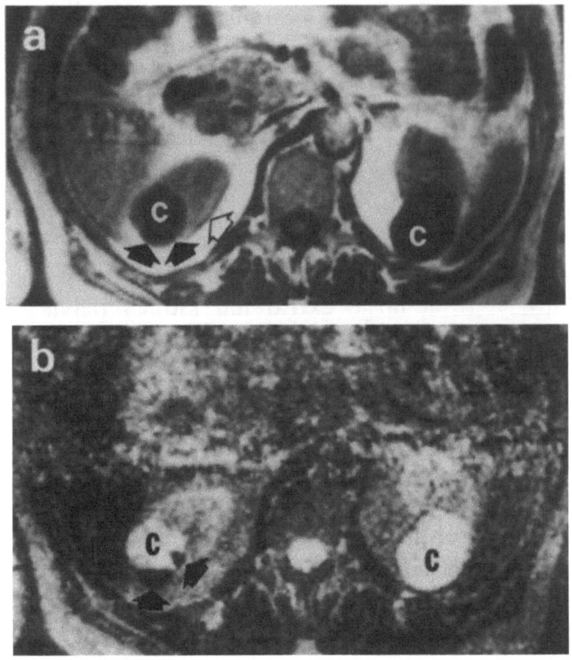

Fig. 6 a, b. Renal cyst containing "milk of calcium." **a** Axial MRI scan (SE 600/45). Cysts (*c*) in both kidneys. There is lack of signal from two small areas along the posterior and medial wall of the cyst in the right kidney (*black arrows*). Note the low intensity artifact along the medial border of the right kidney not to be confused with fluid collection or renal capsule (*open arrow*). **b** On T2 weighted scan (SE 1750/160) with cystic fluid having a very high signal intensity, the lack of signal from calcium is better identified (*arrows*)

calcific fluid layering in the dependent portion of the cyst on all scanning sequences (Fig. 6). This lack of signal is better recognized on T2 weighted scans (Fig. 6b).

In ***polycystic kidneys*** (Figs. 7 and 8) the signal intensity of the cysts may vary greatly depending upon the presence of hemorrhage, or the contents of the cyst, blood, protein concentration, etc. (Fig. 8) [7, 8, 16, 17].

4.4 Renal Abscess

Only a few clinical cases of renal abscess examined with MRI have been reported in the literature [3, 4, 7]. We have investigated the MRI appearance of renal abscess in an experimental animal model [13]. We induced kidney infection by percutaneous injection of *E. coli* culture in rabbit and determined T1 relaxation times of the lesion. The acute renal abscess (with perirenal extension in several animals) had longer T1 relaxation times than normal renal parenchyma, a difference that was statistically significant. The infected kidneys were enlarged and there was loss of corticomedullary demarcation in each case. In clinical cases findings are similar to experimentally induced renal abscess (Fig. 9). However, in some cases the signal intensity differences between normal and abnormal tissues are small, and the lesion is demonstrable only on T2 weighted image. These findings may be difficult or impossible to differentiate from renal tumors.

4.5 Renal Hemorrhage

Traumatic subcapsular hemorrhage presenting as an enlarged kidney or as a renal mass lesion is well demonstrable by MRI (Fig. 10). The sig-

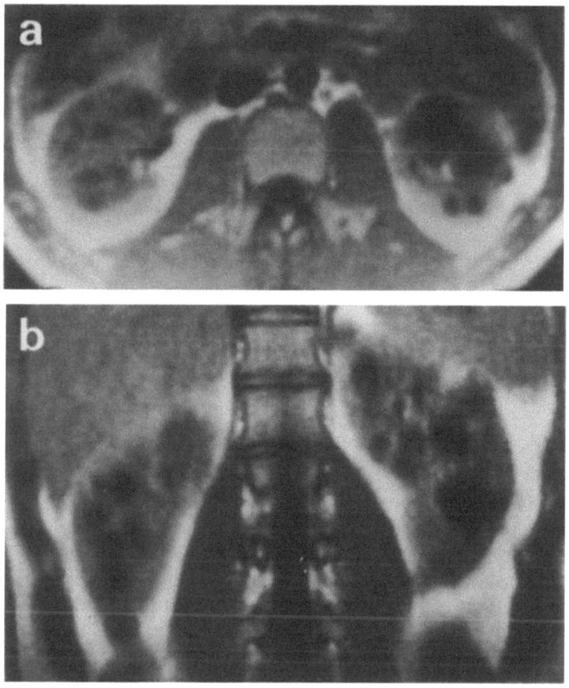

Fig. 7 a, b. Polycystic kidneys **a** axial and **b** coronal T1 weighted MRI scans (SE 500/30). The smallest cysts, all of which are of low signal intensity, are approximately 5 mm in size

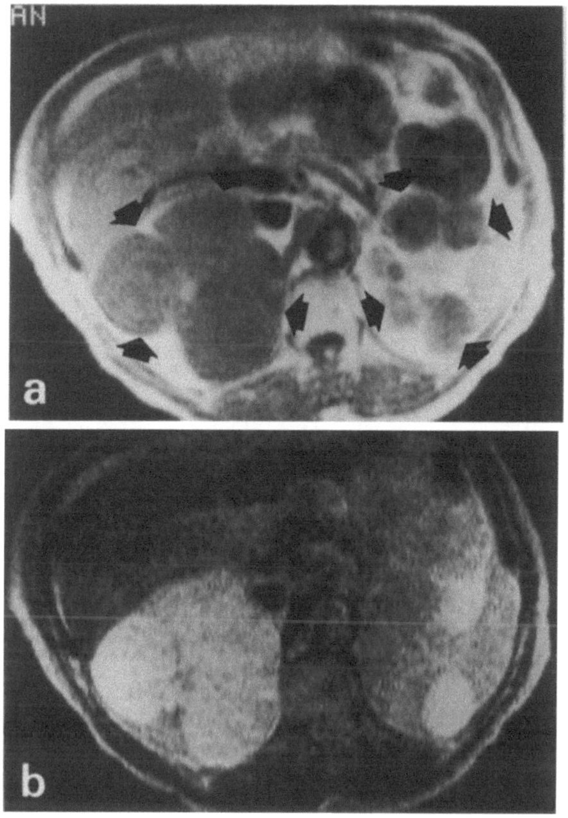

Fig. 8 a, b. Polycystic kidneys. **a** T1 weighted axial MRI scan (SE 500/30). Enlarged kidneys (*arrows*) with multiple cysts of generally low but varied signal intensities, depending upon composition of fluid. **b** T2 weighted scan (SE 2500/90). The signal intensity has increased in most of the cysts

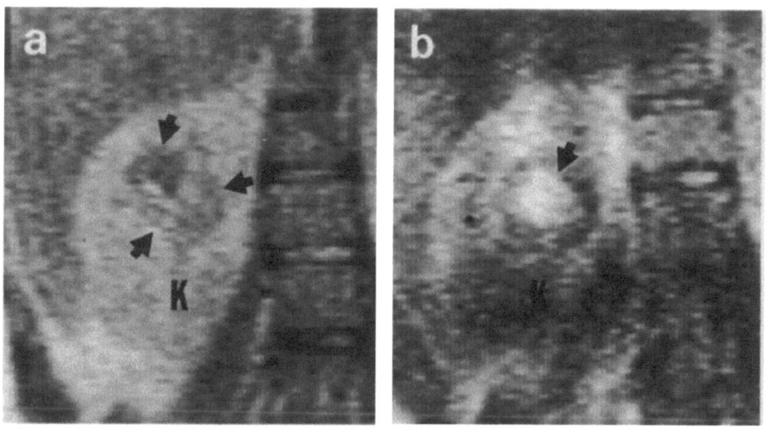

Fig. 9 a, b. Renal-perirenal abscess, coronal MRI multislice/multiecho technique scans of the posterior aspect of the right kidney. **a** The lesion (*arrows*) has mixed but generally lower signal intensity than renal parenchyma (*K*) (SE 2240/30). **b** With delayed echo sequence (SE 2240/60) the signal intensity in part of the lesion (*arrow*) is markedly increased. Histologically xanthogranulomatous infectious process was present

nal intensity of acute hemorrhage may vary depending upon the content of the blood and age of bleeding [18, 19]. It may present as a lesion of relatively low signal intensity on T1 weighted images (Fig. 5a) or as a mass lesion with approximately the same signal intensity as renal parenchyma (Fig. 10a). In some cases the signal intensity of a hemorrhage is mixed (Figs. 11 and 12). With aging of the hemorrhage the signal intensity will increase (short T1) (Fig. 10b), and

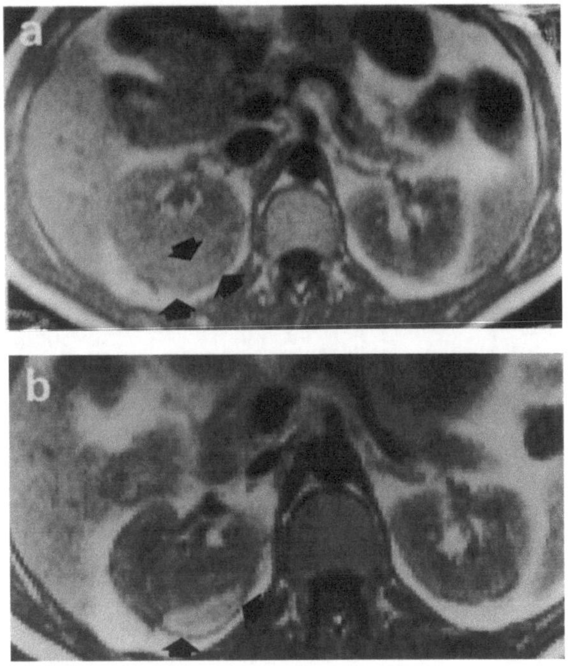

Fig. 10 a, b. Subcapsular renal hemorrhage [12]. **a** Axial T1 weighted MRI scan (SE 500/30). Fresh hemorrhage (a few hours post extracorporeal lithotripsy) (*arrows*) is almost isointense with renal parenchyma. The right kidney is swollen and there is poor differentiation between the renal cortex and medulla. **b** 6 weeks later the hemorrhage is of high signal intensity (*arrows*)

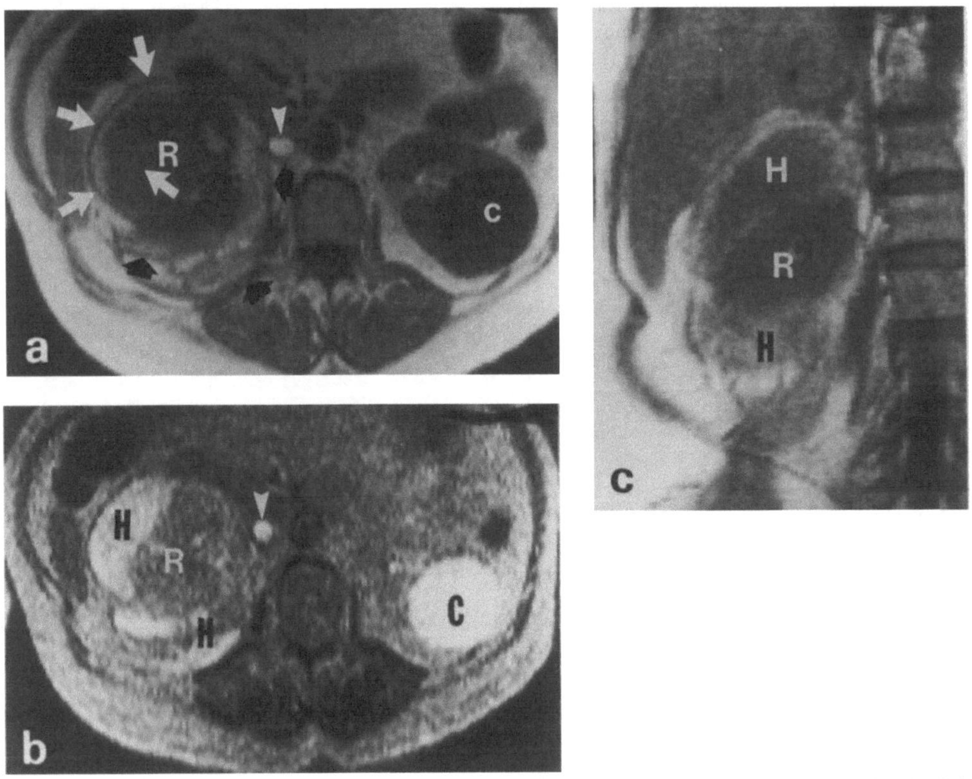

Fig. 11 a–c. Older perirenal hemorrhage (18 days post biopsy of the right kidney). Cyst in the left kidney. **a** Axial T1 weighted MRI scan (SE 500/30). Large mass of mixed intensity posteromedial to the right kidney (*black arrows*). There is also an anterior, well-defined hemorrhage with narrow mass of high signal intensity (clotted blood?) (*white arrows*) anterolateral to the kidney (*R*). *C* cyst. **b** On T2 weighted scan (SE 2500/135) most of the hemorrhage (*H*) as well as the cyst (*C*) has a very high intensity signal. In this case the inferior vena cava (*white arrowhead*) gives a very high intensity signal both on T1 and T2 weighted images. **c** Coronal T1 weighted scan of the right kidney showing the extension of the hemorrhages (*H*) superior and inferior to the kidney (*R*)

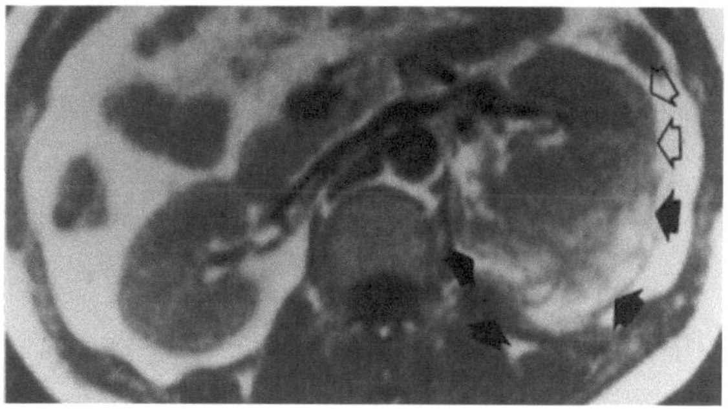

Fig. 12. Subcapsular-perirenal hemorrhage, axial T1 weighted MRI scan (SE 500/30), 24 h post renal biopsy. The left kidney is enlarged and displaced anteriorly by perirenal hemorrhage which dissects into the retroperitoneal fat (*black arrows*). A subcapsular hemorrhage is also present (*open arrows*). The signal intensity of this fresh bleeding has a slightly higher signal than that of renal parenchyma

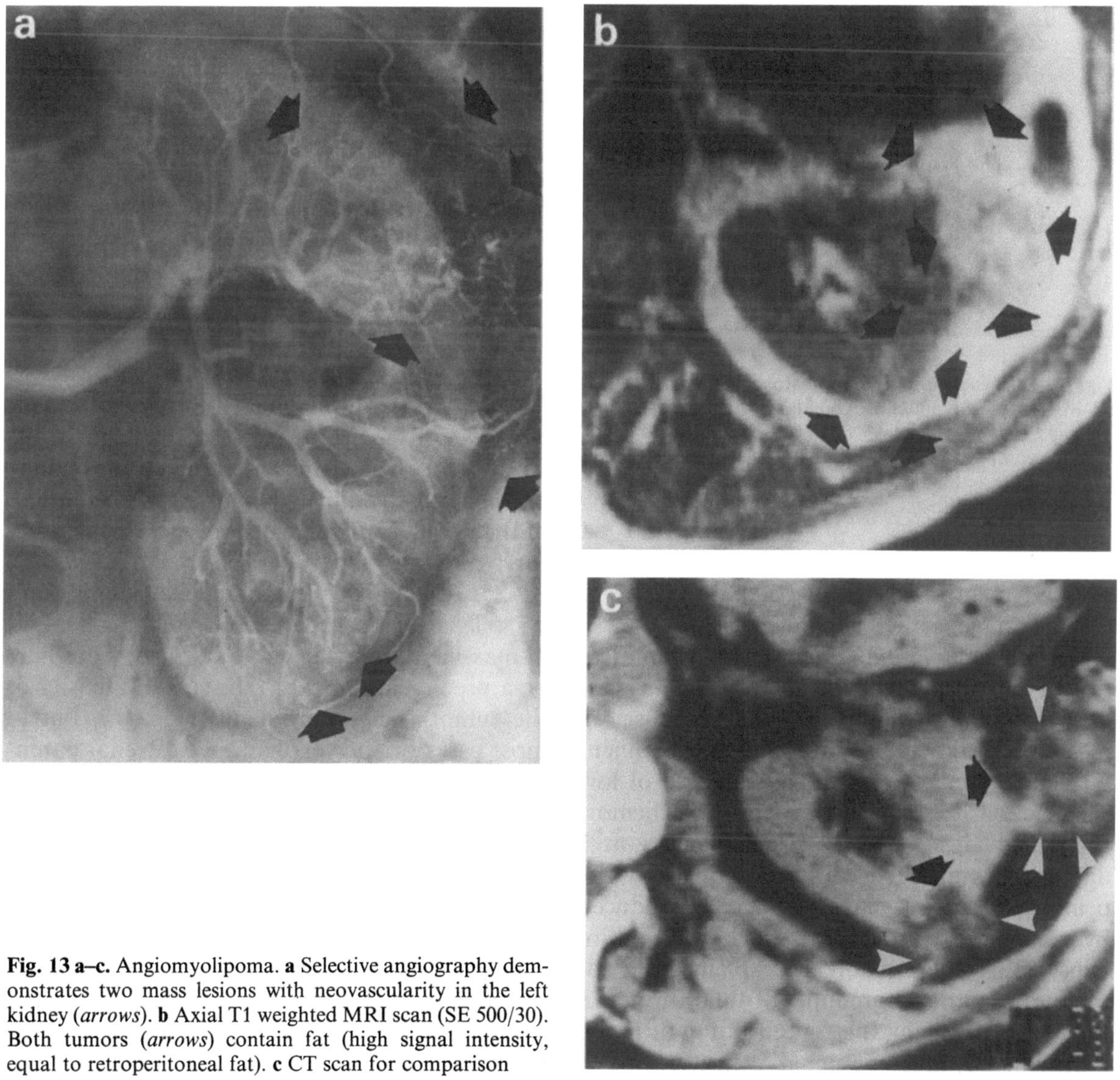

Fig. 13 a–c. Angiomyolipoma. **a** Selective angiography demonstrates two mass lesions with neovascularity in the left kidney (*arrows*). **b** Axial T1 weighted MRI scan (SE 500/30). Both tumors (*arrows*) contain fat (high signal intensity, equal to retroperitoneal fat). **c** CT scan for comparison

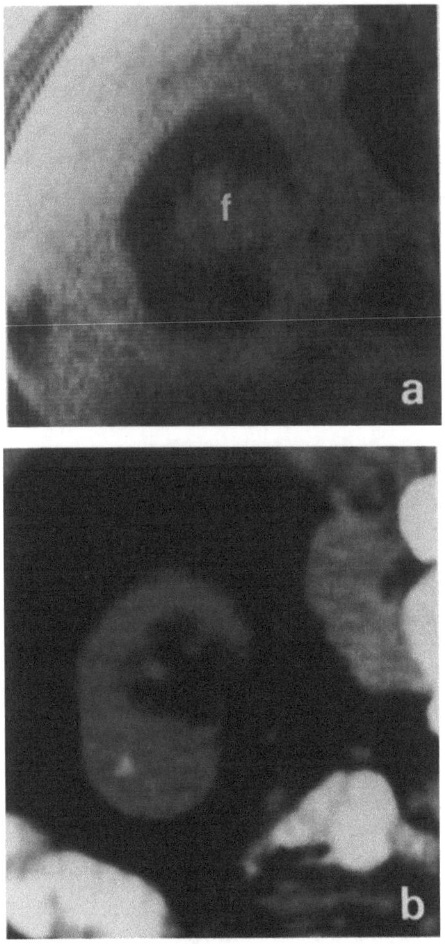

Fig. 14 a, b. Renal sinus fibrolipomatosis. **a** T1 weighted axial MRI scan (SE 500/30). Abundance of sinus fat (*f*) in the right kidney, isointense with retroperitoneal fat. **b** CT scan for comparison. Small renal stones evident on CT are not demonstrated by MRI

on T2 weighted images the signal intensity of a hemorrhage is always high (Fig. 11 b).

Certain reservations against this simplification of diagnosing renal hemorrhage by its higher signal intensity must be made because we have observed acute hemorrhage in experimental animal studies presenting as an area of low signal intensity [20]. This experimental hemorrhage had an even lower signal intensity at 7 days posttrauma. The differences in MRI appearance of a fresh renal hemorrhage produced by trauma (extracorporeal shock wave lithotripsy) [12] can probably be explained by admixture of variable amounts of fluid (urine) to the blood, changing the concentration of blood elements and, thus, the signal intensity.

4.6 Benign Renal Tumors

At the present time only a few benign renal tumors (angiomyolipoma, sclerosing leiomyoma) have been examined with MRI [3, 4, 9, 21]. In angiomyolipoma the fatty components of the tumor have the same high intensity signal as retroperitoneal or renal sinus fat, while the more vascular portions of the tumor, or recent hemorrhage into the tumor, have a lower signal intensity on T1 weighted images [3, 4, 9, 21] (Fig. 13). One single reported case of renal sclerosing leiomyoma [9] presented itself as having a relatively low intensity signal on T1 weighted scans.

4.7 Renal Sinus Fibrolipomatosis

An abundance of renal sinus fat is easily demonstrable by its very high signal intensity on both T1 and T2 weighted images [3] (Fig. 14).

5 Renal Malignancies

5.1 Renal Cell Carcinoma

5.1.1 The Primary Tumor

The diagnosis of malignant tumors of the kidney (Figs. 15–20, 22a, 26, 28, 29) and their differentiation from benign lesions of the kidney become possible through analysis of the outline of the lesion, by involvement of extrarenal structures (nodes, vessels) (Figs. 16b, 17, 19, 20, 23–25, 28), and by the characteristics of T1 and T2 relaxation times. Generally renal cell carcinomas have irregular contours, and there may be a pseudocapsule [9a]. The signal intensity of the tumor is inhomogeneous (Fig. 16), but in most cases it is lower than that of renal parenchyma (long T1) on T1 weighted scans [6, 7, 8] (Fig. 17a). However, renal carcinomas with relatively high signal intensity occur (Figs. 18, 22a) and have been reported in the literature [4, 22, 22a]. The areas of increased intensity may in part be related to prior hemorrhage. Larger renal cell carcinomas present as mass lesions of mixed signal intensity, depending upon the nature of solid, necrotic, or hemorrhagic areas within the tumor (Figs. 16–17). Some tumors,

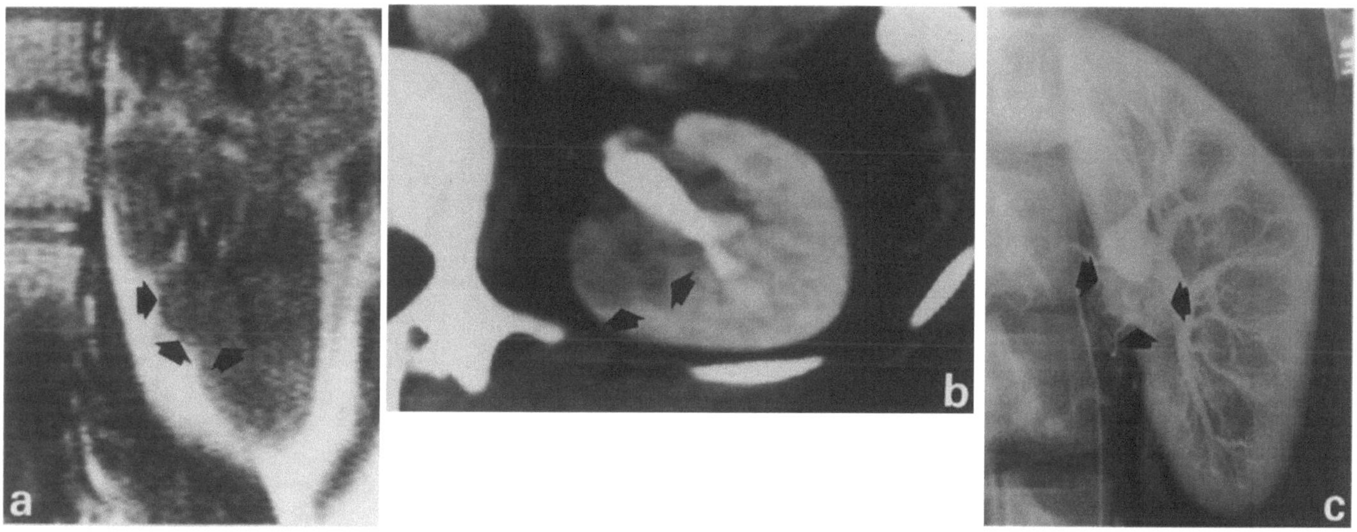

Fig. 15 a–c. Small renal cell carcinoma. **a** MRI coronal T1 weighted scan (SE 500/30) of the left kidney. Small lesion at the kidney hilum (*arrows*). The signal intensity of the lesion is identical to the renal parenchyma. **b** Contrast enhanced CT scan identifies the tumor on the posteromedial aspect of the kidney (*arrows*). **c** Selective angiogram demonstrates neovascularity (*arrows*) at the site of the mass lesion as shown by MRI (**a**)

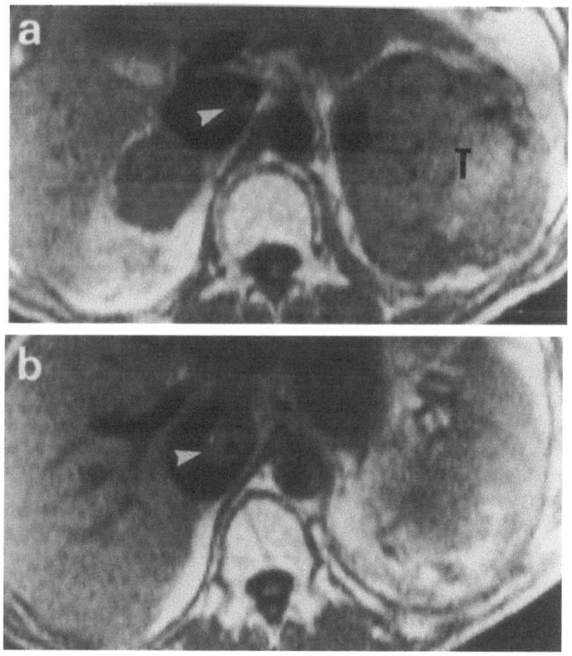

Fig. 16 a, b. Renal cell carcinoma, axial T1 weighted MRI scans (SE 500/30). **a** Large tumor of mixed signal intensity (*T*) of the left kidney. **b** Tumor thrombus in the inferior vena cava (*white arrowhead*)

however, may appear almost isointense with the normal parenchyma of the kidney (Figs. 15a, 19–20). To what extent the vacularity of the tumor may influence the MRI finding remains yet to be determined. In renal cell carcinomas in which we have performed angiography, the signal intensity in most of the tumor has been low on T1 weighted and high on T2 weighted scans (Fig. 17). In two cases, the MRI characteristics have remained unchanged after intra-arterial alcohol embolization of the tumor. These observations indicate that tumor vascularity may not always be an important factor in the MRI appearance of renal cell carcinoma.

5.1.2 Staging and Metastases

The correlation between the MRI staging of renal cell carcinoma and operative findings has been reported with an accuracy of 96% for MRI [6]. Metastatic spread of renal cell carcinoma is well demonstrable by MRI (Figs. 16, 19–25). An interesting observation has been provided by Pettersson [23] indicating that metastatic lesions may have the same T1 and T2 relaxation times as the primary tumor (Fig. 22).

Intravascular tumor thrombi can be outlined exactly by MRI [6, 16, 24, 25] (Figs. 16 and 19). They are characterized by higher intensity signals relative to the flowing blood. Although the signal intensity of the venous blood may vary greatly with the flow velocity, direction of flow, and order in which the multislice images are obtained (Fig. 11), the tumor thrombus is not

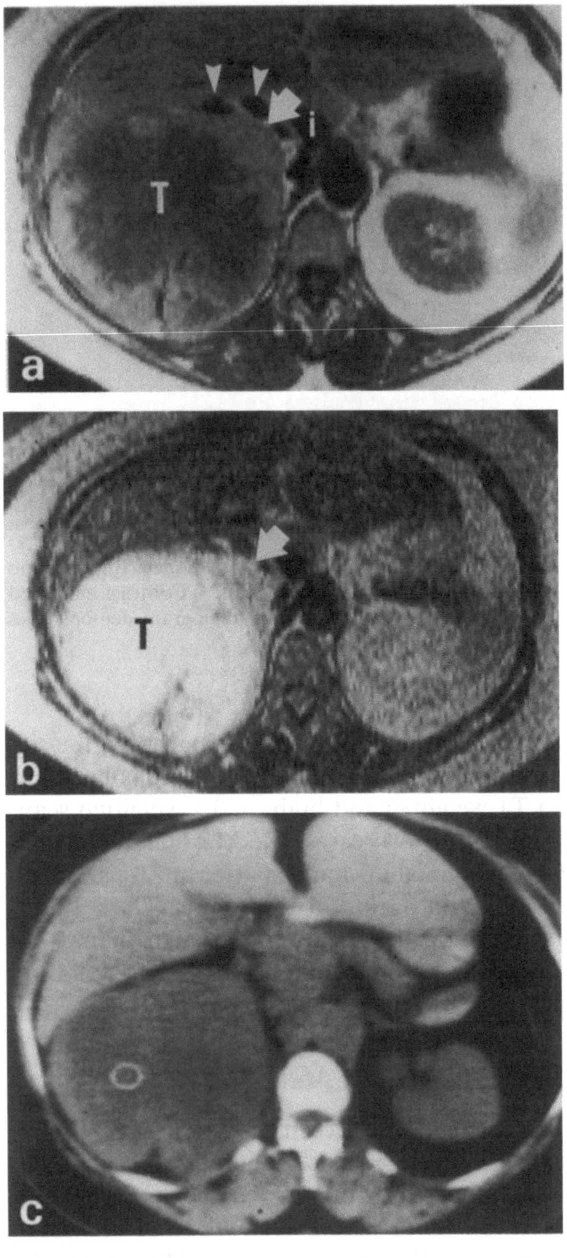

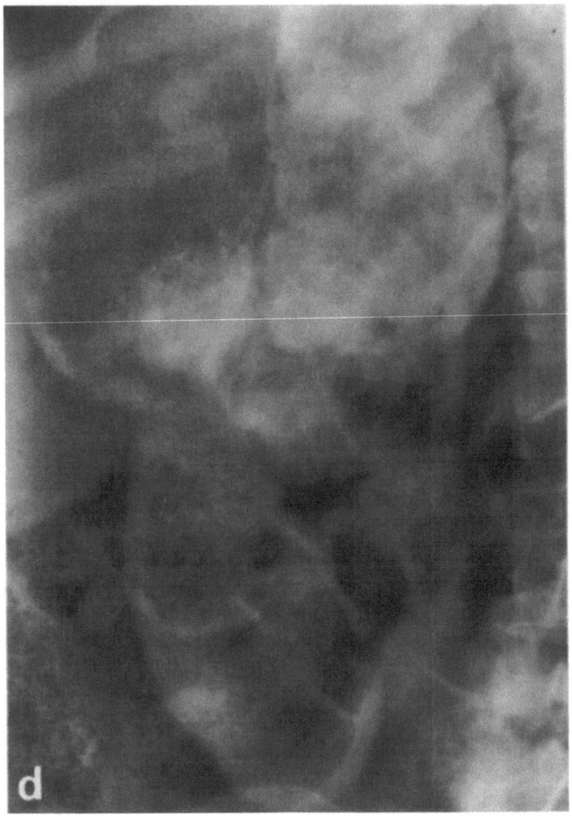

Fig. 17 a–d. Renal cell carcinoma of the right kidney. **a** Axial T1 weighted MRI scan (SE 500/30). Most of the large tumor (*T*) which infiltrates perirenal fat is of lower signal intensity relative to the normal parenchyma (*arrow*) and to the left kidney. The inferior vena cava (*i*) is compressed and displaced. Obstruction of the renal vein is evidenced by the presence of collateral veins (*white arrowheads*). **b** On T2 weighted (axial) scan (SE 2500/120) the signal intensity of the tumor is high. **c** CT scan and **d** angiography for comparison

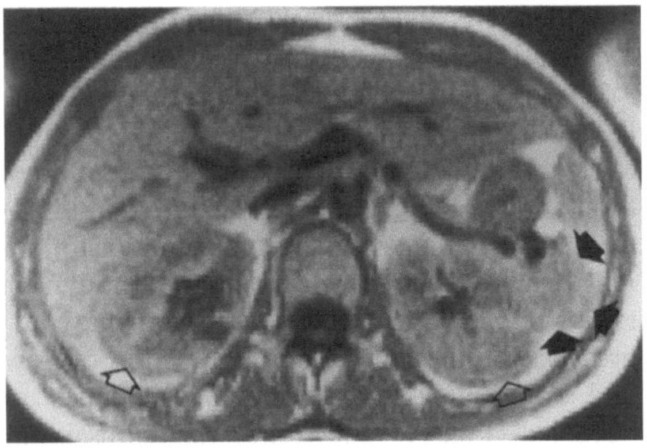

Fig. 18. Renal cell carcinoma, axial T1 weighted MRI scan (SE 500/30). The tumor (*black arrows*) has predominantly extrarenal growth and has relatively high signal intensity (higher than that of the medulla and the same as the signal intensity of renal cortex) (*open arrows*)

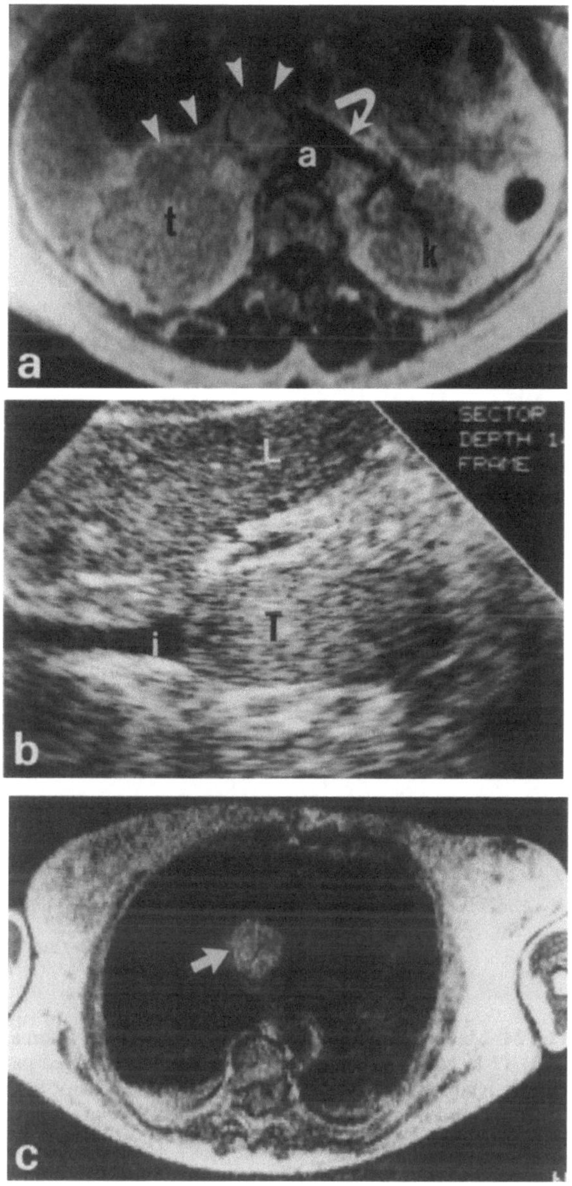

Fig. 19 a–c. Renal cell carcinoma with tumor thrombus in the right renal vein and inferior vena cava. **a** T1 weighted axial MRI scan (SE 500/30). Carcinoma arising from the right kidney (*t*) has a signal intensity which in this case is approximately equal to that of the normal left kidney (*K*). There is continuous growth of the tumor into the right renal vein and inferior vena cava (*white arrowheads*). The left renal vein (curved white arrow) is open. *a*, aorta. **b** Parasagittal real-time ultrasound scan for comparison. Large tumor thrombus (*I*) in the inferior cava (*i*). L, liver. **c** Tumor thrombus (*arrow*) in the right atrium, T2 weighted image (SE 2000/60). Primary tumor in the left kidney (this is a different patient than that presented in **a** and **b**)

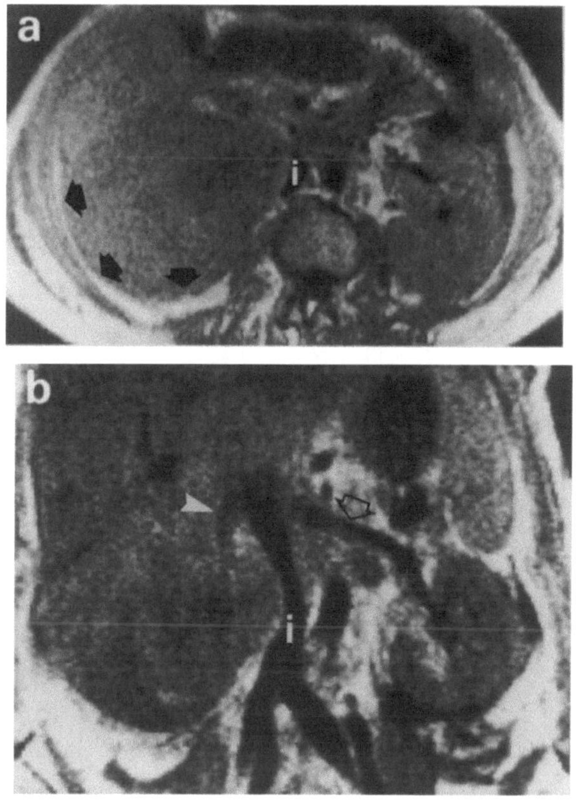

Fig. 20 a, b. Renal cell carcinoma. **a** Axial T1 weighted MRI scan (SE 500/30). The large tumor which is isointense with normal parenchyma displaces and compresses the inferior vena cava (*i*). It is well-defined against the retroperitoneal fat (*arrows*). **b** Coronal T1 weighted scan confirms compression of the inferior vena cava. The right renal vein (*white arrowhead*) is obstructed by the tumor. The left renal vein is patent (*open arrow*)

dependent on these factors and also often enlarges the affected venous structure.

The different intensity signals from lymph nodes (Figs. 23 and 24) and blood vessels permit recognition of metastatic disease without use of contrast medium [26, 27]. The metastatic lesions can be demonstrated best on T1 weighted images (Figs. 21–25). With these echo sequences the signal from the flowing blood is of low intensity and that from the retroperitoneal fat of very high intensity. The metastatic lymph nodes with their intermediate or mixed intensity signal pattern can be separated from the vessels as well as from normal retroperitoneal tissues (Figs. 23 and 24). On T2 weighted images the flowing blood is well demonstrated by keeping its low intensity signal, but the signal intensity from tumorous nodes increases so that they become indistinguishable from retroperitoneal fat. The size of metastatic lymph nodes which can be seen is approximately 1 cm and thus comparable to the size of lymph nodes which are evident

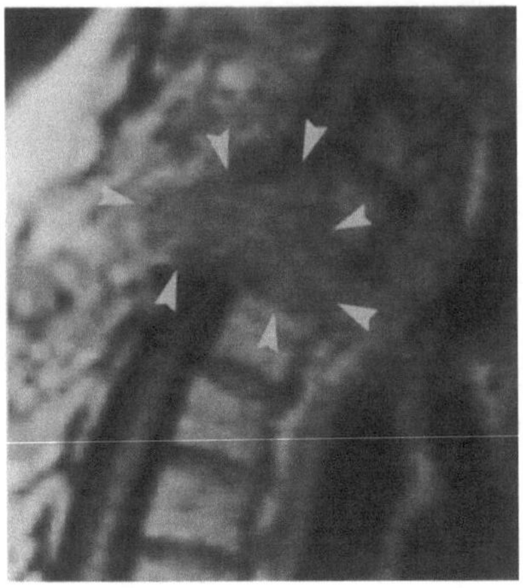

Fig. 21. Metastasis from renal cell carcinoma in the cervical spine (*white arrowheads*), T1 weighted sagittal MRI scan (SE 500/30)

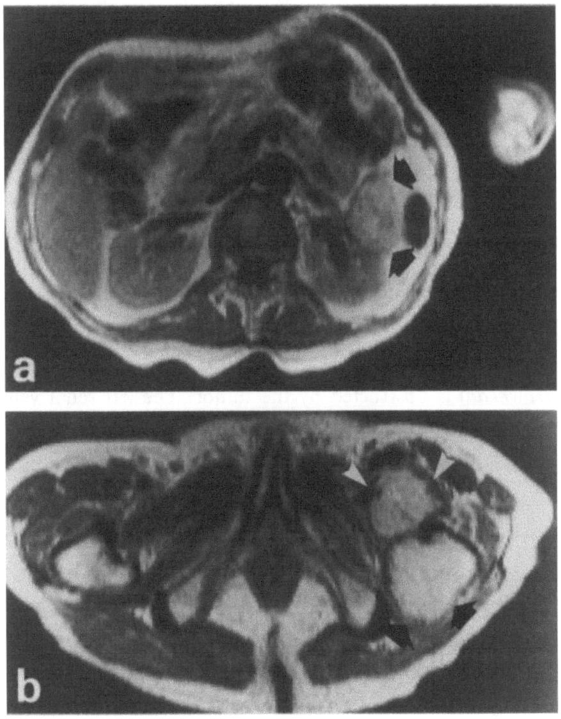

Fig. 22 a, b. Renal cell carcinoma with metastasis, axial MRI scan (SE 650/45) [23] **a** Tumor arising from the anterolateral aspect of the left kidney (*arrows*). **b** Metastatic lesion in the bone (*black arrows*) and soft tissues (*white arrowheads*) of the left hip

on CT scans; however, spatial resolution with MRI is not as good at the present time.

One advantage of MRI over CT in staging of renal malignancies is that scans can be obtained in axial, coronal, and sagittal projection, permitting a 3-dimensional analysis of the ex-

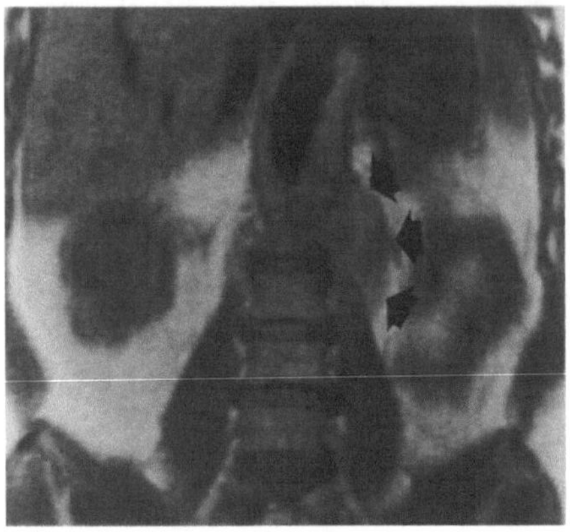

Fig. 23. Retroperitoneal lymph node metastasis from renal cell carcinoma (*arrows*), status post left nephrectomy, coronal T1 weighted MRI scan (SE 500/30)

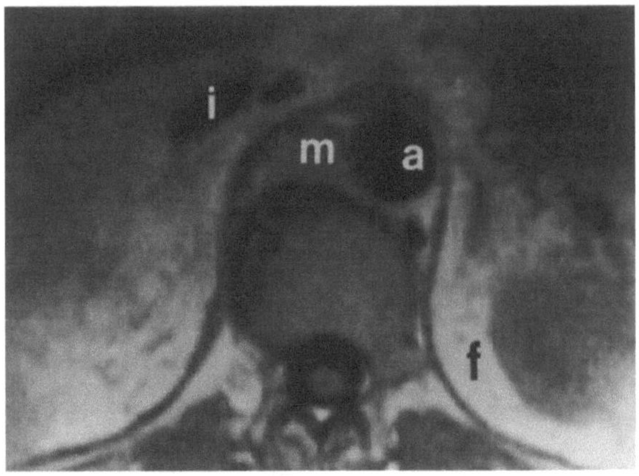

Fig. 24. Metastatic lymph node from renal cell carcinoma, axial T1 weighted MRI scan (SE 500/30). The enlarged paraortic lymph node (*m*) has a higher signal intensity than flowing blood in the aorta (*a*) and the inferior vena cava (*i*), but lower than that of retroperitoneal fat (*f*)

tent of the tumor. Since MRI shows perirenal extension, adjacent organ invasion, involvement of lymph nodes, as well as vessel involvement, its expense may be justified if several other exams are replaced, e.g., dynamic contrast enhanced CT, angiography, and ultrasound.

5.2 Transitional Cell Carcinoma

The information available from technically well-performed excretory urography, occasionally combined with CT, is usually adequate for the diagnosis of a transitional cell carcinoma. The

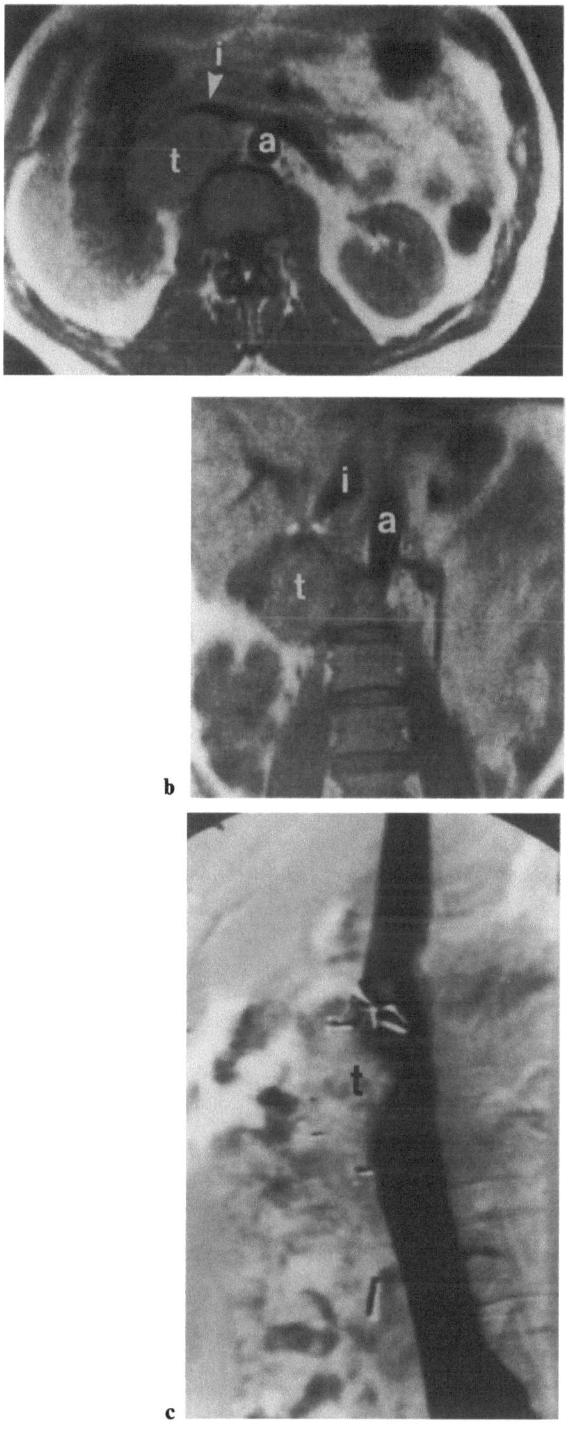

a b c

Fig. 25 a–c. Adrenal metastasis from renal cell carcinoma invading inferior vena cava, status post right nephrectomy. **a** Axial T1 weighted MRI scan (SE 500/30), t, tumor; i, inferior vena cava; a, aorta. The tumor is well outlined against the compressed inferior vena cava. **b** Coronal scan. Note lack of artifacts from surgical clips (**c**) which would have influenced the image quality of the CT scans. **c** Digital angiogram of the inferior vena cava for comparison

number of cases with this malignancy that have been by examined MRI is low [9]. The lesions, when evident on MRI scans, are seen as higher signal intensity masses in the collecting system [9], and the diagnosis can be aided by the presence of caliceal dilatation. However, we were not able to diagnose one histologically verified 2-cm size transitional cell carcinoma with MRI (Fig. 29a).

5.3 Renal Sarcoma

Primary sarcomatous tumors of the kidney are rare and may arise from the renal capsule, sinus, or intrarenal remnants of embryonal tissue. We have been able to examine two patients with sarcomatous renal tumors. One patient had histologically verified malignant fibrous histiocytoma (Fig. 26), and the second patient a metastatic flank lesion from a previously diagnosed leiomyosarcoma of the kidney which had developed after nephrectomy (Fig. 27). As in other malignancies, this metastatic lesion was inhomogeneous with a lower intensity signal relative to retroperitoneal fat. It was surrounded by a capsule or pseudocapsule and well-defined against both normal soft tissue and the liver (Fig. 27). The very poorly vascularized malignant fibrous histiocytoma (Fig. 26d) was indistinguishable from renal cell carcinoma by MRI.

5.4 Renal Lymphoma

Although renal involvement by lymphoma in autopsy materials is found in approximately one-third of cases, its premortem diagnosis is rare [28]. MRI in diffuse renal lymphoma demonstrates enlargement of the kidney with some loss of corticomedullary demarcation and a relatively low signal from the tumor mass (long T1) on T1 weighted scans (Fig. 28).

5.5 Metastatic Renal Tumors

Experience with metastatic lesions to the kidney is limited [16, 22]. The few lesions which have been described have demonstrated low signal in-

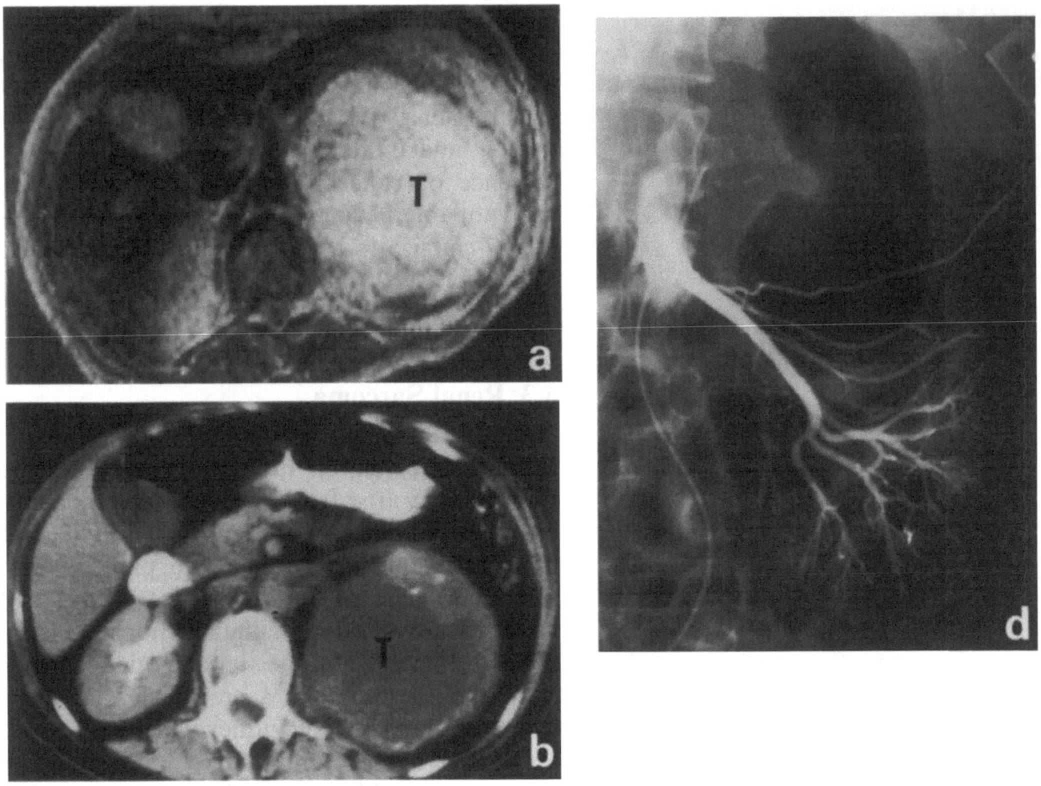

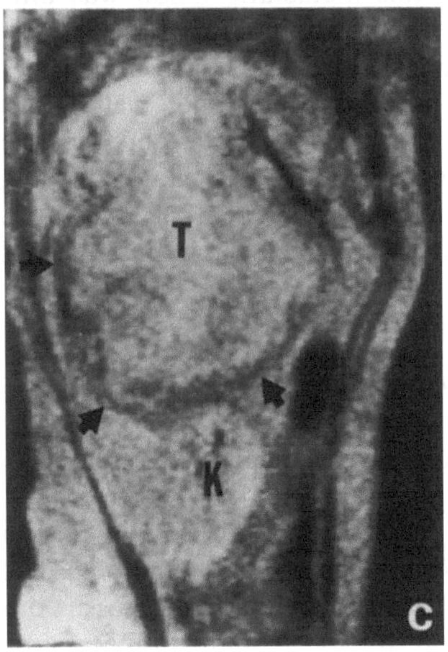

Fig. 26 a–d. Malignant fibrous histiocytoma of the left kidney. **a** Axial T2 weighted MRI scan (SE 2000/60). Large tumor (*T*) of high and mixed signal intensity involving the upper pole of the left kidney. The sarcomatous tumor is indistinguishable from renal cell carcinoma. **b** Contrast enhanced CT shows that the tumor (*t*) is poorly vascularized. **c** The sagittal T2 weighted MRI scan helps to determine the extent of the tumor which is surrounded by a pseudocapsule (*arrows*). K, kidney. **d** Angiogram for comparison. The left kidney is displaced caudad by a poorly vascularized tumor involving the upper pole of the kidney

tensity masses on T1 weighted images. Choykee [22] described two cases where the metastatic renal lesions (from breast and lung carcinoma) were uniformly low in signal intensity. The authors suggested that since well-differentiated adenocarcinomas contain little lipid, it may be possible to differentiate metastatic lesions from primary renal cell carcinomas. Many more cases will be needed to evaluate this hypothesis.

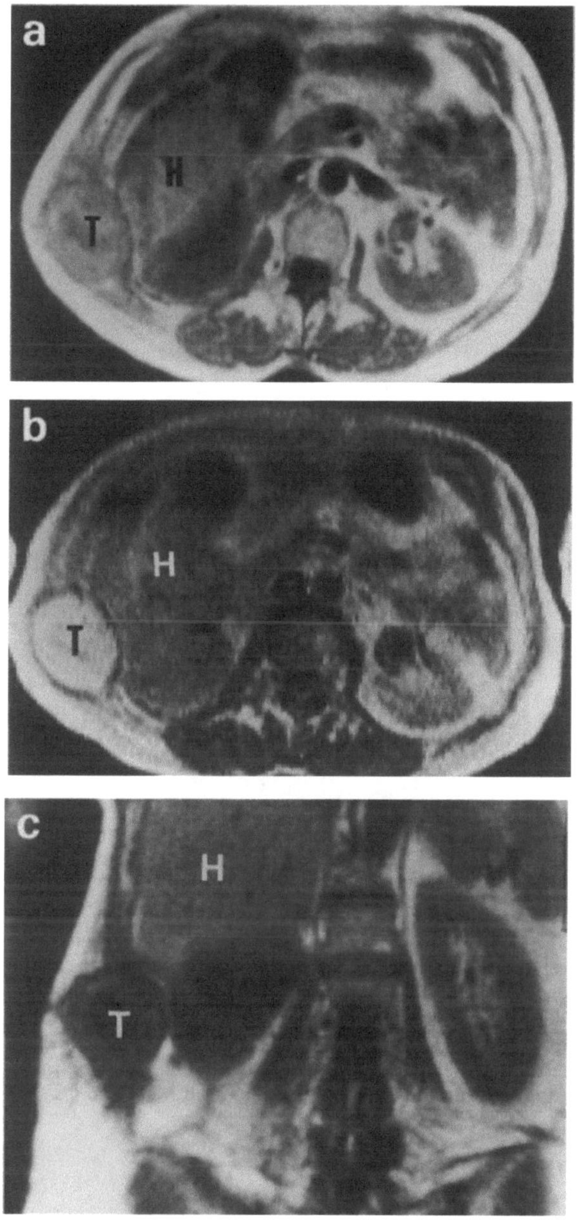

Fig. 27 a–c. Metastatic renal leiomyosarcoma, status post right nephrectomy. The center of the tumor (*T*) in the right flank is necrotic (lower signal intensity). The tumor is outlined by a pseudocapsule and well-defined against the liver (*H*). **a** T1 weighted (SE 500/30), **b** T2 weighted (SE 2000/90) MRI scans, and **c** Coronal T1 weighted scan

6 Differential Diagnosis – Malignant vs Benign Lesions

Unfortunately, MRI has not added much to the specific determination of certain benign from malignant lesions. However, solid renal masses (primary or metastatic) and renal abscesses can readily be differentiated from simple renal cysts using MRI. Current experience suggests that MRI will have an accuracy level comparable to CT in the diagnosis of simple cysts. MRI does show promise in providing more information concerning hemorrhagic cysts and gives some clue to the age of the hemorrhage.

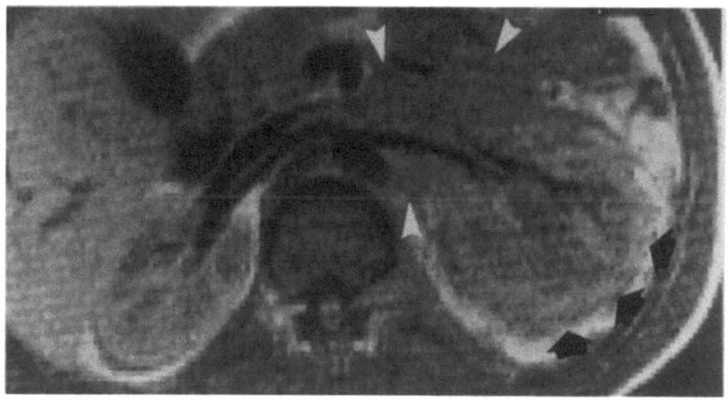

Fig. 28. Renal T-cell lymphoma, axial T1 weighted MRI scan (SE 500/30). The left kidney is enlarged and diffusely infiltrated by the tumor. Corticomedullary demarcation is preserved in the posterior aspect of the kidney (*black arrows*). Retroperitoneal adenopathy is present (*white arrowheads*). Both renal arteries and the right renal vein are well demonstrated on this scan. The right kidney is normal

The ability to differentiate various solid lesions or even determine the malignancy or not of a particular solid lesion is still difficult, even impossible except in a few instances (e.g., angiomyolipoma). One dependable finding regarding renal cell carcinoma or other malignancies when compared with the normal renal parenchyma is a prolonged T1 value for malignant tissue. This assumes that hemorrhagic areas are not included in the area of interest. Other characteristics which support the diagnosis of a malignancy are nonuniform MRI intensities, irregular mass margins, evidence of local invasion, and distant metastases. Tumors which are isointense with renal parenchyma can be diagnosed only when they protrude beyond the renal outline (Fig. 15).

As in CT angiomyolipoma is the only solid tumor which can be accurately diagnosed by MRI (Fig. 13). The high signal intensity of the fat in these lesions on T1 weighted images is characteristic. Hemorrhagic cysts may also have a very high signal intensity but they are very homogenous (Fig. 4). At the opposite end of the scale, no solid lesions to date have demonstrated image intensities as low as those of simple cysts [7, 8].

7 Conclusion

The main impact of MRI in renal imaging most likely will be in the area of staging of renal malignancies [6]. The ability to assess tumor characteristics, evaluate vessel patency without intravenous contrast, and to diagnose local and regional metastasis in several imaging planes in one examination is exciting and may be cost-effective. Nevertheless, further investigations, including studies with experimental animal models and controlled comparisons with other imaging modalities, are needed to determine the exact diagnostic value of MRI in renal tumors.

It is not yet known whether MRI can demonstrate a mass in the kidney which is not demonstrable by CT, ultrasound, or angiography. The smallest malignant renal tumor which we have diagnosed with MRI measured approximately 2 cm (Fig. 15a). The diagnosis in this case was made, however, by contour changes and not by signal intensity differences. These small isointense lesions may be seen better by CT (Fig. 29). The diagnosis of small transitional cell carcinomas is also a problem, as it requires higher resolution and a low signal to noise ratio.

The usefulness of gadolinium in evaluating renal lesions [9] has yet to be determined. Administration of gadolinium-DTPA causes enhancement of vascular tumors by a T1 shortening effect [9, 29, 30], and it may be helpful in diagnosing smaller tumors and assessing tumor vascularity.

We will continue to use MRI in renal mass lesions to gain further experience with it and to supplement the use (due to scheduling problems) of CT. It is of interest to note that referring physicians have come to prefer the MRI because coronal and/or parasagittal scans offer as good an overview in topographic anatomy as they are used to seeing on excretory urography or angiography. It also demonstrates the craniocaudal extent of the disease. This interest by the referring physicians for MRI is important because it has stimulated them to provide the radiologist with more exact clinical histories, which is an important factor in our efforts to differentiate malignancy from inflammatory or traumatic lesions of the kidney.

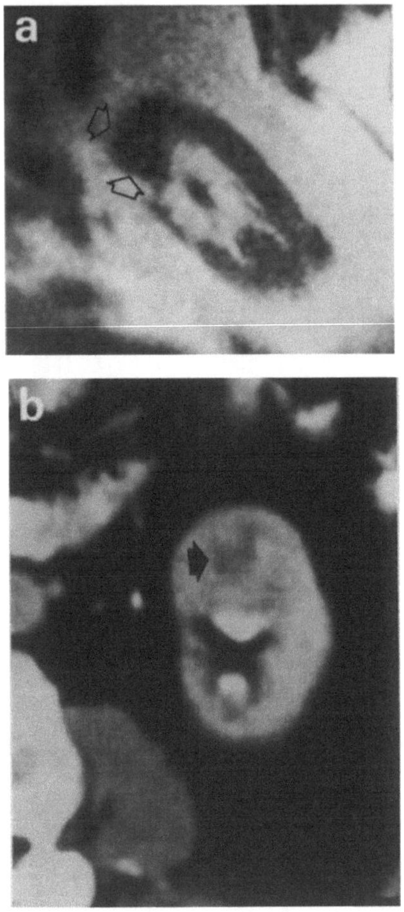

Fig. 29 a, b. Small renal cell carcinoma. **a** Parasagittal T1 weighted MRI scan (SE 500/30). The small tumor in the upper pole of the left kidney is barely demonstrable (*arrows*). Its signal intensity is perhaps slightly lower than that of renal parenchyma. **b** CT scan shows the tumor (*arrow*) better than MRI. (A simultaneously present 2 cm size transitional cell carcinoma was missed by both MRI and CT)

The advantage of a 0.15 T resistive magnet in clinical employment is its cost-effectiveness in comparison to superconductive scanners. The renal lesions we have been able to examine with our 0.15 T unit were all as well-defined as those reported in the literature with the use of higher strength field magnets. However, it is important that a competent staff of radiologists and physicists develop the imaging ability of a low strength field resistive magnet unit to its optimum. This development should include meticulous monitoring of the equipment, design of new software, and special surface coils [31, 32].

References

1. Young IR, Bailes DR, Burl M, Collins AG, Smith DT, McDonnell MJ, Orr JS, Banks LM, Bydder GM, Greenspan RH, Steiner RE (1982) Initial clinical evaluation of a whole body nuclear magnetic resonance (NMR) tomograph. JCAT 6:1–18
2. Alfidi RJ, Haaga JR, El Yousef SJ, Bryan PJ, Fletcher BD, LiPuma JP, Morrison SC, Kaufman B, Richey JB, Hinshaw WS, Kramer DM, Yeung HN, Cohen AM, Butler HE, Ament AE, Lieberman JM (1982) Preliminary experimental results in humans and animals with a superconducting, whole-body nuclear magnetic resonance scanner. Radiology 143:175–181
3. Hricak H, Crooks LE, Sheldon P, Kaufman L (1983) Nuclear magnetic resonance imaging of the kidney. Radiology 146:525–432
4. Hricak H, Williams RD, Moon KL, Moss AA, Alpers C, Crooks LE, Kaufman L (1983) Nuclear magnetic resonance imaging of the kidney: renal masses. Radiology 147:765–772
5. Kressel HY, Axel L, Thickman D, Alavi A, Pollack H, Arger P, Edelstein W, Bottomly P, Redington R, Baum S (1983) NMR imaging of the abdomen at 0.12 T: initial clinical experience with a resistive magnet. AJR 141:1179–1186
6. Hricak H, Demas BE, Williams RD, McNamara MT, Hedgcock MW, Amparo EG, Tonagho EA (1985) Magnetic resonance imaging in the diagnosis and staging of renal and perirenal neoplasms. Radiology 154:709–715
7. Li Puma JP (1984) Magnetic resonance imaging of the kidney. Radiol Clin North Am 22:925–941
8. Li Puma JP, Bryan PJ (1985) MRI of the genitourinary tract, in: Kressels HY (ed) Magnetic resonance annual. Raven, New York, pp 149–196
9. Leung AWL, Bydder GM, Steiner RE, Bryant DJ, Young IR (1984) Magnetic resonance imaging of the kidneys. AJR 143:1215–1227

9a. Fiegler W, Felix R, Nagel R, Schörner W, Clausen C (1984) Die Kernspintomographie bei raumfordernden Nierenprozessen. RÖFO 141:155–159

10. Soila KP, Viamonte M Jr, Starewicz PM (1985) Chemical shift misregistration effect in magnetic resonance imaging. Radiology 153:819–820
11. Kaude JV, Kekomäki M, Walker D, Fitzsimmons JR (1984) Imaging of unilateral hydronephrosis in an experimental animal model – with special reference to magnetic resonance. Acta Radiol Diagn 25:501–506
12. Kaude JV, Williams CM, Millner MR, Scott KN, Finlayson B (1985) Renal morphology and function immediately after extracorporeal shock wave lithotripsy. AJR 145:305–313
13. Hamlin DJ, Ackerman N, Kaude JV, Fitzsimmons JR, Gaskin JM (1985) Magnetic resonance imaging of renal abscess in an experimental animal model. Acta Radiol Diagn 26:315–319
14. Geisinger MA, Risings B, Jordon ML, Zelch MG, Novik AC, George CR (1984) Magnetic resonance imaging of renal transplants. AJR 143:1229–1234
15. Dunbar K, Salomon D, Wingo C, Peterson J, Croker B, Kaude J, Thompson R, Tischer C (1985) Loss of corticomedullary demarcation on magnetic resonance imaging: an index of biopsy-proven acute renal transplant dysfunction. Scientific exhibit, 18th annual meeting. Am Soc Nephrol, New Orleans
16. Kulkarni MV, Shaff MI, Sandler MP, Tishler J, Winfield AC, Patton JA, Wolfe O, Partain CL, James AE (1984) Evaluation of renal masses by MR imaging. J CAT 8:861–865
17. Amendola MA, Glazer GM, Alsen AM, Lande IM (1985) MR imaging of renal masses. Radiology 157(P):384
18. Sipponen JT, Sipponen RE, Sivula A (1983) Nuclear magnetic resonance (NMR) imaging of intracerebral hemorrhage in the acute and resolving phases. J CAT 8:599–607
19. Swensen SJ, Keller PL, Berquist TH, McLeod A, Stephens DH (1985) Magnetic resonance imaging of hemorrhage. AJR 145:921–927
20. Millner MR, Kaude JV, Williams CM, Finlayson B, Newman RC, Hunter PT (1985) Early effects of extracorporeal shock wave lithotripsy on renal function and morphology. Radiology 157(P):385
21. Dooms GC, Hricak H, Sollitto RA, Higgins CB (1985) Lipomatous tumors and tumors with fatty component: MR imaging potential and comparison of MR and CT results. Radiology 157:479–483
22. Choykee PL, Kressel HY, Pollack HM, Arger PM, Axel L, Mamourian AC (1984) Focal renal masses: magnetic resonance imaging. Radiology 152:471–477

22a. Herman SD, Friedman AC, Siegelbaum M, Ramchandani P, Radecki PD (1985) Magnetic resonance imaging of papillary renal carcinoma. Urol Radiol 7:168–171

23. Pettersson H, Springfield D, Hamlin D, Scott K (1985) Magnetic resonance imaging and tissue characterization of a renal cell carcinoma and its osseous metastases. Acta Radiol Diagn 26:193–195
24. Hricak H, Amparo EG, Fisher MR, Crooks LE, Higgins B (1985) Abdominal venous system: assessment using MR. Radiology 156:415–422
25. Amparo EG, Hricak H, Higgins CB (1984) MR evaluation of venous thrombosis and other venous abnormalities associated with neoplasms. Radiology 153(P):168
26. Dooms GC, Hricak H, Crooks LE, Higgins CB (1984) Magnetic resonance imaging of lymph nodes: demonstration by MRI in comparison with CT. Radiology 153:719 728
27. Lee JKT, Heiken JP, Ling D, Glazer HS, Balfe DM, Levitt RG, Dixon WT, Murphy WA (1984) Magnetic resonance imaging of abdominal and pelvic lymphadenopathy. Radiology 153:181–188
28. Richmond J, Sherman RS, Diamond HD, Craver LF (1952) Renal lesions associated with malignant lymphomas. Am J Med 32:184
29. Brasch RC (1983) Work in progress. Methods of contrast enhancement for NMR imaging and potential application. Radiology 147:781–788
30. Strich G, Hagan DL, Gerber KH, Shutsky RA (1985) Tissue distribution and magnetic resonance: open lattice relaxation effects of Gadolinium-DTPA. Radiology 154:723–726
31. Edelman RR, McFuland E, Stark DD, Ferrucci JT, Simeone JF, Wismer GW, White EM, Rosen E, Brady TJ (1985) Surface coil imaging of abdominal viscera. Radiology 157:425–430
32. Fitzsimmons JR, Thomas RG, Mancuso AA (1985) Proton imaging with surface coils on a 0.15 T resistive system. Magnetic Resonance Med 2:180–185

^{125}I Embolotherapy of Renal Tumors

E.K. LANG

1 Introduction

Radical nephrectomy is the procedure of choice for management of (ROBSON) stage 1 and 2 renal cell carcinomas (Table 1) [1–3]. Expanded surgical procedures have made possible the attack and successful removal of tumor extensions into the inferior vena cava and even into the right atrium and ventricle [4–8]. The 5-year survival rate for stage 1 and 2 renal cell carcinomas managed by radical nephrectomy has been reported as 67% and 51% respectively [3]. Even in patients with tumor extension into the inferior vena cava, the infrahepatic segment of the inferior vena cava, or the right atrium, 30–40 percentile 5-year survival rates are reported for surgical procedures extirpating the primary lesion and intravascular tumor extension [6–8].

However, even the most aggressive surgical techniques appear to fail when confronted with metastatic disease to lymph nodes or with multiple distant metastases [9–13]. Theoretically, lymphadenectomy should be capable of controlling spread via the lymphatics; however, some authors report 5-year survival rates as low as 17% in this group of patients [13]. Although resection of presumed isolated metastases and the primary neoplasm has some anecdotal success, the 5-year survival rate is quite low perhaps because of other unrecognized but coexistent metastatic disease [14, 15]. For this reason efforts have been focused on developing adjunctive therapeutic measures for the management of renal cell carcinoma with known lymph node and/or distant metastases [15, 16].

Table 1. Staging of renal cell carcinoma (adapted from [1])

Stage 1:	neoplasm limited to kidney
Stage 2:	neoplasm extending into perirenal space
Stage 3a:	neoplasm extending into renal vein or inferior vena cava
Stage 3b:	neoplasm involving regional lymph nodes
Stage 3c:	neoplasm involving both venous and lymphatic system
Stage 4:	distant metastases

To date chemotherapy has shown only limited success in the treatment of such lesions [17]. Since renal cell carcinoma is a highly immunogenic tumor, immunotherapy should be effective. However, in practice a variety of procedures inducing host immune response (active immunotherapy) as well as passive immunotherapy by infusion of β-interferon have not substantially improved patient survival rates [16, 18–21]. Response to hormone therapy likewise has been inconsistent [22–26].

Transcatheter embolization of the primary tumor and sometimes symptomatic metastases with inert embolic material has been touted as a modality that stimulates the host immune response while ablating tumor volume and reducing tumor burden [26–29]. Despite initial laudatory reports, the results have not been reproducible and definitive improvement of either survival statistics or regression of metastastic disease has not been shown [30].

Transcatheter embolization with radioactive infarct particles has been advocated to accomplish the same goal [31–37]. High dose interstitial radiation therapy reduces the tumor volume while products released from the necrotic tumor serve as an antigenic stimulant of the host immune response mechanism. The mechanism may be akin to the immunostimulation resulting from percutaneously injected irradiated and polymerized tumor cells [38].

2 Concepts Governing Transcatheter Interstitial Radiation Therapy

Although classified as radioinsensitive neoplasm, renal cell carcinoma does respond to high radiation doses in the range from 80–160 Gy. Such radiation therapy results in a significant reduction of tumor volume. Renal cell carcinoma is highly immunogenic. Therefore, once the tumor burden is reduced and the host immune response stimulated and improved, remission and/or stabilization of the metastases may be induced.

External radiation therapy with an attendant high integral dose to the host may adversely affect the host immune response. However, interstitial radiation therapy concentrates absorbed radiant energy almost exclusively into the tumor while keeping the integral dose to the host to a minimum [34–37]. The effective range of radiation is determined by the physical characteristics of the radionuclide used [34, 35]. Thus absorption of radiant energy can be restricted within a determined radius and given volume of tissue.

^{125}I is a radiopharmaceutical ideally suited to this purpose. The low energy levels (27 and 35 keV) guarantee, for practical purposes, absorption of the radiant energy within a few centimeters of tissue thickness. Thus there is a rapid falloff of dose in adjacent tissues. The long half-life (69.6 days) results in sustained irradiation for several months. This increases the probability of irradiating cells during their mitotic phase at which time they tend to be most sensitive to radiation damage [34–37].

An interstitial radioactive implant into the tumor can be created by transcatheter embolization of the tumor's vascular bed with radioactive particles. These particles need be of a size that will be stopped in muscular-sized arteries. Occlusion at such a location permits perfusion of the distal vascular bed via collaterals. The abundant neovascularity of a renal cell carcinoma and the extensive collateral network guarantee adequate oxygenation of the tissues despite these occlusions of the occasional muscular-sized vessel [34–37]. Continued oxygenation is imperative for radiobiologic effectiveness of radiation therapy.

To achieve homogeneous radiation of the tumor the sources must be spaced evenly throughout the volume. Although this is difficult to accomplish by random infarction, techniques capitalizing on preferential flow characteristics can produce such a distribution pattern using fractional infarction.

Sustained radiation reduces the tumor burden. Decay products of the necrotic tumor elements are released into the circulation and provide for antigenic stimulation of the host immune system. This protracted process appears better capable of providing stimulation of the host immune mechanism than the short-lived exposure to such byproducts attendant on transcatheter embolization of renal cell carcinoma with inert embolic material and subsequent surgical resection of tumor and host kidney usually within 1 week [27–37].

3 Technique

Radioactive particles necessary to create an interstitial implant capable of delivering a dose of approximately 160 Gy to the tumor need be deployed. To achieve acceptably homogeneous irradiation the radioactive particles must be spaced evenly throughout the tumor. This could be achieved by superselective embolization of innumerable tumor branch vessels [31–33] (Fig. 1c). However, an equally acceptable distribution of infarct particles results from fractional embolization, deploying the infarct particles during at least three separate sessions. The basis for improved distribution by this modification rests upon induced changes in vascular perfusion.

Infarct particles released into the major tumor supply vessel distribute according to preferential flow. Thus heavily perfused tumor areas will receive more of the radioactive infarct particles. Within 3–4 weeks fibrosis induced by the radiation will substantially alter perfusion characteristics. Tumor components, initially with a low perfusion, will now demonstrate relatively prominent perfusion whereas those areas heavily seeded by the first crop of radioactive infarct particles tend to show marked reduction in vascular perfusion [34–37] (Fig. 1b). A second crop of radioactive infarct particles will therefore distribute to different areas of the tumor. A third or subsequent release of radioactive infarct particles will seek still different locations in the tumor. Thus homogeneity of distribution of infarct particles will be improved by fractional embolization separated adequately en-

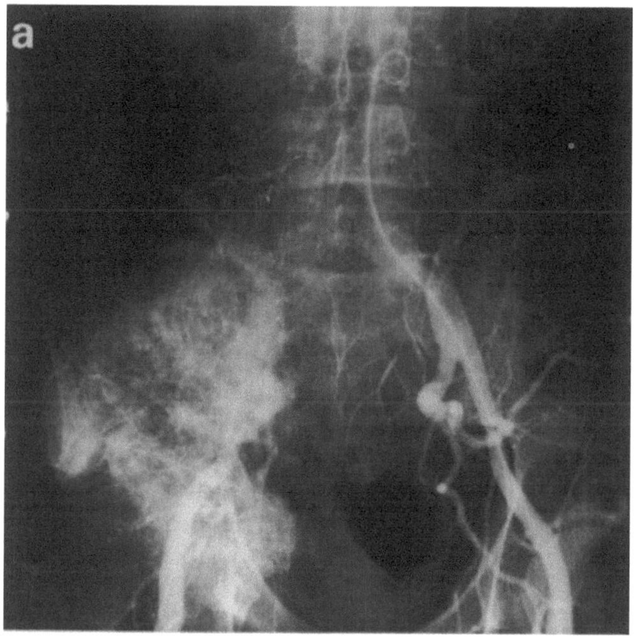

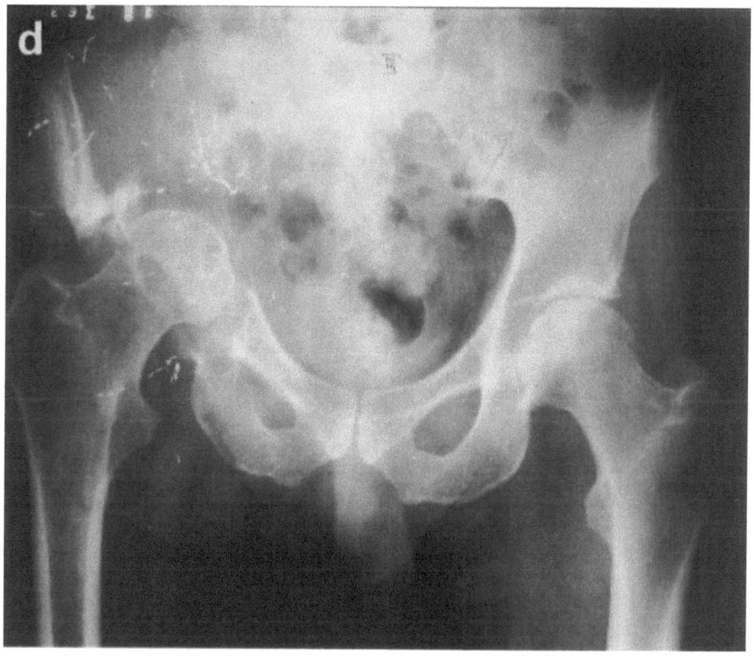

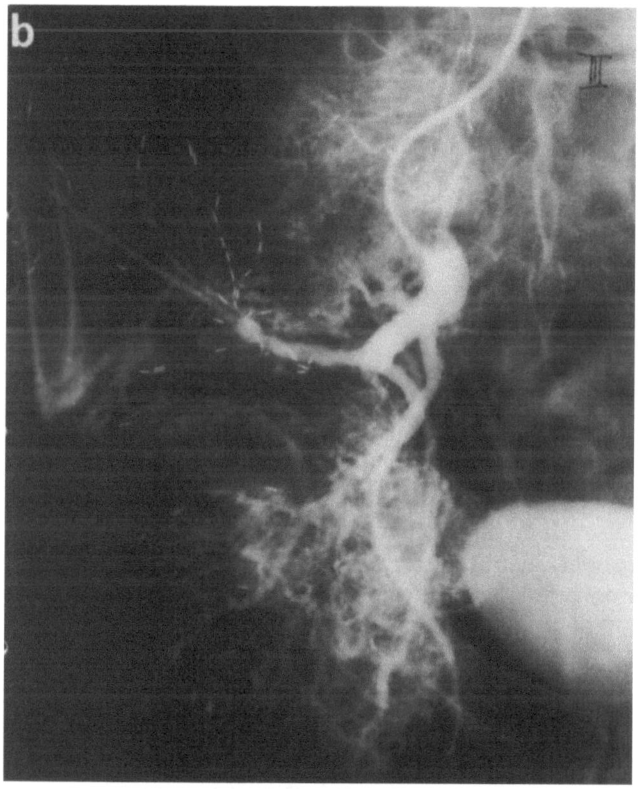

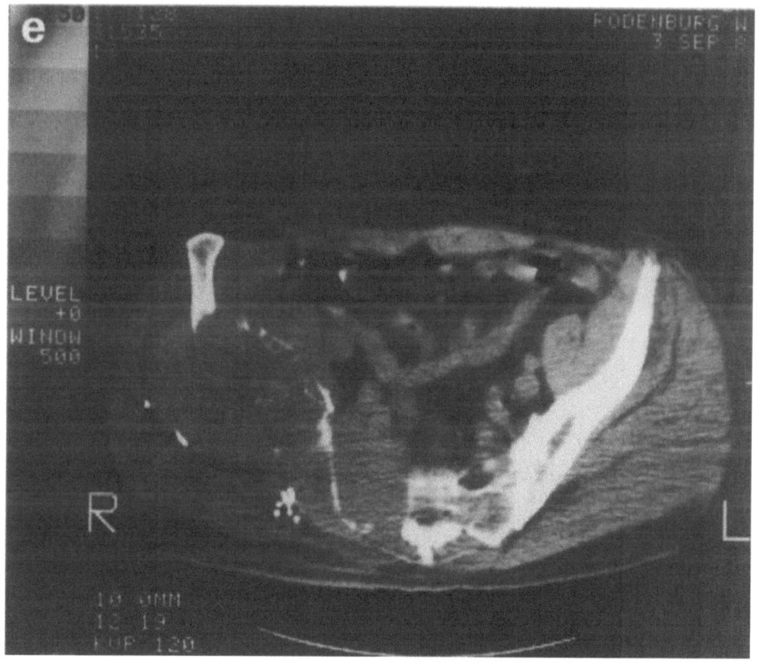

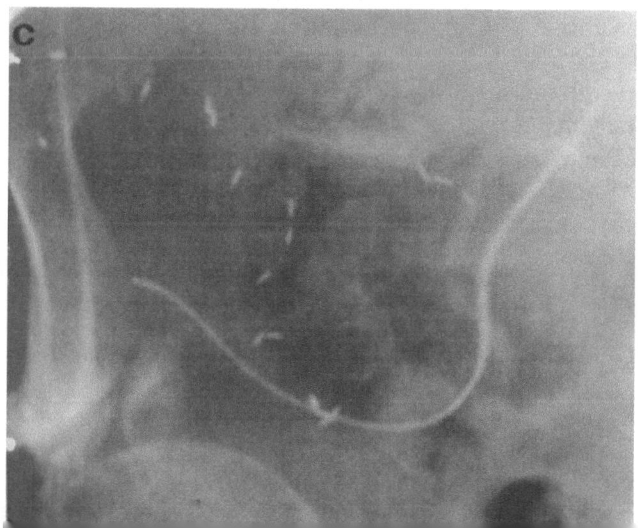

Fig. 1. a A runoff arteriogram demonstrates an enormous hypervascular metastasis destroying the right ilium and acetabulum. **b** A selective hypogastric arteriogram demonstrates residual abundant tumor neovascularity along the sacroiliac joint and the inferior circumference of the acetabulum with prominent tumor masses extending directly into the true pelvis. Note the remarkable change of the peripheral tumor components previously seeded with ^{125}I seeds. **c** Superselective catheterization of tumor branch vessels that have not received radioactive infarct particles during preceeding embolization procedures is carried out. **d** A final film demonstrates salutory distribution of ^{125}I particles throughout the entire tumor-bearing area. **e** Several months after the interstitial infarct implant has been seeded there is marked regression of tumor volume and the beginning of remineralization particularly in the roof of the acetabulum as shown on this CT scan

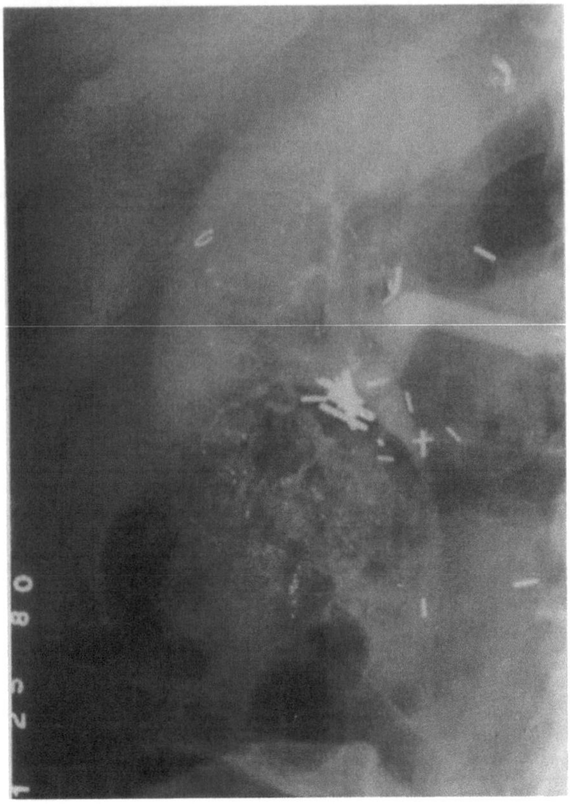

Fig. 2. A satisfactory distribution of radioactive infarct particles is accomplished utilizing fractional embolization techniques in a huge metastasis to the contralateral kidney. Note that the uninvolved cortex of the upper pole of the kidney has been spared, permitting continued satisfactory renal function. Innumerable clips in the hilar area of the kidney refer to a prior, aborted, bench surgery

ough in time to induce changes of flow characteristics within the tumor (Figs. 1a, b, 2).

The then still existing disparity in concentration of seeds in various regions of the neoplasm is not entirely unwelcome since it reflects increased flow to actively growing tumor components; these will attract a higher concentration of seeds.

The size of the radioactive particles, 0.8×4.3 mm, determines the site of lodging. Usually they will lodge in muscular-sized arteries. This location is desirable as it permits retrograde collateral perfusion of the vascular bed distal to the ^{125}I particle. The marked hypervascularity of most renal cell carcinomas safeguards against any appreciable reduction of perfusion following this transcatheter embolization. The oxygen tension in tumor tissues is not diminished, and the radiobiologic effectiveness of radiation therapy is not impaired [34–37].

The dosage in millicuries of ^{125}I necessary to deliver the desired radiation to the tumor is precalculated from Patterson-Parker tables for a tumor volume determined from the CT scan [34–37]. This total dose is distributed in equal fractions to a large number of seeds, from 40 to 100. The larger the number of seeds, the more even the distribution throughout the tumor.

Commercially available ^{125}I seeds fit through a 5.8 French catheter (0.038). The seeds can be loaded with long tweezers into the flared end of the catheter and ejaculated into the tumor circulation with a 0.0038 guide wire or an appropriately adapted implant gun. The location of the seeds is then ascertained on CT scans. Computers calculate the dose as contributed from multiple point sources (i.e., individual ^{125}I seeds) (Fig. 1c).

Progressive shrinkage of the neoplasm results in increased clustering of the individual sources, and recalculation of the dose rate is necessary every 4 weeks [34–37]. The final dose is established as the mean of the interval dose rates (Fig. 3).

4 Clinical Results

While 5-year survival rates for surgically treated stage 1 and stage 2 renal cell carcinomas are in an acceptable range of 50%–66%, the survival rate for stage 4 carcinomas treated similarly is a dismal 13% [3]. Though angioinfarction, subsequent nephrectomy, and postoperative progesterone therapy have significantly improved 1-year survival of patients with pulmonary metastases up to 64%, the 5-year survival for mixed metastases thus treated remains a dismal 10% [29]. The 2-year survival rate for patients treated with a radioactive infarct implant to the primary tumor site and often to metastases is about 40%, the 5-year survival rate 31% (Table 2).

Survival rates, however, vary greatly for different metastatic sites. Of 40 patients with osseous metastases 22 survived 2 years, and 7 of 18 survived 5 years. Conversely there were no 2- or 5-year survivors among patients with brain metastases and only one 5-year survivor among patients with soft tissue metastases (Table 3).

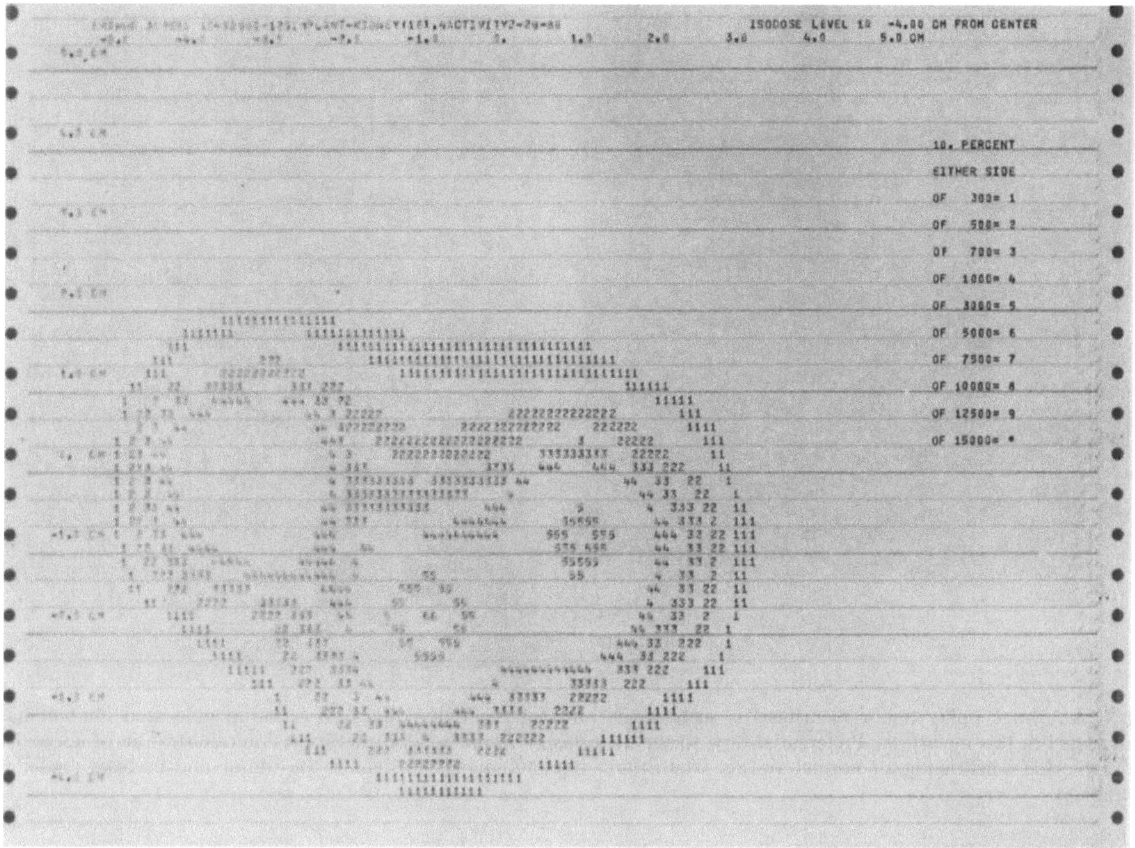

Fig. 3. A computer printout demonstrates the dose rate to the infarcted tumor after one crop of ^{125}I seeds has been sited. Note the rapid falloff of dose rate in the periphery. Progressive shrinkage of the tumor will decrease the distance between the sources and increase the dose rate. This is taken into consideration by subsequent dose calculations

Table 2. Survival of patients treated by transcatheter embolization with ^{125}I and sometimes adjunctive therapy for various stages of metastatic renal cell carcinoma

Stage	Survival		
	2 years	5 years	10 years
$T_4NX_4M_1$	11–28	6–17	1–9
$T_3NX_4M_1$	21–52	7–24	0–13
$T_2NX_2M_1$	1–2	0–1	–/–

Table 3. Survival of patients treated by transcatheter embolization with ^{125}I seeds for metastatic renal cell carcinoma

Location of metastases	Survival		
	2 years	5 years	10 years
Skeletal	7/11	2/5	0/1
Skeletal and pulmonary	8/15	3/8	0/4
Skeletal and others	7/14	2/5	0/2
Pulmonary	2/9	1/5	0/3
Pulmonary and others	2/8	1/4	0/2
Other parenchymal	2/12	1/5	0/3
Central nervous system	0/3	0/2	0/1
Soft tissue	1/5	1/3	0/1

Similarly less than 25% of the patients with pulmonary metastases survived 2 years and less than 20%, 5 years.

Part of the explanation for the better treatment results in patients with skeletal metastases may lie in the aggressive treatment approach towards such metastases. In addition to the primary neoplasm, skeletal metastases were routinely seeded with ^{125}I particles (Figs. 1 b–d). Conversely, central nervous system metastases were never seeded, and only in 2 of 32 patients with pulmonary metastases transcatheter embolization with ^{125}I seeds was attempted.

A significant reduction of tumor volume is appreciated within 90 days after an interstitial

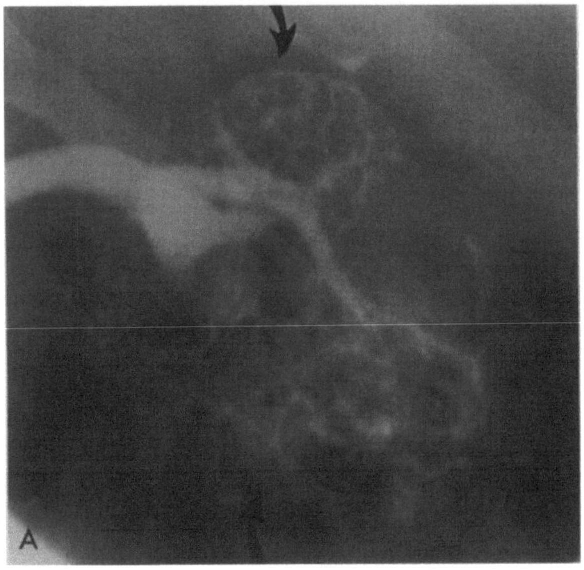

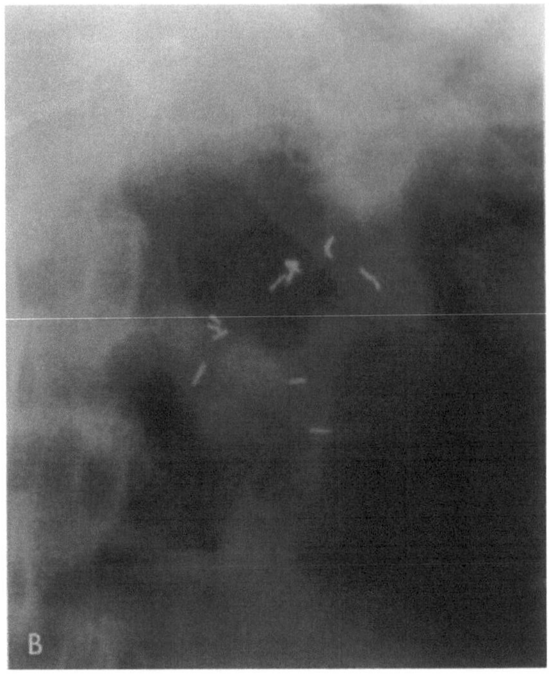

Fig. 4. A A huge bulky tumor metastasis is seen in the hilus of the right kidney. **B** A radon gold seed implant has been seated in this metastasis. Preferential flow to the metastasis was created by intraarterial administration of adrenalin hydrochloride constricting all normal vessels. The infarct implant intends to debulk the tumor and perhaps render it operable

infarct implant has been performed and about 70% of the total dose delivered. After four half-lives have elapsed, 94% of the total dose is delivered and the tumor has regressed maximally, on average to 10% of its original size. Despite the massive regression of the tumor, biopsies tend to reveal viable tumor cell nests surrounded by areas of fibrosis [32, 33].

In addition to the reduction of volume, there is evidence suggesting remission of tumor activity. This is expressed by weight gain, cessation of pain and hematuria, if present, and normalization of laboratory indicators such as erythrocyte sedimentation rate and tumor markers. These plus a rise in the β-interferon levels appear to parallel the course of clinical remission [33–37].

Once again, patients with osseous metastases fared better than patients with metastases to all other locations. Of patients with osseous metastases 55% experienced a prolonged remission of tumor activity for up to 2 years. In 38% of these the remission lasted for 5 years or better (Table 3). The best results were encountered in patients with solitary skeletal metastases. Remission of tumor activity was observed in over 60% for 2 years and in 40% for 5 years. A marked rise in β-interferon levels and an improved response to the blastomyces skin test suggest a potent host immune response.

Despite initial salutory response the neoplasm appeared to ultimately resume its inexorable course. We have observed only one 10-year survivor among some 22 patients at risk who were treated with radioactive infarct implant and other adjuvant therapy.

Strong presumptive evidence (normalization of erythrocyte sedimentation rate, disappearance of tumor markers, and rise of β-interferon levels) suggests an altered and improved host immune response as a major factor in inducing the remission and significantly improving the survival potential. Since this effect depends on sustained stimulation it appears unlikely that a similar beneficial result can be induced and completed within 7 days after total infarction of the tumor with inert embolic material and prior to its surgical resection as advocated by others [27–30].

Transcatheter embolization with ^{125}I and treatment by interstitial radiation therapy appears to be the most effective method for palliating metastatic renal cell carcinoma, particularly skeletal metastases. The addition of adjuvant therapy such as chemotherapy deploying microencapsulated mitomycine c, immunotherapy, or hormone therapy awaits evaluation by clinical trial [17–25].

Lastly, treatment of advanced and bulky primary renal cell carcinoma by interstitial radiation therapy has proven effective for debulking and downstaging the tumor (Figs. 4a, b). A different radionuclide (RN 222) with a short half-life is used for this purpose. This radionuclide permits delivery of the needed dose level in a short period of time. Its short half-life and rapid dissipation of radiant energy make possible resection of the specimen without undue radiation exposure to the surgical team [31, 32].

References

1. Robson CJ, Churchill BM, Anderson W (1969) The results of radical nephrectomy for renal cell carcinoma. J Urol 101:297–301
2. Freed SZ, Feldman JA, Srayragen S (1977) Follow up of patients after nephrectomy for renal cell carcinoma. Urology 9:500–503
3. McNichols DW, Segura JW, DeWeerd JH (1981) Renal cell carcinoma: long term survival and late recurrence. J Urol 126:17–23
4. Kearney GP, Waters WB, Klein LA, Richie JP, Gittes RF (1981) Results of inferior vena cava resection for renal cell carcinoma. J Urol 125:769–773
5. Cummings JB, Li W, Ryan JA, Horton WG, Paton RR (1979) Operative management of renal cell carcinoma with supradiaphragmatic caval extension. J Urol 122:829–832
6. Waters WB, Richie JP (1979) Aggressive surgical approach to renal cell carcinoma: review of 130 cases. J Urol 122:306–309
7. Novick AC, Cosgrove DM (1980) Surgical approach for removal of renal cell carcinoma extending into the vena cava and the right atrium. J Urol 123:947–950
8. Skinner DG, Pfister RF, Colvin R (1972) Extension of renal cell carcinoma into the vena cava: the rationale for aggressive surgical management. J Urol 107:711–716
9. Giuliani L, Martorana G, Giberti C, Pescatore D, Magnani G (1983) Results of radical nephrectomy with extensive lymphadenectomy for renal cell carcinoma. J Urol 130:664–668
10. Peters PC, Brown GL (1980) The role of lymphadenectomy in the management of renal cell carcinoma. Urol Clin North Am 7:705–709
11. O'Dea MJ, Zincke H, Utz DC, Bernatz PE (1978) The treatment of renal cell carcinoma with solitary metastasis. J Urol 120:540–542
12. Fuselier HA, Guice SL, Brannan W, Ochsner MG, Sangisetty KV, Beckman EN, Barnes CA (1983) Renal cell carcinoma. The Ochsner Medical Institution experience (1945–1978). J Urol 130:445–448
13. DeKernion JB, Ramming KP, Smith RB (1978) The natural history of metastatic renal cell carcinoma: a computer analysis. J Urol 120:148–152
14. Middleton RG (1967) Surgery for metastatic renal cell carcinoma. J Urol 97:973–977
15. Barney JD, Churchill EJ (1939) Adenocarcinoma of the kidney with metastasis to the lung: cured by nephrectomy and lobectomy. J Urol 42:269–276

15a. Hrushesky WJ, Murphy JP (1977) Current status of therapy of advanced renal carcinoma. J Surg Oncol 9:277–288

16. DeKernion JB (1983) Treatment of advanced renal cell carcinoma-Traditional methods and innovative approaches. J Urol 130:2–7
17. Nemoto R, Kato T, Iwata K, et al. (1930) Evaluation of therapeutic arterial embolization in renal cell carcinoma using microencapsulated mytomycin-c. Urology 17:315–319
18. Neidhart JA, Murphy SG, Hennick LA, Wise AJ (1980) Active specific immunotherapy of stage IV renal cell carcinoma with aggregated tumor antigen adjuvant. Cancer 46:1128–1134
19. Montie JE, Bukowski RM, James RE, Straffin RA, Stewart BH (1982) A critical review of immunotherapy of disseminated renal adeno-carcinoma. J Surg Oncol 21:5–8

19a. DeKernion JB, Sarna G, Figlin R, Lindner A, Smith RB (1983) The treatment of renal cell carcinoma with human leukocyte alpha-interferon. J Urol 130:1063–1066

20. Quesada JR, Swanson DA, Trindade A, Gutterman JU (1983) Renal cell carcinoma antitumor effective leukocyte interferon. Cancer Res 43:940–947
21. DeKernion JB, Ramming KP (1980) The therapy of renal adenocarcinoma with immune RNA. Invest Urol 17:378–381
22. Morales A, Kiruluta G, Lott S (1975) Hormones in treatment of metastatic renal cancer. J Urol 114:692–693
23. Pierson J, Friedman MA, Hoffman DJ Jr (1981) Hormone receptor in renal cell carcinoma: their utility as predictors of response to endocrine therapy. Cancer Chemother Pharmacol 6:151
24. Nakno E, Tada Y, Fujioka H, Matsuda M, Osafune M, Kotake T, Sato B, Takaha M, Sonoda T (1984) Hormone receptor in renal cell carcinoma and correlation with clinical response to endocrine therapy. J Urol 132:240–245
25. Satomi Y, Takai S, Kondo I, Fukshima S, Furuhata A (1982) Postoperative prophylactic use of progesterone in renal cell carcinoma. J Urol 128:919–922
26. Arkell DJ, Cotter KP, Fitz-Patrick JD, Shaw RE (1978) Preoperative arterial embolisation of renal carcinoma. Br J Urol 50:469–473
27. Wallace S, Chuang VP, Swanson D, Bracken B, Hersh EM, Ayala A, Johnson D (1981) Embolization of renal carcinoma: experience with 100 patients. Radiology 138:563–570
28. Weigel JW, Mebost WK, Forat JD, Nobel MJ, Voptka T, Krishnan EC, Jewell WR (1985) Treatment of renal cell carcinoma with renal infarction delayed nephrectomy, medroxyprogesterone and xenogeneic immune RNA. Urology 25:103–105
29. Swanson DE, Johnson DE, Von Eschenbach AC, Chuang VP, Wallace S (1983) Angioinfarction plus nephrectomy for metastatic renal cell carcinoma – an update. J Urol 130:449–452

30. Gottesman JE, Crawford ED, Grossman HB, Scardino P, McCrecken JD (1985) Infarction – nephrectomy of metastatic renal cell carcinoma. Urology 25:248–250
31. Lang EK (1970) Superselective arterial catheterization of tumors of the urogenital tract: a modality used for perfusion with chemotherapeutic agents and infarction with radioactive pellets. J Urol 104:16–25
32. Lang EK (1971) Superselective arterial catheterization as a vehicle for delivering radioactive infarct particles to tumors. Radiology 98:391–399
33. Lang EK (1975) Local regional treatment of neoplasm by radioactive infarct particles introduced by arterial catheterization. Panminerva Med 17:398–404
34. Lang EK, DeKernion JB (1981) Transcatheter embolization of advanced renal cell carcinoma with radioactive seeds. J Urol 126:581–586
35. Lang EK, Sullivan F, DeKernion JB (1983) Work in progress: transcatheter embolization of renal cell carcinoma with radioactive infarct particles. Radiology 147:413–418
36. Lang EK (1982) Advanced renal cell carcinoma treatment by transcatheter embolization with inert material and radioactive particles. In: Ariel JM (ed) Prog Clin Cancer 8:299–310. Grune+Stratton, NY
37. Lang EK (1984) Transcatheter embolization of renal cell carcinoma. In: Lang EK (ed) Current concepts of uroradiology, Chapter 12. Williams and Wilkins, Baltimore
38. Prager MD, Baechtel FS, Peters PC, Brown GL, Greene CL (1981) Specific immunotherapy of human metastatic renal cell carcinoma. In: Proceedings American association of cancer research. Am Assoc Clin Oncol 22:163 (abstract 647)

Adrenal Mass Lesions in Infants and Children

J.L. Williams and J.V. Kaude

1 Introduction

Lesions of the adrenal glands in the infant and child are rare. The presence of a palpable mass in the flank is often the only presenting clinical sign in the infant. In the older child, however, disorders in specific endocrine functions usually direct attention to the adrenal gland [4]. Once an abnormality is disclosed by serum biochemical studies, identification of the specific site is often necessary for appropriate therapy or follow-up. In this chapter we will first present the imaging options available and discuss the advantages and disadvantages of each. This will be followed by a more detailed discussion of specific pathologic lesions.

2 Imaging Techniques

2.1 Abdominal Radiography

The normal adrenal is not visible on a plain radiograph of the abdomen. Calcium salts within the parenchyma, if present, only indicate that an insult has been applied to the gland. These calcifications may take several forms, and each pattern may suggest a specific pathological process. Peripheral, curved, thin calcifications may suggest resolving hemorrhage in the stressed newborn [15]. Irregular, clumped calcifications with a mass effect may signal the presence of a tumor [16]. Diffuse calcifications within bilaterally enlarged glands suggests a diagnosis of Wolman's disease [18]. Focal, smooth or irregularly marginated calcifications might suggest the presence of an abscess. Thus, the presence of adrenal calcifications can be helpful in formulating a differential diagnosis.

Xeroradiography, as an excellent edge-enhancing technique, would be expected to demonstrate tiny and subtle calcifications within the adrenals. The radiation dose to the patient is increased, however.

2.2 Excretory Urography

The intravenous administration of iodinated contrast agents which are selectively excreted by the kidneys is a common and useful examination. Films obtained during the capillary phase of perfusion (total body opacification phase) may show a hypervascular tumor or a relatively underperfused one. An adrenal mass may displace a normal kidney caudad, producing a flank mass which is actually the palpable lower renal pole. Excretory urography can reveal that the lesion arises from the adrenal gland rather than the kidney. Downward distortion of the upper pole calices by an adrenal neuroblastoma is known as the "drooping lily" effect [4]. It is important to follow such a study with sequential and delayed films to be certain that the mass is not a primary renal lesion such as an obstructed duplication, simple hydronephrosis, or a renal tumor.

2.3 Ultrasound

Real-time sonography is the preferred initial investigative examination in an infant or child suspected of having any retroperitoneal or abdominal mass, although in many cases an abdominal radiograph may have been obtained earlier. Identification of the organ of origin of the mass often directs the choice of subsequent imaging evaluations [14]. Technical improvements in gray-scale, image resolution, transducer arrays, and image processing have combined to produce excellent images of the adrenals in more than 85% of patients [17]. The absence of ionizing radiation is a most attractive feature for the pediatric patient. Most modern units are portable and allow the examination to be done at the bedside. No preparation or sedation of the patient is required, the technique is noninvasive, and video recording of the study permits repeated review. Multiplane imaging is easily obtained for optimal presentation of an adrenal lesion. Smaller scanheads allow imaging to be carried out through rib interspaces and permit the use of 5, 7.5, or even 10 MHz crystals, for excellent spatial resolution and tissue differentiation.

The right adrenal is best displayed with the patient supine. Using the liver and the inferior vena cava as an acoustic window, transverse, longitudinal, and oblique images of the triangular hypoechoic adrenal can be seen [25]. The right adrenal gland lies posterior to the inferior vena cava, and superior and medial to the upper renal pole. The left gland can usually be found with the patient supine, often using a lateral or coronal approach. Fluid in the stomach may permit improved imaging of the more medial left adrenal, particularly if the patient is placed in the left-side-down decubitus position. Occasionally, placing the patient prone and imaging between the ribs will better demonstrate the left gland.

2.4 Computed Tomography

Computed tomography (CT) is currently the most accurate and easily available imaging modality with which to evaluate the adrenal gland and its relationships with adjacent structures [1, 20]. Fine collimation of the interrogating X-ray beam and short individual section scan time together with good tissue differentiation and enhancement techniques allow for demonstration of small lesions within a normal gland, even in the infant. Current software allows the operator to enlarge images, set "windows" to show faint calcifications, and reconstruct in different planes. Intravenous iodinated contrast illustrates the relative vascularity of a lesion and oral contrast is helpful in differentiation of adjacent or distant lymph nodes from loops of bowel. It is often helpful to obtain both a noncontrast and an enhanced study during the initial work-up.

Some of the disadvantages include a moderate ionizing radiation dose and the fairly remote possibility of a contrast reaction. A more serious limiting factor is the absolute innovability of the unit. Transporting a seriously ill infant or child to the scanner, occasionally requiring sedation and thus possibly inducing hypothermia, make the study less than ideal. Careful attention to these details reduces the incidence of complications.

When the lesion has not yet been localized to the adrenal glands, 1 cm contiguous sections from the diaphragm to the pelvic floor are indicated. Thin sections (3–5 mm) of the adrenal lesion may offer some added information about the immediate anatomy and the tissue characteristics.

Cost and available machine time prevent CT from assuming the role of the primary screening modality unless the clinical index of suspicion is very high.

2.5 Radionuclide Imaging

Radioiodinated cholesterol analogues can be used to image the normal or abnormal adrenal gland [12, 16]. Incorporation of the label into hyperfunctioning parenchyma results in increased focal deposition of the radiopharmaceutical in a portion of the gland, throughout the adrenal, or within a functioning metastasis. As the scintigram is dependent upon biochemical incorporation of the labeled cholesterol, delayed imaging for up to 14 days may be required. More rapid and diagnostically more conclusive imaging procedures have generally replaced this time-consuming technique.

2.6 Angiography

Before the era of high resolution CT and ultrasound, angiography was the imaging modality of choice for the final definition of adrenal mass lesions. In more recent years we have utilized angiography only when the other major investigative modalities have failed to determine the origin or vascular nature of an adrenal lesion. A preoperative angiography will illustrate the vascular supply of a tumor or indicate invasion of adjacent structures (liver, kidney, or inferior vena cava) by a large tumor. The major arterial supply of an adrenal tumor may arise from the inferior phrenic artery, aorta, celiac axis, splenic artery, ipsilateral renal artery, or occasionally branches of the pancreatic arteries of the superior mesenteric artery. Variation in vascular anatomy may significantly affect the appropriate surgical procedure.

Venous sampling for hormonal assays is frequently performed at different levels in the inferior vena cava and selectively in the renal and adrenal veins [2, 8]. The left adrenal vein drains into the left renal vein and the right adrenal vein empties into the inferior vena cava. The venous drainage of the adrenal may also be variable, particularly after earlier operations [2].

A percutaneous approach from the femoral artery or vein is generally used. An aortogram defines the larger vessel anatomy and serves as a guide for selective catheterization. In patients with pheochromocytoma, pretreatment with α- and β-adrenergic blocking agents is necessary, as the injection of contrast may precipitate a hypertensive crisis. Intravenous phentolamine is used for the treatment of a hypertensive episode.

2.7 Magnetic Resonance Imaging

In the last few years MRI has become clinically available [6, 21, 23]. Its most obvious advantage is that images may be reconstructed in almost any plane. Pulse-imaging sequences are variable and illustrate anatomy excellently with acceptable spatial resolution as well as indicating tissue characteristics that separate most abnormal tissue from normal parenchyma.

Our experience derives from a 0.15 Tesla resistive magnet (Technicare, Cleveland, Ohio). Standard vendor-supplied small coils and site-fabricated receiver coils are used, depending upon the region of interest and the physical size of the part to be examined. We utilize three routine spin echo (SE) data acquisitions for imaging of the abdomen. The first T-1 weighted transaxial scans are obtained with a pulse repetition time (TR) of 500 ms and echo delay time (TE) of 30 ms (SE 500/30). A second series of transaxial images is obtained with a multislice-multiecho technique (TR = 2000–2500 ms; TE = 30, 60, 90, 120 ms or TE = 45, 90, 135, 180 ms) for T-2 weighted images to illustrate specific abnormal tissue response. Each of the sections is contiguous and has a slice thickness of 0.6–1 cm. Additional T-1 weighted images (SE 500/30) are usually obtained in the coronal and sometimes sagittal planes.

A major disadvantage of MRI is that the complete examination is long, requiring 8–13 min acquisition time for each sequence, depending upon the pulse-imaging technique chosen. Sedation of the infant or young child is often necessary as motion seriously degrades the image. A lack of paramagnetic response results in nonvisualization of small calcium deposits; larger accretions are inferred by loss of any signal response.

Currently, the accumulated experience of MRI in the adrenal lesions of the infant and young child is limited. Its exact role with respect to ultrasound and CT has yet to be defined.

3 Normal Adrenal Glands

The normal adrenal gland in the newborn (Fig. 1) may be up to one-third to one-half the size of the kidney [4]. This enlargement is normal, and involution occurs over the course of the next few weeks. The gland has an inverted "Y" or "V" shape as it caps the upper pole of the kidney. The normal gland measures from 1–4 cm in length and each limb varies from 0.2–0.5 cm in thickness [17].

The typical ultrasound appearance shows a central medullary echodensity surrounded by a thick hypoechoic cortex. At birth the cortex is mostly composed of a more central fetal cortex that involutes, leaving behind the normal thin (peripheral) adult cortex. The absence of periadrenal fat in the infant favors ultrasound imaging, while the deposition of fat in the older child permits good imaging with CT.

With CT the normal right adrenal is found as a thin sliver of dense tissue adjacent to the right diaphragmatic crus, just behind the inferior vena cava. The left adrenal is located between the anterior aorta and medial left diaphragmatic crus. The radiographic density of the gland is relatively homogeneous, showing less of the cortico-medullary differentiation than is seen with an ultrasound examination.

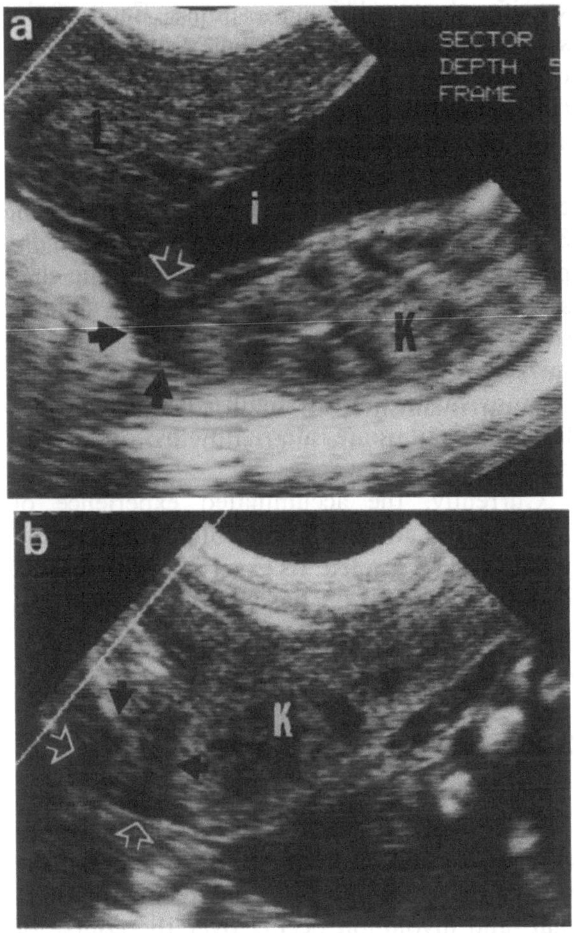

Fig. 1 a, b. Parasagittal real-time sonograms (7.5 MHz transducer) of normal adrenals in a two-week-old infant. **a** right and **b** left adrenal (*arrows*). *K*, kidney; *i*, inferior vena cava; *L*, liver

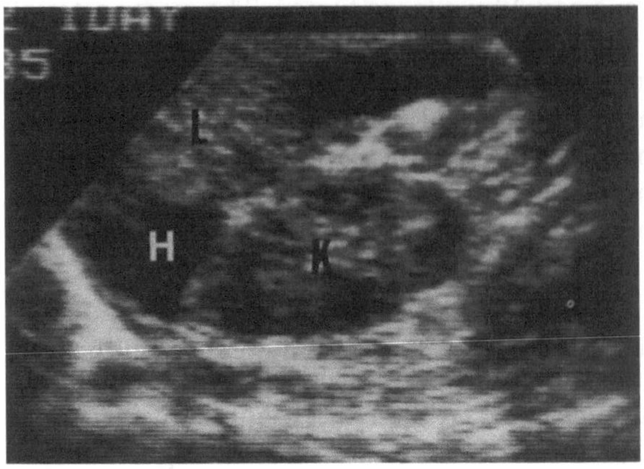

Fig. 2. Parasagittal real-time sonogram (7.5 MHz transducer) of adrenal hemorrhage in a one-day-old infant. This fresh hemorrhage (*H*) is hypoechoic relative to the kidney (*K*) and the liver (*L*)

4 Pathological Lesions

4.1 Congenital Adrenal Hyperplasia

The clinical manifestations of congenital adrenal hyperplasia reflect hyperandrogenism. In the male there is precocious puberty (macrogenitosomia precox), while in the female virilization occurs. If the hyperplasia occurs before birth, distortions in the development of the urogenital sinus or pseudohermaphroditism can be seen in the female infant [4].

Bilateral symmetric enlargement has been found in a newborn infant [9]. The normal cortico-medulla ultrasound pattern is preserved. Treatment with cortisone produces a return to normal adrenal size. In the older child, the cortex is enlarged with the medulla remaining normal. CT illustrates this bilateral nonnodular enlargement well. A recent report indicates that these patients are at increased risk for the development of sarcomatous lesions [7].

4.2 Adrenal Hemorrhage

Hemorrhage into the adrenal gland (Figs. 2–6) is a relatively common event in the newborn period. There is an association with birth trauma, shock, sepsis, diabetic mothers, and intravascular clotting [11]. The hemorrhage occurs within the first week of life and the infant may present with prolonged jaundice or even a palpable flank mass. Massive retroperitoneal hemorrhage is rare and often the adrenal hemorrhage goes unrecognized until later in life when the lesion has calcified (Figs. 4–6) [4]. The right adrenal gland is more often involved (70%) but hemorrhage can be bilateral (10%) [12]. Calcification of the hematoma may be seen within 10 days and show either flocculent central or linear peripheral patterns of calcification.

The initial imaging examination should be an ultrasound examination (Figs. 2 and 3). The acute hemorrhage is usually, but not always, echogenic. For several days following the hemorrhage, lysis of the clot occurs, and the sonographic appearance is anechoic. Later the hem-

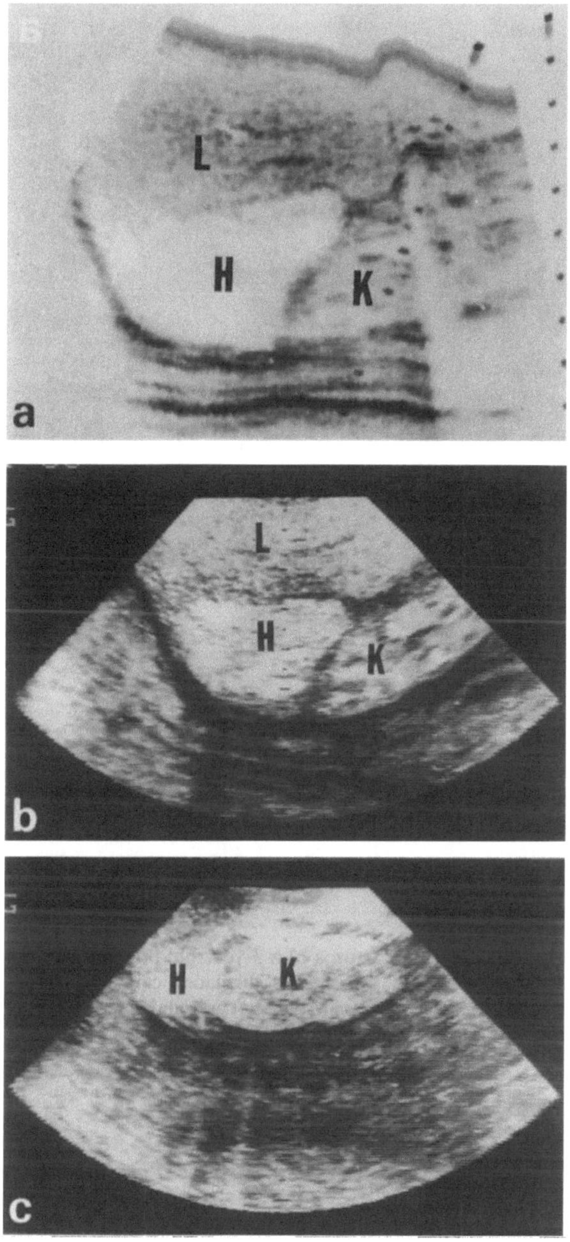

Fig. 3 a–c. Parasagittal sonograms of an adrenal hemorrhage. **a** Large anechoic mass (*H*) of the right adrenal in a 7-day-old infant. *K*, kidney; *L*, liver. **b** At 14 days the hemorrhage contains low intensity echoes. **c** A smaller adrenal hemorrhage is also present on the left [14]

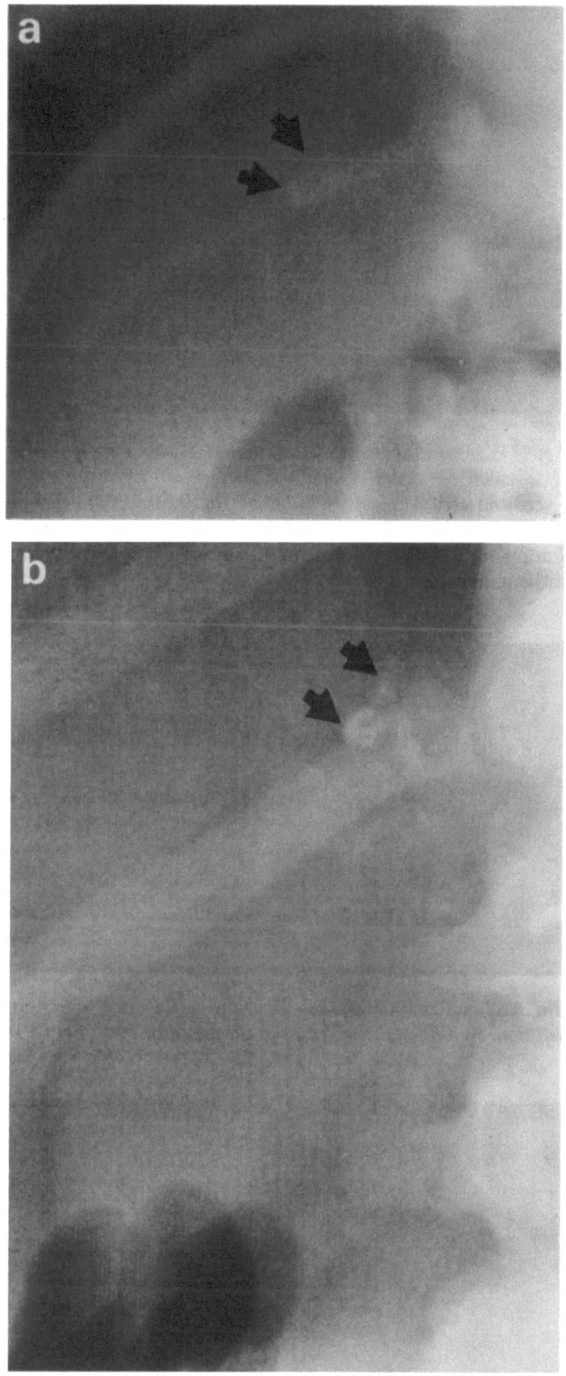

Fig. 4 a, b. Calcified adrenal hemorrhage (*arrow*) in an asymptomatic child **a** at the age of 1 month and **b** at the age of 9 years

orrhage becomes organized and contains low intensity echoes (Fig. 3b). No other imaging procedures are necessary for diagnosis, particularly if the mass becomes smaller or the lesions are bilateral.

The differential diagnoses should include an abscess of the adrenal or a duplex anomaly of the kidney with dilatation of the upper pole system. Less common is a cystic or necrotic neuroblastoma. Lymphoma, histoplasmosis, and tuberculosis are rare causes of an adrenal mass in the young.

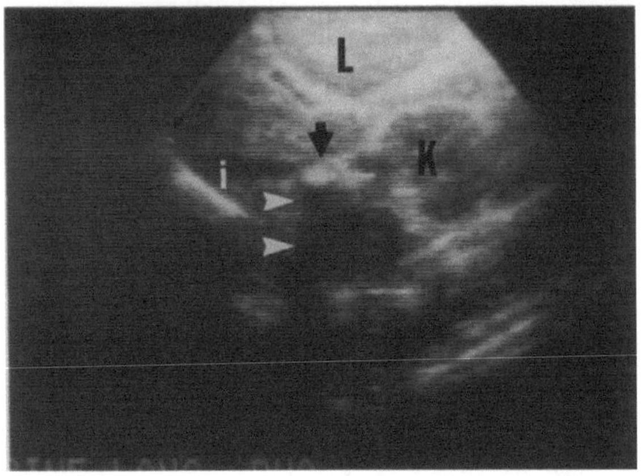

Fig. 5. Parasagittal real-time sonogram (5 MHz transducer) of a calcified adrenal hemorrhage in an asymptomatic 6-year-old girl. The calcification of the right adrenal (*black arrow*) prevents echo transmission and produces acoustic shadowing (*white arrowheads*). *K*, kidney; *L*, liver; *i*, inferior vena cava

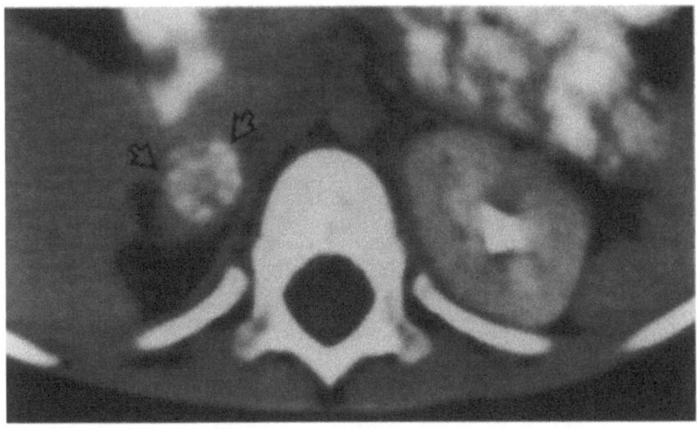

Fig. 6. Posthemorrhagic calcification (*arrows*) of the right adrenal on a CT scan of an asymptomatic infant

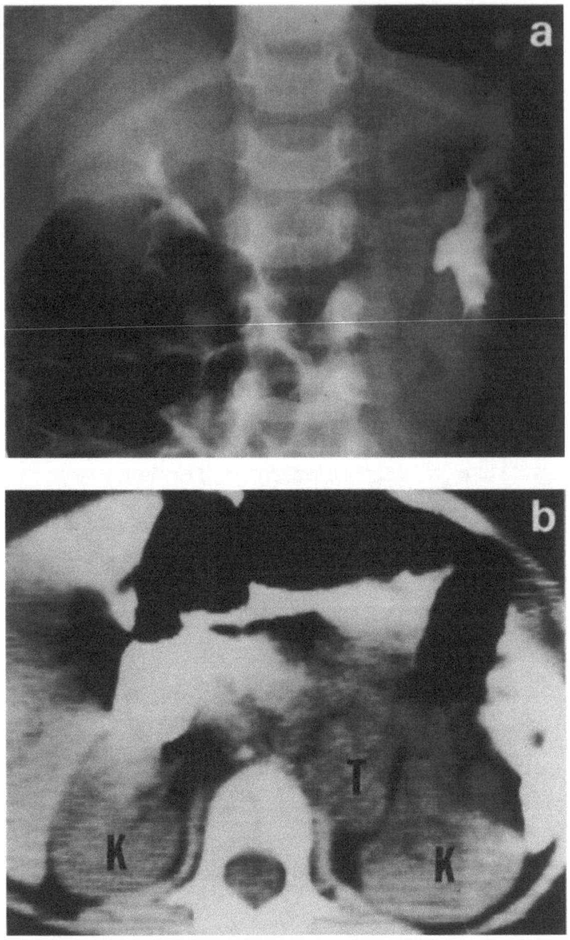

Fig. 8 a, b. Neuroblastoma of a 3-year-old boy. **a** Excretory urography. The left kidney is displaced caudally and its axis is tilted by a noncalcified left adrenal mass. **b** CT of the tumor (*T*). *K*, kidneys

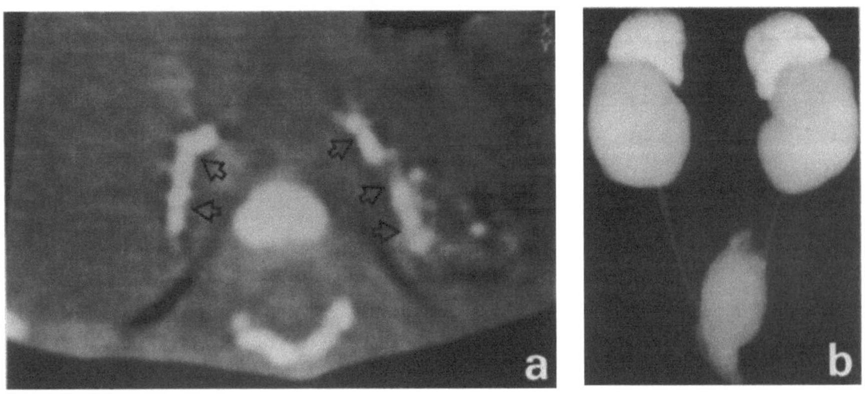

Fig. 7 a, b. Wolman's disease. **a** Extensive calcification of both adrenals (*arrows*) on a CT scan in a child with Wolman's disease. **b** Enlarged, heavily calcified adrenals (autopsy specimen of another child)

4.3 Wolman's Disease

Wolman's disease (Fig. 7) is a disorder of lipid metabolism which results in deposition of triglycerides and cholesterol in an enlarged adrenal. Failure to thrive and hepatosplenomegaly are early manifestations of this lethal xanthomatosis [18]. Each adrenal is symmetrically enlarged. The fine punctate calcification are usually distributed throughout both glands although

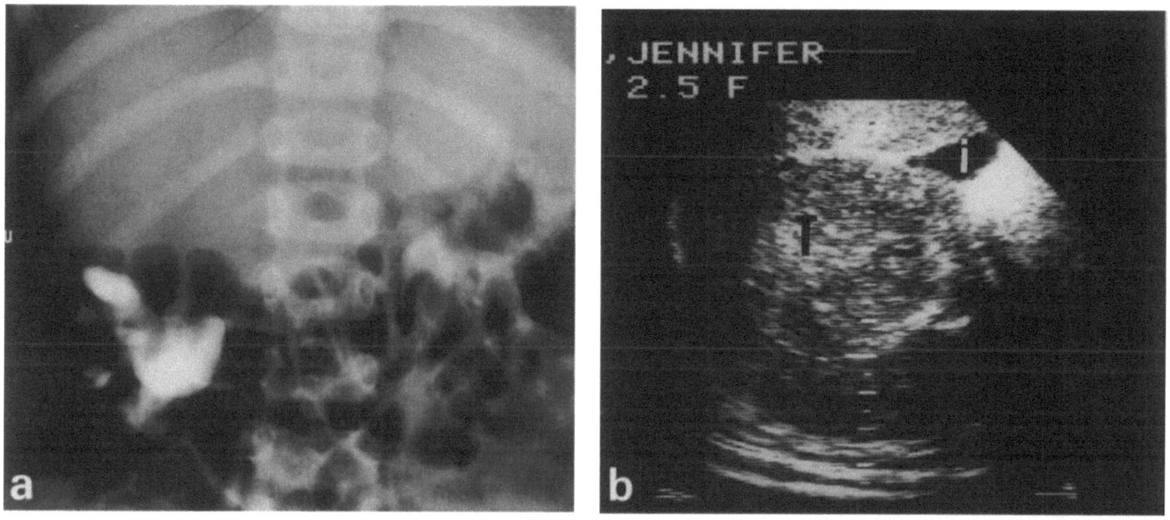

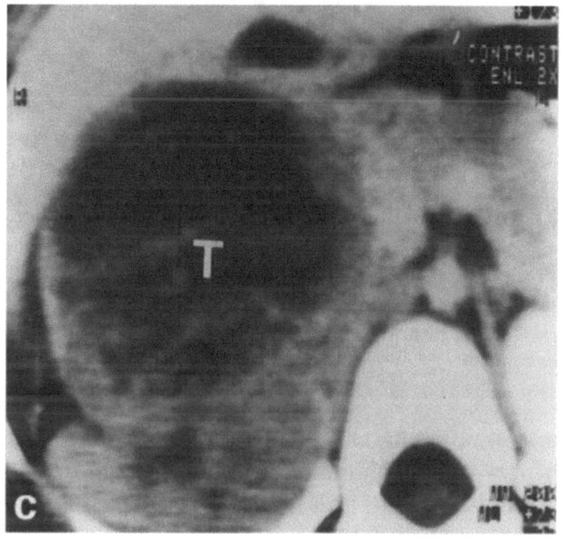

Fig. 9 a–c. Neuroblastoma in a 2.5-year-old girl. **a** Excretory urography. A suprarenal mass has displaced the right kidney caudad. **b** Parasagittal real-time sonogram (sector scanner, 7.5 MHz transducer). The mass is a solid tumor (*T*) obstructing the inferior vena cava (*i*). **c** Contrast-enhanced CT shows necrotic nature of the tumor (*T*)

early deposition is sometimes seen in the medulla. Little distortion of the kidney is present and the adrenals maintain their normal shape.

Niemann–Pick disease is clinically similar but shows no adrenal calcifications. Neuroblastoma often exhibits punctate calcifications but in a more irregular pattern. The calcifications from hemorrhage are coarser and tend to be more curvilinear and peripheral. Infection and the Waterhouse–Friderichsen syndrome show irregular calcifications in a small gland.

4.4 Neuroblastoma

Neuroblastoma (Figs. 8–11) is the most common abdominal neoplasm in childhood [4]. The tumor may arise from the adrenal medulla or any portion of the sympathetic chain. Only about one-half of the intra-abdominal tumors originate from the adrenal. Thin, curvilinear or coarse, irregular clumps of calcification occur within the tumor, secondary to necrosis from rapid growth (Figs. 10 and 11 b). Displacement or involvement of adjacent structures is dependent upon size (Figs. 8 a, 9 a, b, 10 b, 11 a), and metastasis to skin, bone, or central nervous system (Fig. 12) is present in over half the patients at the time of presentation. Marrow invasion is common, and narrow is often the tissue removed for diagnosis. Hydronephrosis (Fig. 9 a) or hematuria are quite rare when the tumor arises from an adrenal, although, when large enough, its separation from a primary exophytic

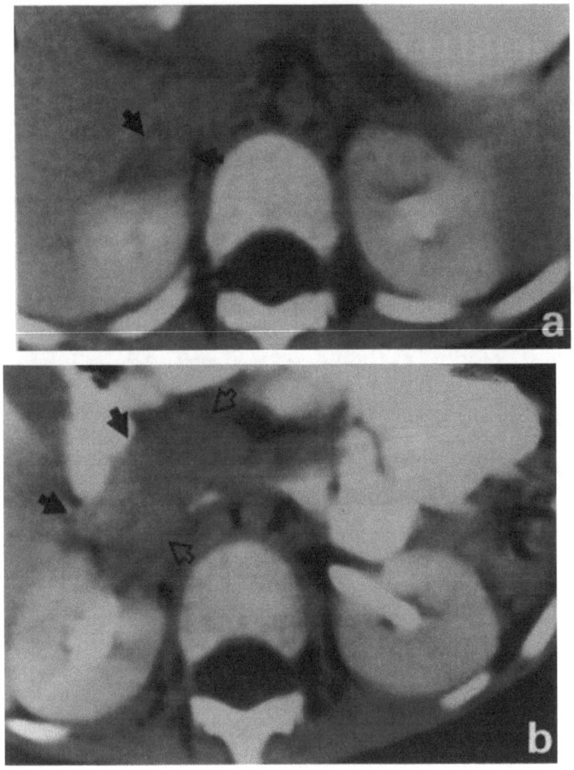

Fig. 10 a, b. Neuroblastoma in a 2-year-old boy. **a** The tumor of the right adrenal contains faint calcifications (*arrows*). **b** The tumor grows continuously caudal in the retroperitoneum

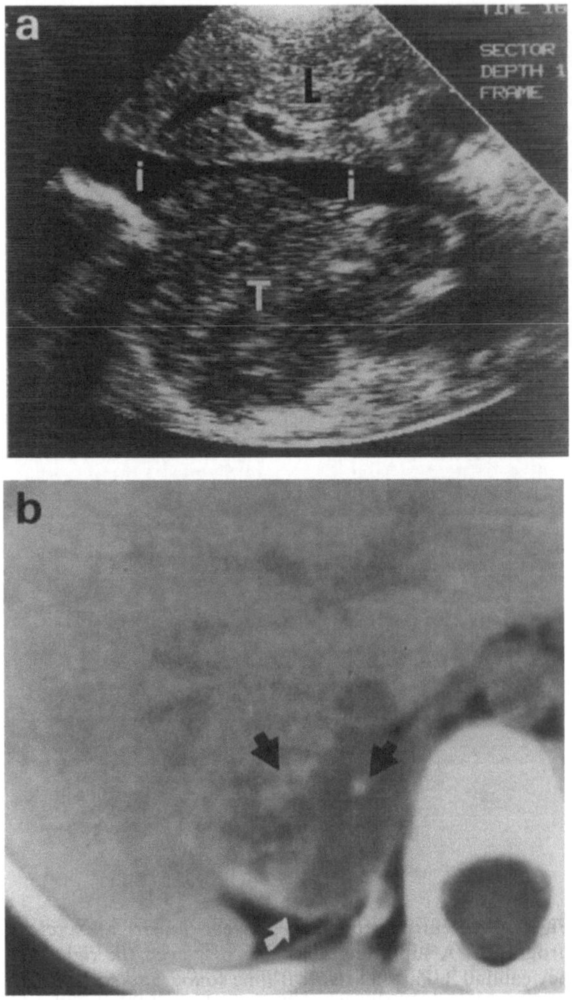

Fig. 11 a, b. Neuroblastoma in a 5-year-old boy. **a** Parasagittal real-time sonogram (7.5 MHz transducer) of a large adrenal tumor (*T*) with compression of the inferior vena cava (*i*). *L*, liver. **b** CT scan demonstrates small calcifications within the tumor (*arrows*)

renal lesion can be difficult (Fig. 13). Serum and urinary catecholamines are very useful in the initial diagnosis and for indicating the presence of recurrent disease.

Ultrasound is the most common and useful imaging modality to show the point of origin, the size, and the amount of local spread of the tumor (Figs. 9b and 11a) [19]. Focal or diffuse metastasis to the liver is often present and is hyperechoic. The primary tumor typically shows mixed echogenicity, with areas of cystic degeneration or necrosis. A cleavage plane is usually present between the primary adrenal lesion and the kidney although the demarcation from the liver is often less distinct. Radionuclide skeletal imaging and CT of the abdomen are used to illustrate the peripheral and local extent of the disease. In our institution MRI has recently been found to be very effective in demonstrating the extent of the tumor, particularly if invasion of the spinal canal is suspected (Fig. 12). Even if CT or MRI have been used for the primary diagnosis, follow-up examinations during therapy should be performed with ultrasound as it is the most practical and cost-effective imaging modality to illustrate regression or recurrence of tumor growth.

4.5 Adrenocortical Tumors

Adrenocortical adenomas and carcinomas may elaborate androgens, cortisol and related substances, aldosterone, or rarely estrogens. A recent multi-institutional review revealed over 100 cases of primary adrenal tumors [12]. The mean age of presentation was 5 years, and more females were affected than males. The right and

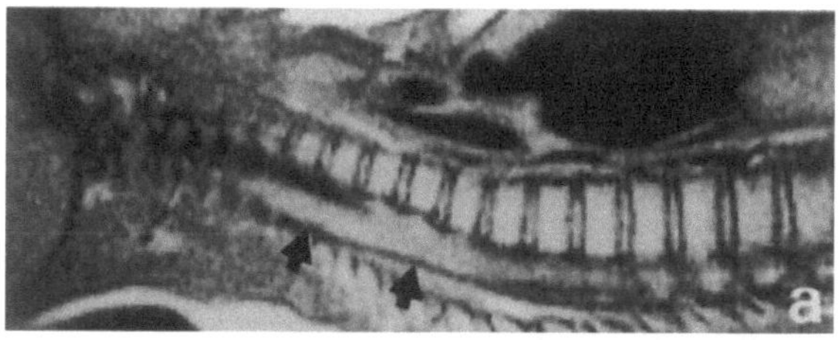

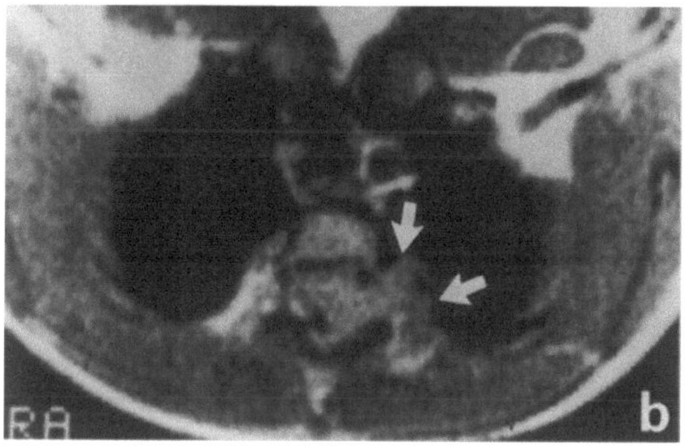

Fig. 12 a, b. Metastatic neuroblastoma. **a** Parasagittal MRI (SE 50/30) indicating a high intensity lesion of the thoracic cord (*arrows*). **b** Transaxial MRI (SE 500/30). The tumor is eroding the vertebra and penetrating the paravertebral space (*arrows*)

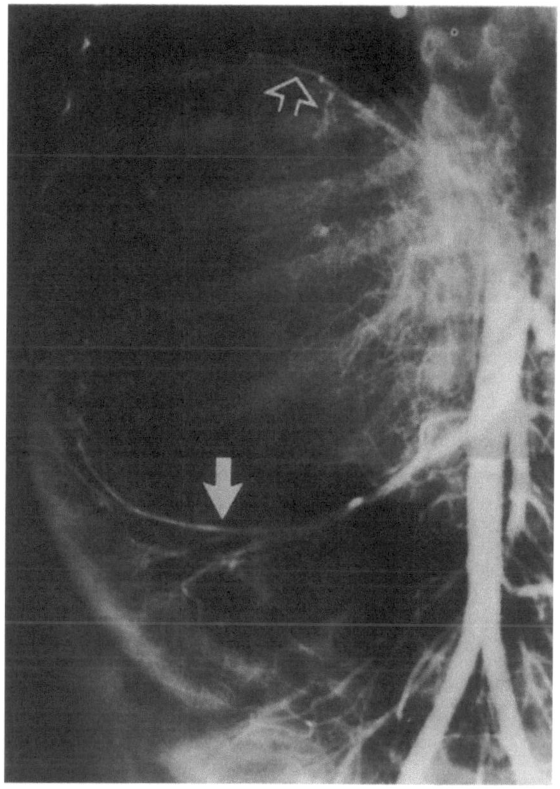

Fig. 13. Aortogram of a Wilms' tumor simulating an adrenal mass. The tumor in the right suprarenal location displaces the renal (*white arrow*) and inferior phrenic arteries (*open arrow*)

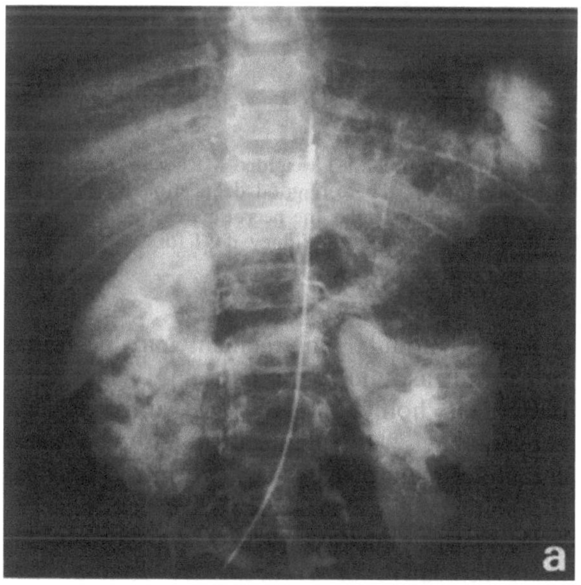

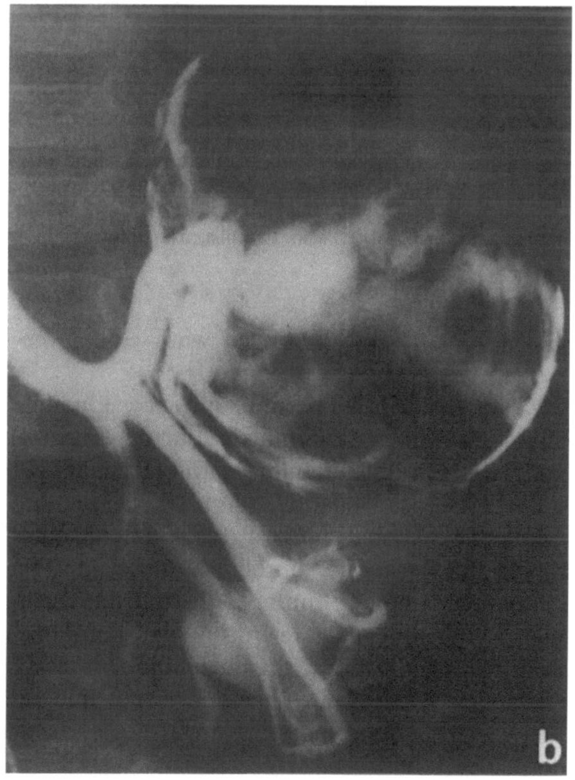

Fig. 14 a, b. Adrenal virilizing cortical carcinoma in a 10-month-old girl. **a** Aortogram of a well-defined, poorly vascularized tumor of the left adrenal with depression of the left kidney. **b** Selective left adrenal venography showing grossly dilated veins in the tumor (film with 1.8-fold geometric magnification, 0.3 mm focal spot) [5]

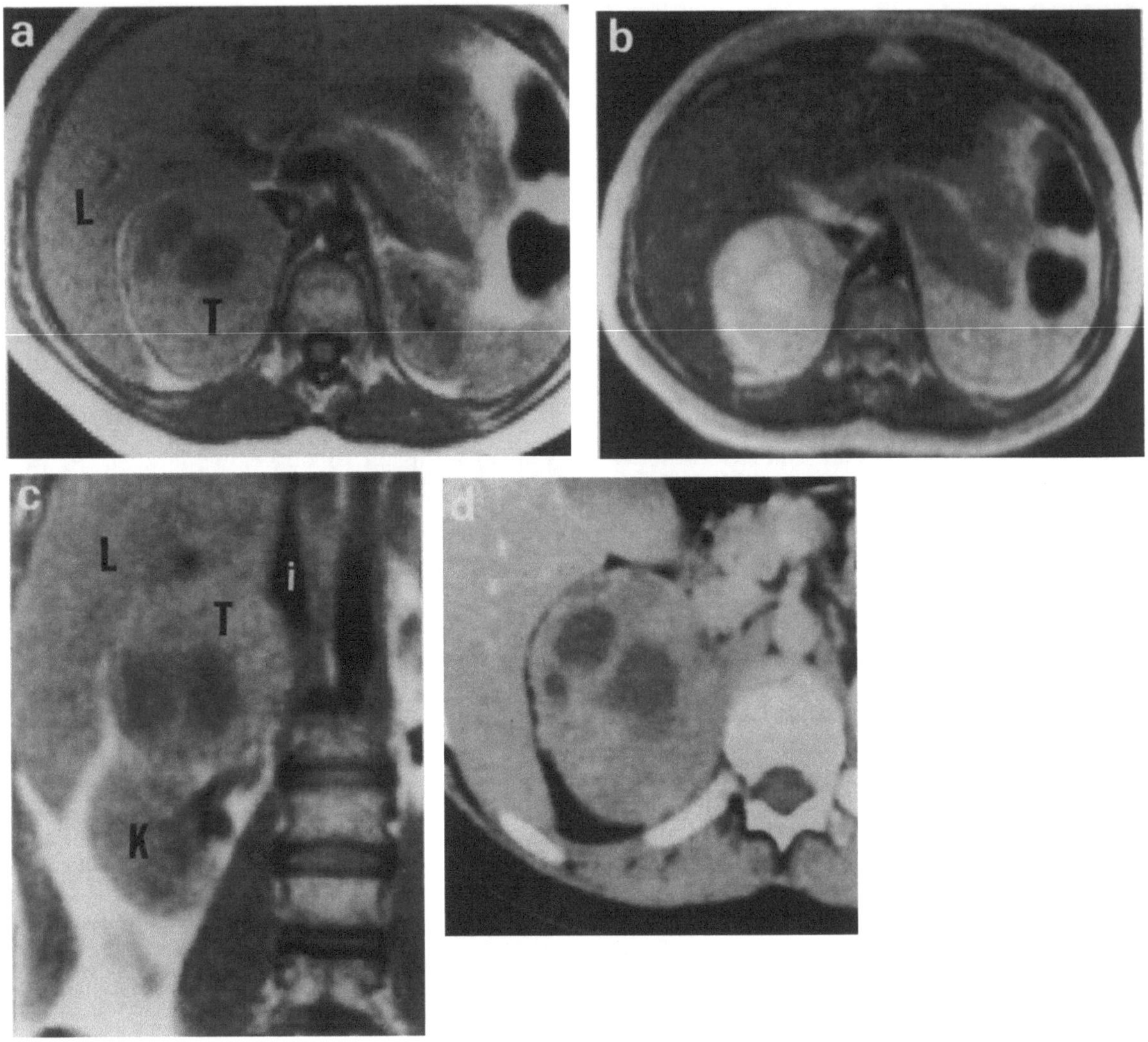

Fig. 15 a–d. Pheochromocytoma of the adrenal gland in a 15-year-old boy. **a** Axial T-1 weighted MRI scan (SE 500/30). There are three low intensity areas (probably necrotic) within the tumor (*T*). There is good delineation of the tumor against the liver (*L*). **b** T-2 weighted MRI scan (SE 2500/60). The tumor, in particular the necrotic area, has high signal intensity. **c** Coronal MRI scan demonstrates compression of the inferior vena cava (*i*). *K*, kidney. **d** CT for comparison

left adrenals were involved with equal frequency.

Adenomas tend to be small and have a benign histology, while carcinomas are larger (Fig. 14) and demonstrate malignant histological changes such as necrosis, local or regional invasion, and frequent abnormal mitoses. Blood and urinary biochemical tests are unreliable in designating benign or malignant tumors. Virilization, Cushing's syndrome, aldosteronism, and feminization are usually found in descending order of frequency. Most of the Cushing's syndrome patients show some degree of virilization, however.

A focal nodular enlargement may be found by an ultrasound examination [3]. The echo pattern is homogenous, solid, and with no acoustic back wall enhancement. Adenoma and carcinoma cannot be separated on the basis of the sonographic characteristics of a single lesion. The presence of calcification, however, is more indicative of a carcinoma than an adenoma. The high sensitivity of CT for calcification is helpful. In addition, similar nodular lesions in adjacent lymph nodes or the liver can be best excluded by CT as their presence indicates malignancy [1]. Iodinated cholesterol scintigraphy shows accumulation in adenomas,

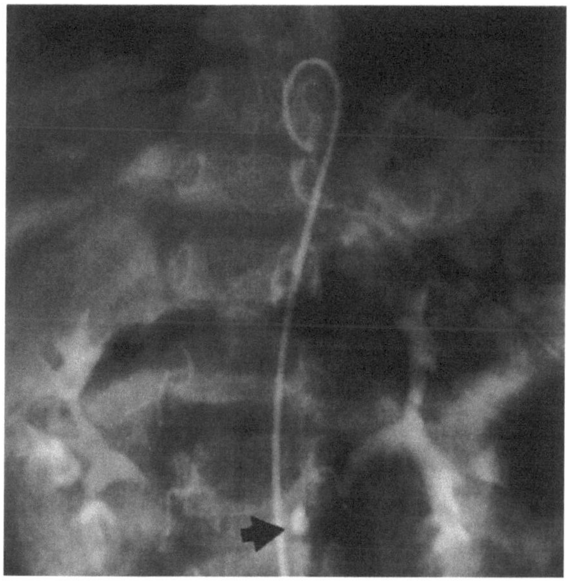

Fig. 16. Pheochromocytoma in a 6-month-old infant with hypertension. Aortogram demonstrates a small hypervascular lesion arising from the para-aortic sympathetic chain (*arrow*) [13]

while little accumulation is seen in carcinomas. Adenomas tend to be hypervascular on angiography and venous sampling may help to distinguish a functioning adenoma from bilateral hyperplasia [12]. The utility of MRI in differentiating adenoma from carcinoma is yet to be defined. In carcinoma angiography will demonstrate neovascularity, which in larger (necrotic) tumors is sparsely present, and grossly abnormal adrenal veins [5].

4.6 Pheochromocytoma

This tumor (Figs. 15 and 16) is rare in infants and young children and is more common in males. Bilateral adrenal or multiple sites are found in 10% or less of the patients [12]. The majority of the tumors arise from the chromaffin tissue within the adrenal medulla and only one third arise from extra-adrenal chromaffin tissue (paragangliomas). The most common presenting symptom in pheochromocytoma is sustained hypertension. The elevation in blood pressure is due to hypersecretion of epinephrine, norepinephrine, and catecholamines.

An ultrasound examination of the adrenal for a focal mass is indicated as an initial study [24]. The tumors tend to be more echogenic than the surrounding adrenal, probably secondary to hypervascularity. Thin section CT may disclose a bilateral lesion or, if the ultrasound examination is negative, offers a more complete search of the paraspinal chromaffin chain [22]. In the search for a pheochromocytoma, CT or MRI have generally replaced angiography; the last is indicated only when other imaging modalities have failed to demonstrate the tumor, the presence of which is strongly suspected either clinically or by biochemical assay. While in these cases multiple venous sampling may indicate the location of a tumor, the demonstration of a very small pheochromocytoma can be obtained only by angiography (Fig. 16) [13].

Summary

In this chapter we have given an overview of the use and usefulness of different imaging modalities which can be employed in the diagnosis of these lesions.

It is important to recognize the normal appearance of relatively large adrenals in infancy so that the examiner is not misled to a false positive diagnosis of adrenal hemorrhage or another mass lesion. Also, adrenal calcifications may be present both in benign conditions without any clinical significance and in malignancies requiring prompt treatment. With the variety of imaging modalities available, a (pediatric) radiologist must act as consultant to the clinician for the selection of the correct type of examination to reveal the greatest amount of diagnostic information and to be cost-effective for the primary diagnosis and follow-up studies. Therefore, the (pediatric) radiologist should not only be acquainted with but able to master all available diagnostic equipment and examination techniques from plain radiography to magnetic resonance imaging (MRI) and angiography. As in all diagnostic radiology, fragmentation of the diagnostic work-up of adrenal mass lesions in children into machine-oriented services may confuse the referring physician, result in unnecessary examinations, and delay the diagnosis.

References

1. Adams JE, Johnson RJ, Rickards D, Isherwood I (1983) Computed tomography in adrenal disease. Clin Radiol 34:39–49

2. Agee OF, Kaude JV, Lepasoon J (1973) Preoperative localization of pheochromocytoma. Acta Radiol Diagn 14:545–560
3. Bernardino ME, Goldstein HM, Green B (1978) Gray scale ultrasonography of adrenal neoplasms. AJR 130:741–744
4. Caffey J (1978) Pediatric x-ray diagnosis, 7th edn. Year Book Medical, Chicago, pp 817, 943–948, 1797–1807
5. Craig WP, Hawkins IF Jr, Kaude JV (1975) Selective adrenal venography in an infant with virilizing adrenal cortical carcinoma. Pediatr Radiol 3:53–54
6. Davis PL, Hricak H, Bradley WG Jr (1984) Magnetic resonance imaging of the adrenal glands. RCNA 22:891–895
7. Duck SC (1981) Malignancy associated with congenital adrenal hyperplasia. J Pediatr 99:423–424
8. Geisinger MA, Zelch MG, Bravo EL, Risius BF, O'Donovan PB, Borkowski GP (1983) Primary hyperaldosteronism: comparison of CT, adrenal venography and venous sampling. AJR 141:299–302
9. Ghiacy S, Dubbins PA, Baumer H (1985) Ultrasound demonstration of congenital adrenal hyperplasia. J Clin Ultrasound 13:419–420
10. Guerin CK, Wahner HW, Gorman CA, Carpenter PC, Sheedy PF (1983) Computed tomographic scanning versus radioisotope imaging in adrenocortical diagnosis. Am J Med 75:653–657
11. Hayman S, Treves S (1979) Adrenal hemorrhage in the newborn: scintigraphic diagnosis. J Nucl Med 20:521–523
12. Humphrey GB (ed) (1984) Adrenal and endocrine tumors in children. Martinus Nijhoff, Boston
13. Kaude JV (1979) Preoperative localization of Pheochromocytoma. In: Loehr E (ed) Renal and adrenal tumors. Springer, Berlin Heidelberg New York, pp 258–267
14. McInnis AN, Felman AH, Kaude JV, Walker D (1982) Renal ultrasound in the neonatal period. Pediatr Radiol 12:15–20
15. Mittelstaaedt CA, Volberg FM, Merten DF, Brill PW (1979) The sonographic diagnosis of neonatal adrenal hemorrhage. Radiology 131:453–457
16. Older RA, Van Moore A Jr, Glenn JF, Hidalgo HJ (1984) Diagnosis of adrenal disorders. RCNA 22:433–454
17. Oppenheimer DA, Carroll BA, Yousem S (1983) Sonography of the normal neonatal adrenal gland. Radiology 146:157–160
18. Queloz JM, Capitanio MA, Kirkpatrick JA (1972) Wolman's disease. Radiology 104:357–359
19. Saks JB, Bryan PJ, Yulish BS, Gauderer MWL, Haaga JR (1985) Comaprison of computed tomography and ultrasound in the evaluation of abdominal neuroblastoma. J Clin Ultrasound 13:641–645
20. Sample WF, Sarti DA (1978) Computed tomography and gray scale ultrasonography of the adrenal gland: a comparative study. Radiology 128:377–383
21. Schultz, CL, Haaga JR, Fletcher BD, Alfidi RJ, Schultz MA (1984) Magnetic resonance imaging of the adrenal glands: a comparison with computed tomography. AJR 143:1235–1240
22. Welch TJ, Sheedy PF II, van Heerden JA, Sheps SG, Hattery RR, Stephens DH (1983) Pheochromocytoma: value of computed tomography. Radiology 148:501–503
23. White EM, Edelman RR, Stark DD, Simeone JF, Mueller PR, Brady TJ, Wittenberg J, Butch RJ, Ferrucci JT (1985) Surface coil MR imaging of abdominal viscera. Part II. The adrenal glands. Radiology 157:431–436
24. Wicks JD, Mettler FA Jr (1983) Sonography of adrenal lesions causing hypertension. Urol Radiol 5:99–102
25. Yeh H-C (1980) Sonography of the adrenal glands: normal glands and small masses. AJR 135:1167–1177

Computed Tomography of the Adrenal Glands

A.A. Moss and W.P. Shuman

1 Introduction

Shortly after the introduction of abdominal computed tomography (CT), its value as a noninvasive adrenal imaging technique became apparent. Normal-sized adrenal glands could be imaged in 85%–99% of patients and virtually all adrenal masses larger than 1.0 cm in diameter were routinely demonstrated [1–4]. CT successfully characterized a variety of adrenal abnormalities and became the imaging procedure of choice to guide fine needle adrenal biopsies [5–14].

Technical advancements have permitted faster scans, greater spatial resolution, better density discrimination, reformatting of images, and dynamic scanning techniques to be routinely employed. Compared to other adrenal imaging procedures CT has proven to have sensitivity, specifity, and accuracy rates as high or higher than ultrasonography, radionuclide examinations, and angiography [15–20]. Because of its high overall accuracy, patient acceptance, and general availability, it has become the preferred imaging procedure for evaluating patients with suspected adrenal abnormalities.

2 Techniques of Examination

To achieve the highest level of diagnostic accuracy, there must be meticulous attention to CT technique, knowledge of adrenal gland embryology and anatomy, and thorough understanding of the CT appearance of the normal adrenal glands and the alterations produced by adrenal pathology.

All adult patients are given 480–750 ml of a 2% sodium diatrizoate or barium sulfate solution 30 min before scanning, and another 250 ml just prior to scanning. This regimen outlines the small bowel and duodenum and thus permits the adrenal glands to be easily differentiated from adjacent bowel. Pediatric patients are given a volume commensurate with their age and weight.

CT scans are usually performed using the small or medium calibration fields, with the patient supine, and the CT gantry at 0° angulation. Technical factors are chosen to ensure maximal spatial resolution without excessive radiation exposure. Spatial resolution using 3–5 mm thick sections is superior to sections 8–10 mm thick. Contiguous nonoverlapping scans are usually sufficient; the distance between scans should never be greater than 1 cm.

While many patients can be successfully scanned without intravenous contrast administration, contrast injection often provides improved characterization of adrenal gland pathology and better delineation of the adrenals from adjacent structures (Fig. 1). Injection of 150 cc of 60% meglumine diatrizoate over 2–3 min provides excellent contrast enhancement of adrenal lesions and adjacent structures.

Reformatting axial CT images into coronal, sagittal, or oblique configurations give additional anatomic information (Fig. 2) but is essential in only a small percentage of patients. Ultrathin (1.5–2 mm thick) sections are useful when subtle adrenal abnormalities are suspected; however, their routine use has not proven necessary. Magnifying the CT study 1.2- to 2.0-fold makes it easier to view the adrenal glands and to delineate subtle contour abnormalities.

3 Anatomy

Embryologically the adrenal gland is derived from two sources. The cortex is formed in the

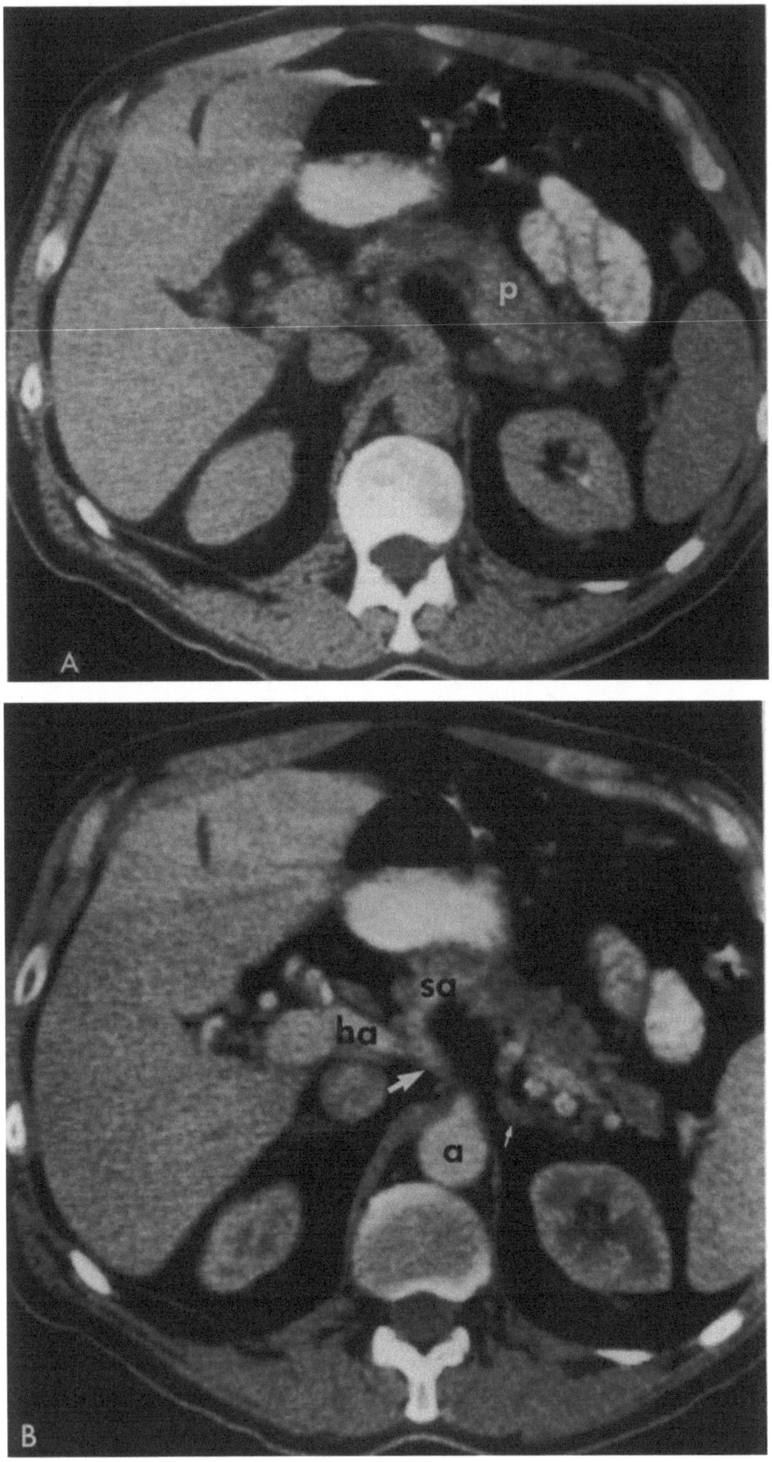

Fig. 1. A CT scan after contrast infusion demonstrates the tail of the pancreas (*p*), but separation of left adrenal from splenic vessels is difficult. **B** CT study after bolus injection of contrast reveals aorta (*a*), hepatic artery (*ha*), splenic artery (*sa*), celiac axis (*large arrow*). The left adrenal (*small arrow*) is readily identified dorsal to the splenic vessels

6th week of life from a proliferation of mesodermal coelomic epithelial cells medial to the mesonephros. One week later the adrenal medulla is formed by ectodermal neural crest cells migrating from sympathetic ganglia. Once formed, the adrenals descend caudally to meet the ascending kidney [21].

Each adrenal gland lies within Gerota's fascia in the perinephric space, embedded in adipose tissue, and surrounded by a tough fibroelastic

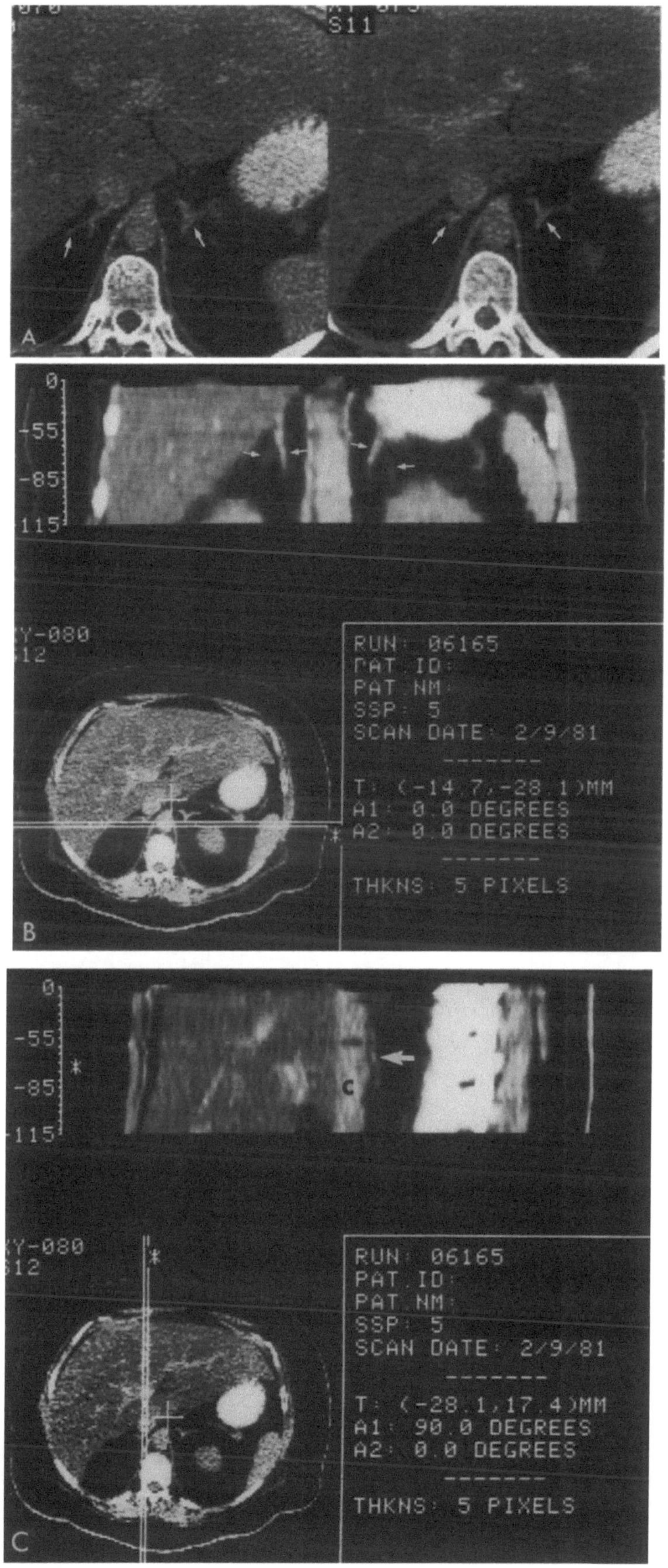

Fig. 2 A–C. Normal adrenal glands. **A** Axial CT scans 5 mm apart. **B** Coronal and **C** sagittal reformation of adrenal glands. Both limbs of each adrenal gland (*arrows*) are seen on the coronal image. The right adrenal (*large arrow*) is shown just dorsal to the inferior vena cava (*c*)

capsule that penetrates the cortex, dividing the gland into distinct columns [22]. The superior pole of each gland is anchored to Gerota's fascia by strong fibrous bands.

4 Location

4.1 Right Adrenal Gland

The right adrenal gland is positioned just dorsal to the inferior vena cava at the level of its intra- and extrahepatic portions (Fig. 3). The body extends slightly laterally and dorsally for a few millimeters along its long axis. The prominent medial limb of the gland extends dorsally in the fat between the liver laterally and the diaphragm medially. The medial limb frequently courses parallel to the crus of the diaphragm and may extend to the lateral posterior margin of the vertebral body [2]. Most right adrenal glands are cephalic to the right kidney; the most caudal extent is almost always cephalad to the renal vessels.

4.2 Left Adrenal Gland

The medial portion of the left adrenal gland is lateral to the crus of the left diaphragm, but its course is not as parallel to the diaphragm as the medial limb of the right adrenal. Over 90% of left adrenals are anterior to the anterior vertebral margin, and virtually all are posterior to the aortic tangent [2]. The base of the left adrenal touches the left kidney. The most cephalad portion of the left adrenal is related to the dorsal margin of the stomach. The body of the left adrenal splits into medial and lateral limbs at an acute angle. While these limbs are often equal in length, when unequal the lateral is usually slightly longer.

The upper pole of the adrenal is located at the same level (51%), higher (15%), or lower (34%) than the right gland (Fig. 3) [3]. The tail of the pancreas is usually (96%) seen on at least one section with the left adrenal and therefore serves as an aid in locating the left adrenal [2].

The location of the adrenal glands is extremely constant. Adrenal ectopia is very rare and the adrenal glands remain in their expected location even in patients with renal ectopia and/or other congenital renal anomalies [23].

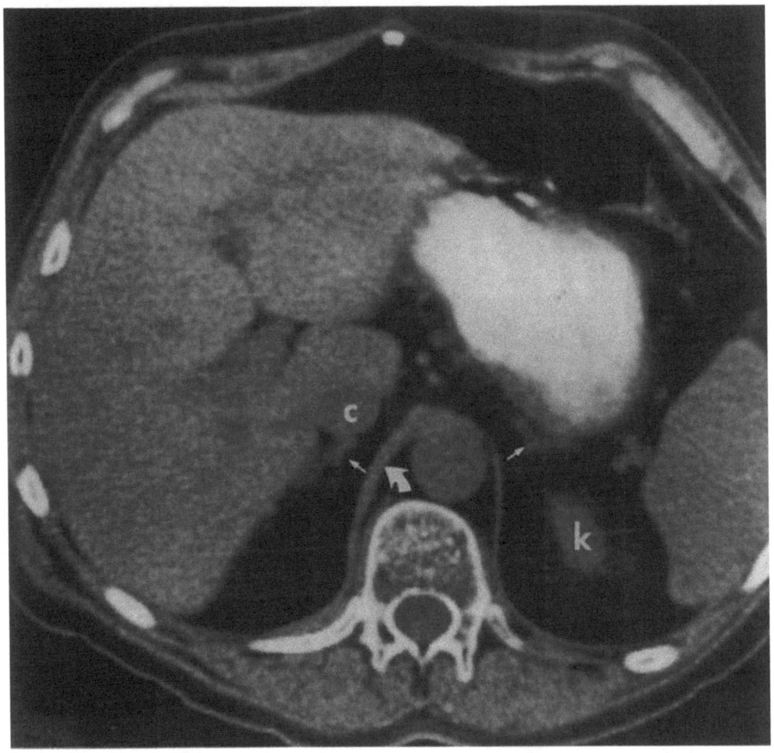

Fig. 3. Normal adrenal gland location. The right adrenal gland (*arrow*) is just dorsal to the inferior vena cava (*C*) at the level of its intra- and extrahepatic portions. The left gland (*arrow*) is seen at the same level as the upper pole of the left kidney (*K*), *large arrow* CTUS of diaphragm

5 Morphology

Normal adrenal glands have a variety of cross-sectional configurations (Fig. 4) [1–4, 16, 21–24]. The right adrenal is commonly revealed as having a linear (80%) or short inverted V (10%) shape. The lateral limb of the right gland is frequently shorter than the medial limb; it usually courses roughly parallel to the medial limb but may be directed laterally at a right angle, appear as a horizontal linear structure, or have a K- or X-shaped appearance (Fig. 5) [4, 16].

The shape of the left adrenal also varies considerably (Fig. 5). It most often has an inverted V (50%) or Y (32%) shape but can appear linear, triangular, crescentic, or V-shaped. Due to the polymorphic shape of the adrenal glands and differences in rotation about the longitudinal or transverse axis, the CT appearance of each adrenal varies depending on the particular CT section (Fig. 6).

6 Size

Normal adrenal glands average 3–5 g in weight and are approximately 4 × 3 × 1 cm in size [3, 21, 24]. The exact length, width, and thickness can be calculated according to the method of MONTAGNE et al. [3] (Fig. 7). Length is determined by counting the number of contiguous CT scans in which the gland can be identified. Thickness is the greatest dimension perpendicular to the gland's long axis, and width is the greatest ventral–dorsal dimension. Measurements of adrenal size determined by CT are in agreement with measurements of pathologic specimens [3, 4, 22, 25, 26].

7 Pathology

7.1 Cortical Abnormalities

7.1.1 Cushing's Syndrome

Patients with Cushing's syndrome have a constellation of symptoms and physical findings produced by continued exposure to elevated plasma corticosteroid levels. Most patients have truncal and facial obesity with thin extremities (centripetal obesity), hypertension, purple stria, oligo- or amenorrhea, tendency to bruise easily, and weakness. Chemical studies confirm the diagnosis by demonstrating (a) an absence of corticosteroid response to insulin-induced hypoglycemia, (b) loss of normal corticosteroid circadian rhythm, and (c) resistance to corticosteroid suppression by a low dose of dexamethasone [27]. Cushing's syndrome is 3–4 times more common in females and occurs most frequently between the ages of 25 and 35 years [28].

It is essential to separate those patients with Cushing's syndrome secondary to an adrenal tumor from those with adrenal cortical hyperplasia as a result of excessive pituitary adrenocorticotropic hormone (ACTH) or excess ACTH from ectopic, nonendocrine tumors. While

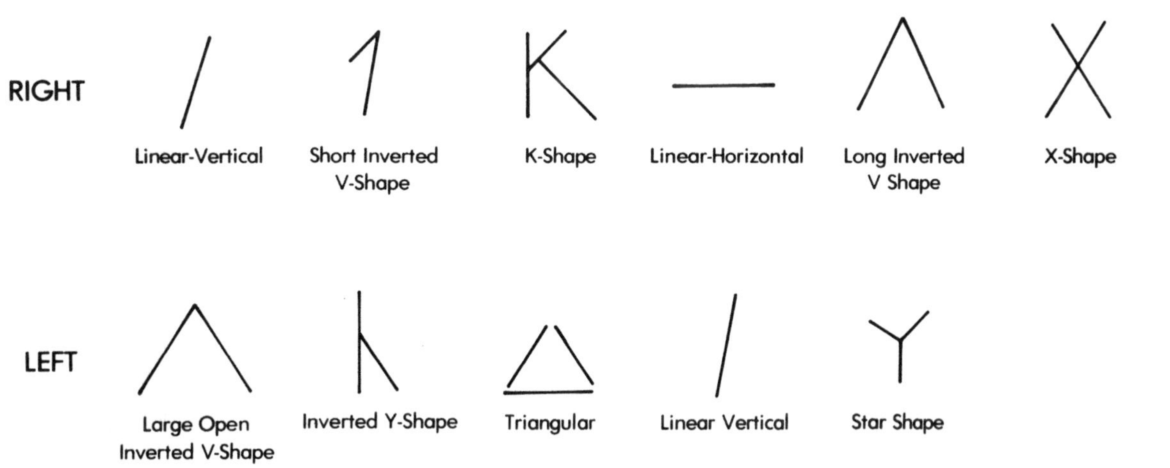

Fig. 4. Some of the adrenal shapes seen on computed tomography

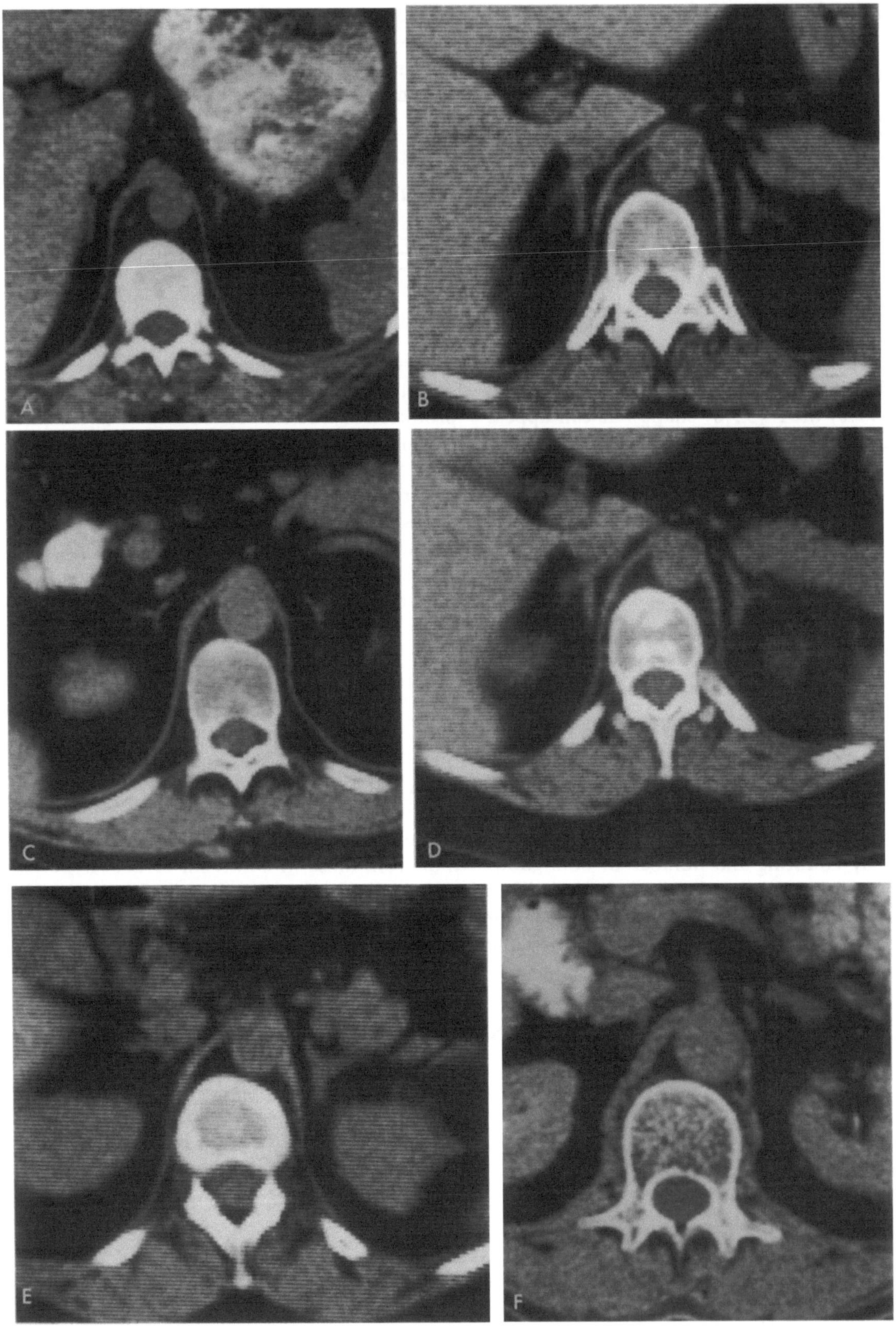

Fig. 5 A–F. Various shapes of adrenal glands in different patients

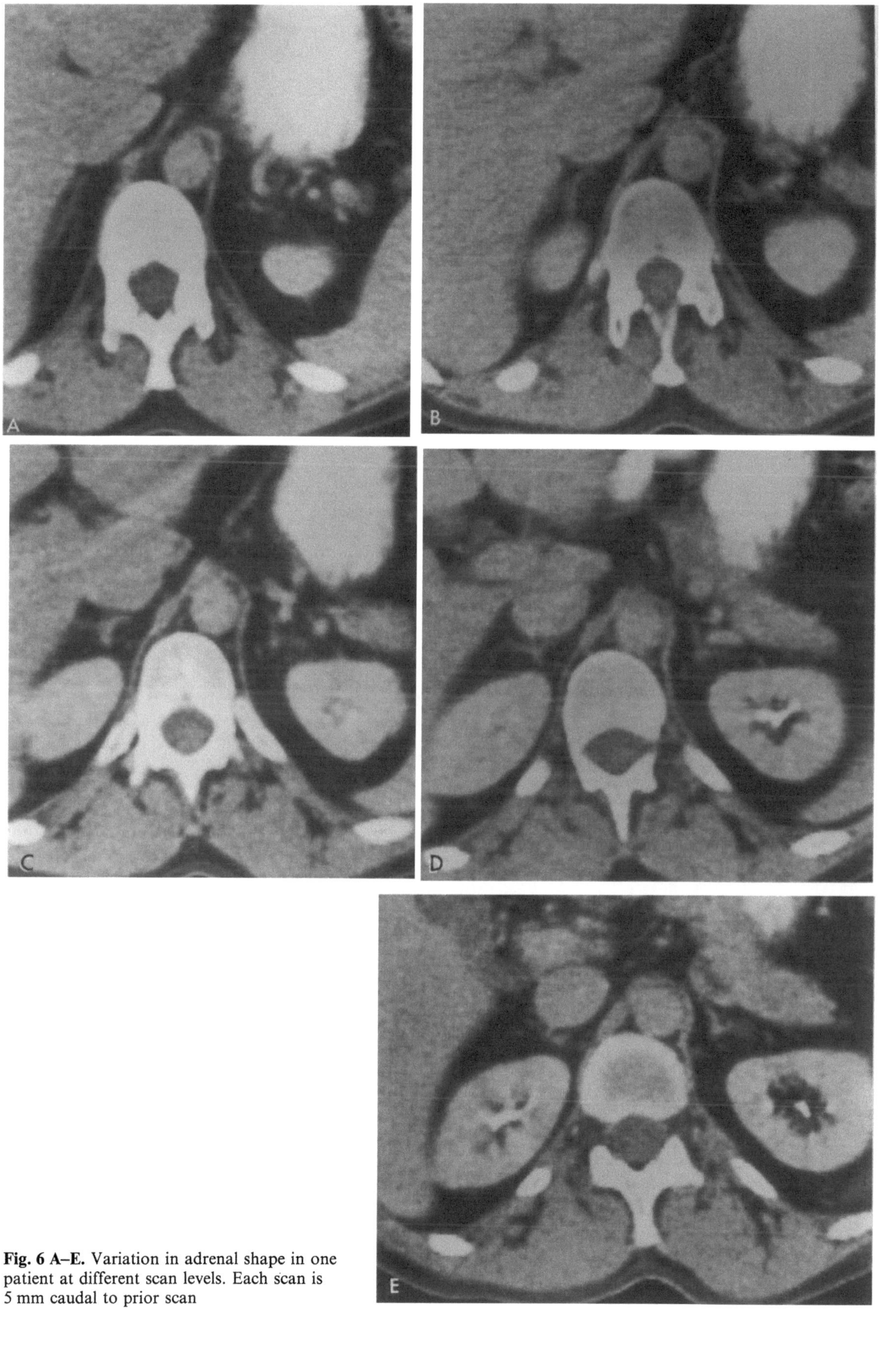

Fig. 6 A–E. Variation in adrenal shape in one patient at different scan levels. Each scan is 5 mm caudal to prior scan

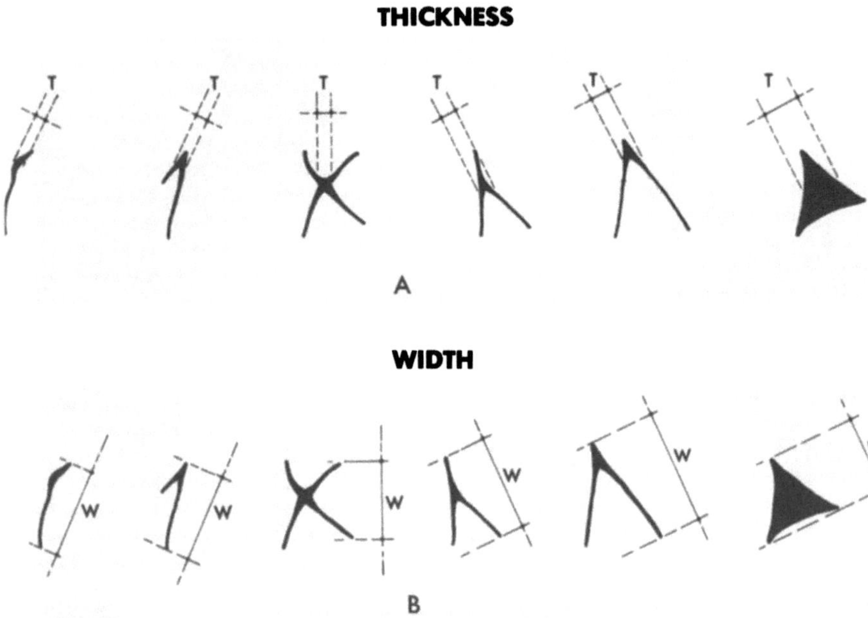

Fig. 7 A, B. Methods of measuring adrenal thickness (A) and width (B)

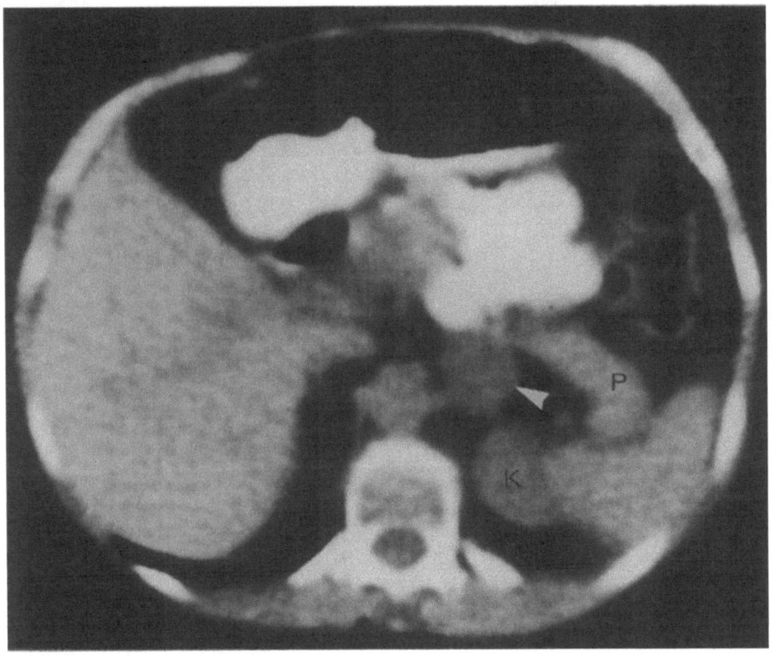

Fig. 8. Left adrenal adenoma (*arrow*). The top of the left kidney (*K*) and pancreatic tail (*P*) serve as reference points to locate the mass within the left adrenal gland. The CT attenuation value of the adenoma is the same as the left kidney

chemical studies can be used to make this distinction, the results may be equivocal. CT has been shown to accurately differentiate ACTH-dependent Cushing's syndrome from that caused by an adrenal neoplasm [1, 5, 6, 7, 12–14, 21, 29–32].

A benign adrenal cortical adenoma is found in 10%–15% of patients and adrenal carcinoma in approximately 5% of patients with Cushing's syndrome [33]. In less than 10% of patients the adenoma is bilateral. On CT the majority of functioning adrenal tumors appear as solid mass lesions ranging from 2–10 cm in diameter (Fig. 8). Adrenal adenomas and carcinomas are not distinguishable unless metastatic disease or vascular extension of the neoplasm is demonstrated [29]. Intravenous administration of contrast does not aid in the distinction of benign from malignant adrenal neoplasia. The usual CT attenuation range of adrenal lesions is

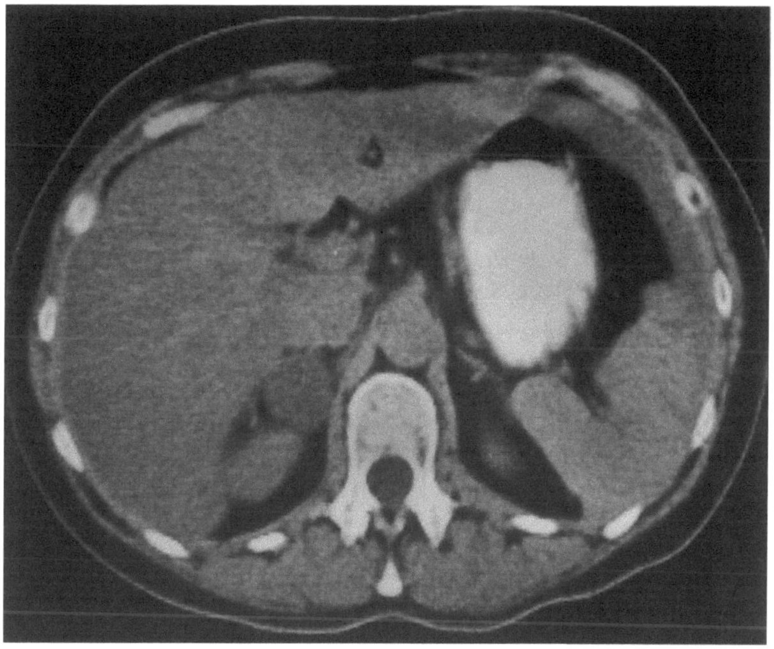

Fig. 9. Right adrenal adenoma having a low attenuation value (18 H) due to a high fat content

30–50 H, but adenomas having a high lipid content have been shown to have lower attenuation values, and calcification has been shown in both adrenal adenoma and carcinoma (Fig. 9) [1, 6, 11, 28].

In patients with Cushing's syndrome secondary to overproduction of ACTH, the CT findings may reveal normal adrenal glands, diffuse, bilateral adrenal enlargement with preservation of shape, or a form of adrenal hyperplasia where single or multiple small nodules are found in a diffusely enlarged gland (Fig. 10) [5, 16, 30].

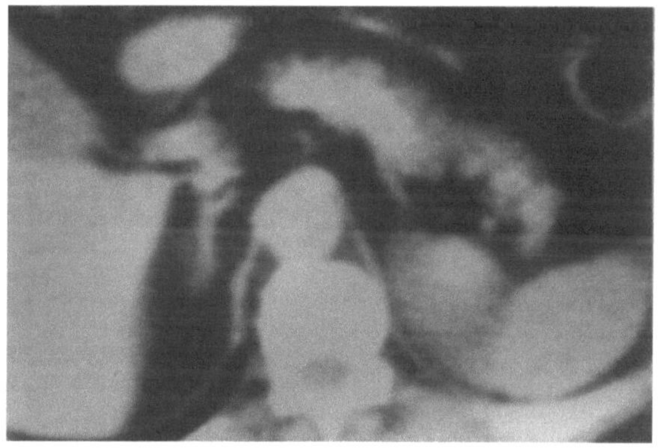

Fig. 10. CT scan in a patient with Cushing's syndrome due to a pituitary tumor reveals diffusely thickened adrenal glands that maintain a normal shape

Pathologic studies have shown that some patients with ACTH-dependent Cushing's syndrome have adrenal glands that are grossly and histologically normal [34, 35]. This would explain the CT finding of normal adrenal glands in some patients with proven syndrome. Although CT can never exclude a diagnosis of ACTH-dependent Cushing's disease, it can differentiate ACTH-dependent Cushing's syndrome from that due to an adrenal neoplasm in greater than 90% of instances [1, 5, 6, 7, 12–14, 21, 29–32].

An abnormally low attenuation value of the liver due to fat deposition within it is an associated CT finding in Cushing's syndrome [13]. CT may demonstrate atrophy of the contralateral adrenal gland in a patient with a functioning cortical adenoma [21], and following pituitary surgery [16], demonstrate the return of the diffusely enlarged adrenal glands to normal.

7.1.2 Primary Aldosteronism (Conn's Syndrome)

Primary aldosteronism results from excessive autonomous production of aldosterone [36] and is characterized by mild hypertension, hypocalcemia, headache, sodium retention, and reduced or absent plasma renin [8, 33]. It is the cause of hypertension in approximately 1% of pa-

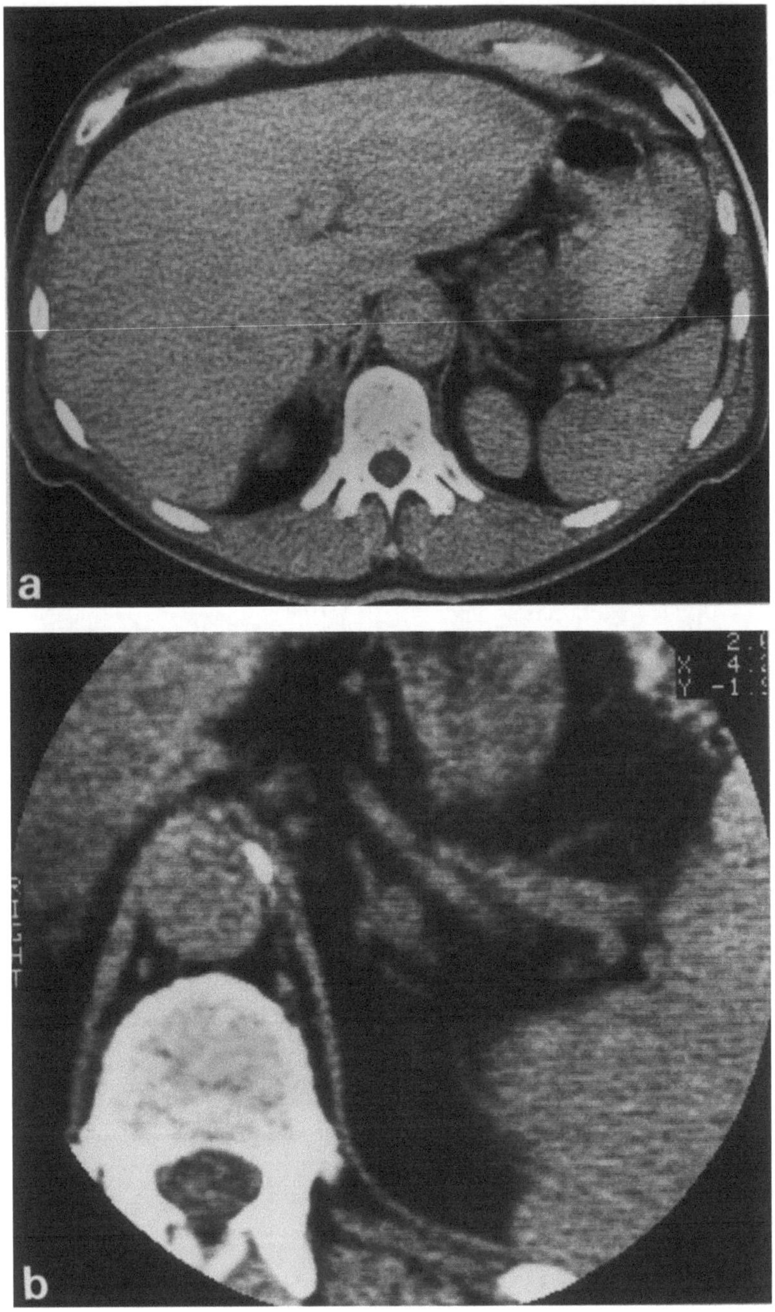

Fig. 11. a Aldosterone producing adenomas. A small adenoma arises from the medial limb of the right adrenal. **b** A lateral limb, left adrenal adenoma less than 1 cm in size

tients, affects males twice as frequently as females, and is most often diagnosed between the ages of 30–50 years [33].

Approximately 75% of patients have a unilateral adrenal cortical adenoma, located twice as frequently on the right. The tumor is often less than 2 cm in greatest dimension and rarely exceeds 4 cm (Fig. 11) [8, 33, 37]. The majority of the remaining patients have "idiopathic aldosteronism" due to nodular, bilateral, adrenal cortical hyperplasia. In these patients the adrenal glands may be slightly nodular and thickened or normal in size and shape. It is in these patients that the thinnest CT sections and highest resolution studies will be rewarding [35]. In pediatric patients with primary aldosteronism, bilateral, adrenal, cortical nodular hyperplasia is more common than functioning adenomas [33]. Adrenal carcinoma is an extremely rare cause of primary aldosteronism [33].

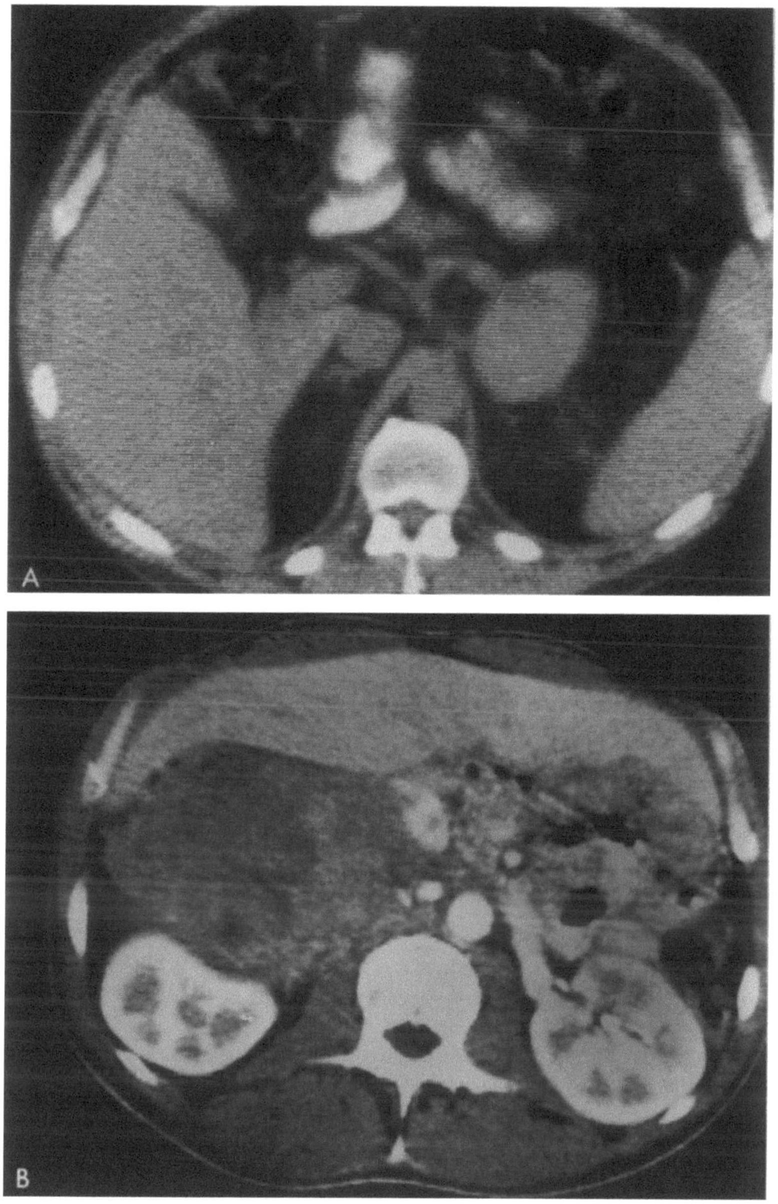

Fig. 12 A, B. Nonfunctioning adrenal tumors. **A** Left adrenal adenoma appearing as a solid, oval-shaped mass. **B** A large right adrenal carcinoma displacing the inferior vena cava. The tumor has an inhomogeneous CT density

The diagnosis of primary aldosteronism can be confirmed by finding an elevated rate of aldosterone secretion and a clinical response to spirolactone therapy. Adrenal adenomas tend to produce higher urinary and plasma aldosterone levels than found in patients with bilateral hyperplasia [8]. Resection of solitary adenomas will restore normal aldosterone production and alleviate a patient's hypertension. However, adrenal surgery, even bilateral adrenalectomy, may fail to affect the hypertension in patients with bilateral cortical nodular hyperplasia [6, 9, 38].

The presence and location of an adenoma can also be confirmed by arteriography [39, 40, 41], venography [34, 39, 42], adrenal venous sampling [43], and radionuclide scintigraphy [44–46]. However, the risks and limitations of angiographic and radionuclide techniques have currently made CT the preferred initial imaging procedure. High resolution CT usually demonstrates a small solid mass arising from one limb of the adrenal gland. Adenomas as small as 0.5 cm can be identified, with more than 83% accuracy [6–8]. Adenomas may contain as much as 5% fat and thus have CT attenuation values

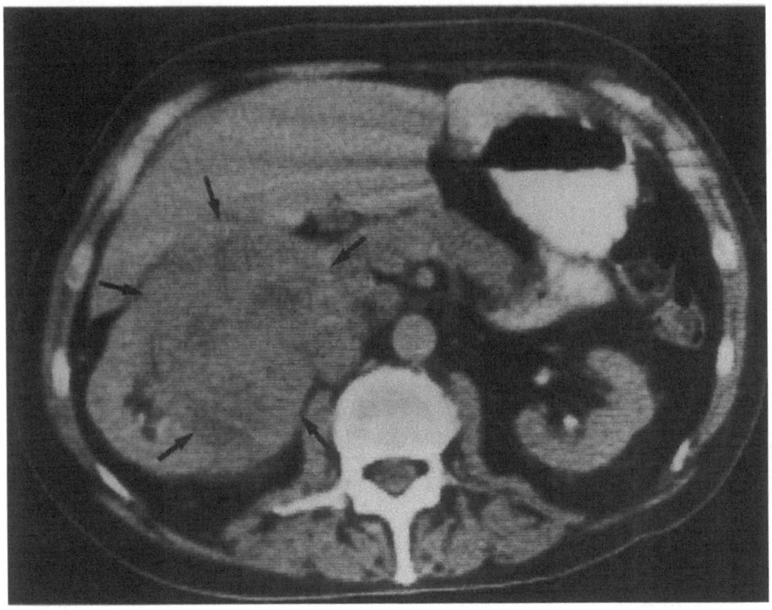

Fig. 13. A large adrenal carcinoma (*arrows*) involving the right kidney

significantly lower than adjacent organs [6]. Calcification in aldosteronomas occurs but is decidedly rare, and intravenous contrast administration may help to distinguish a small aldosterone-producing adenoma from hyperplasia and thus determine the most effective mode of therapy.

7.1.3 Nonfunctioning Adrenal Adenoma and Carcinoma

Adrenal adenomas and adenocarcinomas are demonstrated as unilateral or bilateral solid mass lesions by computed tomography (Fig. 12) [5, 16, 21, 24]. Adenomas are most frequently unilateral and less than 3 cm in diameter, whereas carcinomas are more frequently bilateral and larger. Both lesions grow slowly and can become extremely large before producing symptoms. Calcification is more common in carcinomas but adenomas also contain calcium [47]. It is not possible using CT alone to distinguish between these two lesions unless there is evidence of metastatic disease or direct tumor extension into adjacent organs (Fig. 13) [29].

At autopsy nonfunctioning adenomas are found in 2%–9% of adults [48]. Therefore, it is not surprising that using state-of-the-art CT equipment, small adrenal masses are frequently detected. Recent articles have reported that for masses less than 3 cm in size found in patients without evidence of malignancy or adrenal dysfunction, the incidence of metastatic or primary adrenal malignancy is low [48]. Currently it is recommended that either a fine needle aspiration biopsy or follow-up CT scan in 3–6 months be performed instead of a surgical procedure. In patients with masses larger than 3 cm the incidence of carcinoma is greater, and immediate biopsy is recommended.

7.1.4 Myelolipoma and Adenolipoma

Myelolipomas are rare tumors (0.8% of all autopsies) of the adrenal cortex that contain varying proportions of bone marrow elements and fat [49]. Calcification occurs in approximately 20% of cases [50]. Adenolipomas are extremely rare adrenal tumors, being composed predominantly of adipose tissue in which varying stages of degeneration, hemorrhage, fibrosis, and calcification are found. Both tumors are usually asymptomatic unless they become extremely large or undergo abrupt internal hemorrhage [32].

The typical CT appearance of both lesions is that of a well-circumscribed adrenal mass having an attenuation value of fat and frequently containing areas of calcification (Fig. 14). While CT permits a diagnosis of a fat-containing adrenal tumor, it is not patho-

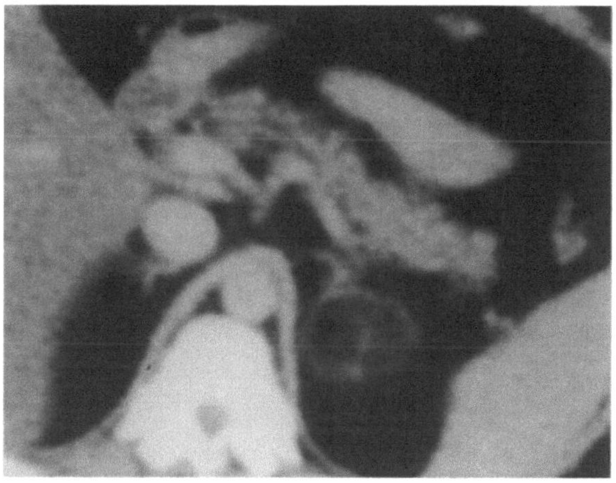

Fig. 14. Myelolipoma of the left adrenal gland. The CT attenuation value was −30 H indicating considerable fat within the tumor

gnomonic of a myelolipoma or adenolipoma, as cortical adenomas and aldosteronomas may appear similar due to their high fat content [6, 32].

7.2 Medullary Abnormalities

7.2.1 Pheochromocytoma

Pheochromocytomas are tumors which secrete abnormal amounts of catecholamines. Paroxysmal attacks of hypertension, diaphoresis, tachycardia, and anxiety are the most frequent clinical manifestations of the tumor [51].

Pheochromocytomas are derived from chromaffin cell nests, which may arise anywhere along the autonomic ganglia chain, or from chromaffin bodies such as the adrenal medulla and organs of ZUCKERKANDL [13, 52–54, 56]. They are located in the adrenal glands in 90% of cases, but can be found anywhere along the axial skeleton from the base of the skull to the lower rectum. Most are solitary and have a predilection for the right adrenal, but approximately 10% are bilateral and 10% ectopic. In children the right over left predominance increases to 2:1, and 20% are bilateral. Multiple and ectopic locations are also much more common [13].

Pheochromocytomas are commonly associated with medullary thyroid carcinomas and parathyroid disease. This triad, termed MEA II or Sipple's syndrome, has a 40% incidence of bilateral pheochromocytoma, which increases to more than 70% when familial pheochromocytoma is associated with medullary carcinoma of the thyroid [13, 52, 57]. Pheochromocytomas are also associated with multiple endocrine adenomatosis type I (Wermer's syndrome). Components of MEA I syndrome include pancreatic islet cell tumor, hyperplasia or tumor of the pituitary and/or parathyroid glands, gastrointestinal or bronchial carcinoid, von Hippel–Lindau syndrome, and neurofibromatosis [13, 52]. Not all components in either syndrome are always present, and the two syndromes can overlap. Pheochromocytomas in the MEA syndromes are almost exclusively adrenal in origin but are frequently unsuspected as the patients are usually normotensive. The detection of pheochromocytoma in patients with MEA syndromes is important because surgery for the associated tumors may precipitate a hypertensive crisis [52].

In 91 cases of proven pheochromocytomas evaluated by CT, the overall accuracy rate was 96% [16, 57, 58]. Most frequently CT identified a unilateral adrenal mass with an attenuation value of 6–70 H and a normal contralateral gland (Fig. 15).

Pheochromocytomas are usually larger than 2 cm in diameter when detected, and while they may be solid lesions, often they contain both cystic and solid components and infrequently are entirely cystic (Figs. 15 and 16). Calcification is uncommon but does occur. They are vascular lesions, and intravenous injection of contrast media makes the nonhomogeneity of some more apparent and helps differentiate the tumor from the inferior vena cava and kidney.

Of the approximately 10% of pheochromocytomas that are malignant, one-third are extra-adrenal [52]. Multiple primary pheochromocytomas (Fig. 17), recurrent benign pheochromocytomas, or other primary tumors appearing later must be distinguished from malignant pheochromocytoma. Distinguishing multiple benign para-aortic pheochromocytomas from lymph node metastases may be difficult with CT, and differentiating a malignant from a benign pheochromocytoma is not always possible on microscopic criteria alone. If a pheochromocytoma is found on CT, additional CT sections through the liver and lungs to exclude metastases are recommended. When normal adrenal

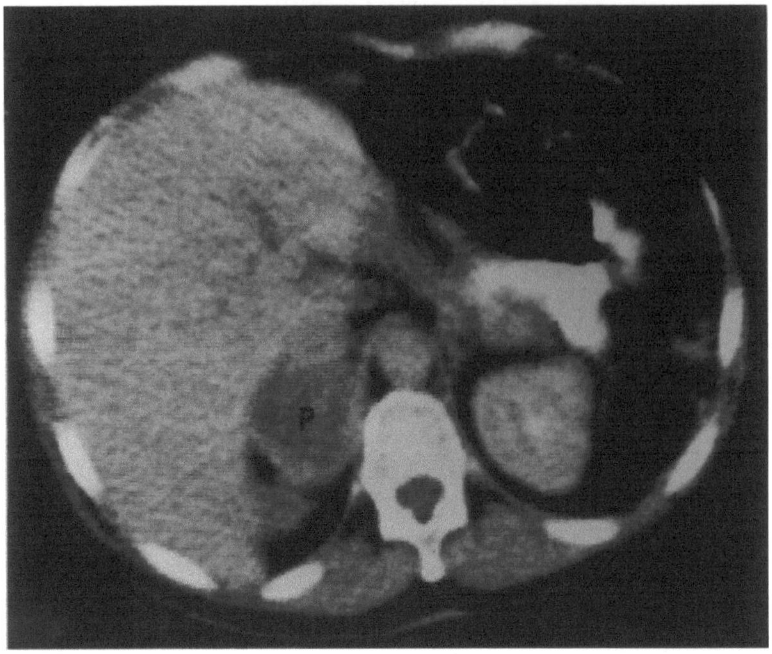

Fig. 15. A right adrenal pheochromocytoma (*P*) having a lower CT density than liver or adjacent muscle

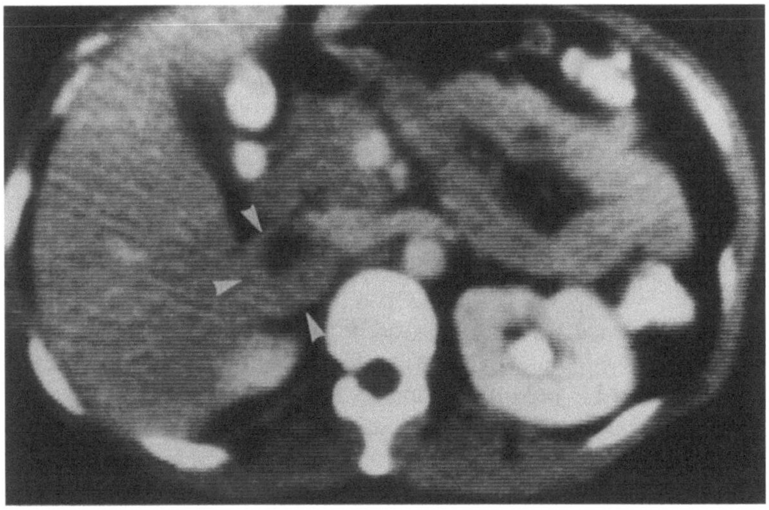

Fig. 16. A right adrenal pheochromocytoma (*arrows*) shown as a nonhomogeneous mass having a solid peripheral component and a central region of cystic degeneration

glands are found in a patient with a strong clinical suspicion of pheochromocytoma, the remaining portion of the abdomen and pelvis should be scanned. Ectopically positioned pheochromocytomas may be identified as mass lesions in the retroperitoneum, pelvis, bladder, or mediastinum.

7.2.2 Neuroblastoma

Neuroblastoma is the second most frequent abdominal malignancy in childhood. While most neuroblastomas arise from the adrenal glands, tumors may originate anywhere along the sympathetic chain from the cervical region to the pelvis [59, 60]. The histologic features range from highly malignant (sympathicogonioma), to the slightly less malignant neuroblastoma, to benign ganglioneuroma [28, 59, 61]. The term neuroblastoma is commonly used to refer to the various malignant grades, and ganglioneuroma to the benign forms. Neuroblastomas are more frequent in males, while ganglioneuromas are more common in females [60, 61].

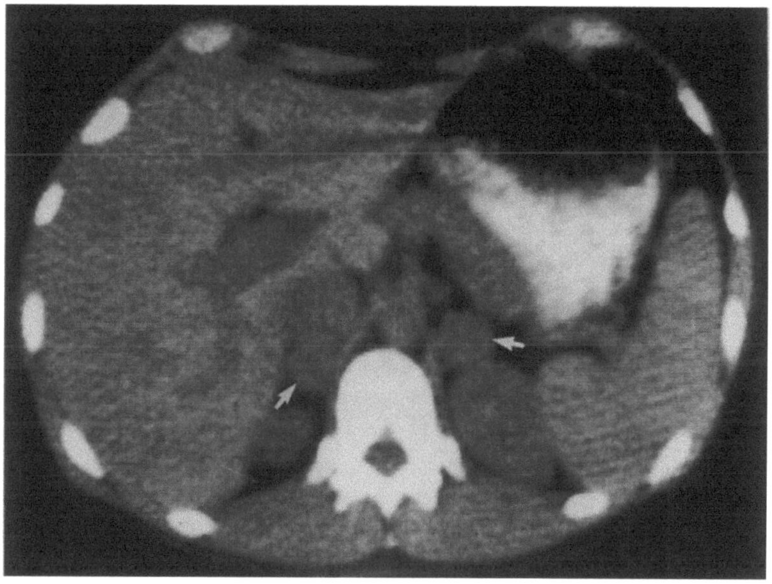

Fig. 17. Bilateral pheochromocytomas in a patient with multiple endocrine adenomatosis Type II (Sipple's syndrome)

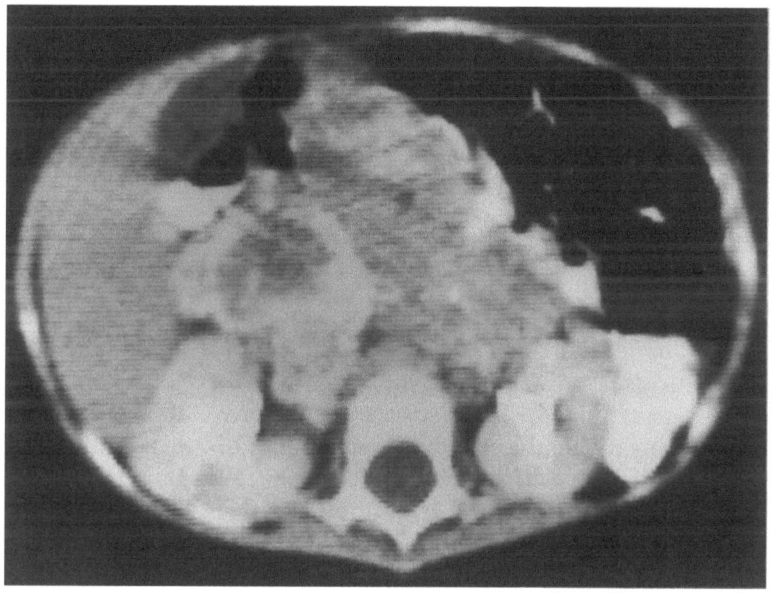

Fig. 18. Right adrenal neuroblastoma containing confluent and ring calcification

Neuroblastomas are more frequent on the left side of the body, and approximately 80% of lesions occur in children younger than 3 years old. These small, round cell tumors metastasize early, with 60%–75% of patients having metastases when initially diagnosed [60–64]. Bone marrow, skeletal, liver, lymph node, and skin metastases are common, but lung metastases are rare and generally occur only late in the course of the disease.

In 85% of primary neuroblastomas, CT demonstrates calcification (Fig. 18). Most frequently the calcifications are scattered irregularly throughout the neuroblastoma, but large solid and ring calcifications surrounding areas of low attenuation within the tumor are also frequent findings [62–64]. The areas of low attenuation probably represent areas of hemorrhage or necrosis within the rapidly growing tumor. Detection of calcifications permits differentiation of a neuroblastoma from Wilms' tumor or other renal or suprarenal masses.

Treatment for neuroblastoma varies depending upon the stage of the tumor when diag-

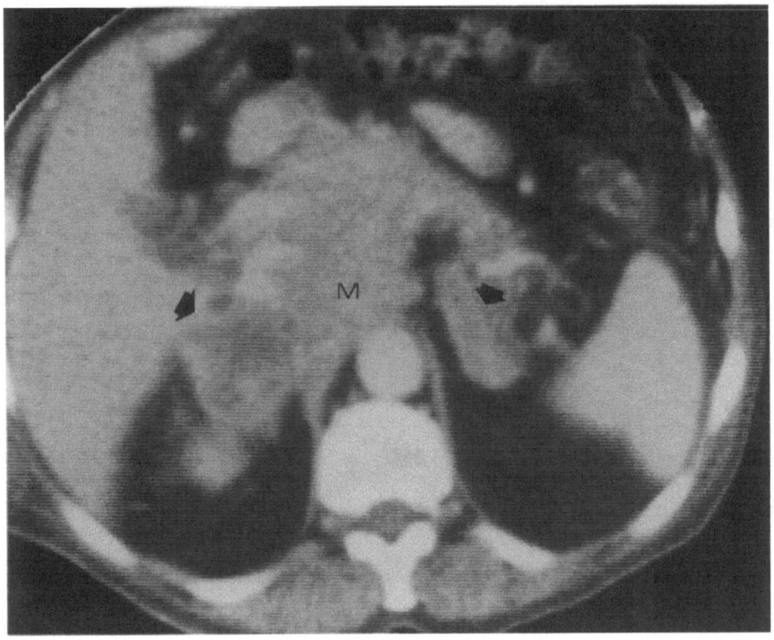

Fig. 19. Bilateral adrenal metastases (*arrows*) from lung carcinoma. A para-aortic mass (*M*) is also present

nosed. Although a variety of imaging techniques can be employed to stage neuroblastoma, to date CT appears to be the most accurate single staging procedure [62, 63]. CT clearly delineates the nature and extent of the primary lesion and simultaneously defines nodal liver metastases, spread of tumor across the diaphragm or midline, and bone destruction. However, CT has proven to be less accurate than bone scintigraphy or bone marrow aspirates in detecting spread of disease to the bone marrow prior to bone destruction [64]. Bone scintigraphy therefore remains a valuable procedure in staging of neuroblastoma. It is likely that nuclear magnetic resonance will be a valuable addition in this staging.

7.3 Secondary Neoplasms

The adrenal glands are the fourth most frequent site of blood-borne metastatic disease [16]. Carcinoma of the lung is the most common, followed by breast, thyroid, colon, and melanoma [13, 47]. Metastasis produces circumscribed mass lesions within the adrenal gland that alter the glands contour (Fig. 19) [5, 10, 13, 47]. They may be unilateral but often are bilateral. The attenuation coefficient of the metastasis is usually close to or identical to the normal adrenal gland, but if tumor necrosis has occurred, the lesion may be nonhomogeneous or even cystic. Metastases are usually relatively small (1–4 cm) but may reach enormous size (Fig. 20). By CT features alone an adrenal metastasis cannot be distinguished from nonfunctioning adrenal tumors. A CT-directed aspiration biopsy or a follow-up CT study in 3–6 months is recommended if it is critical to determine whether an adrenal mass is metastatic [65].

Usually adrenal metastases produce no symptoms and are detected when CT is performed to assess another clinical problem. Rarely a clinical picture of hypoadrenalism will be produced by adrenal metastasis, most frequently by carcinoma of the lung. It is therefore important to evaluate all patients with idiopathic hypoadrenalism to exclude metastatic disease as the etiologic factor.

As nonfunctioning adenomas are extremely common in the general population, one should not assume that an adrenal mass lesion in a patient with a known malignancy represents an adrenal metastasis. Pagani [66] demonstrated that only 17% of glands biopsied were positive for metastatic disease in a series of patients with small cell lung carcinoma. Barnardino et al. [67] also showed that fine needle aspiration in patients with adrenal masses and known malignancy yielded positive results in only 46% of patients. Thus it is clear that not all adrenal masses in patients with carcinoma are malig-

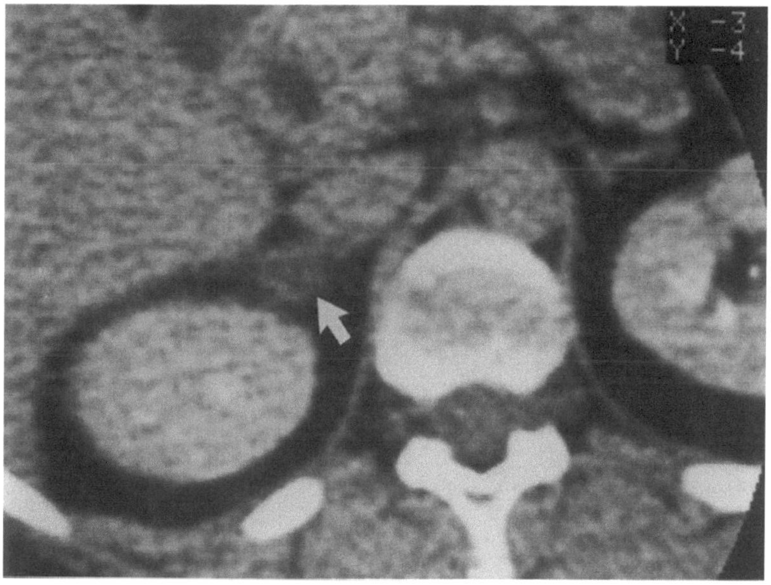

Fig. 20. A small right adrenal metastases (*arrow*) from a gastrin-producing tumor

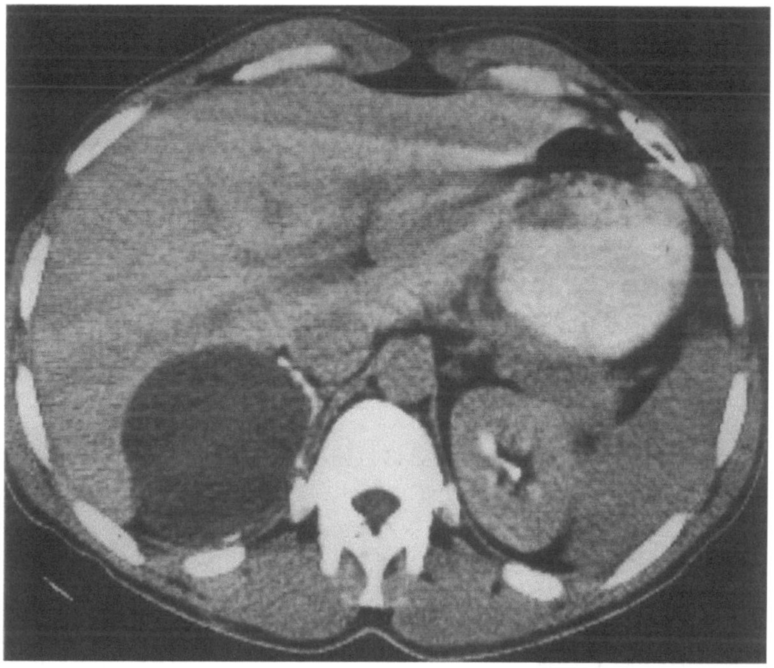

Fig. 21. A large right adrenal cyst with a partially calcified wall

nant, nor does the lack of identification of an adrenal mass preclude a microscopic metastasis being present.

7.4 Unusual Primary Tumors

Adrenal tumors can originate from any of the cellular components of the adrenal gland. Benign tumors such as lymphangiomas, hemangiomas, fibromas, neurofibromas, myomas, and hamartomas as well as malignant degeneration of these tumors can occur [13, 28, 29, 33, 68]. The incidence of these lesions is extremely rare, and their CT appearance have not been described. A single case report of an adrenal hemangioma showed a rounded soft tissue mass containing central calcification [68].

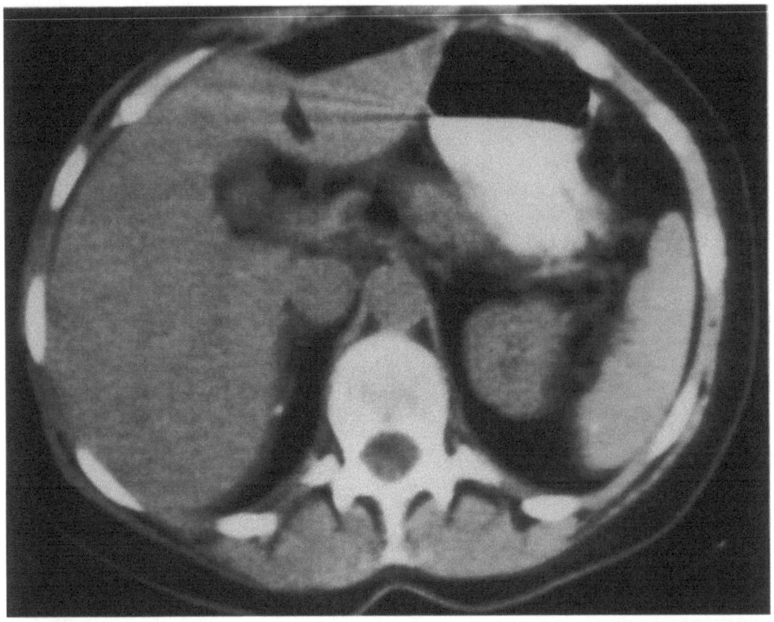

Fig. 22. A partially calcified right adrenal gland due to histoplasmosis

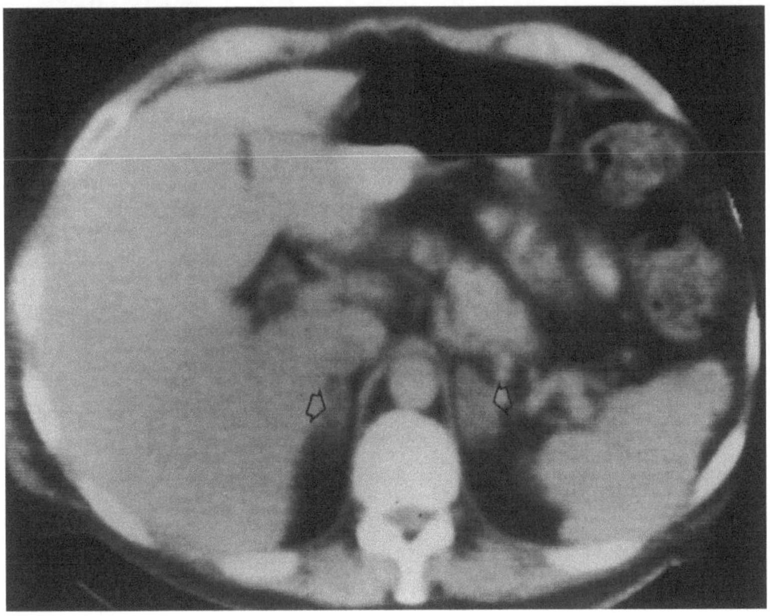

Fig. 23. Hypoadrenalism due to bilateral adrenal hemorrhage. Both adrenal glands (*arrows*) are diffusely enlarged but maintain a normal configuration

7.5 Adrenal Cysts

Cysts of the adrenal may be classified as parasitic, epithelial, endothelial (lymphangiectatic), angiomatous, hamartomatous, and pseudocystic resulting from degenerative necrosis and hemorrhage into the adrenal masses [10, 28]. Of these, pseudocysts and lymphangiectatic cysts are the most common. Cysts may range from small to very large in size and are unilateral in greater than 80% of instances. They are usually asymptomatic and appear on CT as rounded, low density, mass lesions within the adrenal gland. A rim of calcification is present in 15% of cases (Fig. 21) [69, 70]. The diagnosis can be confirmed by surgery or cyst puncture.

7.6 Miscellaneous Abnormalities

7.6.1 *Infection*

A variety of infectious agents can affect the adrenal glands [10, 28, 71], of which tuberculosis [71], histoplasmosis [16], meningococcus, and echinococcus are the most frequent (Fig. 22). The most common radiologic and CT appearance of bilateral adrenal tuberculosis is adrenal calcification, which can be diffuse or localized and punctate. However, tuberculosis can be calcified and result in a unilateral, rounded mass of homogeneous density [71]. Administration of contrast may result in inhomogeneities within the lesion being detected. Without calcification the appearance would be similar to that of a necrotic tumor.

7.6.2 *Hypoadrenalism*

In patients with acute hypoadrenalism secondary to adrenal hemorrhage, CT demonstrates bilaterally enlarged adrenal glands that may maintain a normal configuration (Fig. 23) [16, 72]. Small- to normal-sized adrenal glands have been identified in patients with hypoadrenalism secondary to pituitary irradiation or long-term steroid therapy [5].

7.6.3 *Acromegaly*

The adrenal glands in acromegalic patients are larger than normal but maintain a normal shape and configuration. Adrenal function is normal.

References

1. Karstaedt N, Sagel SS, Stanley RJ, Melson GL, Levitt RG (1978) Computed tomography of the adrenal gland. Radiology 129:723
2. Brownlie K, Kreel L (1978) Computer-assisted tomography of normal supradrenal glands. J Comput Assist Tomogr 2:1
3. Montagne J-P, Kressel HY, Korobkin M, Moss AA (1978) Computed tomography of the normal adrenal glands. AJR 130:963
4. Wilms G, Baert A, Marchal G, Goddeeris P (1979) Computed tomography of the normal adrenal glands: correlative study with autopsy specimens. J Comput Assist Tomogr 3:467
5. Korobkin M, White EA, Kressel HY, Moss AA, Montagne J-P (1979) Computed tomography in the diagnosis of adrenal disease. AJR 132:231
6. Schaner EG, Dunnick NR, Doppman JL, Strott CA, Gill JR Jr, Javadpour N (1978) Adrenal cortical tumors with low attenuation coefficients: a pitfall in computed tomography diagnosis. J Comput Assist Tomogr 2:11
7. Epstein AJ, Patel SK, Petasnick JP (1979) Computerized tomography of the adrenal gland. JAMA 242:2791
8. White EA, Schambelan M, Rost CT, Biglieri EG, Moss AA, Korobkin M (1980) Use of computed tomography in diagnosing the cause of primary aldosteronism. N Engl J Med 303:1503
9. Eghrari M, McLoughlin MJ, Rosen IE, St Louis EL, Wilson SR, Wise DJ, Yeung HPH (1980) The role of computed tomography in assessment of tumoral pathology of the adrenal glands. J Comput Assist Tomogr 4:71
10. Hauser H, Battikba JG, Wettstein P (1981) Pathology of the adrenal glands: common and uncommon findings on computed tomography. Eur J Radiol 1:215
11. Behan M, Martin EC, Muecke EC, Kazam E (1977) Myelolipoma of the adrenal: two cases with ultrasound and CT findings. AJR 129:993
12. Dunnick NR, Schancer EG, Doppman JL, Strott CA, Gill JR, Javadpour N (1979) Computed tomography in adrenal tumors. AJR 132:43
13. Reynes CJ, Churchill R, Moncada R, Love L (1979) Computed tomography of adrenal glands. Radiol Clin North Am 17:91
14. Curtis JA, Brennan RE, Kurtz AB (1980) Evaluation of adrenal disease by computed tomography. Comput Tomogr 4:165
15. Abrams HL, Siegelman SS, Adams DF, Sanders R, Finkerg HJ, Hessel SJ, McNeil BJ (1982) Computed tomography versus ultrasound of the adrenal gland: a prospective study. Radiology 143:121
16. Moss AA (1983) Computed tomography of the adrenal glands. In: Moss A, Gamsu G, Genant H (eds) Computed tomography of the body. Saunders, Philadelphia, pp 837–876
17. Sample WF (1977) A new technique for the evaluation of the adrenal gland with gray-scale ultrasonography. Radiology 124:463
18. Yeh HC, Mitty HA, Rose J, Wolf BS, Gabrilove JL (1978) Ultrasonography of adrenal masses: unusual manifestations. Radiology 127:475
19. Bernardino ME, Goldstein HM, Green B (1978) Gray-scale ultrasonography of adrenal neoplasms. AJR 130:741
20. Yeh H-C (1980) Sonography of the adrenal glands: normal glands and small masses. AJR 135:1167
21. Kenney PJ, Berlow ME, Ellis DA (1984) Current imaging of adrenal masses. Radiographics 4:743
22. Meschan I (1978) Synopsis of radiologic anatomy with computed tomography. Saunders, Philadelphia, pp 534 538
23. Symington T (1969) Functional pathology of the human adrenal gland. Livingston, Edinburgh, pp 13–16
24. Buck J, Reiser V, Heuck F (1982) Computed tomography of the adrenal glands. Eur J Radiol 2:52
25. Herbut PA (1952) Urologic pathology, vol 2. Lea and Febiger, Philadelphia, pp 693–696
26. Soffer LS (1951) Diseases of the endocrine glands. Lea and Febiger, Philadelphia, pp 163–164
27. Besser GM, Edwards CRW (1972) Cushing's syndrome. Clin Endocrinol Metab 1:451
28. McAlister WH, Koehler PR (1967) Diseases of the adrenal. Radiol Clin North Am 2:205
29. Dunnick NR, Doppman JL, Geelhoed GW (1980) Intravenous extension of endocrine tumors. AJR 135:471
30. Federle MP, Moss AA (1979) Adrenal abnormalities. CT/T Clinical symposium, vol 1, no 4. General Electric, Milwaukee
31. Ganguly A, Prott JH, Yune HY, Grim CE, Weinberger MH (1979) Detection of adrenal tumors by computerized tomographic scan in endocrine hypertension. Arch Intern Med 139:589

32. Costello P, Clouse ME, Kane RA, Paris A (1977) Problems in the diagnosis of adrenal tumors. Radiology 125:335
33. Bethune JE (1974) The adrenal cortex. Upjohn, Kalamazoo
34. Mitty HA, Nicolis GL, Gabrilove JL (1973) Adrenal venography: clinical roentgenographic correlation in 80 patients. AJR 119:564
35. Neville AM, MacKay AM (1972) The structure of the human adrenal cortex in health and disease. Clin Endocrinol Metab 1:361
36. Conn JW, Cohen EL, Rouner DR (1964) Suppression of plasma activity in primary aldosteronism: distinguishing primary from secondary aldosteronism in hypertensive disease. JAMA 190:213
37. Linde R, Coulam C, Barttino R, Rhamy R, Gerlock J, Hollifield J (1979) Localization of aldosterone-producing adenoma by computed tomography. J Clin Endocrinol Metab 49:462
38. Biglieri EG, Schambelan M, Burst N, Chang B, Hogan M (1974) Plasma aldosterone concentration: further characterization of aldosterone producing adenomas. Circ Res 34 [Suppl I]:I-183
39. Kahn PC, Killeher MD, Egdahl RH, Melby JC (1971) Adrenal arteriography and venography in primary aldosteronism. Radiology 101:71
40. Kahn PC, Nickrosz LV (1967) Selective angiography of the adrenal glands. AJR 101:739
41. Alfidi RJ, Gili WM Jr, Klein HJ (1969) Arteriography of adrenal neoplasms. AJR 106:635
42. Bookstein JJ, Conn J, Reuter SR (1968) Intraadrenal hemorrhage as a complication of adrenal venography in primary aldosteronism. Radiology 90:778
43. Melby JC, Spark RF, Dale SL, Egdahl RH, Kahn PC (1967) Diagnosis and localization of aldosterone-producing adenomas by adrenal-vein catheterization. N Engl J Med 277:1050
44. Troncone L, Galli G, Salvo D, Barbareno A, Bonoma L (1977) Radioisotopic study of the adrenal glands using ^{131}I-19 iodocholesterol. Br J Radiol 50:340
45. Hogan MJ, McRae J, Scharmbelan M, Biglieri EG (1976) Location of aldosterone producing adenomas with ^{131}I-19 iodocholesterol. N Engl J Med 294:410
46. Miles IM, Wahner HW, Carpenter PC, Salassa RM, Northcutt RC (1979) Adrenal scintiscanning with NP-59, a new radioiodinated cholesterol agent. Mayo Clin Proc 54:321
47. Bosniak MA, Siegelman SS, Evans JA (1976) The adrenal retroperitoneum and lower urinary tract. In: Hodes PJ (ed) Atlas of tumor radiology. Year Book Medical, Chicago
48. Glazer HS, Weyman PJ, Sagel SS, Levitt RG, McClennan BL (1982) Nonfunctioning adrenal masses: incidental discovery on computed tomography. AJR 139:81
49. Olsson CA, Krane RJ, Klugo RC, Selikowitz SM (1973) Adrenal myelolipoma. Surgery 73:665
50. Fink DW, Wurtzebach LR (1980) Symptomatic myelolipoma of the adrenal: report of a case with computed tomographic evaluation. Radiology 134:451
51. Engleman K (1977) Phaeochromocytoma. Clin Endocrinol Metab 6:709
52. Thomas JL, Bernardino ME (1981) Pheochromocytoma in multiple endocrine adenomatosis: efficacy of computed tomography. JAMA 245:1467
53. Thomas JL, Bernardino ME, Samaan VA, Hickey RC (1980) CT of pheochromocytoma. AJR 135:477
54. Foley WD (1980) Ectopic pheochromocytoma. CT/T Clinical symposium, vol 3, no 10. General Electric, Milwaukee
55. Zelch JV, Meany TF, Belhobek GH (1974) Radiographic approach to the patient with suspected pheochromocytoma. Radiology 111:279
56. Laursen K, Damgaard-Pedersen K (1980) CT for pheochromocytoma diagnosis. AJR 134:277
57. Chok J, Freier DT, McCormick TL, Nishiyama RH, Forrest ME, Kaufman A, Borlaza GS (1980) Adrenal medullary disease in multiple endocrine neoplasia type II. AJR 134:23
58. Stewart GH, Bravo EL, Haaga J, Meany TF, Tarazi R (1978) Localization of pheochromocytoma by computed tomography. N Engl J Med 299:460
59. McLaughlin JE, Ulrich H (1977) Maturing neuroblastoma and ganglion neuroblastoma: a study of four cases with long survival. J Pathol 121:19
60. Brasch RC, Korobkin M, Gooding CA (1978) Computed body tomography in children: evaluation of 45 patients. AJR 131:21
61. Dominick HC, Bachmann KD (1979) Neuroblastoma. In: Lohr E (ed) Renal and adrenal tumors. Springer, Berlin Heidelberg New York, pp 302–310
62. Stark DD, Moss AA, Brasch RC, deLorimier AA, Albin AR, London DA, Gooding CA (1983) Neuroblastoma: diagnostic imaging and staging. Radiology 148:101
63. Stark DD, Brasch RC, Moss AA, deLorimier AA, Ablin AR, London DA, Gooding CA (1983) Recurrent neuroblastoma: the role of CT and alternative imaging tests. Radiology 148:107
64. Podrasky AE, Stark DD, Hattner RS, Gooding CA, Moss AA (1983) Radionuclide bone scanning in neuroblastoma: skeletal metastases and primary tumor localization of ^{99m}TCMDP. AJR 141:469
65. Heaston DK, Handel DB, Ashton PR, Korobkin M (1982) Narrow gauge needle aspiration of solid adrenal masses. AJR 138:1143
66. Pagani JJ (1983) Normal adrenal glands in small cell lung carcinoma: CT-guided biopsy. AJR 140:949
67. Bernardino ME, Walther MM, Phillips VM, Graham SD, Sewell CW, Giedgaudas-McClees K, Baumgartner BR, Torres WE, Erwin BC (1985) CT-guided adrenal biopsy: accuracy, safety, and indications. AJR 144:67
68. Lee WJ, Weinreb J, Kumari S, Phillips G, Pochaczeusky R, Pillari G (1982) Adrenal hemangioma. J Comput Assist Tomogr 6:392
69. Palubinskas AJ, Christensen WR, Harrison JH, Sosman MC (1959) Calcified adrenal cyst. AJR 82:853
70. Daffener RH (1979) Evaluation of suprarenal mass. CT/T Clinical symposium, vol 1, no 3. General Electric, Milwaukee
71. Wilms GE, Baert AL, Kint EJ, Pringot JH, Goddeeris PG (1983) Computed tomographic findings in bilateral adrenal tuberculosis. Radiology 146:729
72. Albert SG, Wolverson MK, Johnson FE (1982) Bilateral adrenal hemorrhage in an adult: demonstration by computed tomography. JAMA 247:1737

Scintigraphic Studies of Renal and Adrenal Function*

M.D. GROSS and B. SHAPIRO

1 Introduction

Scintigraphic localization of renal and adrenal tumors is based upon the selective accumulation and excretion of specific radiopharmaceuticals designed to take advantage of the unique and multiple biologic characteristics of these tissues. In this regard the radiodiagnostic probes used to image the kidneys, adrenal cortex, and medulla are singular for each purpose. Their metabolism and pharmacology allow a glimpse into the functional status of their respective target tissues. The quantitative scintigraphic map created by the distribution of these radiopharmaceuticals represents a multifaceted approach to the determination of anatomy and function that cannot be achieved by other static, noninvasive, radiographic methods. The efficacy has been repeatedly confirmed.

With the increasing sensitivity of biochemical analysis, the diagnosis of disease has become more dependent upon the recognition of abnormal function. In many instances, even high spatial resolution modalities of this approach of localization may fail to depict subtle changes in anatomy that are functionally manifest. The role of scintigraphy in demonstrating the functional state of the target tissue has become very important in the diagnostic evaluation of renal and adrenal disease, especially in multimodality imaging. Thus, scintigraphy complements the anatomic detail afforded by ultrasonography, computed tomography, and, potentially, that from nuclear magnetic resonance imaging.

* Supported by NCI(CA-09015), the NIAMDD(RO1-AM-21477-RAD), the GCRX(HEW 3M01-RR-0042-21CLR), the Nuclear Medicine Research Fund, and the Veterans Administration Research Service

2 Radiopharmaceuticals

The agents used to image the kidneys are broadly characterized as those that depict glomerular filtration or tubular secretion, or those that bind to parenchymal elements. Each category of agents has its own special characteristics necessary to provide particular information. Thus, there is no single "ideal" renal imaging agent; a spectrum of radiopharmaceuticals exist that can define a specific facet(s) of renal function(s) and be used in concert to depict renal activity and to perform differential function analysis. Optimal agents for glomerular filtration are those that are gamma-labeled, excreted rapidly after injection, and are neither metabolized nor bound to plasma proteins. Optimal agents for the study of tubular secretion share the same characteristics, but must be excreted by active tubular function. Anatomic definition of the kidneys is best depicted by agents that bind to the renal parenchyma with high affinity and are labeled with gamma emitters with short half-lives, e.g., ^{99m}Technetium.

Adrenal imaging agents to date have been limited to precursor compounds in adrenal cortical imaging, e.g., iodocholesterol, and antiadrenergics with structural similarity to the neurotransmitter hormone norepinephrine for chromaffin tissue imaging. The accumulation of the iodocholesterol derivatives depicts adrenal function and with appropriate pharmacologic manipulation, patterns of uptake can be further compartmentalized to allow analysis of all three zones of the adrenal cortex in glucocorticoid, androgen, and mineralocorticoid dysfunction. Accumulation of the adrenergic imaging agent, metaiodobenzylguanidine (mIBG) depicts the adrenergic nature of tumors. The uptake of the agent is affected by manipulations and drugs known to modify catecholamine secretion, neuronal storage, and re-uptake. Sufficiently avid uptake of mIBG has allowed therapeutic doses of radiation to be delivered to some primary and metastatic lesions.

2.1 Renal Imaging Agents

^{99m}Technetium-labeled radiopharmaceuticals have replaced most of the radioiodine-containing renal imaging agents. These include:

1. Agents cleared by glomerular filtration: diethylenetriaminepentaacetic acid (DTPA), glucoheptonate (GLH);
2. Agents cleared by tubular secretion: orthoiodohippurate (OIH); and
3. Agents with parenchymal retention: 2,3-dimercaptosuccinic acid (DMSA) and GLH.

Their individual renal clearance rates dictate their use in the study of renal anatomy and function: those that are more rapidly excreted are employed primarily for functional analysis, while those retained for longer intervals are used to depict renal anatomy. The retention times also influence dosimetry as those agents that are cleared rapidly expose the bladder wall to a greater amount of radiation than those which are cleared more slowly (Table 1). The most useful agents are DTPA [1], GLH [2], DMSA [3].

The radioiodinated renal imaging agent OIH is rapidly cleared by the renal tubules (>90%) and has been the agent of choice for the evaluation of tubular function [4]. Moreover, as the clearance of this agent approximates that of para-aminohippurate, it is the only radiopharmaceutical used to assess and quantify effective renal plasma flow. The availability of ^{123}Iodine for these compounds provides a gamma emitter with a short half-life for renal tubular functional analysis that obviates the problems inherent using ^{131}Iodine (Table 1) [5]. Of the three ^{99m}Technetium-labeled agents, GLH has been used most generally for renal imaging. GLH demonstrates prompt renal excretion (<1 h) so renal anatomy can be defined. A more important characteristic of GLH is that pelvicaliceal collecting system imaging, critical in the evaluation of obstructive uropathy, can be easily performed [2]. DTPA is used primarily as an agent for the study of glomerular filtration [1]. The agent is rapidly cleared and provides optimal images of the pelvicaliceal collecting system. In contrast to GLH, however, the rapid clearance of DTPA does not allow optimal cortical imaging in evaluation of renal parenchymal disease. DMSA is cleared by the cortex more slowly than either DTPA or GLH and is used to depict anatomic abnormalities of the kidneys. Moreover, as a result of its slow plasma clearance, it is not an optimal radiopharmaceutical for delineating the pelvicaliceal collecting system [3].

Table 1. Dosimetry of the radiopharmaceuticals for renal imaging under conditions of normal renal function (rad/mCi)

	^{99m}Tc-DTPA	^{99m}Tc-GLH	^{99m}Tc-DMSA	^{131}I-OIH	^{123}I-OIH
Kidney	0.04	0.2	0.6	0.07	0.02
Bladder	0.6	0.8	0.3	8.0	0.7
Total body	0.016	0.007	0.016	0.020	0.008

2.2 Adrenal Imaging Agents

The radiopharmaceuticals used to image the adrenals depict adrenal function by specific receptor-dependent mechanisms of uptake. The agents are quite dissimilar; derivatives of radiocholesterol are used to image the functions of the adrenal cortex, while derivatives of the benzylguanidines are used to image abnormal tissues of adrenergic origin.

2.2.1 Adrenal Cortical Imaging Agents

The agents available for adrenal cortical imaging include ^{131}I-19-iodocholesterol, ^{131}I-6β-iodomethyl-19-norcholesterol (NP-59) and ^{75}Se-selenomethylnorcholesterol (Table 2; Fig. 1) [6]. All are accumulated by the adrenal cortex via

Table 2. Dosimetry of the radiopharmaceuticals for adrenal gland imaging (rad/mCi)

	^{131}I-NP-59	^{75}Se-selenomethylnorcholesterol	^{131}I-mIBG	^{123}I-mIBG
Adrenal	30	24.4	100	0.8
Liver	2.4	14.0	0.4	0.05
Heart	–	–	0.7	0.03
Spleen	–	0.4	1.6	0.14
Ovary	8.0	7.6	1.0	0.06
Testes	2.3	–	–	0.06
Total body	1.2	5.6	0.1	0.02

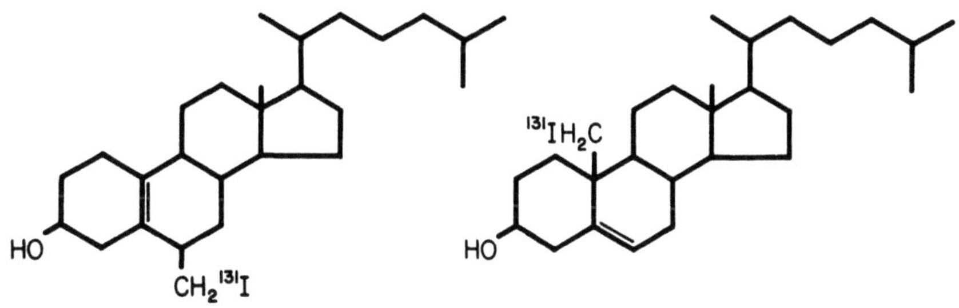

^{131}I-NP-59
(6β-^{131}I-IODOMETHYL-19-NOR CHOLEST-5(10)-EN-3β-OL)

^{131}I-19-IODOCHOLESTEROL
(^{131}I-19-IODOCHOLEST-5(6)-EN-3β-OL)

Fig. 1. Structural formulae of ^{131}I-NP-59 (6β-^{131}I-iodomethyl-19-norcholest-5(10)-en-3β-ol) and ^{131}I-19-iodocholesterol (^{131}I-19-iodocholest-5(6)-en-3β-ol)

receptor-dependent processes [7]. Once injected, these agents are packaged in the liver into lipoproteins, particles that allow their solubilization in the blood [8]. In man the lipoprotein responsible for substrate acquisition by the adrenals has a characteristic apoprotein located on its surface, and the specific particle created has a characteristic density [7]. These adrenal "specific" particles are of the low density type (LDL) and are recognized by a specialized portion of the adrenocortical cell membrane, the LDL receptor [8]. Accumulation of cholesterol substrate necessary for steroid hormone biosynthesis and of radiocholesterol for imaging is dependent upon LDL receptor activity [7]. Modulation of LDL receptor number and avidity for LDL results in reciprocal changes in LDL-derived cholesterol and radiolabeled cholesterol adrenal uptake [8]. The tropic hormones, adrenocorticotropin (ACTH), and angiotensin-2 affect LDL-derived cholesterol receptor-mediated adrenal cortical uptake [7]. Conversely, suppression of ACTH by exogenous steroid hormones, expanded plasma volume following salt loading, and, potentially, inhibitors of gonadotropins result in decreases of LDL-derived cholesterol and radiocholesterol adrenal cortical uptake [7]. Furthermore, the levels of circulating LDL-derived cholesterol and intra-adrenal cortical cholesterol affect LDL-derived cholesterol (and radiocholesterol) uptake by the adrenal cortex [7, 8]. Thus, a complex mechanism functions to supply substrate cholesterol to the adrenal that can have profound effects upon the uptake of radiocholesterol in both health and disease.

As a result of the more avid adrenal cortical uptake of the 6β-norcholesterol derivative, NP-59 and the ^{75}Selenium-labeled cholesterol analogue (Scintidren) have become the adrenal cortical imaging agents of choice. Although distributed rapidly into LDL, the clearance of radiocholesterol is slow, and to reach favorable target to background radioactivity ratios for adequate adrenal cortical imaging requires from 72 to 96 h after injection [10]. High background radioactivity persists as a result of hepatic uptake and there is an enterohepatic circulation of radiocholesterol with persistent bowel radioactivity. These characteristics are responsible for the radiation dosimetry of these compounds (Table 2).

Once localized within the adrenal cortex, there is little if any metabolism of these agents [11]. Radiolabeled steroid metabolites are not evident, and the biological half-life of the agent once localized in the adrenal parallels the physical half-life of the radiolabel.

2.2.2 Adrenal Medulla Imaging Agents

Although many radiolabeled compounds have shown selective accumulation in catecholamine-secreting tissues, none has demonstrated the sufficient uptake necessary for in vivo imaging until the introduction of the guanethidine analogue, metaiodobenzylguanidine (mIBG) [12]. Avid and specific uptake of mIBG has been reported in pheochromocytomas, neuroblastomas, and other neoplasms that share characteristics of adrenergic tissues [13–15].

The structural similarity of mIBG to the neurotransmitter norepinephrine probably accounts for the kinetics of mIBG uptake into adrenergic tissues (Fig. 2) [16]. Like norepinephrine, mIBG is accumulated by a specific,

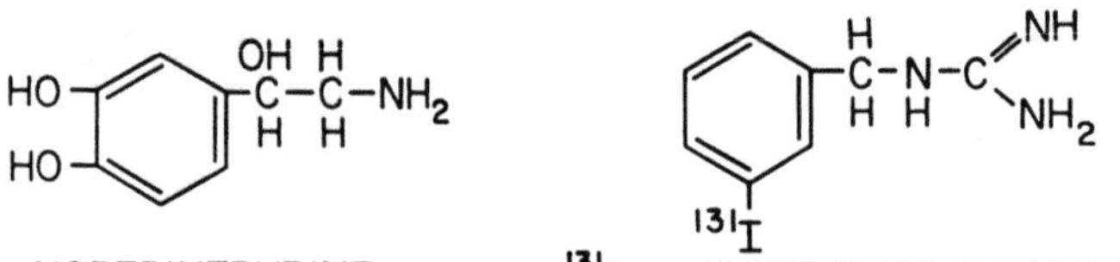

NOREPINEPHRINE ^{131}I-m-IODOBENZYLGUANIDINE

Fig. 2. Structural formulae of norepinephrine and ^{131}I-m-iodobenzylguanidine

energy dependent process within adrenergic cells, the so-called uptake 1 mechanism [17]. mIBG appears to be stored within the neurosecretory granules of these tissues. Like a norepinephrine analogue, pharmacologic manipulations using maneuvers known to block catecholamine uptake, e.g., reserpine, result in a decrement of mIBG uptake [18]. Conversely, agents known to deplete neurosecretory catecholamine granules facilitate mIBG egress, e.g., insulin hypoglycemia [18].

Although ^{131}I-mIGB is distributed widely its uptake into adrenergic tumors is rapid and with high affinity. The dosimetry of mIBG, even radiolabeled with ^{131}I, is not excessive and is in a range acceptable for screening procedures (Table 2). The rapid clearance and minimal deiodination make ^{123}I-mIBG imaging possible, and single photon emission tomography (SPECT) may be a useful adjunct to localization of adrenergic neoplasms [19]. Furthermore, its rapid accumulation within malignant pheochromocytomas and neuroblastomas in many patients has allowed therapeutic levels of radiation to be delivered to these neoplasms without significant adverse systemic effects [20].

3 Functional Scintigraphy of the Kidneys

A simplified view of renal function is that of a three-component system wherein blood is filtered at the glomerulus, various electrolytes and metabolites are selectively absorbed and secreted, concentration of urine in the tubular system, and excretion into the pelvicaliceal system. Each of the processes can be depicted and functionally characterized using the appropriate scintigraphic approach; specific radiopharmaceuticals can be administered and by virtue of their renal handling, provide a qualitative and quantitative glimpse into this anatomically and functionally complex organ.

3.1 Measurement of Glomerular Filtration

The dynamic process of glomerular filtration provides for the creation of an ultrafiltrate of plasma that begins the process of urine formation. The rate of glomerular filtration (GFR) is an integrated value composed of and dependent upon multiple factors including glomerular and tubular membrane hydrostatic pressures, oncotic pressures, capillary wall permeability, and the effective surface area of the filtration membrane [21]. Calculation of GFR is dependent upon the knowledge of the volume of urine created of a substance in a given time interval. This is done using the well-described mathematical formula $GFR = UV/P$ where U is the concentration of a given indicator in the urine, V is the volume of urine excreted (unit/time), and P is the plasma concentration of the substance [22]. The ideal agent for this purpose has been inulin, an agent that is not metabolized or bound to plasma proteins, and does not experience significant renal tubular secretion or reabsorption.

Radiotracer studies of GFR were initially performed using multiple sampling of blood radioactivity levels. GFR calculations compared favorably to those utilizing inulin, but were cumbersome to perform. The application of ^{99m}Tc-labeled compounds, particularly ^{99m}Tc-labeled DTPA, has allowed rapid and reliable measurements of GFR from individual kidneys (the relative proportion of the overall GFR contributed by each kidney), information that is not available with traditional methods (creatinine clearance calculation) [23, 24]. The recent introduction of single injection algorithms and sampling available on many computer software packages allows split GFR calculations with absolute quantitation. These techniques have clinical utility in the evaluation of renal transplant function and the pre- and postoperative evaluation of asymmetric renal dysfunction (Fig. 3). The actual calculations and methods used are outside the scope of this chapter; however,

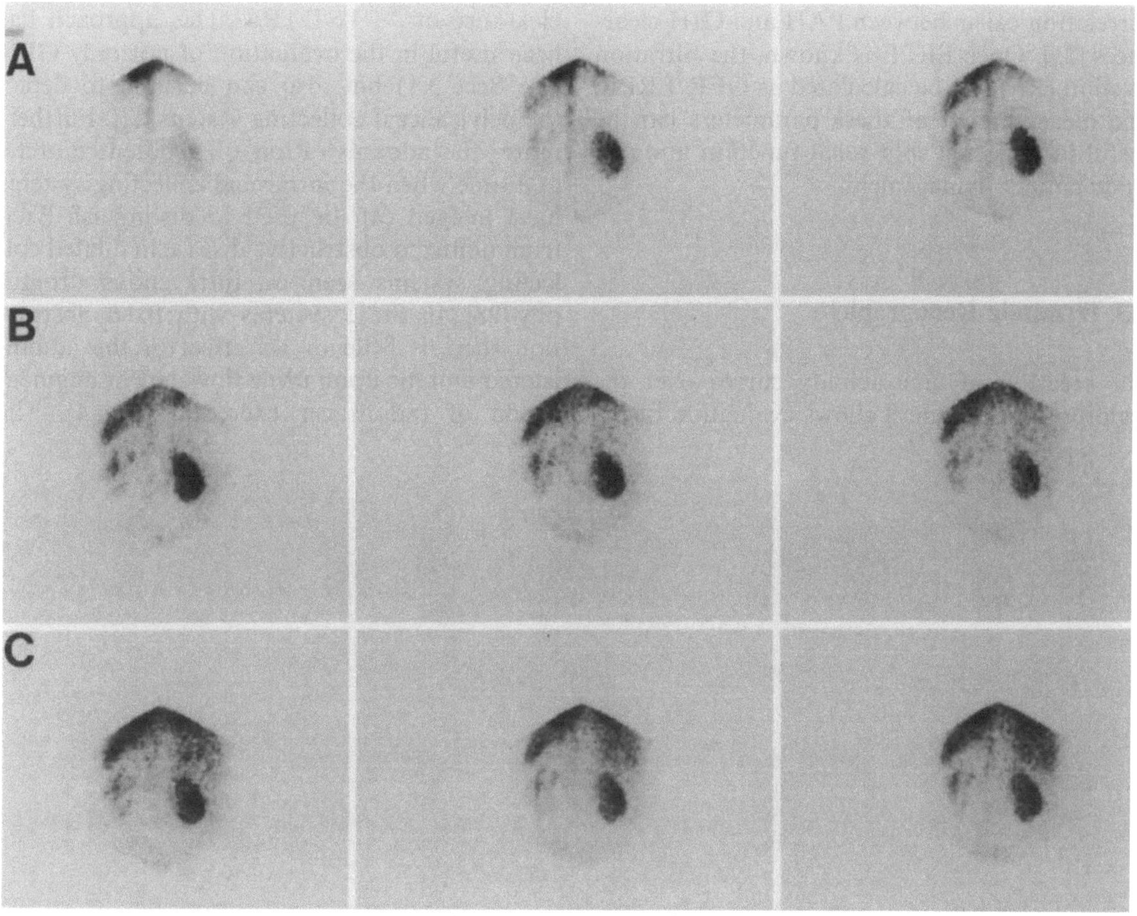

Fig. 3 A-C. Selected images from a posterior ^{99m}Tc-DTPA sequential renal scan demonstrating marked asymmetric renal function. **A** The arterial phase of the tracer wherein minimal left-sided adrenal activity is shown. **B** Confirmation of the marked absence of left-sided renal activity (5-7 min postinjection). **C** Continued absence of significant left-sided renal activity in a patient with severe renal vascular disease and renal infarction (25-35 min postinjection)

many excellent monographs are available for the interested reader [23, 24].

3.2 Renal Tubular Function Studies

A complex series of events occurs within the renal tubules where the ultrafiltrate of plasma passes through a specialized system of tubule membranes, each having a set of special function(s). In the proximal convoluted tubule extensive reabsorption of water, chloride, sodium, bicarbonate, glucose, and amino acids occurs. The process then moves to the loop of Henle, where there is continued resorption of sodium and chloride in the descending limb, and resorption of potassium in the ascending limb. Once the urine has passed out of the descending limb of the loop of Henle, it is further concentrated in the distal convoluted tubule and in the renal collecting system. These last two sites are affected by antidiuretic hormone (ADH) and aldosterone [25].

Estimation of tubular function demands agents that are neither metabolized nor protein bound, but are completely secreted by the tubules. The traditional agent used to study tubular function is para-aminohippuric acid (PAH). The radiopharmaceutical used for tubular function analysis has been OIH labeled with either ^{131}I or ^{123}I [26]. An assessment of effective renal plasma flow (ERPF) can be obtained using single injection compartmental analysis. The methods used are outside the scope of this chapter, but suffice it to say that a very close correlation exists between PAH and OIH clearances [25]. Once ERPF is known, the filtration fraction (FF) can be calculated as GFR/ERPF. The measurement of these parameters can be useful in assessing split renal function and can guide patient management.

3.3 Dynamic Renography

The creation of time activity curves over the region of both kidneys allows evaluation of the clearance of ^{99m}Tc-DTPA. This approach has been useful in the evaluation of not only GFR (see Sect. 3.1) but also can be used to depict the pelvicaliceal collecting system [27]. Furthermore, the administration of a potent diuretic at a time when the intrarenal collecting systems have imaged can be used to distinguish fixed from nonfixed obstructive disease in dilated collecting systems seen on intravenous urography [28]. In those systems with fixed obstruction there is little or no effect of the administered diuretic upon urine flow and/or augmentation of radiotracer excretion (Fig. 4). The

A

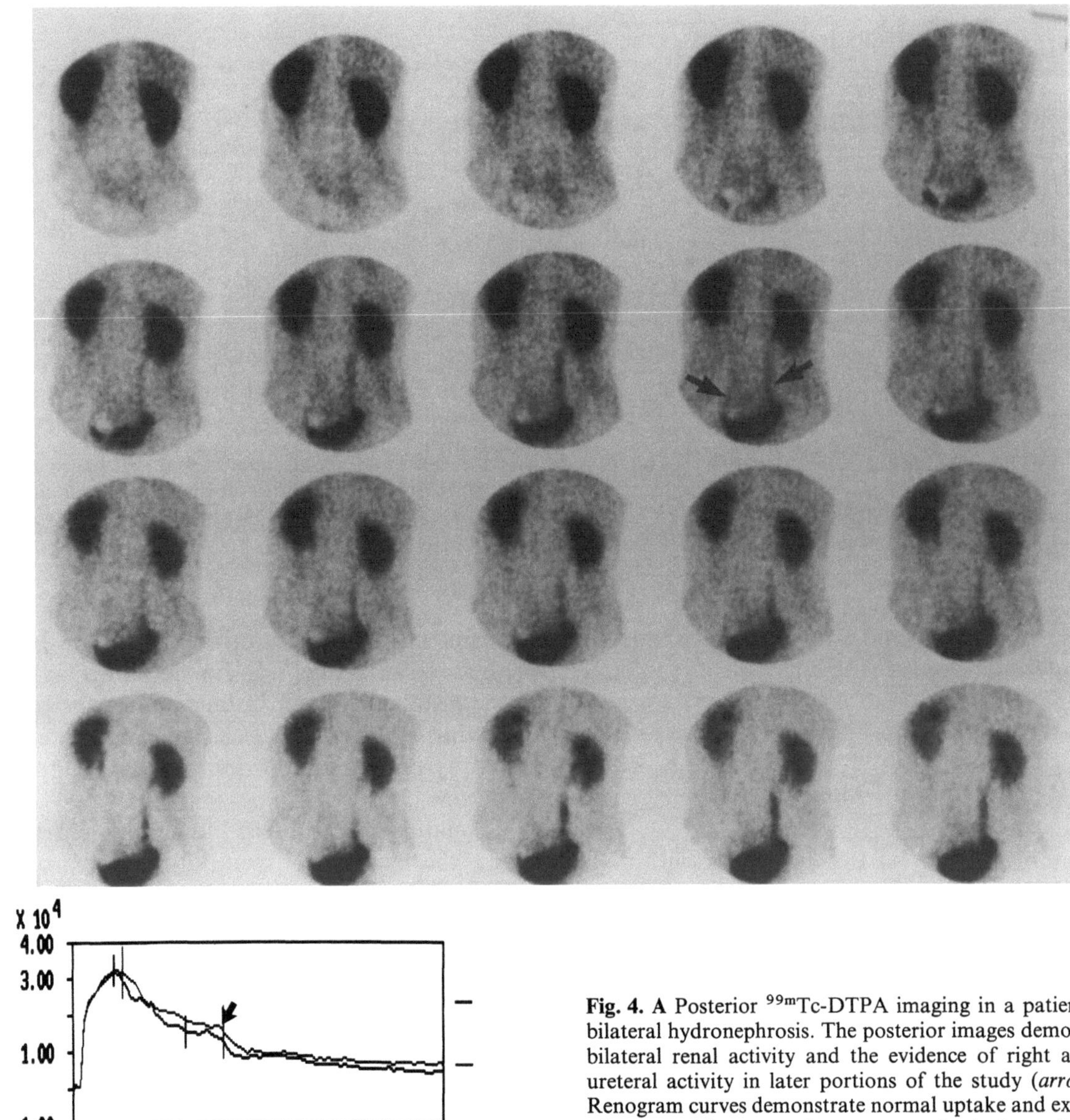

B

Fig. 4. A Posterior ^{99m}Tc-DTPA imaging in a patient with bilateral hydronephrosis. The posterior images demonstrate bilateral renal activity and the evidence of right and left ureteral activity in later portions of the study (*arrows*). **B** Renogram curves demonstrate normal uptake and excretion of tracer with a normal response to Lasix (*arrow*) in this patient with dilated but otherwise normally functioning kidneys and no evidence of fixed obstruction

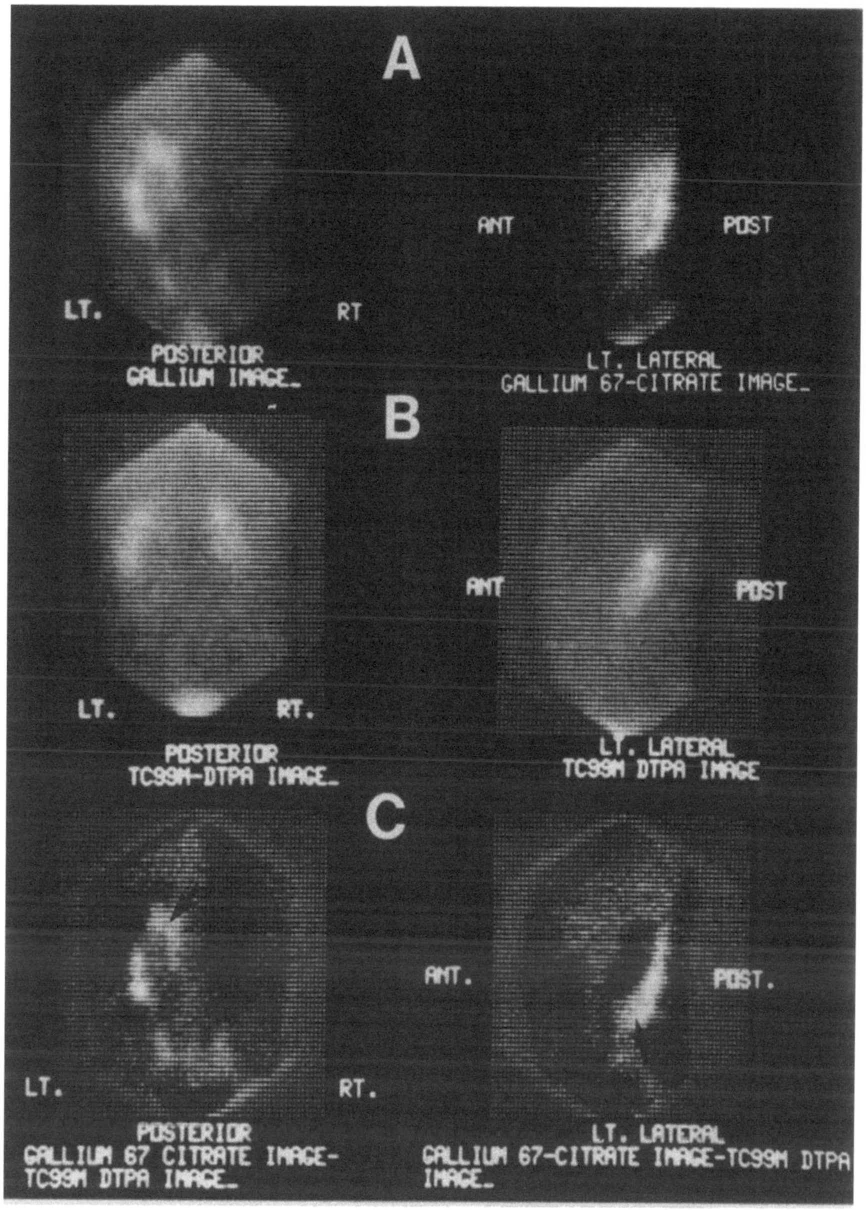

Fig. 5 A-C. Composite study of a patient with a left-sided perinephric abscess. **A** Posterior and left lateral gallium citrate images demonstrating increased uptake in the region of the left kidney. **B** Posterior and left lateral ^{99m}Tc-DTPA images for renal localization. **C** Posterior and left lateral gallium citrate minus ^{99m}Tc-DTPA image localizes the abscess to the posterior perinephric region (*arrows*)

study allows for determination of split excretion dynamics and has considerable utility in a preoperative assessment to ensure that only those patients with fixed obstructions are selected for drainage procedures. This examination is not as useful in those patients with markedly abnormal renal function as sufficient renal function is necessary to accumulate radiotracer within the collecting systems that can be augmented by diuretics to demonstrate urine flow. An alternative approach involves mathematical analysis, using deconvolution to obtain renal parenchymal and whole kidney (parenchymal and collecting system) transit times [29]. In this technique the time activity curve of the tracer in the vascular compartment is mathematically converted into an instantaneous pulse input function (the equivalent of administering the tracer by very rapid injection directly into the renal artery). The same procedure is performed on the renogram curves for the kidney as a whole and for a region of interest over the renal parenchyma alone. From these the parenchymal and whole kidney time activity curves transit times are derived. Normal kidneys will have rapid tracer transit times through the parenchyma

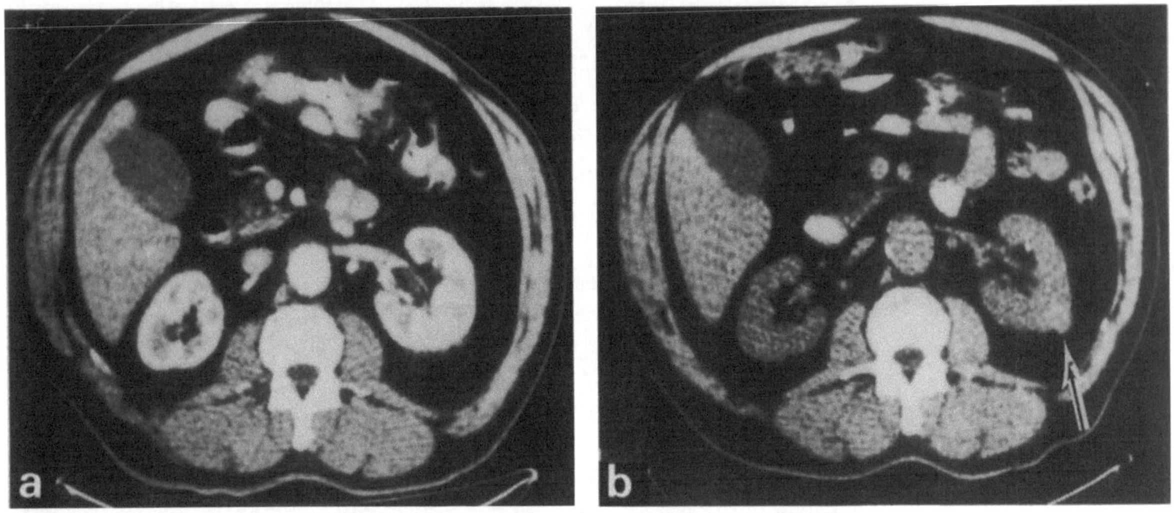

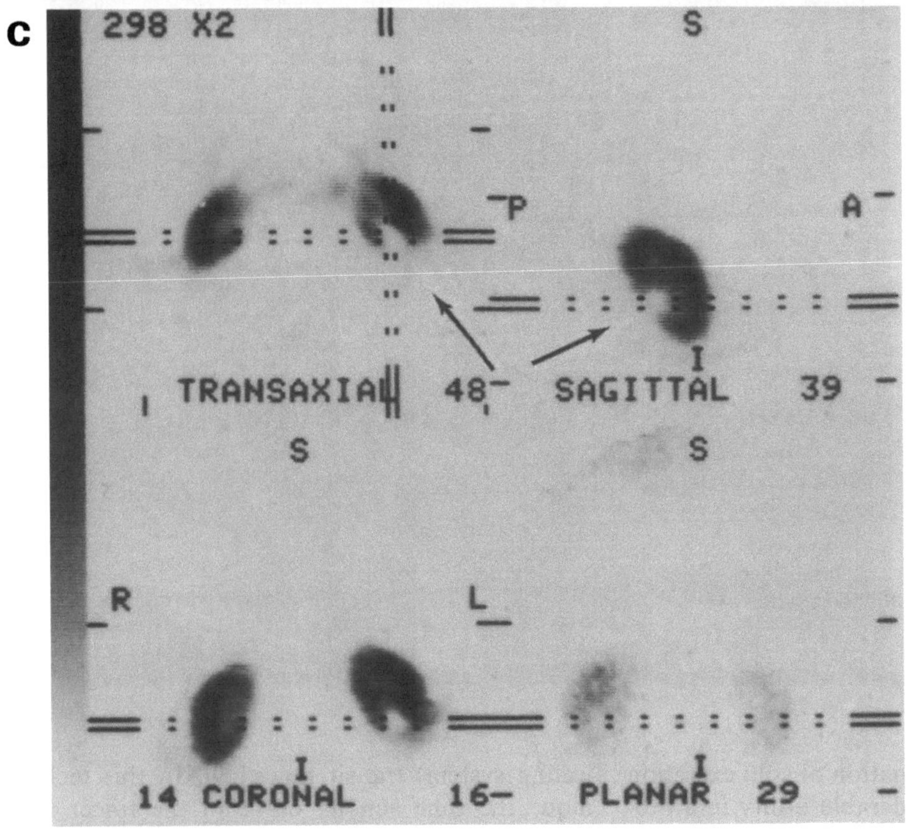

Fig. 6. **a** Contrast-enhanced CT; no renal masses detected. **b** Noncontrast-enhanced CT; cortical mass showing projection beyond cortex (*arrow*). **c** ^{99m}Tc-GLH single photon emission tomographic renal scan demonstrating a cortical mass (*arrow*) on both the transaxial and sagittal sections which was not detected with other imaging procedures. With permission: Eur J Nucl Med (1985) 11:217-220

and the pelvicaliceal system (and thus the kidney as a whole). Kidneys with dilated but patent collecting systems will have normal parenchymal transit times but delayed whole kidney transit times. In contrast those kidneys with significant obstruction of the collecting systems have prolonged parenchymal whole kidney transit times [19].

3.4 Radionuclide Renal Localization

Evaluation of renal anatomy by the scintigraphic approach has not had the same acceptance as that by CT or ultrasound. The radiotracer studies lack the high spatial resolution of the other modalities. Lacking specific radiopharmaceuticals for tumor imaging, radionuclide studies of renal anatomy rely upon the identification of photopenic regions to localize most neoplasms [30]. There is some benefit in the identification of functioning but abnormal anatomic renal parenchyma, e.g., column of Bertin or fetal lobulation, but this is not a commonly encountered problem. Scintigraphy has been used in renal parenchymal disease to detect: primary mass lesions, both benign (functional) and malignant, metastases, vascular lesions, renal trauma, collecting system disorders such as obstruction, renal infarction, inflammation, and congenital disorders. Renal and perirenal infections can be localized with ^{67}Gallium citrate and occasionally can be separated from parenchymal processes by a computer subtraction approach (Fig. 5). The introduction of SPECT imaging of the kidneys has allowed improved localization and spatial resolution (Fig. 6). Traumatic injuries to the renal parenchyma can also be imaged using the scintigraphic, noninvasive approach [30]. Hematomas and lacerations are visualized as "cold" defects. Rapid sequence imaging following intravenous ^{99m}Tc-DTPA injection may be very helpful in demonstrating partial or complete vascular avulsion and may be performed in the emergency room using a mobile gamma camera. The same tracer may also be helpful in demonstrating urine leaks following accidental or surgical trauma.

4 Adrenal Cortical Scintigraphy

The adrenal cortex is composed of three concentric rings of tissue each with a separate principal steroid hormone product. Control of hormone secretion from the zones is unique and permits their manipulation by pharmacologic means. The outer zone of the cortex, the zona glomerulosa, is responsible for synthesis and secretion of the hormone aldosterone, which is the principle mineralocorticoid responsible for sodium and potassium exchange in the distal nephron. Secretion of aldosterone is under the influence of the renin-angiotensin system in which renin, an enzyme produced by the kidney, circulates to the lung where it catalyzes the degradation of angiotensinogen to angiotensin 1. Angiotensin 1 is then cleaved by a converting enzyme to angiotensin 2. Angiotensin 2 circulates to the adrenal where it stimulates the release of aldosterone. Other effectors of aldosterone secretion are hyperkalemia, plasma volume depletion (probably acting through the recently described cardiac hormone, atrial natriuretic factor), and ACTH [31].

The steroid hormones produced by the two inner adrenal cortical zones, the zona fasiculata and zona reticularis, are cortisol and androgens, respectively. Both zones respond to ACTH stimulation and exogenous suppression with glucocorticoids. As yet there is no separate factor apart from ACTH that stimulates adrenal androgens, but in some patients suppression of gonadotropins, e.g., LH, has resulted in suppression of adrenal androgen secretion [31].

As a result of the complex nature of the adrenal cortex, pharmacologic manipulation of adrenal secretagogues is an important adjunct in the successful determination of adrenal dysfunction and is critical for the scintigraphic localization of adrenal cortical tumors [31].

4.1 Normal Adrenal Imaging

Adrenal cortical scintigraphy is performed using 1 mCi of NP-59 administered intravenously after thyroid blockade with a suitable stable iodide-containing compound [32]. As a result of high background radioactivity images are best obtained after 72 h, with most optimal imaging occurring at 5 days or later. Normal images show bilateral and symmetric NP-59 uptake. These images depict the normal cephalocaudal and anteroposterior adrenal asymmetry; the right adrenal lies more superior and posterior than the left. This asymmetry must be recognized if scintiscans are to be correctly interpreted [33].

4.2 Quantification of Adrenal Gland Radiocholesterol Uptake

The level of NP-59 accumulation by the adrenal cortex can be used in addition to the scintiscan (pattern of imaging) to characterize adrenal function. The presence of abnormal function (excessive hormone production) is accompanied

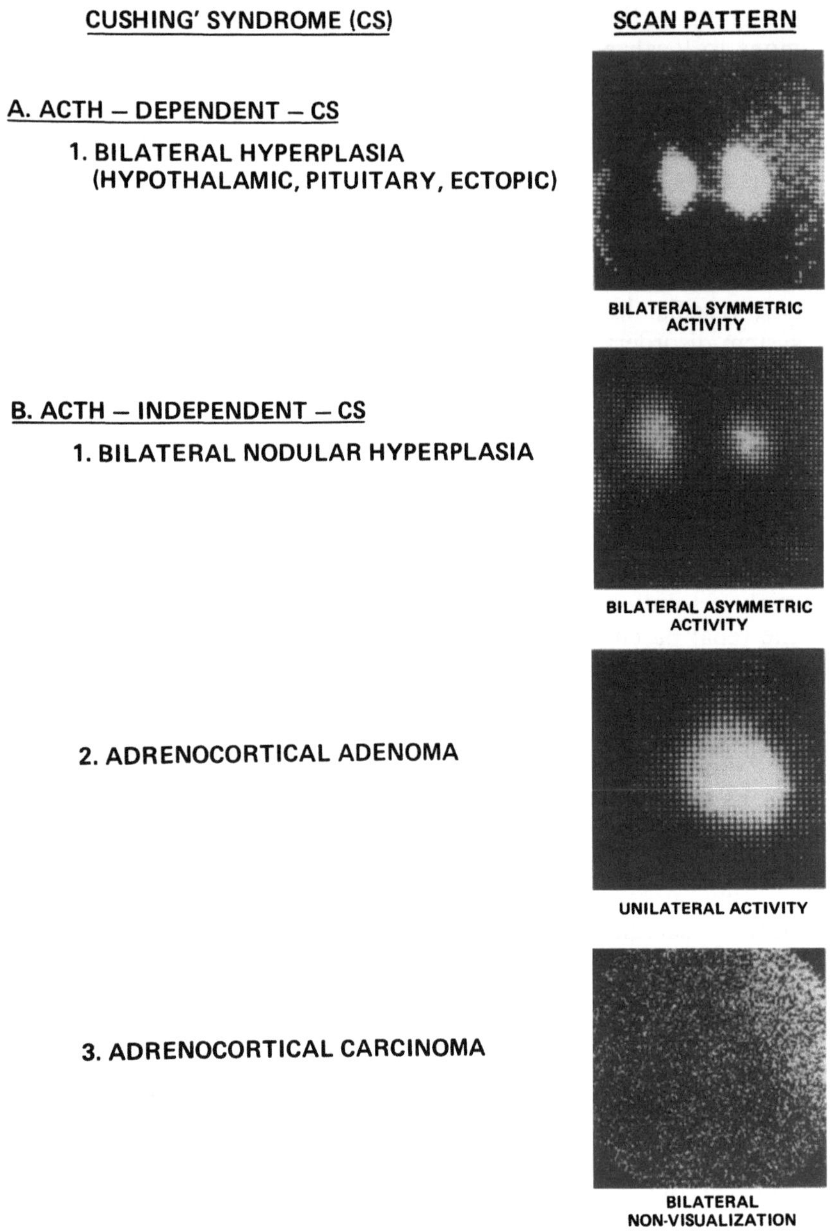

Fig. 7. Scan patterns in Cushing's syndrome. With permission: Urol Radiol (1982) 3:241-244

by elevated NP-59 uptake by the adrenal gland. The method utilized is a semi-operator-independent computer algorithm in which the "center" point of each adrenal is selected from the computer display [34]. The algorithm then iterates over the "adrenal area," selecting points of maximum count density drop. A two-point pixel displacement edge surrounding each adrenal is used to estimate local background radioactivity. Radioactive decay and depth attenuation are taken into account in the calculation of uptake. Normal adrenal cortical uptake is 0.16% with a standard deviation of 0.05% [33]. The uptakes generated in this manner can be used to confirm diagnostic impressions; it has not, however, been found useful in making diagnostic decisions [35]. With this approach the apparent adrenal asymmetry can be reduced, eliminating much of this uncertainty, and it is important in research applications relating adrenal NP-59 uptake to adrenal function.

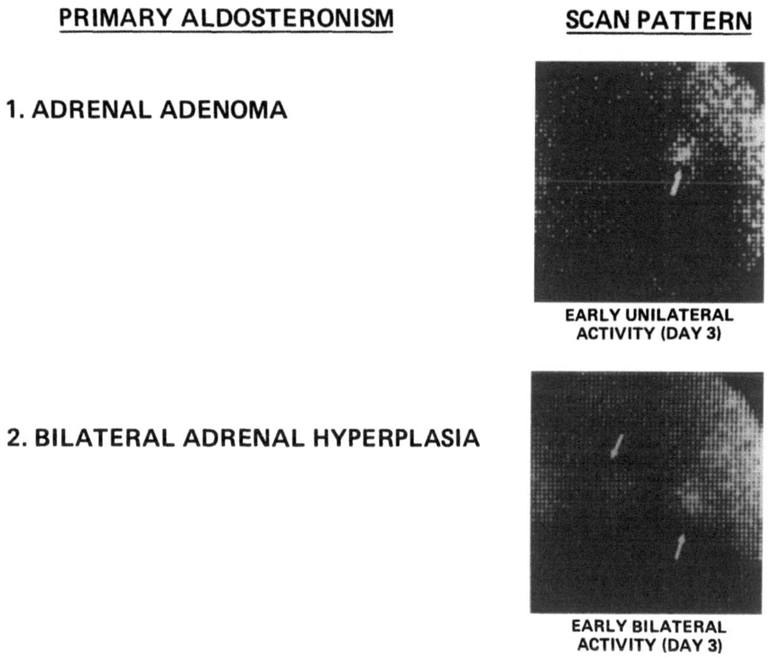

Fig. 8. Scan patterns in primary aldosteronism. With permission: Urol Radiol (1982) 3:241-244

4.3 Adrenal Cortical Tumor Imaging

The hallmark of adrenal tumor localization is the presence or absence of significant lateralization of NP-59 uptake. Accurate preimaging biochemical diagnosis and, when appropriate, pharmacologic manipulations of adrenal secretagogues, e.g., ACTH, serve to improve the diagnostic yield in the majority of cases.

4.3.1 Lesions Producing Cushing's Syndrome

Glucocorticoid excess can be the result of excessive adrenal secretion either as a result of a primary adrenal process or due to secretagogue excess [36]. Elevated ACTH can develop from excessive secretion from the pituitary due to adenoma or hyperplasia (hypothalamic dysfunction), or be the result of ectopic ACTH production from a tumor located elsewhere, e.g., thymoma or pancreatic carcinoma (Fig. 7) [37]. Of the tumorous etiologies for adrenal Cushing's syndrome, abnormalities can arise from adenoma, carcinoma, or an unusual variant of ACTH-independent disease, bilateral nodular hyperplasia. The former conditions manifest themselves as elevated plasma and/or urinary cortisol, and suppressed or low plasma ACTH levels. More sophisticated biochemical tests show absent responses to exogenous steroids. Adrenal scintiscans separate adenoma from carcinoma. The latter, although producing excessive glucocorticoids, has too low an uptake of NP-59 for imaging; the glucocorticoid-producing carcinoma causing Cushing's syndrome suppresses the normal contralateral cortex but does not itself image [37]. The adrenal adenoma also results in Cushing's syndrome and suppresses ACTH and contralateral NP-59 uptake, but in contradistinction to the adrenal cortical carcinoma, images with NP-59 (Fig. 7). The unusual variant, bilateral nodular hyperplasia, can present with variable biochemistry: ACTH levels may not necessarily be suppressed, and there may be some degree of suppression of glucocorticoids with exogenous steroid administration [36]. These confusing findings can be resolved with scintigraphy as the pattern of imaging is bilateral, but often markedly asymmetric. The scan is of particular importance as CT can be misleading and may not identify the bilateral nature of this form of Cushing's syndrome (Fig. 7). The efficacy of scintigraphy in localizing the abnormal adrenals in Cushing's syndrome approaches 100% [37].

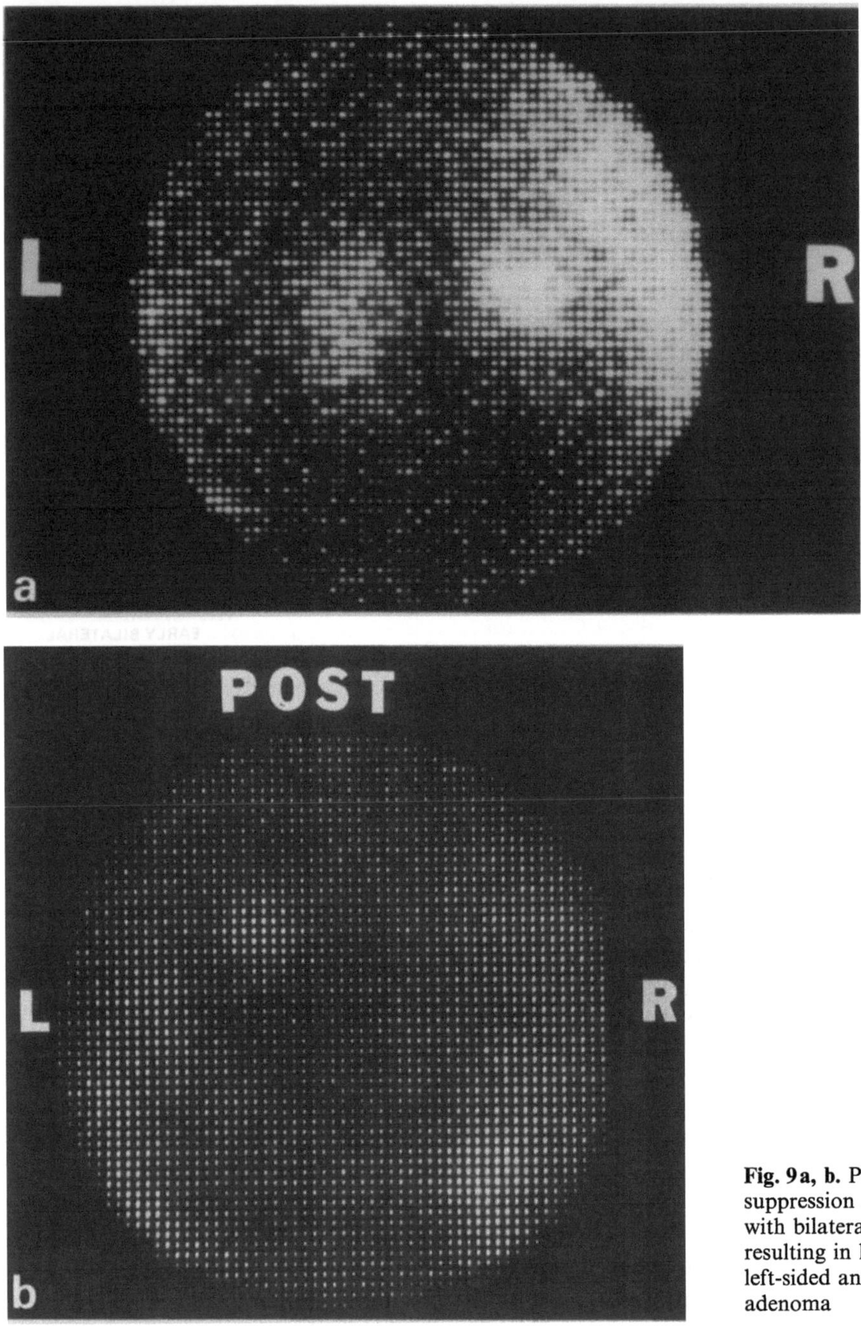

Fig. 9a, b. Posterior dexamethasone suppression adrenal scintiscans. **a** Patient with bilateral adrenal cortical hyperplasia resulting in hyperandrogenism. **b** Unilateral left-sided androgen-producing adrenal adenoma

4.3.2 Adrenal Lesions Producing Aldosteronism

The constellation of hypertension, hypokalemia, suppressed or low plasma renin activity, and elevated plasma and/or urinary aldosterone levels heralds the presence of primary aldosteronism. In this context it is particularly important to distinguish primary adrenal from other secondary etiologies of aldosterone excess. As the output of aldosterone is considerably less than that of the other hormones from the adrenal cortex, suppression of ACTH levels (and thus cortisol and androgen output) allows for improved diagnostic efficacy. Dexamethasone suppression (1 mg every 6 h) is given for 7 days prior to NP-59 injection and for a 5-day post-injection imaging interval [38]. Stable iodide is given orally to suppress the thyroidal uptake of free radioiodine. Normal adrenals image on

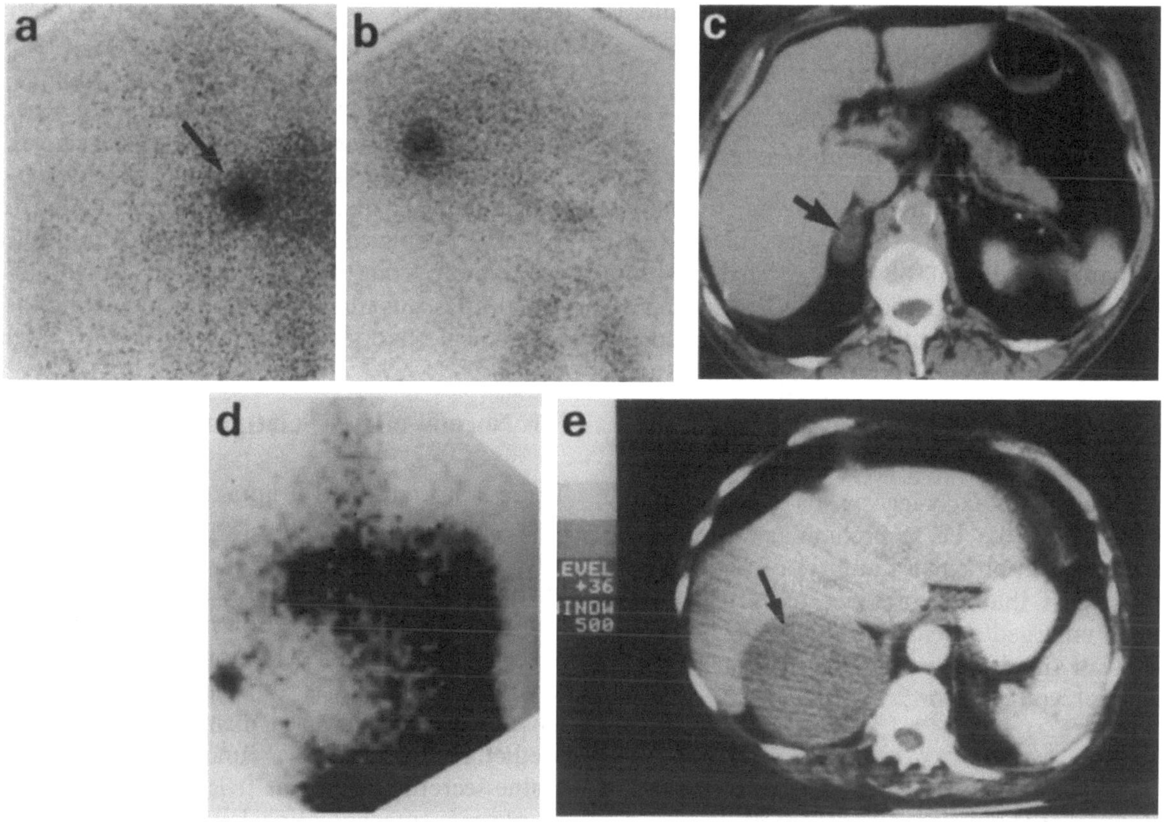

Fig. 10. **a** Posterior adrenal scintiscan in a patient with a right-sided adrenal mass demonstrates marked lateralization of uptake to the region of the right adrenal (*arrow*). No significant uptake is observed in the left adrenal gland. **b** Left lateral scintiscan identifies the area of uptake as the adrenal. **c** CT scan of the abdomen demonstrates a right adrenal mass (*arrow*). **d** Posterior adrenal scintiscan demonstrating bilateral adrenal cortical uptake with an abnormal configuration of the right adrenal. **e** A large right periadrenal mass is observed on the CT (*arrow*). This was later shown to be a right adrenal hematoma

day 5 or later; thus, diagnostic imaging is performed from day 3 through day 5.

Tumorous aldosteronism is distinguished from nontumorous adrenal etiologies on scintiscans as early unilateral uptake of NP-59 (Fig. 8) [39]. Adrenal carcinomas producing aldosteronism have shown variable degrees of NP-59 uptake [40]. Bilateral early (<5 day) imaging is compatible with nontumorous disease and is not amenable to surgical therapy (Fig. 8). Suppression scintigraphy for primary aldosteronism has a proven efficacy that is greater than CT [39]. Moreover, the scintiscan positively identifies both adenomas and hyperplasia where other modalities often show hyperplasia only as the absence of an recognizable anatomic abnormality. When used in tandem, scintigraphy and CT positively diagnose adrenal lesions in primary aldosteronism in many patients and eliminate the necessity for more invasive approaches such as arteriography and venous sampling.

4.3.3 Adrenal Lesions Producing Hyperandrogenism

Scintigraphic manifestations of androgen excess are not unlike those seen in primary aldosteronism [41]. While under constant dexamethasone suppression of ACTH, adrenal adenomas image as unilateral foci of increased NP-59 uptake (Fig. 9). Bilateral adrenal cortical imaging is compatible with hyperplasia (Fig. 9); bilateral nonvisualization in a patient with an adrenal mass on dexamethasone suppression or on unilateral imaging on the opposite side to an adrenal mass is compatible with an androgen-secreting adrenal carcinoma. Nonadrenal etiologies resulting in hyperandrogenism are from ovarian and testicular sources. Reports of imaging of tumors in these organs can found in the literature [10].

4.3.4 *Scintigraphic Evaluation of Clinically Silent Adrenal Masses*

High resolution adrenal imaging frequently identifies small masses or adrenal enlargements in patients without obvious adrenal dysfunction [42]. These "incidentally discovered" masses can be functionally characterized by their accumulation of NP-59 [43]. Initial studies suggest that the presence of NP-59 uptake in these lesions predicts normal function (at least in the sense of having NP-59 uptake), while the absence of uptake suggests space-occupying lesions (Fig. 10). These preliminary impressions are based upon small numbers of patients, but it appears that the presence of NP-59 uptake in an enlarged adrenal suggests that the probability of an adrenal malignancy (primary or metastatic) would be low.

5 Adrenal Medulla Scintigraphy

The principal secretory products of the adrenal medulla are epinephrine and to a lesser degree norepinephrine. Norepinephrine is also a neurotransmitter hormone produced in the sympathetic nervous system. As a structural analogue of norepinephrine, mIBG will depict lesions of adrenergic origin and localize these as focal collections of mIBG. Many drugs have profound effects upon catecholamine release and uptake by sympathetic nervous tissues, e.g., reserpine, cocaine, phenylpropanolamine, and tricyclic antidepressants, and consideration must be given to their exclusion prior to mIBG imaging to protect against false negative studies. It is fortunate that neither α- nor β-adrenergic blockade substantially affects the accumulation of mIBG, and both phenoxybenzamine and propranolol can be administered concurrently to protect patients with suspected pheochromocytomas from the potentially deleterious effects of excessive catecholamine secretion [16].

^{131}I-mIBG studies are performed with a gamma camera interfaced to a digital minicomputer. Serial, composite, total body images are obtained from the base of the skull to the lower pelvis at 24, 48, and 72 h (or later) after tracer administration. Stable iodide preparations are given orally to block the uptake of free radioactive iodine. Complementary imaging with other radiopharmaceuticals, e.g., ^{99m}Tc-bone, renal, liver, blood pool, and/or ^{201}Thallium-myocardial imaging agents, can be used to further localize these neoplasms that are found at multiple sites remote from the adrenal glands. mIBG directed CT scans may be helpful in depicting the anatomical relations of lesions.

5.1 Normal mIBG Scintigraphy

There is normal mIBG uptake observed in the liver, spleen, bladder, and less frequently in the lung and colon [44]. Salivary gland uptake is particularly prominent and is a reflection of the rich sympathetic innervation of these glands. It is seen in almost all patients studied (Fig. 11). Myocardial uptake is a frequent finding, and its presence can be used in many instances to predict the absence of a functioning catecholamine-secreting tumor as it is inversely related to plasma catecholamine levels [45]. Late discernable adrenal uptake of mIBG has been noted in approximately one-fifth of patients studied; the uptake is low and usually does not cause difficulty in the interpretation of scans in patients with documented hypercatecholamenia [44].

5.2 Scintigraphic Localization of Lesions Resulting in Catecholamine Excess

The documentation of elevated plasma and/or urinary catecholamines in the presence of signs and symptoms compatible with pheochromocytoma is sufficient to prompt attempts at localization. Therapy should be started to protect the patient, and as it does not interfere with either CT or scintigraphic studies, it is a prudent first step in expectant management of pheochromocytoma. Some information from plasma and/or urinary catecholamine studies can be used to guide attempts at localization in the early stages. The presence of elevated epinephrine or its metabolites whether or not accompanied by elevated norepinephrine levels suggests

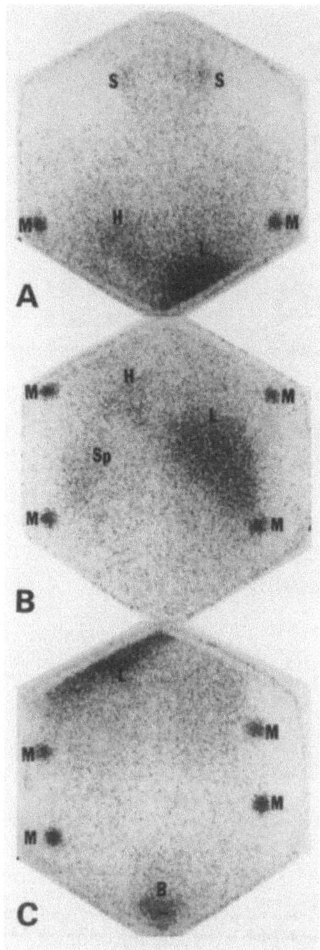

Fig. 11 A-C. Overlapping ^{131}I-mIBG images 48 h after injection in a typical normal patient. **A** Posterior head and chest; **B** posterior midabdomen; **C** anterior lower abdomen. Note accumulations of ^{131}I-mIBG in the salivary glands (*S*), heart (*H*), liver (*L*), spleen (*Sp*), and urinary bladder (*B*). *M* indicates markers on the body surface. With permission: J Nucl Med (1983) 24:672-682

an intra-adrenal pheochromocytoma, as extra-adrenal neoplasms lack the enzymes necessary for the methylation of norepinephrine to epinephrine. The presence of elevated norepinephrine and epinephrine metabolites helps little in localization for pheochromocytomas can be intra-adrenal, extra-adrenal, multiple, and/or metastatic. Furthermore, the localization of one neoplasm does not guarantee that there are not others (10% of cases), and histologic studies are unreliable as to the malignant potential (10% of cases) of a given lesion(s) [46].

Neuroblastomas present usually as large intra-abdominal masses in the pediatric patient. They are frequently metastatic and have a predilection for bone marrow or skeletal involvement. Catecholamines can be elevated but usually are moderately so, blood pressure is usually normal, and there may not be "spells" as seen in patients with pheochromocytomas [47].

5.2.1 Localization of Pheochromocytomas

Scintigraphy with mIBG depicts the sporadic, intra-adrenal pheochromocytoma as a solitary focus of markedly increased uptake (Fig. 12). Extra-adrenal tumors are problematic as they can occur anywhere throughout the sympathetic nervous system from the base of the skull to the pelvic floor. Any significant focus of activity on an mIBG scan, except for those sites of normal uptake (vide supra), can be an extra-adrenal neoplasm (Fig. 12) [13]. Metastatic pheochromocytoma is portrayed as multiple sites of uptake with a predilection for skull, spine, and diaphyses of the long bones of the leg. The arm, liver, lung, and lymph nodes are often less frequent sites of metastases (Fig. 13) [48]. The potential for the development of pheochromocytoma in the adrenals of patients with multiple endocrine neoplasia type II can be identified with mIBG [49]. The increasing accumulations of the radiotracer may identify susceptible family members prior to the development of the full-blown picture of bilateral pheochromocytomas seen in this syndrome. This pattern can also be seen in patients with other neurocristopathies such as the von Hippel–Lindau and neurofibromatosis syndromes where there is a strong association with the development of pheochromocytoma (Fig. 14) [50]. The overall sensitivity of mIBG scintigraphy in pheochromocytoma has been found to be about 85% with a specificity of almost 100% in the appropriate clinical setting.

5.2.2 Localization of Neuroblastomas

Neuroblastoma is a common malignancy of childhood that can be identified using mIBG [14]. There is usually a large primary intra-abdominal mass or less often intrathoracic mass with multiple metastases to bone marrow, lungs, liver, and bone (Fig. 15). Although not all the involvement may be depicted by mIBG,

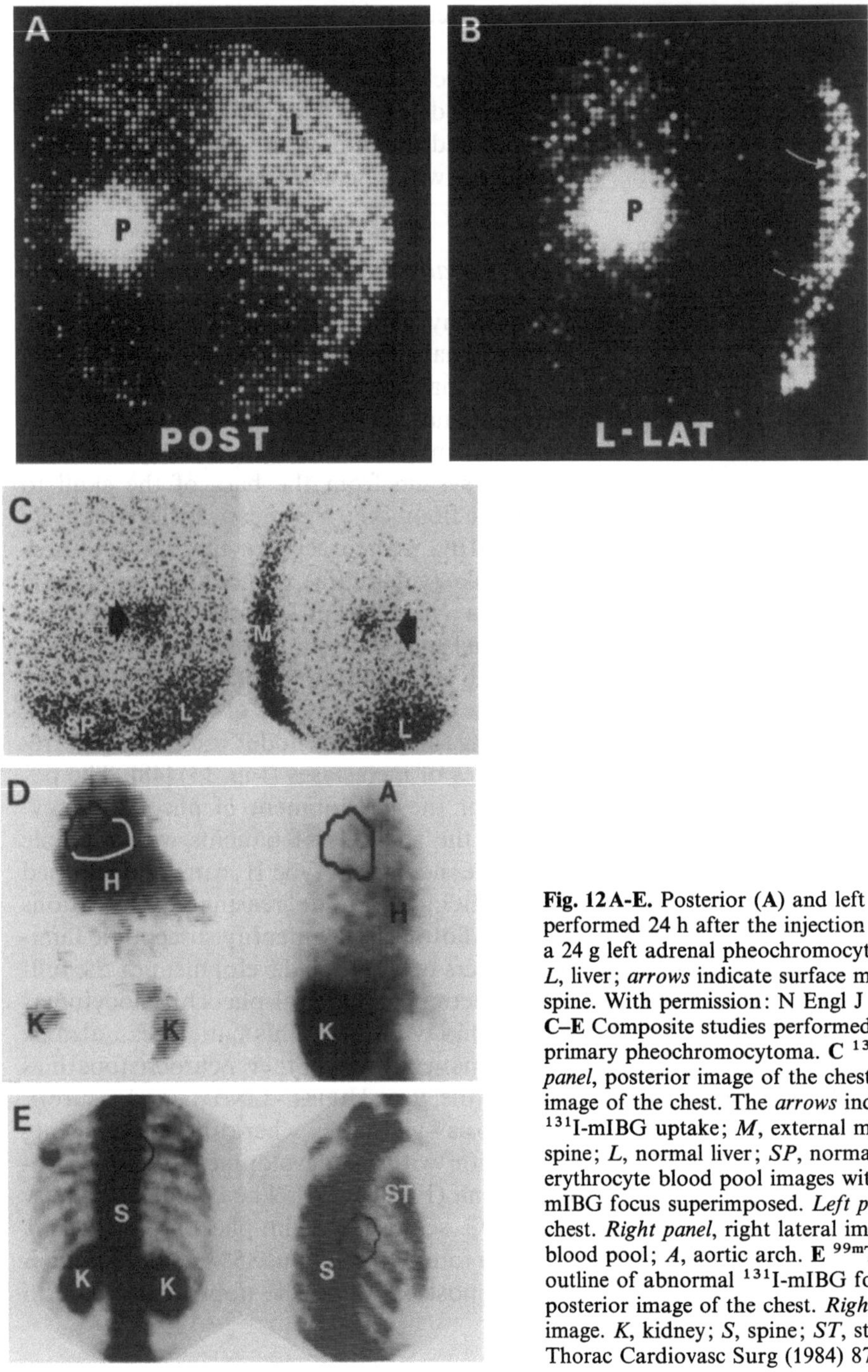

Fig. 12 A-E. Posterior (**A**) and left lateral (**B**) adrenal scintiscans performed 24 h after the injection of ^{131}I-mIBG in a patient with a 24 g left adrenal pheochromocytoma. *P*, pheochromocytoma; *L*, liver; *arrows* indicate surface markers on the patients lumbar spine. With permission: N Engl J Med (1981) 305:12-17. **C–E** Composite studies performed in a patient with a left atrial primary pheochromocytoma. **C** ^{131}I-mIBG scintigraphy. *Left panel*, posterior image of the chest. *Right panel*, right lateral image of the chest. The *arrows* indicate the focus of abnormal ^{131}I-mIBG uptake; *M*, external marker placed along the lumbar spine; *L*, normal liver; *SP*, normal spleen. **D** ^{99m}Tc-labeled erythrocyte blood pool images with outline of abnormal ^{131}I-mIBG focus superimposed. *Left panel*, anterior image of the chest. *Right panel*, right lateral image. *K*, kidney; *H*, cardiac blood pool; *A*, aortic arch. **E** ^{99m}Tc-MDP bone scan with the outline of abnormal ^{131}I-mIBG focus superimposed. *Left panel*, posterior image of the chest. *Right panel*, right posterior oblique image. *K*, kidney; *S*, spine; *ST*, sternum. With permission: J Thorac Cardiovasc Surg (1984) 87:814-820

the diffuse nature of the process can be characterized. Scintigraphy with mIBG may be most helpful in staging the disease and monitoring the response to therapy. In selected cases sufficiently avid uptake has prompted therapy doses of mIBG with variable degrees of success [47].

5.3 Scintigraphic Localization of Lesions Other Than Adrenergic Tumors

Accumulation of mIBG sufficient for imaging has been reported in a number of lesions that share characteristics of adrenergic tumors, e.g., neurosecretory granules. The cells in these le-

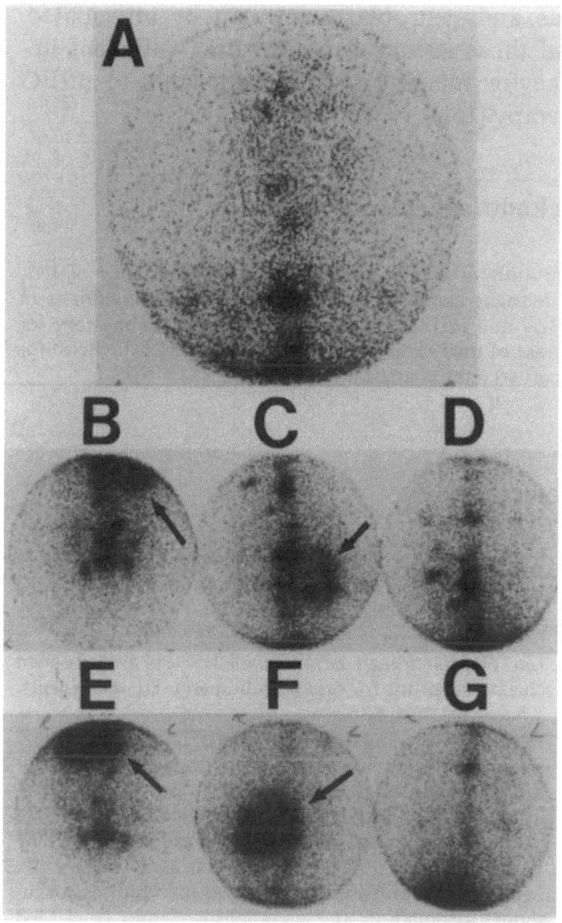

Fig. 13A-G. An example of a patient with extensive metastases from a malignant pheochromocytoma. **A** anterior head and neck; **B** posterior pelvis; **C** posterior abdomen; **D** posterior chest; **E** anterior pelvis; **F** anterior abdomen; **G** anterior chest. The *arrows* indicate a large right adrenal primary tumor with a necrotic center appearing as a "halo." With permission: Clin Endocrinol (1986) 20:189-203

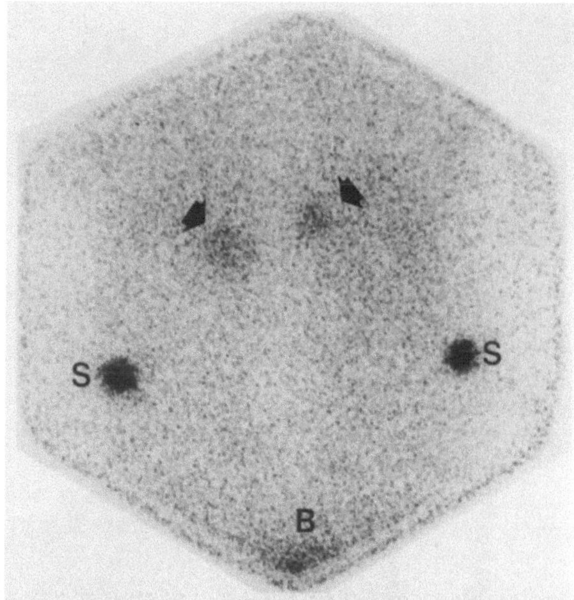

Fig. 14. Posterior ^{131}I-mIBG scintiscan in a patient with neurofibromatosis and bilateral pheochromocytomas. Abnormal uptake in the adrenal pheochromocytomas are indicated by *arrows*. *S*, Surface markers; *B* radioactivity observed in the urinary bladder. With permission: Arch Intern Med (1982) 142:2092-2098

sions have been loosely described as demonstrating amine recursor uptake and decarboxylation (APUD) [15]. These so-called APUDomas probably accumulate mIBG by mechanisms of amine uptake, and in so doing, image. As with other tumors demonstrating mIBG uptake, a biochemical evaluation is a critical first step in the process of accurate diagnosis and localization.

5.3.1 Localization of Carcinoid Tumors

The elaboration of 5-hydroxyindoleacetic acid and other serotoninergic compounds with the characteristic signs and symptoms (this is dependent upon the site(s) of the primary and the total amount of tumor present) suggests this type of APUD tumor. Moreover, it is not unusual for these neoplasms to elaborate more than one type of hormone(s) or precursor product(s) which can serve to confuse and confound biochemical diagnosis. The site(s) in which carcinoids can be seen include: the bronchus of the lung, the pancreas, and the gut. Each has its own particular constellation of signs and symptoms. Examination with mIBG portrays carcinoid tumors as focal collections of ^{131}I radioactivity [51]. CT is particularly useful in further localization of the abnormal foci of mIBG. Studies suggest that over 50% of these lesions will image, and mIBG may in the future be used to contribute to the diagnosis and therapy of these tumors [51].

5.3.2 Localization of Medullary Carcinoma of the Thyroid

Medullary carcinoma of the thyroid (MCT) arises from the c-cells (parafollicular) of the thyroid follicle. These cells produce the hormone calcitonin whose principle effect is lowering of serum calcium levels. The neoplasms associated with MCT can be sporadic or familial (part of

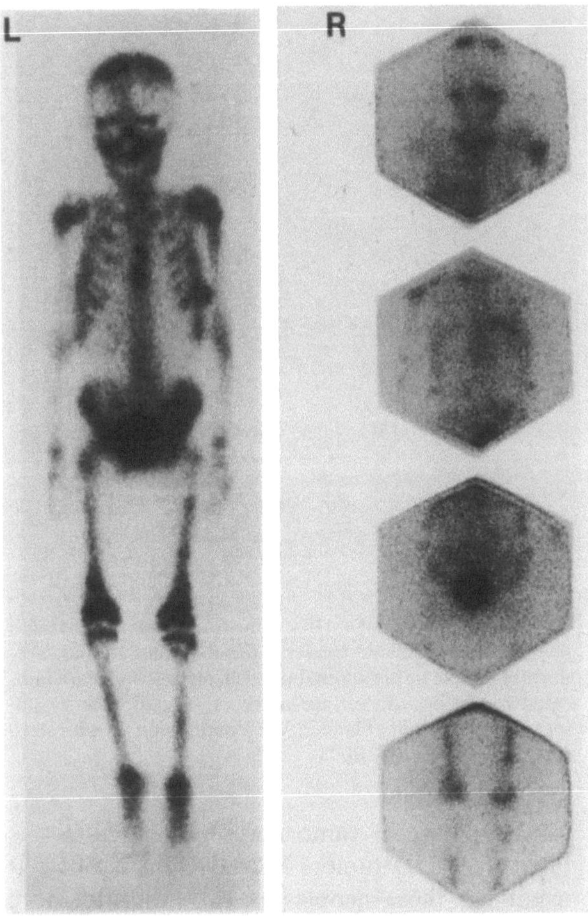

Fig. 15. *L*, ^{99m}Tc-MDP bone scan showing multiple skeletal foci of neuroblastoma. *R*, ^{131}I-mIBG scan showing extensive skeletal and bone marrow deposits of neuroblastoma to a greater extent than the ^{99m}Tc-MDP bone scan. With permission: J Nucl Med (1985) 26:736-742

the multiple endocrine neoplasia type syndrome). With metastatic disease calcitonin levels are usually elevated, but with lesser degrees of involvement stimulatory tests with pentagastrin and/or calcium infusion may be necessary to identify affected patients. Metastatic disease has been identified with mIBG in some patients [52].

5.3.3 Other Tumors Imaged with mIBG

Reports of other APUD-like tumors that image with mIBG continue to appear. Recently a Merkel cell tumor of the skin has been depicted. With more widespread use of the agent, greater success at localization with tumors demonstrating histology characteristic of pheochromocytomas and neuroblastomas can be anticipated, and those lesions demonstrating sufficient uptake for imaging may be amenable to mIBG therapy [15].

Acknowledgements

The authors wish to acknowledge the assistance of Drs. T. Mangner and H. Anderson-Davis for the synthesis of NP-59 and mIBG, the Phoenix Memorial Laboratory for the use of their radiochemistry facilities, and L.C. Beird for expert secretarial assistance.

References

1. Richards P, Atkins HL (1967) Technetium-99m labeled compounds. Jpn J Nucl Med 7:165-170
2. Arnold RW (1975) Comparison of Tc-99m complexes for renal imaging. J Nucl Med 16:357-367
3. Lin TH, Khentigan A, Winchell HS (1974) A Tc-99m chelate substitute for organoradiomercurial renal agents. J Nuc Med 15:34-35
4. Burbank MK, Tauxe WN, Maher FT, Hunt JC (1961) Evaluation of radioiodinated hippuran for the estimation of renal plasma flow. Mayo Clin Proc 36:372-386
5. Thakur ML, Chauser BM (1975) Synthesis of I-123 orthoiodohippurate. Int J Appl Radiat Inst 26:319-320
6. Beierwaltes WH, Wieland DM, Yu T, Swanson DP, Mosley S (1978) Adrenal imaging agents: rationale, synthesis, formulation and metabolism. Semin Nucl Med 8:5-21
7. Gross MD, Swanson DP, Wieland DM, Beierwaltes WH (1982) The mechanisms of localization, specificity and metabolism of adrenal gland imaging agents. In: Billinghurst MW (ed) Studies of cellular function using radiotracers. CRC, Boca Raton, pp 189-224
8. Brown MS, Goldstein JL (1976) Receptor mediated control of cholesterol metabolism. Science 191:150-153
9. Brown MS, Goldstein JL (1975) Regulation of the activity of the low density lipoprotein receptor in human fibroblasts. Cell 6:307-310
10. Gross MD, Thrall JH, Beierwaltes WH (1980) The adrenal scan: a current status report on radiotracers, dosimetry and clinical utility. In: Freeman LM, Weissman HS (eds) Nuclear medicine annual 1980. Raven, New York, pp 127-175
11. Fukushi K, Irie T, Nozaki T, Ido T, Kasida Y (1979) Adrenal affinity and plasma lipoprotein binding of radiohalogen derivatives of cholesterol. J Labeled Comp 16:49-51
12. Wieland DM, Wu JL, Brown LE, Mangner T, Swanson DP, Beierwaltes WH (1980) Radiolabeled adrenergic neuron blocking agents: adrenal medulla imaging with (^{131}I)iodobenzylguanidine. J Nucl Med 21:349-353
13. Sisson JC, Frager MS, Valk TW, Gross MD, Thompson N, Beierwaltes WH (1981) Scintigraphic localization of pheochromocytoma. N Engl J Med 305:12-17
14. Geatti O, Shapiro B, Sisson JC, Hutchinson RJ, Mallette S, Eyre P, Beierwaltes WH (1985) 131-I-metaiodobenzylguanidine (131-I-mIBG) scintigraphy for the loca-

tion of neuroblastoma: preliminary experience in 10 cases. J Nucl Med 26:736-742
15. Shapiro B, Sisson JC, Geatti O, Eyre P, Lynn M, Beierwaltes WH (1986) The scintigraphic imaging of pheochromocytoma by means of metaiodobenzylguanidine (mIBG) (1986) In: Winkler C (ed) Nuclear medicine in clinical oncology. Springer, Berlin Heidelberg New York Tokyo, pp 129-137
16. Shapiro B, Wieland DM, Brown LE, Nakajo M, Sisson JC, Beierwaltes WH (1984) ^{131}I-meta-iodobenzylguanidine (mIBG) adrenal medullary scintigraphy: interventional studies. In: Spencer RP (ed) Interventional nuclear medicine. Grune and Stratton, New York, pp 451-482
17. Tobes MC, Jacques S Jr, Wieland DM, Sisson JC (1985) Effect of uptake-one inhibitors on the uptake of norepinephrine and meta-iodobenzylguanidine. J Nucl Med 26:897-907
18. Nakajo M, Shapiro B, Swanson DP, Beierwaltes WH (1982) Mechanism of I-131-metaiodobenzylguanidine accumulation in the salivary glands. Clin Res 30:721 A
19. Lynn MD, Shapiro B, Sisson JC, Swanson DP, Mangner TJ, Wieland DM, Meyer LJ, Glowniak JV, Beierwaltes WH (1985) Improved visualization of pheochromocytomas and normal adrenal medullae with ^{123}I-mIBG scintigraphy. Radiology 156:789-793
20. Sisson JC, Shapiro B, Beierwaltes WH, Glowniak JV, Nakajo M, Mangner T, Carey T, Swanson D, Copp JE, Satterlee WG, Wieland DM (1984) Radiopharmaceutical treatment of malignant pheochromocytoma. J Nucl Med 25:197
21. Smith HW (1951) The kidney structure and function in health and disease. Oxford University Press, New York
22. Tauxe WN (1985) Glomerular filtration in nuclear medicine. In: Tauxe WN, Dubovsky GV (eds) Clinical urology and nephrology. Appleton-Century-Crofts, Norwalk, Conn, pp 61–76
23. Fischer M, Veall N (1975) Glomerular filtration rate estimation based upon a single blood sample. Br J Med 2:542-547
24. Gates GF (1982) Glomerular filtration rate: estimation from functional renal accumulation of 99m Tc-DTPA. AJR 138:565-570
25. Tauxe WN (1985) Tubular function in nuclear medicine. In: Tauxe WN, Dubovsky EV (eds) Clinical urology and nephrology. Appleton-Century-Crofts, Norwalk, Conn, pp 78-82
26. Tauxe WN, Maher FT, Taylor WF (1971) Effective renal plasma flow: estimation from theoretical volumes of distribution of intravenously injected 131I-orthoiodohippurate. Mayo Clin Proc 46:524-531
27. Koff SA, Thrall JH, Keyes JW Jr (1979) Diuretic radionuclide urography: a noninvasive method for evaluating nephroureteral dilatation. J Urol 122:451-455
28. Thrall JH, Koff SA, Keyes JW (1981) Diuretic radionuclide urography in the differential diagnosis of hydroureteronephrosis. Semin Nucl Med 11:89-122
29. Britton KE, Nimmon CC, Whitfield HN, Hendry WR, Wickham JEA (1979) Obstructive nephropathy; successful evaluation with radionuclides. Lancet I:905-907
30. Taylor A Jr (1985) Renal imaging with diuerocaptosuccinic acid in nuclear medicine. In: Tauxe WN, Dubovsky EV (eds) Clinical urology and nephrology. Appleton-Century-Crofts, Norwalk, Conn, pp 287-303
31. Gross MD, Valk TW, Swanson DP, Thrall JH, Grekin RJ, Beierwaltes WH (1981) The role of pharmacologic manipulation in adrenal cortical scintigraphy. Semin Nucl Med 11:128
32. Thrall JH, Freitas JE, Beierwaltes WH (1978) Adrenal scintigraphy. Semin Nucl Med 8:23-41
33. Freitas JE, Thrall JH, Swanson DP, Rafai A, Beierwaltes WH (1978) Normal adrenal asymmetry: explanation and interpretation. J Nucl Med 19:149-154
34. Koral KF, Abukhadra H, Tuscan M, Beierwaltes WH (1982) Computing adrenal uptakes with compact, fixed-sized regions. Comput Prog Biomed 15:73-78
35. Gross MD, Shapiro B, Freitas JE (1985) The limited significance of assymetric adrenal visualization on dexamethasone suppression scintigraphy. J Nucl Med 26:43-47
36. Gross MD, Shapiro B (1984) Pharmacological intervention: strategies for adrenocortical imaging. In: Spencer RP (ed) Interventional nuclear medicine. Grune and Stratton, New York, pp 483-518
37. Gross MD, Shapiro B, Beierwaltes WH (1983) The functional characterization of the adrenal cortex by quantitative scintigraphy. In: Lawrence JH (ed) Recent advances in nuclear medicine, vol VI. Grune and Stratton, New York, pp 83-115
38. Gross MD, Freitas JE, Swanson DP, Brady T, Beierwaltes WH (1979) The normal dexamethasone suppression adrenal scintiscan. J Nucl Med 20:1131-1135
39. Gross MD, Shapiro B, Grekin RJ, Freitas JE, Glazer G, Beierwaltes WH, Thompson NW (1984) The scintigraphic localization of the adrenal lesion in primary aldosteronism. Am J Med 77:839-845
40. Shenker Y, Gross MD, Shapiro B, Grekin R (1986) Scintigraphic localization of mineralocorticoid producing adrenal carcinoma. J Endocrinol Invest 9:115–120
41. Gross MD, Freitas JE, Swanson DP, Woodbury MC, Steingart DE, Beierwaltes WH (1981) Dexamethasone suppression adrenal scintigraphy in hyperandrogenism. J Nucl Med 22:12–17
42. Glazer HS, Weyman PJ, Sagel SS, Leutt RG, Mc Clennan BL (1983) Nonfunctioning adrenal masses: incidental discovery on computed tomography. AJR 139:81–85
43. Gross MD, Wilton G, Shapiro B, Smid A, Bouffard A, Glazer G, Francis IR (1986) Adrenal Scintigraphy in the evaluation of the clinically silent adrenal mass. J Nucl Med 27:908 (ABST)
44. Nakajo M, Shapiro B, Copp JE, Kalff V, Gross MD, Sisson JC, Beierwaltes WH (1983) The normal and abnormal distribution of the adrenomedullary imaging agent m-[I-131] iodobenzylguanidine (I-131-mIBG) in man: evaluation by scintigraphy. J Nucl Med 24:672-679
45. Nakajo M, Shapiro B, Glowniak J, Sisson JC, Beierwaltes WH (1983) Inverse relationship between cardiac accumulation of meta [^{131}I] iodobenzylguanidine (I-131-mIBG) and circulating catecholamines in suspected pheochromocytoma. J Nucl Med 24:1127-1134
46. Manger WM, Gifford RW Jr (1982) Hypertension secondary to pheochromocytoma. Bull N Y Acad Med 58:139-158
47. McEwan AJ, Shapiro B, Sisson JC, Beierwaltes WH, Ackery DM (1985) Radioiodobenzylguanidine for the scintigraphic location and therapy of adrenergic tumors. Semin Nucleic Med 15:132-153
48. Shapiro B, Sisson JC, Lloyd RV, Nakajo M, Satterlee

W, Beierwaltes WH (1984) Malignant pheochromocytoma: clinical, biochemical and scintigraphic characterization. Clin Endocrinol 20:189-203
49. Valk TW, Frager MS, Gross MD, Sisson JC, Wieland DM, Swanson DP, Mangner TJ, Beierwaltes WH (1981) Spectrum of pheochromocytoma in multiple endocrine neoplasia: a scintigraphic portrayal using 131-I-metaiodobenzylguanidine. Ann Intern Med 94:762-767
50. Kalff V, Shapiro B, Lloyd RV, Sisson JC, Holland K, Nakajo M, Beierwaltes WH (1982) The spectrum of pheochromocytoma in hypertensive patients with neurofibromatosis. Arch Intern Med 142:2092-2098
51. Munkner T (1985) ^{131}I-metaiodobenzylguanidine scintigraphy of neuroblastomas. Semin Nucleic Med 15:154-160
52. Fischer M, Kamanabroo D, Sonderkamp M, Proske T (1984) Scintigraphic imaging of carcinoid tumors with 131-I-MIBG. Lancet 2:165

Surgical Management of Renal Cell Carcinoma

H. BEHRENDT

1 Radical Nephrectomy

In the absence of distant metastases, radical nephrectomy is the treatment of choice for renal carcinoma. The operative procedure has been described by CHUTE et al. [12] and FOLEY et al. [19]. It includes preliminary ligation of the artery and vein of the tumor-bearing kidney, with subsequent en bloc removal of the kidney and the perinephric fat, the intact Gerota's capsule, and the ipsilateral adrenal gland. The rationale for this widely accepted surgical strategy is based on data obtained by ROBSON et al. [64]. They were able to demonstrate that radical nephrectomy increased the 5-year survival rate to 52%, compared with 33% for simple nephrectomy, and the 10-year survival rate from 7.1% to 49%. FUSELIER et al. [21], however, did not find any differences in long-term survival after radical or simple nephrectomy.

Early identification and control of the renal vascular pedicle is necessary for a safe and bloodless radical nephrectomy. The operative approach depends upon the size and site of the tumor and its local extension, and upon the surgeon's experience (Figs. 1 and 2). We prefer a transverse subcostal incision (Chevron), which allows a good transperitoneal approach to the renal pedicle and to the adjacent organs.

The thoracoabdominal approach was used by CHUTE [12] to resect large renal cell carcinomas. More recently, it has been popularized by SKINNER. It is mandatory only for special situations, such as when a tumor involves the inferior vena cava above the level of the diaphragm, or when a very large tumor is present at the upper pole of the kidney.

The thoracoabdominal approach is contraindicated in severe pulmonary lesions associated with respiratory failure and in high-risk patients [25].

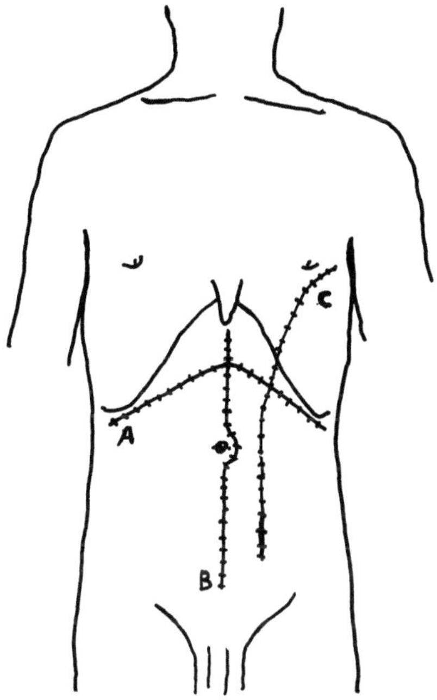

Fig. 1. Transperitoneal approach to the kidney. *A*, Subcostal transverse incision; *B*, median laparotomy; *C*, thoracoabdominal incision

The operative mortality of radical nephrectomy is 2%–5% [28, 29, 47, 75]. The most frequent intraoperative complication is injury to the spleen, which may occur in up to 12% of cases [75].

2 Preoperative Embolization

"Therapeutic" embolic infarction of renal cell carcinoma has become a widely accepted procedure since its initial description by ALMGÅRD et al. [2]. KLIMBERG et al. [38] performed preoperative infarction using absolute ethanol (first

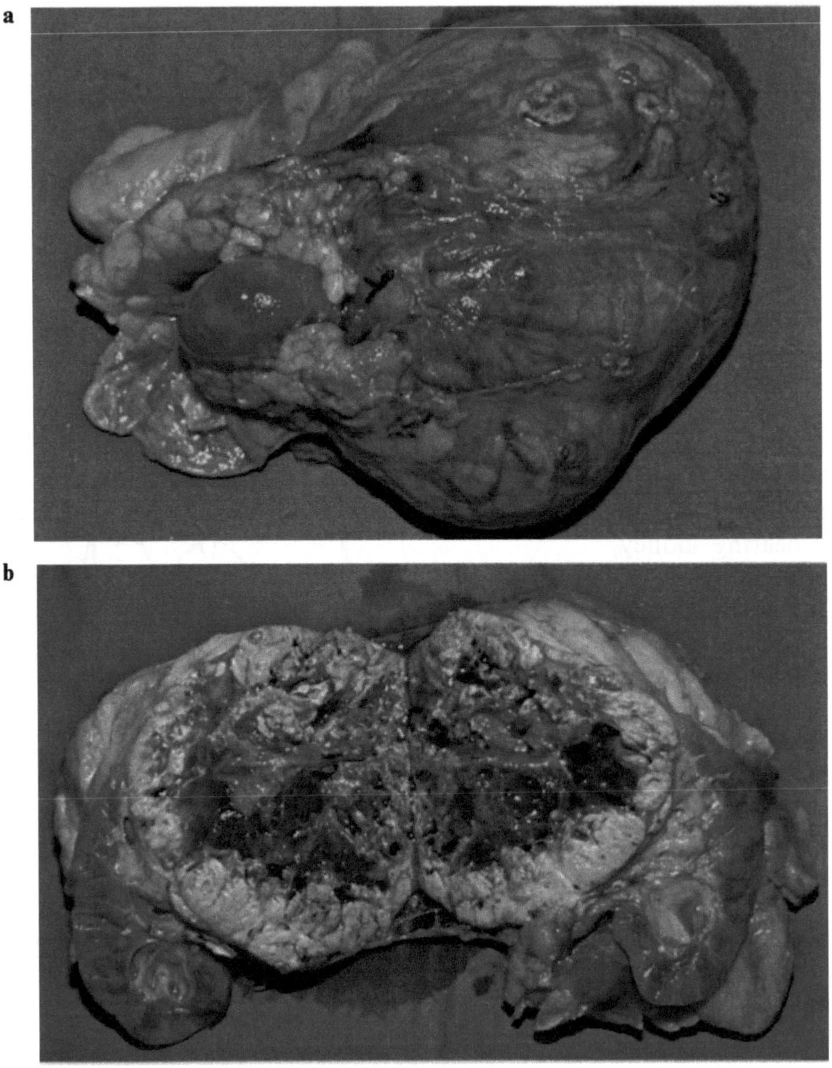

Fig. 2. Renal cell carcinoma (weight 1450 g)

described by Ellman et al. [17], and found that subsequent surgical dissection was facilitated, particularly with large tumors. Christensen et al. [11], however, were not able to observe any advantages due to embolization of the tumor-bearing kidney. There was no statistically significant difference with respect to blood loss or survival between patients treated with or without preoperative embolization. As to our opinion there are only a few patients, those with very large tumors and especially with hilar involvement, who may benefit from this procedure. Such cases are the only instances in which we perform preoperative renal artery occlusion at present.

There are, however, some observations which may indicate an improvement of the immunologic response to the tumor when infarction is performed 8–10 days before radical nephrectomy [16, 76, 35, 79]. Swanson et al. [76] observed in disseminated disease after preoperative embolization and postoperative progesterone therapy an overall response of 28% (7% complete response, 8% partial response, 13% stable for at least 1 year). Of the patients with parenchymal pulmonary metastases alone, 64% survived for at least 1 year, 33% for 2 years, and 20% for 3 years. Giuliani et al. [23] could not find any beneficial effect on prognosis due to embolization. The real value of preoperative embolization is still unclear [4]. On the other hand the procedure has a remarkably high morbidity (20% incidence of postembolization syndrome), and a mortality of 3% [46].

3 Regional and Radical Lymphadenectomy

The incidence of lymph node metastases due to renal cell carcinoma is 2%–32.6% (Table 1). This wide variation may be attributed to the extent of the lymphadenectomy performed and the precision of the pathologic examination of the removed lymph nodes. The ipsilateral lumbar nodes are the usual sites of metastases, but isolated lymph node metastases can occur in the supraclavicular and iliac regions [31, 26]. Most patients with positive nodes have microscopic involvement which will be overlooked unless a meticulous lymphadenectomy is performed. Although those with microscopic disease would appear to be the patients most likely to be cured after lymph node dissection, the therapeutic value of lymphadenectomy for renal cell carcinoma is as yet unproven [9, 7, 23] and its pros and cons are controversial. The prognostic value of lymphadenectomy is limited by the fact that metastases may spread via the blood stream without involving the lymphatic system. The recent literature on survival of patients with positive lymph nodes after radical nephrectomy (Table 2) clearly reveals that metastatic spread to the lymph nodes has a very negative impact upon prognosis.

A limited lymphadenectomy along the ipsilateral great vessels is easily performed and gives some useful prognostic information [15, 21]. An extensive retroperitoneal lymph node dissection is advocated by Robson et al. [64], Angerwall and Wahlquist [3], and Herrlinger et al. [28], whereas de Kernion and Berry [15] recommend regional lymphadenectomy in order to facilitate correct staging. Marshall and Powell [43] defined the normal extrarenal lymphatic drainage of the kidney on the basis of anatomical studies and delineated the extent of regional lymphadenectomy to be performed with radical nephrectomy. According to their observations, right radical nephrectomy should include dissection of the lateral caval, pre- and postcaval, and interaortocaval nodes. Left radical nephrectomy should include the left lateral aortic nodes, the left diaphragmatic nodes, and the pre- and postaortic nodes. Herrlinger et al. [28] found after facultative lymph node dissection an uncorrected 5-year survival rate of 50% ± 9% compared with 60% ± 11% when systematic radical lymph node dissection was performed. Determination of the status of the regional lymph nodes will be much more important when effective adjuvant chemotherapy for renal cell carcinoma becomes available.

Table 1. Frequency of metastases involving lymph nodes in renal cell carcinoma

Reference	%	
[18]	25.0	
[31]	32.0	
[64]	22.7	
[62]	8.0	
[72]	8.1	
[52]	11.0	
[3]	22.0	
[50]	2.0	
[9]	7.7	
[23]	32.6	
[28]	16.0	(after facultative lymphatic dissection)
	23.0	(after systematic lymphatic dissection)
[57]	18.0	
[6]	12.3	

Table 2. Survival of patients with lymph node metastases in renal cell carcinoma

Reference	*n*	Survival rate	
		(%)	(years)
[18]	21	14.0	5
[64]	20	35.0	3
[62]	16	25.0	5
[71]	19	16.0	5
[52]	7	29.0	5
[69]	9	11.0	5
[23]	15	34.6	5
[57]	11	8.0	5
[6]	31	7.0	5

4 Tumor Extension into the Inferior Vena Cava

Of the patients with renal cell carcinoma, 7%–9% have a tumor thrombus extending into the inferior vena cava [49] most of them with a right-sided tumor. The only effective therapy is radical nephrectomy and complete removal of the tumor thrombus. Operative mortality for these patients has ranged from 4% to 14% [1, 67, 13, 36]. The prognostic implications of tumor thrombus extension into the inferior vena cava has been a point of controversy in the literature [50, 10]. It is clear, from a number of studies, that involvement of the inferior vena cava itself without evidence of metastatic disease does not have the same negative prognostic impact as the finding of positive lymph nodes. SKINNER et al. [72] studied 309 patients and found no significant difference in the survival of patients with renal vein or inferior vena caval involvement compared to those with tumor confined to the kidney, providing there were no positive lymph nodes or perinephric fat involvement at the time of surgery. The 5-year survival rate was 54%. Comparable results were published by SCHEFFT et al. [67], KEARNEY et al. [36], and SOGANI et al. [74].

HENEY and NOCKS [27] investigated the influence of perinephric fat involvement on survival in patients with renal cell carcinoma extending into the inferior vena cava. In patients with involvement of only the inferior vena cava, these authors found a mean survival time of 75 months (5-year survival rate, 67%), compared to 17 months (5-year survival rate, 0%) when the tumor additionally extended into the perinephric fat. Survival rates have also been poor in patients with inferior vena caval tumor and distant metastases. These patients should not be treated surgically [49, 74].

The involvement of the inferior vena cava by tumor thrombus is managed surgically by controlling the inferior vena cava above and below the level of the thrombus and also controlling the uninvolved renal vein. The inferior vena cava is incised and the thrombus extracted. The operative procedure is more difficult when tumor thrombus extends above the level of the hepatic veins. Then, for proximal control of the inferior vena cava the liver can be mobilized by incising the falciform, coronary, and triangular ligaments. Extension of tumor thrombus to the right atrium may require the application of extracorporal circulation during removal of the tumor [44]. To prevent pulmonary thromboembolism from the tumor during operation, placement of a Greenfield filter or of a Moretz inferior vena caval clip above the level of the thrombus may be useful [59, 74, 66].

When tumor invasion of the inferior vena cava wall is present, simple removal of the tumor thrombus is not possible. Surgical resection of the involved inferior vena cava is required [48, 59]. In the presence of an extensive collateral drainage of the left renal vein, often seen in patients with suprarenal inferior vena caval obstruction due to a tumor thrombus from a right-sided renal cell carcinoma, the ligation of the left renal vein is possible during resection of the inferior vena cava. The right renal vein lacks collateral drainage and cannot be ligated without danger of renal insufficiency. Caution should be exercised especially in children, in whom inadequate collateral drainage may lead to complete renal failure [53].

According to CLAYMAN et al. [13] and ORTENBERG et al. [59] it is possible to test whether the ligation of the left renal vein will be possible without serious danger to the kidney. The pressure in the unaffected renal vein is determined with the inferior vena cava clamped above the thrombus. If this pressure is more than 40 mm Hg, there is a danger of renal congestive proteinuria and possible renal failure. The second test is done with additional clamping of the artery of the tumor-bearing kidney. After intravenous application of 5 ml indigo carmine, blue urine should appear in the bladder drainage system within 12 min.

5 Partial Nephrectomy in Renal Cell Carcinoma

Bilateral tumors, synchronous or asynchronous, occur in 1.8% to 3.8% of renal carcinoma patients [49]. In simultaneous bilateral renal cell carcinomas, the usual treatment is radical nephrectomy of the kidney bearing the larger tumor and partial nephrectomy on the contralateral side. An organ-preserving operation is also performed in patients with a tumor in a solitary kidney or in patients suffering from renal insuffiency. Because of the morbidity and mortality associated with chronic renal failure and its treatment, the goal of therapy for such patients should be the removal of carcinoma with preser-

Table 3. Survival after partial nephrectomy or enucleative surgery in renal cell carcinoma

Reference	*n*	Survival rate (%)
[61]	21	23.8 (5 years)
[56]	17	65.0 (3 months–10 years)
[68]	62	77.0 (mean follow-up: 45.7 months)
[42]	72	78.0 unilateral disease (5 years) 48.0 bilateral synchronous disease (5 years) 38.0 bilateral asynchronous disease (5 years)
[40]	19	68.0 (3 years)
[32]	61	61.0 (5 years)
[73]	37	64.0 (>1 year)
[33]	15	60.0 (9–49 months follow-up: NED)

vation of enough renal tissue to support life without dialysis. PENN [60] reported on 26 patients with bilateral renal cell carcinoma or with a tumor in a solitary kidney. These patients underwent radical surgery and were made anephric. After varying intervals on chronic hemodialysis, the patients each received a renal allograft. The overall survival rate was 35%.

When metastases are not present at the time of diagnosis, partial nephrectomy offers a reasonable survival expectancy (Table 3). Bench surgery with subsequent autotransplantation is not mandatory but is sometimes necessary when the tumor is located in the central part of the kidney [5].

There has been some discussion in the literature as to whether simple enucleation of the tumor is a sufficient treatment [56, 24, 8], or whether removal of a wide margin of the adjacent renal parenchyma is mandatory [65]. Renal cell carcinoma is often enclosed in a characteristic pseudocapsule. This capsule seems sometimes to allow simple enucleation with protection of the vessels and optimal preservation of the healthy renal parenchyma. Survival for up to 5 years without evidence of recurrent disease after this operative procedure has been reported [24]. JACOBS et al. [32] observed a local tumor recurrence in 10% of their patients; NOVICK et al. [56] described the same development in 4 of 17 patients. Two of 15 patients reported by JAEGER et al. [33] suffered pulmonary metastases after tumor enucleation.

ROSENTHAL et al. [65] examined the relationships of renal cell carcinomas to their pseudocapsules and to the adjacent renal parenchyma using microangiographic and histopathologic techniques. The pseudocapsule of every tumor was invaded by neoplastic cells and the surrounding renal parenchyma was often infiltrated by the carcinoma, even around some of the smallest tumors. On the basis of these results it may be possible to treat smaller (less than 6 cm) tumors with partial nephrectomy including resection of a sufficiently wide margin of adjacent renal parenchyma. When, because of the size of a tumor in a solitary kidney or in both kidneys, partial nephrectomy is impossible, unilateral or bilateral nephrectomy with subsequent hemodialysis and renal transplantation remains an option. Renal allotransplantation performed after a 15-month waiting period from the time of radical nephrectomy has resulted in long-term survival [60].

6 Surgery for Disseminated Disease

For patients with only a single metastasis at the time of diagnosis, or in whom a single metastasis develops after nephrectomy, the treatment of choice is tumor nephrectomy and surgical removal of the metastasis. About 2.5%–3.23% of patients with renal cell carcinoma fall into this category (McDONALD 1982). Five-year survival rates of about 35% have been reported [51, 58], however, HUBMER et al. [30] observed a mean survival of only 18.5 months (2–48 months) for 14 patients with surgically treated solitary metastasis.

7 Adjunctive Nephrectomy

There are very few indications for palliative nephrectomy, because the primary tumor seldom produces symptoms requiring surgical intervention. The occasional spontaneous remission after tumor nephrectomy in patients with metastatic disease has been regarded as an indication for nephrectomy, which was said to stimulate the immune response to the tumor. The rate of spontaneous remission in these patients is only 0.8%, whereas operative mortality is

2%–5%. Nephrectomy per se does not improve the survival of patients with disseminated disease [34, 54, 14].

Adjunctive nephrectomy is sometimes combined with "specific" [11] or "non-specific" [55] immunotherapy. There seems to be little improvement in survival from this treatment [20]. Only $^1/_3$ of the patients in our institution with disseminated renal carcinoma treated by radical nephrectomy and subsequent active "specific" immunotherapy ($n=30$) survived more than 2 years, most of them with tumor progression. Embolization of inoperable renal carcinoma has no significant effect on tumor progression and survival. The only indications for this procedure are massive hematuria, severe local pain due to the tumor, and life-endangering tumor endocrine activity.

8 Future Prospects

The excellent survival rates reported after enucleative surgery or partial nephrectomy (Table 3) raise some doubt about the need for radical nephrectomy for small peripheral renal carcinoma in the presence of a normal contralateral kidney. Survival rates after partial nephrectomy approximate those after radical nephrectomy for unilateral disease [6]. An argument could thus be made for the use of partial nephrectomy for pT1+2 N0 M0 renal cell carcinoma especially when the lesion is at a renal pole [73]. Routine use of ultrasound and computerized tomography has led to earlier diagnosis, therapy at a lower stage of tumor development, and better prognosis in incidentally diagnosed cases of renal cell carcinoma [39]. In the next few years it must be determined whether early detection of low-stage tumors will justify organ-preserving surgery.

References

1. Abdelsayed M, Bissada N, Finkbeiner A, Redman J (1978) Renal tumors involving the inferior vena cava: plan for management. J Urol 120:153
2. Almgård L, Fernström J, Haverling M, Ljungquist A (1973) Treatment of renal adenocarcinoma by embolic occlusion of the renal circulation. Br J Urol 45:474
3. Angervall L, Wahlquist L (1978) Follow-up and prognosis of renal carcinoma in a series operated by perifascial nephrectomy combined with adrenalectomy and retroperitoneal lymphadenectomy. Eur Urol 4:13
4. Bakke A, Goethlin J, Hoisaeter P (1985) Renal malignancies: outcome of patients in stage 4 with or without embolization procedure. Urology 26:541
5. Banowsky L (1982) Renal in situ surgery, partial nephrectomy and renal autotransplantation. In: Crawford E, Borden T (eds) Genitourinary cancer surgery. Lea and Febiger, Philadelphia, p 52
6. Bassil B, Dosoretz D, Prout G Jr (1985) Validation of the tumor, nodes and metastasis classification of renal cell carcinoma. J Urol 134:450
7. Boileau M (1982) Cancer of the kidney: overview. In: Johnson RE, Boileau MA (eds) Genitourinary tumors; fundamental principles and surgical techniques. Grune and Stratton, p 293
8. Carini M, Selli C, Muraro G, Trippitelli A, Masini G, Turini D (1981) Conservative surgery for renal cell carcinoma. Eur Urol 7:19
9. Chatelain C (1982) Results of radical nephrectomy without lymphadenectomy in renal cell carcinoma. In: Küss R, Murphy G, Khoury S, Karr J (eds) Renal tumors: proceedings of the first international symposium on kidney tumors. Alan R Liss, New York, p 475
10. Cherrie R, Goldman D, Lindner A, de Kernion J (1982) Prognostic implications of vena caval extension of renal cell carcinoma. J Urol 128:910
11. Christensen K, Dyreborg U, Anderson J, Nissen H (1985) The value of transvascular embolization in the treatment of renal carcinoma. J Urol 133:191
12. Chute R, Soutter L, Kerr W Jr (1949) The value of the thoraco-abdominal incision in the removal of kidney tumors. New Engl J Med 241:951
13. Clayman R, Gonzalez R, Fraley E (1980) Renal cell cancer invading the inferior vena cava: clinical review and anatomical approach. J Urol 123:157
14. de Kernion J, Ramming K, Smith R (1978) The natural history of metastatic renal cell carcinoma: a computer analysis. J Urol 120:148
15. de Kernion J, Berry D (1980) The diagnosis and treatment of renal cell carcinoma. Cancer 45:1947
16. Dreikorn K, Terweg B, Drings P, Horsch R, Palmtag H, Rössler W (1983) Complete regression of multiple pulmonary metastases in a patient with advanced renal cell carcinoma treated by occlusion of the renal artery with subsequent radical nephrectomy and progesterone. Eur Urol 9:254
17. Ellman B, Green C, Eigenbrodt E, Garriott J, Curry T (1980) Renal infarction with absolute ethanol. Invest Radiol 15:318
18. Flocks R, Kadesky M (1958) Malignant neoplasms of the kidney: an analysis of 353 patients followed five years or more. J Urol 79:196
19. Foley F, Mulvaney W, Richardson E, Victor J (1952) Radical nephrectomy for neoplasm. J Urol 68:39
20. Fowler J Jr (1986) Failure of immunotherapy for metastatic renal cell carcinoma. J Urol 135:22
21. Fuselier H Jr, Guice S, Brannan W, Ochsner M, Sangisett K, Beckman E, Barnes C (1983) Renal cell carcinoma: The Ochsner medical institution experiences (1945–1978). J Urol 130:445
22. Gilloz A, Tostain J (1982) Comparative study of actuarial survival rates in stage II and III renal cell carcinoma managed by radical nephrectomy alone or associated with formal retroperitoneal lymph node dissection. In:

Küss R, Murphy G, Khoury S, Karr J (eds) Symposium on kidney tumors. Alan R Riss, New York, p 489

23. Giuliani L, Martorana G, Giberti C, Pescatore D, Magnani G (1983) Results of radical nephrectomy with extensive lymphadenectomy for renal cell carcinoma. J Urol 130:664
24. Graham S Jr, Glenn J (1979) Enucleative surgery for renal malignancy. J Urol 122:546
25. Grégoir W (1982) Thoracophrenolaparotomy. In: Küss R, Murphy G, Khoury S, Karr J (eds) Renal tumors: proceedings of the first international symposium on kidney tumors. Liss, New York, p 453
26. Hellstein S, Berge T, Linell F (1983) Clinically unrecognised renal carcinoma: aspects of tumor morphology, lymphatic and haematogenous metastatic spread. Br J Urol 55:166
27. Heney N, Nocks B (1982) The influence of perinephric fat involvement on survival in patients with renal cell carcinoma extending into the inferior vena cava. J Urol 128:18
28. Herrlinger A, Sigel A, Giedl J (1984) Methodik der radikalen transabdominalen Tumornephrektomie mit fakultativer oder systematischer Lymphdissektion und deren Ergebnisse an 381 Patienten. Urologe A 23:267
29. Holland J (1973) Cancer of the kidney – natural history and staging. Cancer 432:1030
30. Hubmer G, Guad H, Vilits P (1984) Renal carcinoma with solitary distant metastasis. Urol Int 39:46
31. Hulten L (1969) Rosencrantz M, Seeman T, Wahlquist L, Ahren C (1969) Occurrence and localization of lymph node metastases in renal carcinoma. Scand J Urol Nephrol 3:129
32. Jacobs S, Berg R, Lawson K (1984) Synchronous bilateral renal cell carcinoma: total surgical excision. Cancer 46:2341
33. Jaeger N, Weissbach L, Vahlensieck W (1985) Value of enucleation of tumor in solitary kidneys. Eur Urol 11:369
34. Johnson D, Kaesler K, Samuels M (1975) Is nephrectomy justified in patients with metastatic renal carcinoma. J Urol 114:27
35. Kaisary A, Williams G, Riddle P (1984) The role of preoperative embolization in renal cell carcinoma. J Urol 131:641
36. Kearney G, Waters W, Klein L, Richie J, Gittes R (1981) Results of inferior vena cava resection for renal cell carcinoma. J Urol 125:769
37. Khoury S (1982) Lumbar flank approach. Küss R, Murphy G, Khoury S, Karr J (eds) Renal tumors: proceedings of the first international symposium on kidney tumors. Liss, New York, p 457
38. Klimberg J, Hunter P, Hawkins F, Drylie D, Wajsman Z (1985) Preoperative angioinfarction of localized renal cell carcinoma using absolute ethanol. J Urol 133:21
39. Konnak J, Grossman H (1985) Renal cell carcinoma as an incidental finding. J Urol 134:1094
40. Küss R (1982) Conservative surgery in renal cell carcinoma. In: Küss R, Murphy G, Khoury S, Karr J (eds) Renal tumors: proceedings of the first international symposium on kidney tumors. Liss, New York, p 519
41. Malek R, Utz D, Culp O (1976) Hypernephroma in the solitary kidney: experience with 20 cases and review of the literature. J Urol 116:553
42. Marberger M, Pugh R, Auvert J, Bertermann H, Costantini A, Gammelgaard P, Petterson S, Wickham J (1981) Conservative surgery of renal carcinoma. The EIRSS experience. Brit J Urol 53:528
43. Marshall F, Powell K (1982) Lymphadenectomy for renal cell carcinoma: anatomical and therapeutic considerations. J Urol 128:677
44. Marshall R, Reitz B, Diamond D (1984) A new technique for management of renal cell carcinoma involving the right atrium: hypothermia and cardiac arrest. J Urol 131:103
45. Marshall F, Reitz B (1985) Supradiaphragmatic renal cell carcinoma tumor thrombus: indications for vena caval reconstruction with pericardium. J Urol 133:266
46. Marx F, Chaussy C, Moser E (1982) Grenzen und Gefahren der palliativen Embolisation inoperabler Nierentumoren. Urologe A 21:206
47. Mazeman E, Wemeau L (1975) Les limites du traitement chirurgical du cancer du rein. J Urol Nephrol 80:82
48. McCullough D, Gittes R (1974) Vena cava resection for renal cell carcinoma. J Urol 112:162
49. McDonald M (1982) Current therapy for renal cell carcinoma. J Urol 127:211
50. McNichols D, Segura J, De Weerd J (1981) Renal cell carcinoma: long-term survival and late recurrence. J Urol 126:17
51. Middleton R (1967) Surgery for metastatic renal cell carcinoma. J Urol 97:973
52. Middleton R, Presto A (1973) Radical thoracoabdominal nephrectomy for renal cell carcinoma. J Urol 110:36
53. Miedema B, Stubenbord W (1984) Irreversible renal failure following right nephrectomy and left renal vein ligation. J Urol 132:335
54. Montie J, Stewart B, Straffon R, Banowsky L, Hewitt C, Montague D (1977) The role of adjunctive nephrectomy in patients with metastatic renal cell carcinoma. J Urol 117:272
55. Morales A, Wilson J, Pater J, Loeb M (1982) Cytoreductive surgery and systemic bacillus calmette-guerin therapy in metastatic renal cancer: a phase II trial. J Urol 127:230
56. Novick A, Stewart B, Straffon R, Banowsky L (1977) Partial nephrectomy in the treatment of renal adenocarcinoma. J Urol 118:932
57. Nurmi M (1984) Prognostic factors in renal carcinoma. An evaluation of operative findings. Br J Urol 56:270
58. O'Dea M, Zincke H, Utz D, Bernatz P (1978) The treatment of renal cell carcinoma with solitary metastases. J Urol 120:540
59. Ortenberg J, Novick A, Stewart B (1982) Clinical problems involving the inferior vena cava. In: Novick A, Straffon R (eds) Vascular problems in urologic surgery. Saunders, Philadelphia
60. Penn J (1977) Transplantation in patients with primary renal malignancies. Transplantation 24:424
61. Puigvert A (1976) Partial nephrectomy for renal tumour: 21 cases. Eur Urol 2:70
62. Rafla S (1970) Renal cell carcinoma. Cancer 25:26
63. Robson C, Churchill B, Anderson W (1968) The result of radical nephrectomy for renal cell carcinoma. Am Assoc Genitourin Surg 60:122
64. Robson C, Churchill B, Anderson W (1969) The results of radical nephrectomy for renal cell carcinoma. J Urol 101:297
65. Rosenthal C, Kraft R, Zingg E (1984) Organ-preserving surgery in renal cell carcinoma: tumor enucleation versus partial kidney resection. Eur Urol 10:222

66. Rosenthal D, Gershon C, Rudderman R (1985) Renal cell carcinoma invading the inferior vena cava: the use of the Greenfield filter to prevent tumor emboli during nephrectomy. J Urol 134:126
67. Schefft P, Novick A, Straffon R, Stewart B (1978) Surgery for renal cell carcinoma extending into the inferior vena cava. J Urol 120:28
68. Schiff M Jr, Bagley D, Lytton B (1979) Treatment of solitary and bilateral renal carcinoma. J Urol 121:581
69. Siminovitch J, Montie J, Straffon R (1982) Lymphadenectomy in renal adenocarcinoma. J Urol 127:1090
71. Skinner D, Colvin R, Vermillion C, Pfister R, Leadbetter W (1971) diagnosis and management of renal cell carcinoma. A clinical and pathological study of 309 cases. Cancer 28:1165
72. Skinner D, Pfister R, Colvin R (1972) Extension of renal cell carcinoma into the vena cava: the rationale for aggressive surgical management. J Urol 107:711
73. Smith R, de Kernion J, Ehrlich R, Skinner D, Kaufman J (1984) Bilateral renal cell carcinoma and renal cell carcinoma in the solitary kidney. J Urol 132:450
74. Sogani P, Herr H, Bains M, Whitmore W Jr (1983) Renal cell carcinoma extending into inferior vena cava. J Urol 130:660
75. Swanson D, Borges P (1983) Complications of transabdominal radical nephrectomy for renal cell carcinoma. J Urol 129:704
76. Swanson D, Johnson D, von Eschenbach A, Chuang V, Wallace S (1983) Angioinfarction plus nephrectomy for metastatic renal cell carcinoma – an update. J Urol 130:449
77. Tykkä H, Oravisto K, Lehtonen T, Sarna S, Tallberg T (1978) Active specific immunotherapy of advanced renal cell carcinoma. Eur Urol 4:250
78. Waters W, Richie J (1979) Aggressive surgical approach to renal cell carcinoma: review of 130 cases. J Urol 122:306
79. Weigel J, Mebust W, Foret J, Noble M, Votapka T, Kirshnan E, Jewell W (1985) Treatment of renal cell carcinoma with renal infarction, delayed nephrectomy, medroxyprogesterone, and xenogenic immune RNA. Urology 15:103
80. Wickham J (1975) Conservative renal surgery for adenocarcinoma. The place of bench surgery. Br J Urol 47:25

Operative Therapy of Nephroblastoma

R. HARTUNG

1 Introduction

1.1 Incidence, Age, and Sex Distribution

The incidence rate is about seven cases per one million children less than 15 years of age per year [30, 50, 49]. This figure varies a little bit in different countries; the highest rate observed was 10.4 cases per million per year among American black males [63] and the lowest, 4.9 cases among males in England [7]. At the time of diagnosis 64% of the children are 4 years old or younger. The average age is between 3 and 4 years. The frequency is about equal between the sexes. The first National Wilms' Tumor Study (NWTS) showed a ratio of 0.97:1.0 (male:female) [1].

1.2 Pathology

Wilms' tumors are composed of three elements, blastemic, epithelial, and stromal [5]. For therapeutic reasons it is necessary to identify the different parts of the tumor as precisely as possible. Today the histologic subdivision of Wilms' tumors is known, which allows us to speak of favorable and unfavorable histology (Table 1) [9, 34, 41].

Table 1. Histologic subdivision of Wilms' tumors [30]

Favorable histology		Unfavorable histology	
Mixed	232 (55.3%)	Anaplastic	
Epithelial predominant	49 (12.9%)	Focal	15 (3.6%)
		Diffuse	9 (2.1%)
Blastemic predominant	95 (22.6%)	Sarcomatous	
		Rhabdoid	8 (1.9%)
		Clear cell	11 (2.6%)
	376 (89.8%)		43 (10.2%)

1.3 Presentation and Clinical Symptoms

The clinical manifestations of Wilms' tumor disease are widely discussed in earlier chapters. Most common is a painless abdominal swelling or the presence of an abdominal mass. This asymptomatic tumor swelling is the first symptom in 50%–60% of the cases. Other symptoms are obstipation, hematuria, altered urinary frequency, and hypertension [3, 55]. Weight loss is rare and even rarer is dyspnea due to pulmonary metastases.

Table 2. National Wilms' Tumor Study staging system

Stage I	Tumor limited to kidney and completely excised. The surface of the renal capsule is intact. The tumor was not ruptured before or during removal. There is no residual tumor apparent beyond the margins of resection.
Stage II	Tumor extends beyond the kidney but is completely excised. There is regional extension of the tumor, i.e., penetration through the outer surface of the renal capsule into the perirenal soft tissues. The vessels outside the kidney substance are infiltrated or contain tumor thrombus. The tumor may have been biopsied. There may be local spillage of tumor confined to the flank. There is no residual tumor apparent at or beyond the margins of excision.
Stage III	Residual nonhematogenous tumor confined to the abdomen. Any one or more of the following occur: (a) lymph nodes in the renal hilus, the para-aortic chains, or beyond, are found on biopsy to be involved; (b) there has been diffuse peritoneal contamination by tumor such as by spillage beyond the flank before or during surgery, or by tumor growth that has penetrated through the peritoneal surface; (c) implants are found on the peritoneal surfaces; (d) the tumor extends beyond the surgical margins either microscopically or grossly; (e) the tumor is not completely excisable because of local infiltration into vital structures.
Stage IV	Hematogeneous metastases. Deposits beyond stage III, e.g., in the lung, liver, bone, and/or brain.
Stage V	Bilateral renal involvement at diagnosis.

Table 3. Clinical TNM classification of Wilms' tumor

T 0	No evidence of primary tumor (palpation and X-ray)
T 1	Unilateral tumor area of kidney and tumor in the intravenous pyelogram (IVP) is smaller than 80 cm^2
T 2	Unilateral tumor area of kidney and tumor in the IVP is larger than 80 cm^2
T 3	Ruptured tumor (before therapy) or clinically and X-ray proven infiltration of neighbouring organs in the abdomen
T 4	Bilateral tumor before therapy
T x	No adequate information about primary tumors
N 0	No evidence of lymph node metastases (clinically, sonography, IVP, CT)
N 1	Evidence of regional lymph node disease
N x	No adequate information about lymph node involvement
M 0	No evidence of distant metastases
M 1	Evidence of distant metastases
M x	No adequate information about distant metastases

1.4 Tumor Stages

A precise staging is mandatory nowadays to evaluate therapy and prognosis. The classification of the NWTS is recommended (Table 2) [25] and internationally accepted.

For clinical purposes the TNM classification is also important, which includes postoperative data. This staging is usually done pre- and postoperatively and may be corrected after intraoperative findings. A preoperative staging is important in those cases in which preoperative therapy may be necessary (Table 3).

1.5 Diagnostic Procedures

Intravenous pyelography, sonography [24, 27, 48], computerized tomography [10, 20, 42a, 47],

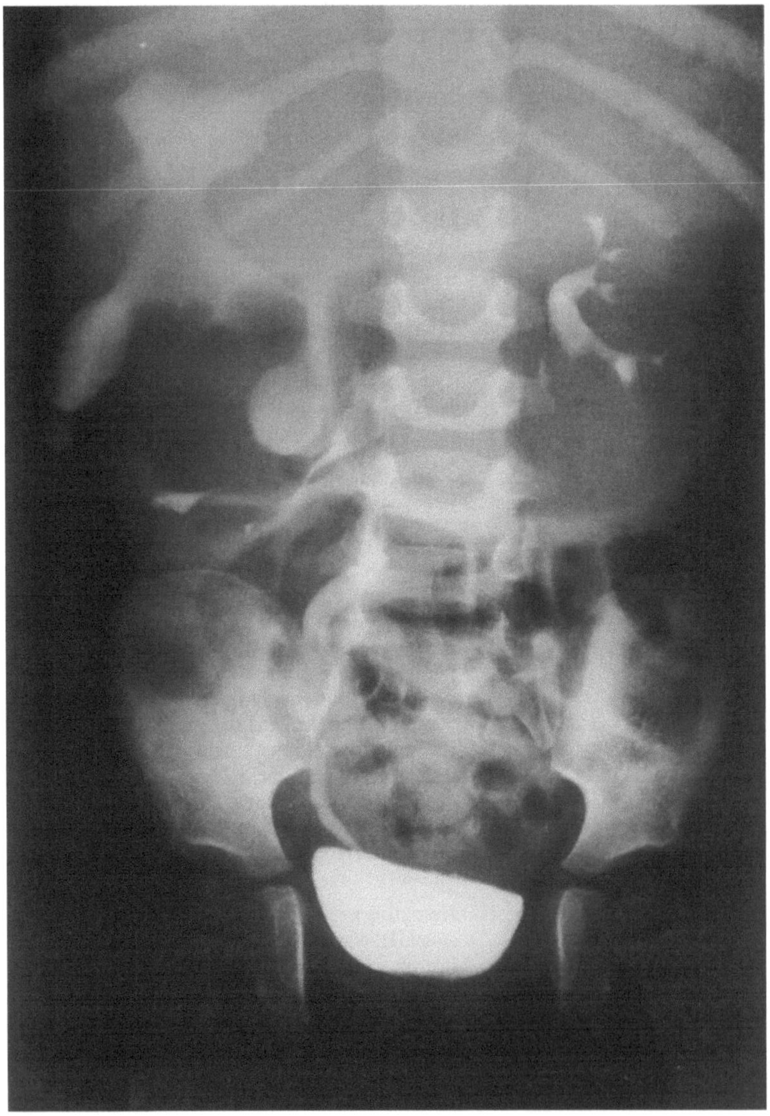

Fig. 1. Intravenous pyelogram of a right-sided tumor with a distended pelvic system representing a large kidney

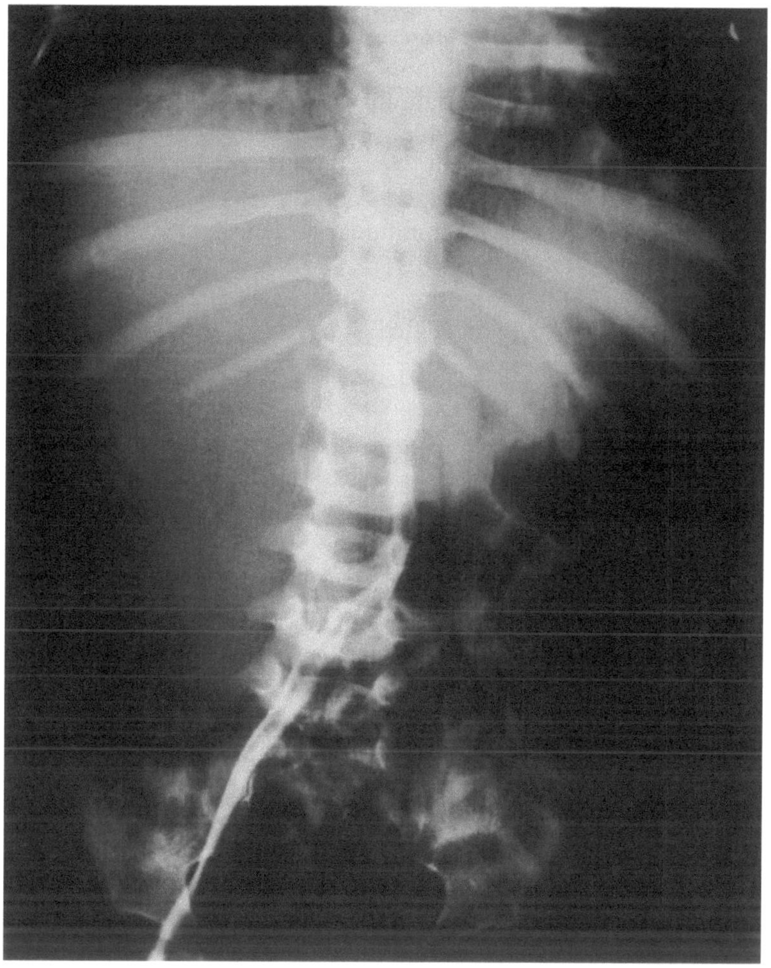

Fig. 2. Cavography shows lateralization of the vena cava to the left side with a clear impression

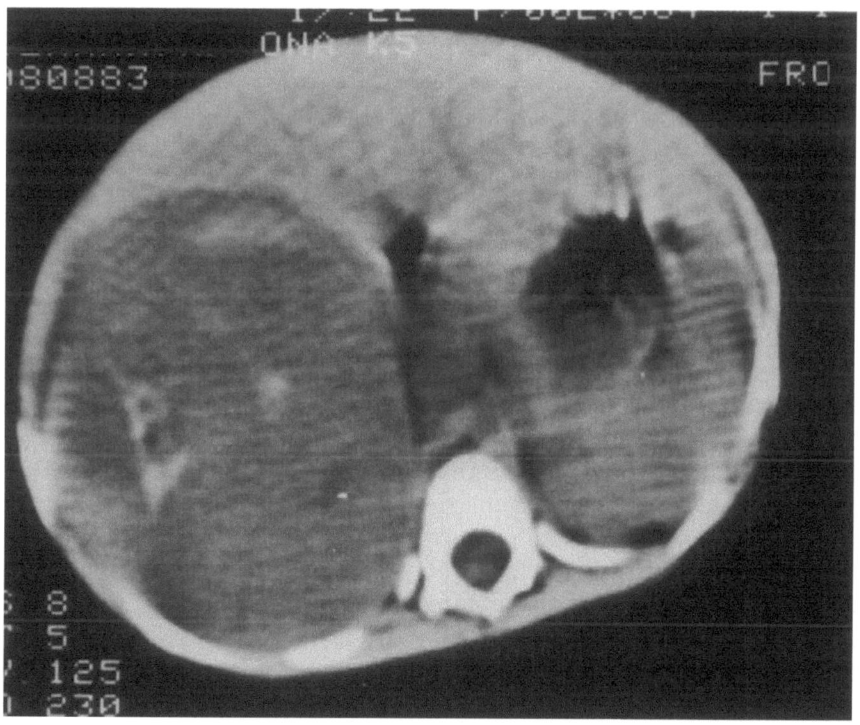

Fig. 3. CT scan shows large Wilms' tumor with impression, but not infiltration of the liver

and, if indicated in special cases, cavography and DSA are the techniques to establish the extension of most abdominal tumors. Sonography is also very important for examining the contralateral kidney in cases in which CT shows a very large mass on one side and does not clearly identify the other kidney. A plain chest X-ray is mandatory to check for pulmonary metastases [17, 18].

The figures 1–3 show an example of a 2.5-year-old girl with a right-sided tumor.

2 Treatment

Treatment of Wilms' tumor consists of surgery, radiotherapy, and chemotherapy, all of which are effective [31, 39, 42, 44, 60]. Multicenter studies, such as the NWTS and the SIOP (Société Internationale d'Oncologie Pédiatrique), support this treatment [21, 22, 46]. Wilms' tumor therapy consists of particular combination of these techniques according to the diagnosed tumor stage and the histologically proven tumor subtype.

Clinical stages I and II and perhaps stage III (NWTS classification) in all children under 2 years of age should undergo surgery directly.

In cases of metastatic disease or a large tumor mass which is also infiltrating neighbouring organs, preoperative treatment should be carried out in all children over 2 years of age. This preliminary treatment is necessary for downstaging for later surgery [11, 36, 43, 57, 59].

Tumors of all stages should have postoperative treatment. The recommended regimens of radiotherapy and chemotherapy are presented in a later chapter (Havers, this volume).

2.1 Preoperative Treatment

Stages III and IV need preoperative treatment such as chemotherapy and perhaps also radiotherapy [2, 4, 46, 53]. These preoperative treatments improve the situation for surgery in many cases [13]; in our experience preoperative chemotherapy led to a lower incidence of intraoperative tumor bursting than preoperative radiotherapy. Bilateral tumor disease, which appears in about 4% of all cases, may require an individual approach [29, 37, 38, 45].

The aim of therapy must be to make the tumor operable and to prevent a situation arising in which a previously undiscovered inoperable condition is found during surgery, leading to further chemo- and radiotherapy and to a delayed, second-look procedure. Those situations should be preventable by exact staging and precise selection of the therapeutic modality.

2.2 Operative Technique

Before starting surgery the diagnostic imaging must have supplied clear information about extension of a tumor thrombus to the vena cava [16]. This should not be diagnosed intraoperatively and necessary steps for treating the thrombus should be considered preoperatively. In the rare cases of a very extensive tumor thrombus, which can reach as far as the right atrium of the heart, a thoracoabdominal approach is necessary, and the urologist should cooperate with a cardiovascular surgeon.

The aim of operative therapy should be radical surgery [54, 56]. This is possible in most cases of unilateral tumor, even very large ones, with or without preoperative treatment. We prefer a transverse subcostal incision; very rarely a thoracoabdominal incision is necessary (Fig. 4).

The operation starts with opening the retroperitoneum, dissecting the renal artery and vein carefully, and clamping them before mobilizing the tumor. An en bloc dissection should be the aim, including the tumor and the entire fatty capsule around it. If possible, the adrenal gland should be included. In all cases of tumor involvement of the vena cava, loop vessels should be placed inferior and cranial to the tumor extension and on the contralateral kidney vein. The vena cava should be dissected carefully; a partial resection of it is mandatory in cases of tumor thrombus (Fig. 5) [12].

The contact areas with neighbouring organs at which adhesions might be seen should be considered. Biopsies of those areas should be taken separately. For ligating little vessels we use titan-clips, as these do not disturb the CT-imaging in later follow-ups. An intraoperative tumor

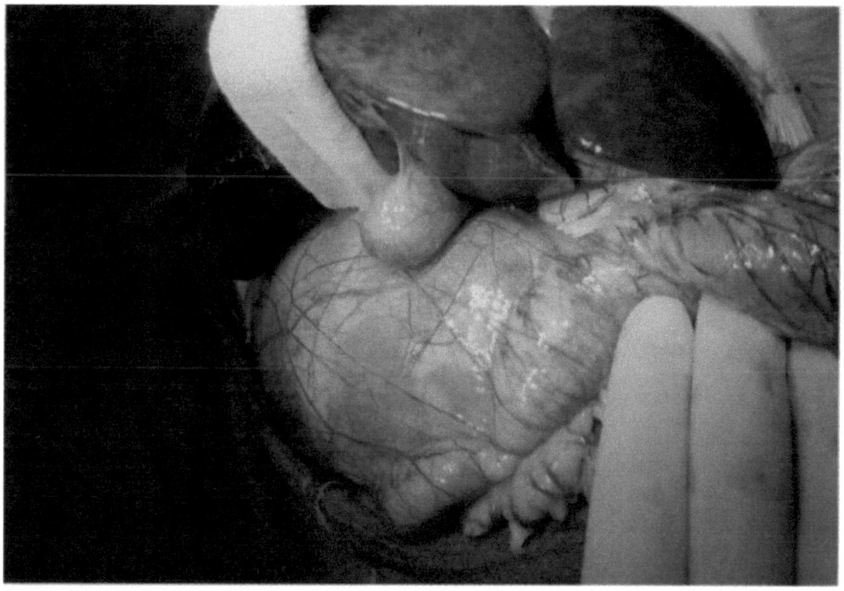

Fig. 4. Situation of the right-sided tumor

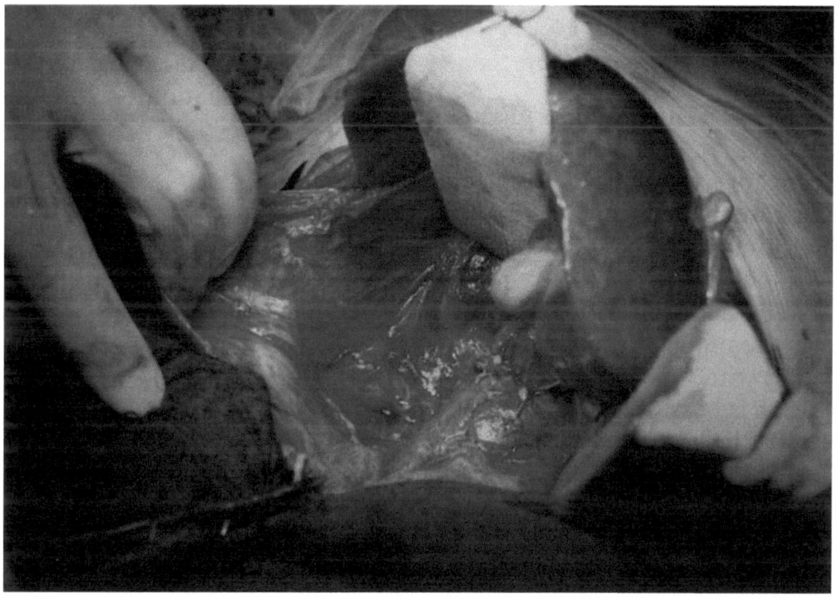

Fig. 5. Situation after radical nephrectomy, adrenalectomy, and lymphadectomy

burst should be prevented; if it occurs the tumor must be upstaged for later postoperative therapy.

The paracaval and para-aortic lymph nodes must be inspected and dissected as well. A lymph node dissection should be performed routinely in all cases, even in those in which lymph nodes appear not to be involved [12, 14, 40]. The lymph node dissection may take more time than the tumor nephrectomy, especially in those cases in which extensive involvement is evident. Lymph node dissection should run from the bifurcation up to the truncus coeliacus and also to the area of the contralateral renal vein. The contralateral kidney should be palpated. Owing to better imaging techniques with ultrasound and CT, nowadays it is not necessary to free the contralateral kidney from the fascia in order to have direct manual or optical control.

The exact intraoperative status has to be described, and the removed tumor volume measured precisely. These data are necessary for the evaluation of additional postoperative treatment (Fig. 6).

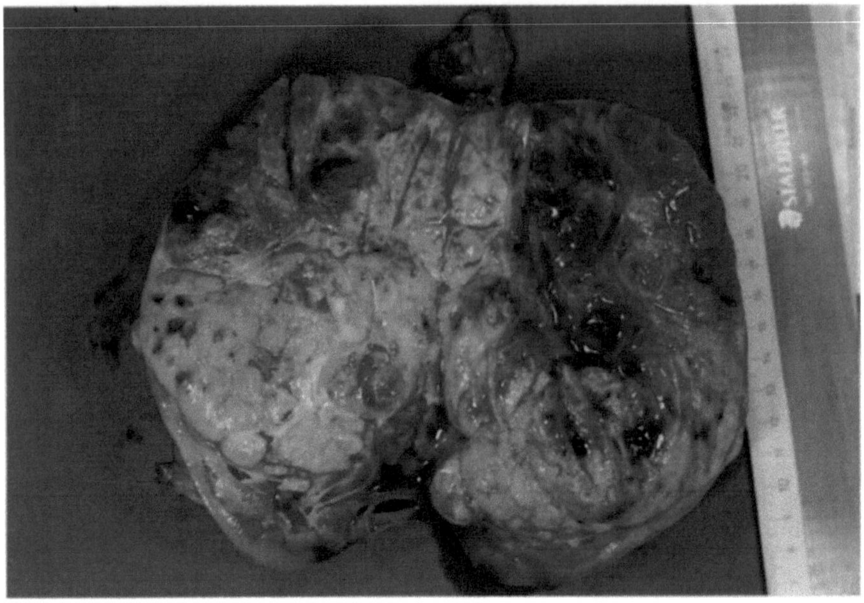

Fig. 6. The tumor specimen

2.2.1 *Tumor Enucleation*

In cases of bilateral tumor disease the situation may arise that at least one organ can be preserved for satisfactory kidney function. Tumor enucleation, heminephrectomy, or partial nephrectomy may be applied [8, 32, 61]. In all cases the renal artery and vein must be dissected carefully and held with vessel loops for temporary clamping. We have used simple bulldog clamps without complications. This tumor enucleation is possible in cases treated preoperatively with chemotherapy or radiotherapy. The tumor can be removed by blunt dissection and the larger vessels sutured or ligated. All borders have to be biopsied to be sure that no part of the tumor is left. This technique is not more difficult in children than partial resection of hypernephroma in the adult. In our experience tumor enucleation with bilateral tumors is preferred to radical nephrectomy with subsequent dialysis [52]. This operative therapy is followed by effective postoperative treatment which guarantees good long-term results because of the organ-preserving surgery [15, 33, 58].

2.2.2 *Extrarenal Wilms' Tumors*

These are very rare cases with locations in the inguinal canal, scrotum, retroperitoneum, and chest wall. Surgery is concerned with local tumor resection and may be combined with local radiation or combination chemotherapy [6, 24, 28, 35].

2.2.3 *Surgery of Metastases*

Metastases to the liver may require to partial resection of the liver; those to the lung in special cases wedge resection or segmental resection. The surgery of metastatic disease follows the guidelines of surgical techniques for other tumor metastases; here treatment is always combined with radiotherapy and/or chemotherapy [26, 51].

2.2.4 *Intraoperative Complications*

Major complications which may happen are tumor burst and bleeding. Even in very large tumors the dissection of the tumor vessels is in most cases quite possible. They can be safely ligated, so that bleeding from larger vessels can be avoided. Also, in very impressive bulky disease cases, the tumor can generally be moved aside, facilitating the approach to the major vessels. There may be bleeding from the suprarenal vein, but normally with careful operative technique, this does not present a problem.

If the tumor infiltrates neighbouring organs such as the liver or spleen, surgery can be difficult and include local bleeding. These cases should have preoperative treatment. Partial resection of the neighbouring organs may be necessary.

Tumor rupture or burst of involved lymph nodes require a careful wash-out of the abdominal cavity.

2.2.5 *Postoperative Complications*

Postoperative bleeding requiring intervention within the first 12 h is rare. Intra-abdominal adhesions may lead to symptoms of subileus or ileus which can be treated conservatively.

2.3 Postoperative Treatment

Postoperative treatment varies according to the tumor stage. Stage I and II tumors should have chemotherapy after tumor resection. Stage III and IV tumors, which have already had preoperative treatment, should also undergo postoperative chemo- and radiotherapy. Details of these treatment protocols are presented elsewhere. Patients with metastases to the lungs, brain, bone, or liver need individual treatment; only in selected cases will metastatic surgery be required as described above.

2.3.1 *Follow-up*

The follow-up of all stages higher than stage II involves regular radiological examinations including bone scan, X-ray of the lung, and computerised tomography [17, 18, 19, 62].

2.3.2 *Recurrent Disease*

Local recurrent disease may lead to further surgical procedures. Distant metastases may be treated by surgery, chemo- and/or radiotherapy.

References

1. Allerton SE, Bierle JW, Powars DR, Bavetta LA (1970) Abnormal extracellular components in Wilms' tumor. Cancer Res 30:679
2. Alzen G, Gutjahr P (1982) Präoperative Wilmstumorbehandlung (Stadium III): die Rolle der Sonographie. Kinderarzt 13:348
3. Aron BS (1974) Wilms' tumor. A clinical study of 81 cases. Cancer 33:637
4. Bachmann KD (1976) Das Nephroblastom (Wilms-Tumor) bei Kindern. Dtsch Ärztebl 73:647
5. Beckwith JB, Palmer NF (1978) Histopathology and prognosis of Wilms' tumor. Cancer 41:1937
6. Bhajekar AB, Joseph M, Bhat HS (1964) Unattached nephroblastoma. Br J Urol 36:187
7. Birch JM, Marsden HB, Swindell R (1980) Incidence of malignant disease in childhood: a 24-year review of the Manchester children's tumor registry data. Br J Cancer 42:215
8. Bishop HC, Tefft M, Evans AE (1977) Survival in bilateral Wilms' tumors – review of 30 national Wilms' tumor study cases. J Pediatr Surg 12:631
9. Bolande RP, Brough AJ, Isant RJ Jr (1967) Congenital mesoblastic nephroma of infancy. A report of eight cases and the relationship to Wilms' tumor. Pediatrics 40: 272
10. Boldt DW, Reilly BJ (1977) Computed tomography of abdominal mass lesions in children. Radiology 124:471
11. Bracken RB, Sutow WW, Jaffe N, Ayala A, Guarda L (1982) Preoperative chemotherapy for Wilms' tumor. Urology 19:55
12. Breslow NE, Palmer NF, Hill RL, Buring J, D'Angio GJ (1978) Wilms' tumor: prognostic factors for patients without metastases at diagnosis. Cancer 41:1577
13. Bürger D, Moorman-Voestermans CGM, Mildenberger H, Lemerle J, Voute PA, Tournade MF, Rodary C, Delemarre JFM, Sandstedt B, Sarrazin D, Burgers JMV, Bey P, Carli M, de Kraker J (1985) The advantages of preoperative therapy in Wilms' tumour. A summarised report on clinical trials conducted by the International Society of Paediatric Oncology (SIOP). Z Kinderchirur 40:170
14. Cassady JR, Tefft M, Filler RM, Jaffe N, Hellman S (1973) Considerations in the radiation therapy of Wilms' tumor. Cancer 32:598
15. de Chadarevian J-P, Fletcher BD, Chatten J, Rabinovitch JJ (1977) Massive infantile nephroblastomatosis. Cancer 39:2294
16. Clayman RV, Sheldon CA, Gonzales R (1982) Wilms' tumor: an approach to vena caval intrusion. Prog Pediatr Surg 15:285
17. Cohen M, Provisor A, Smith WL, Weetman R (1981) Efficacy of whole lung tomography in diagnosing metastases from solid tumors in children. Radiology 141:375
18. Cohen M, Smith WL, Weetman R, Provisor A (1981) Pulmonary pseudometastases in children with malignant tumors. Radiology 141:371
19. Cohen MD, Siddiqui A, Weetman R, Baehner R, Weber T, Grosfeld JL (1982) A rational approach to the radiologic evaluation of children with Wilms' tumor. Cancer 50:887
20. Damgaar-Pederson K (1980) CT and IVU in the diagnosis of Wilms' tumour. Pediatr Radiol 9:207
21. D'Angio GJ, Evans AE, Breslow N, Beckwith B, Bishop H, Feigl P, Goodwin W, Leape L, Sinks LF, Sutow WW, Tefft M, Wolff J (1976) The treatment of Wilms' tumor – results of the National Wilms' Tumor Study. Cancer 38:633
22. D'Angio GJ, Beckwith JB, Breslow NE (1980) Wilms' tumor – an update. Cancer 45:1791
23. Edelstein G, Webb RS Jr, Romsdahl MM, Arboit JM (1965) Extrarenal Wilms' tumor. Am J Surg 109:509
24. Farah J, Lofstrom JE (1968) Angiography of Wilms' tumor. Radiology 90:775
25. Farewell VT, D'Angio GJ, Breslow N, Norkool P (1981) Retrospective validation of a new staging system for Wilms' tumor. Cancer Clin Trials 4:167

26. Filler RM, Tefft M, Vawter GF (1966) Hepatic lobectomy in childhood: effects of x-ray and chemotherapy. J Pediatr Surg 4:31
27. Folin J (1969) Angiography in Wilms' tumour. Acta Radiol (Diagn) 8:201
28. Gaikwad KD, Patil PS, Bhavthankar AG, Dave VB, Chavan SB (1977) Extrarenal Wilms' tumour. Ind Pediatr 14:657
29. Garett RA, Donohue JP (1978) Bilateral Wilms' tumor. J Urol 120:586
30. Green DM (1985) Diagnosis and management of malignant solid tumors in infants and children. Nijhoff, Boston
31. Gross TE, Neuhnauser EBD (1950) Treatment of mixed tumors of the kidney in childhood. Pediatrics 6:843
32. Gruner M, Chaouachi B, Bitker M (1982) Surgical aspects of simultaneous bilateral Wilms' tumors. Prog Clin Biol Res 100:155
33. Haddy TB, Bailie MD, Bernstein J, Kaufman DB, Rous SN (1977) Bilateral, diffuse nephroblastomatosis: report of a case managed with chemotherapy. J Pediatr 90: 784
34. Harms D, Gutjahr P, Hohenfellner R, Willke E (1980) Fetal rhabdomyomatous nephroblastoma. Eur J Pediatr 133:167
35. Ho J, Ma L, Wong KC (1981) An extrarenal Wilms' tumour arising from an undescended testis. Pathology 13:619
36. Jacobsen R, Rubenson A, Hanson G, Sorensen S-E, Hagberg S (1979) Regression of Wilms' tumor after preoperative chemotherapy. Acta Paediatr Scand 68:763
37. Jagasia KH, Thurman WG, Pickett E, Grabstaldt H (1964) Bilateral Wilms' tumors in children. J Pediatr 65: 371
38. Jereb B (1971) Bilateral nephroblastoma. Acta Radiol Ther Phys Biol 10:417
39. Jereb B, Eklund G (1973) Factors influencing the cure rate in nephroblastoma. Acta Radiol 12:84
40. Jereb B, Tournade MF, Lemerle J, Voute PA, Delemarre JF, Ahstrom L, Flamant R, Gerard-Marhant R, Sandstedt B (1980) Lymph node invasion and prognosis in nephroblastoma. Cancer 45:1632
41. Joshi VV, Banerjee DK, Yadav K, Pathak IC (1977) Cystic, partially differentiated nephroblastoma. A clinico-pathologic entity in the spectrum of infantile renal neoplasia. Cancer 40:789
42. Klapproth HJ (1959) Wilms' tumor: a report of 45 cases and an analysis of 1351 cases reported from 1940–1958 in the world literature. J Urol 81:633
42a. Kuhn JP (1981) CT in the evaluation of pediatric abdominal abnormalities. CRC Crit Rev Diagn Imaging 16:125
43. Kumar APM, Wrenn EL Jr, Fleming ID, Hustu HO, Pratt CB, Pinkel D (1975) Preoperative therapy for unresectable malignant tumor in children. J Pediatr Surg 10:657
44. Ladd WE (1938) Embryoma of the kidney (Wilms' tumor). Ann Surg 108:885
45. Leen RLS, Williams IG (1971) Bilateral Wilms' tumor. Cancer 28:802
46. Lemerle J, Voute PA, Tournade MF, Delemarre JFM, Jereb B, Ahstrom L, Flamant R, Gerard-Marchant R (1976) Preoperative versus postoperative radiotherapy, single versus multiple courses of actinomycin D, in the treatment of Wilms' tumor. Preliminary results of a controlled clinical trial conducted by the International Society of Paediatric Oncology (SIOP). Cancer 38:647
47. Masselot J, Couanet D, Nihoul-Fekete C, Passail G, Piekarsky J-P, Vanel D (1979) Computed tomography in the study of abdominal mass in pediatry. In: Lamarque JL, Bruel JM (eds) Abdominal computerized tomography. Excerpta Medica, Amsterdam, p 341
48. McDonald P, Hiller HG (1968) Angiography in abdominal tumours in childhood with particular reference to neuroblastoma and Wilms' tumor. Clin Radiol 19:1
49. McWhirter WR, Bacon JE (1981) Incidence of childhood tumors in Queensland. Br J Cancer 44:637
50. Pastore G, Magnani C, Zanetti R, Terracini B (1981) Incidence of cancer in children in the province of Torino (Italy) 1967–1978. Eur J Cancer 17:1337
51. Price JB Jr, Schullinger JN, Santulli TV (1982) Major hepatic resections for neoplasia in children. Arch Surg 117:1139
52. Ringert R-H, Hartung R, Havers W (1983) Interdisciplinary treatment of Wilms' tumour. Brit J Urol 55:347
53. Rusche C (1951) Treatment of Wilms' tumor. J Urol 65:950
54. Sieber WK, Dibbins AW, Wiener ES (1979) Retroperitoneal tumors. In: Ravitch MM, Welch KJ, Benson CD, Aberdeen E, Randolph JG (eds) Pediatric surgery. Yearbook Medical, Chicago, p 1082
55. Silva-Sosa M, Gonzales-Cerna JL (1966) Wilms' tumor in children. Progr Clin Cancer 2:323
56. Simone JV, Cassady JR, Filler RM (1982) Cancers of childhood. In: DeVita VT Jr, Hellman S, Rosenberg SA (eds) Cancer: principles and practice of oncology. Lippincott, Philadelphia, p 1288
57. Sullivan MP, Sutow W, Cangir A, Taylor G (1967) Vincristine sulfate in management of Wilms' Tumor. JAMA 202:381
58. Telander RL, Gilchrist GS, Burgert EO Jr, Kelalis PP, Goellner JR (1978) Bilateral massive nephroblastomatosis in infancy. J Pediatr Surg 13:163
59. Wagget J, Koop CE (1970) Wilms' tumor: preoperative radiotherapy and chemotherapy in the management of massive tumors. Cancer 28:338
60. Weisel W (1943) Wilms' tumor of the kidney: a clinicopathological study of 44 proved cases. J Urol 50:399
61. Wiener ES (1976) Bilateral partial nephrectomies for large bilateral Wilms' tumors. J Pediatr Surg 11:867
62. Wilimas JA, Hammond E, Douglas EC, Champion J, Parvey L, Coburn T (1984) The value of computerized tomography as a routine follow-up procedure for patients with Wilms' tumor. Med Pediatr Oncol 12:221
63. Young JL Jr, Miller RW (1975) Incidence of malignant tumors in U.S. children. J Pediatr 86:254

Nonoperative Treatment of Renal Cell Carcinoma

R.-D. MÜLLER, E. SCHERER and C. WIRTZ

1 Introduction

Nonoperative treatment of hypernephroma comprises irradiation and transfemoral catheter embolization of advanced, inoperable, and symptomatic primary tumors; as well as chemotherapy for metastases, using cytostatic substances, hormones, and immunotherapeutic agents.

Of all malignancies in man, 2%–3% are renal tumors. Hypernephroma has the highest incidence of these, with 70%–80% in all age groups and 90% in adults. The other malignant renal tumors are epithelial carcinomas of the renal pelvis, followed in incidence by tumors of mesodermal and mesenchymal tissues (mainly nephroblastoma in children), and metastases from other tumors, e.g., carcinoma of the lung, testis, or thyroid.

There has been some uncertainty regarding the natural history of hypernephroma. Because of its site of origin – it is commonly found immediately beneath the renal capsule – and its cellular morphology, GRAWITZ [33] assumed that this tumor was caused by ectopic tissue of the suprarenal gland. He named it "Struma lipomatodes aberratae renis." In Zollinger's opinion it originates from the inner part of the renal blastema. KANTOR [34] suggested a de novo origin from the proximal parts of the convoluted tubular epithelium. Other authors surmise that this tumor develops slowly from adenomatous hyperplastic parenchyma.

Histologically, hypernephroma can be differentiated into clear cell, granular cell, and mixed cell types. The clear cell type is two to three times more common than the granular cell type. In contrast to the usually expressed opinion that the clear cell type is more differentiated and thus prognostically more favorable [86, 135, 34], a study of the proliferation kinetics by RABES [106] found that there was no significant, prognostically useful difference between these two cellular types. On the other hand, histological grading permits a prognosis [48, 83, 35]. Apart from the usual signs of malignancy, particularly useful criteria for categorisation are the structure of the nuclei (condensed, pleomorphic, irregular) and the tissue structure (papillary, tubular, solid) [4, 75, 134]. The morphological assessment of hypernephroma is difficult because heterogeneous tissue structures are often found close together within the same tumor [106, 18]. An attempt to introduce greater objectivity into the histological grading has been carried out by BAISCH [5] and by OTTO et al. [93] with a determination of DNA content using flow cytometry. They found a close correlation between chromosome ploidy, nuclear morphology (grade), and incidence of metastasis. HERMANEK et al. [42], MEISTER [84] and MCNICHOLS [83] consider the combination of malignancy grade with clinical staging to permit a more accurate prognosis.

Hypernephroma generally becomes manifest after the age of 40 with a peak incidence between the 6th and 7th decades, and a rapid drop in incidence thereafter [83, 34, 44].

In children and adolescents, the tumor is rare [96, 147]. PATEL and LAVENGOOD [98] reported on 186 cases from the literature, the youngest of which was a child of 3 months. The occurrence of hypernephroma in 89 young adults between 20 and 40 years of age is described by LIEBER et al. [71]. The clinical course of the disease in children does not seem to differ from that in adults, particularly with respect to the prognosis [70].

A more recent, large-scale epidemiological study by RITCHIE et al. [117] shows an increase of 36% in the incidence of hypernephroma in men over the period from 1967 to 1979. In 74–84 year-old men, the incidence doubled. On the other hand, the incidence of hypernephroma among women has remained constant. The predominance of this tumor among men has already been described by KANTOR [61]. He found that this disease was three times commoner in men below 40 years of age than in women below 40 years of age, and twice as common over the age of 40 years. Despite some reports in the literature [6, 139], a familial disposition has not been proved.

The right and left kidneys are affected equally often. Bilateral hypernephroma is rare. It occurs in less than 2% of all reported cases [57]. Approximately 150 bilateral cases have been reported [144, 7, 136–137]. In these, a conservative operation, allowing retention of organ function with either tumor enucleation or partial resection of the kidney has been recommended. Bilateral nephrectomy requiring subsequent dialysis or kidney transplantation should be carried out only as the treatment of last resort.

Hypernephroma is spread via local invasion and infiltration into the blood and the lymphatic system of the kidney. The larger the primary tumor at the time of diagnosis, the greater is the probability that it has already metastasized [134]. About one-third of patients have metastases at the time of diagnosis. Predominant sites are the regional lymph nodes, lungs, liver, and skeletal system [60, 98, 26, 141].

At operation, tumor invasion of, or tumor thrombus in the renal vein is found in 40%–62% of hypernephromas [145, 53, 26, 30, 119]. Others have reported that in as many as 22%, renal vein infiltration has occurred [98, 148, 39, 132, 90]. The tumor thrombus may occasionally extend into the right atrium. Blockage of the hepatic vein by the tumor is also possible, mimicking Budd-Chiari syndrome with ascites. In 50% of all patients with metastatic disease, lung involvement is found, with the tumor mass invading a bronchus. This may lead to hemoptysis and coughing up of pieces of tumor.

Of those patients dying from hypernephroma, 32% have skeletal metastases. Initially, only isolated oval foci with osteolytic changes are found. Tumor cells enter the circulation via the vertebral venous plexus, then spread into the axial skeleton and also, typical of hypernephroma, into the periphery of the extremities, e.g., the calcaneus.

Liver metastases are seen at autopsy in 33% of cases. Metastases to the brain are found more often than expected, but metastases to the thyroid, heart, stomach, eye, vagina [3, 98, 35], and pancreas [146] have been reported. Direct spread into neighboring organs, such as the colon, liver, spleen, and diaphragm, is present in 9% of patients. Infiltration into the adrenal gland is seen in 6%–10% of the surgical specimens [118]. Metastatic spread of hypernephroma is especially favored by the kidney's close proximity to major elements of the lymphatic system. Knowledge of the lymphatic drainage of the kidney is of decisive importance for specifying therapy [89]:

> The lymphatic drainage of the renal parenchyma is via lymphatics which, after encompassing the glomeruli and tubuli, gather as lymphatic capillaries at the pyramids. Across the hilus of the kidney three large bundles of lymphatics run, parallel to the renal blood vessels, to the para-aortic and paracaval lymph nodes. Here they join the lymphatics lying to the right and left sides of the aorta and vena cava. There is some crossing of lymphatics from the right to the left side. This plexus extends caudally to the aortic bifurcation. In addition, a few lymphatics drain the renal capsule, especially the perirenal fat. These travel partially via the diaphragm to the mediastinal lymph nodes but also have direct connections to the liver and peritoneum. Moreover, lymphatics drain the lower portion of the renal capsule into the lymph nodes between the renal vein and the inferior mesenteric artery. The lymphatic drainage along the ureters, originating from the renal pelvis and extending down to the iliac lymph nodes, should also be taken into consideration.

Reports of the incidence of disease in the lymph nodes vary from 2.8% [83] to 32.6% [39]. HERRLINGER et al. [44] in his review of the literature found that the most common values given lay between 15% and 25%. The probability of detecting positive lymph nodes is dependent on both the operative technique and the thoroughness of the histological examination. SIGEL et al. [133], operating through a transabdominal approach, found 4%–14% increase in positive lymph nodes compared with the previously used flank approach. After the systematic removal of all para-aortic and paracaval lymph nodes from the aortic bifurcation to the diaphragm, a further increase in the percentage of positive lymph nodes from 7% to 15% could be demonstrated [133, 44]. Using this technique, HERRLINGER [44] established that in 44% the cancer growth in the lymph nodes consisted of micrometastases and was thus subclinical.

Some authors [63, 26, 24, 85] recommend the radical removal of the regional lymph nodes only on the basis of an exact staging, whereas others [119, 39, 44] recommend this on therapeutic grounds, as they found that this leads to an increase in the 5-year survival rate.

RICHES [112, 113] analyzed the fate of patients who received no therapy. Only 4.4% of these patients survived for 3 years, and 1.7% lived 5 years. Even then, after radical removal of a locally infiltrating tumor, one can expect somewhat less than half of these patients to present later with metastases [58, 102]. The postmortem examination of operatively untreated patients revealed metastases in over 80% [125]. Local recurrence and metastases occur relatively soon after treatment, 80%–90% within 3 years [122, 115]. However, even 5 years after operation, metastases could be established [24].

A very late recurrence of the tumor after more than 10 years of freedom from disease was observed by MCNICHOLS et al. [83] in 3% of his patients.

Once distant metastases occur, 5-year survival is reduced to below 10% [134, 12]. BOXER et al. [15] calculated an average survival of 1.1 years after presentation of the first metastases. However, as hypernephroma does not cause any characteristic early symptoms, it is very often diagnosed only in an advanced stage. The triad of macrohematuria, flank pain, and palpable tumor, caused by local tumor spread, which was regarded as a classic feature of hypernephroma, occurs in only 10%–15% of patients; however, at least one of these symptoms is present in 65%. When these symptoms are observed, 47% of patients have metastatic disease [85]; the triad is to be regarded as a late sign of advanced disease. In 10% of all patients the presenting symptoms are due to distant metastases alone, and are not due to renal involvement [26].

An increased erythrocyte sedimentation rate (ESR) is a frequent and prognostically significant finding [91]. For those patients with a preoperative ESR below 10 mm in the first hour, a 5-year survival rate of 80% can be expected. On the other hand, an ESR above 50 mm in the first hour suggests a 5-year survival of about 30% [60, 48, 12].

The introduction of ultrasound screening gives rise to the hope that, in this disease for which survival is very much stage dependent, early detection will bring about increased survival.

2 Radiotherapy

The radiosensitivity of a tumor is generally the same as that of the cells from which it originates. Therefore, the radiosensitivity of hypernephroma can be assumed to be the same as that of renal tubular elements. The tubular epithelial cells of the kidney are long-living postmitotic cells, which are regarded as being comparatively radioresistant [142]. This resistance is probably increased by hypoxia in the central parts of a given tumor. As well, the technique used in conventional radiotherapy does not allow irradiation of the retroperitoneum with an adequate dose without causing considerable damage to the neighbouring organs. These reservations prompted some authors [135, 21, 28, 98, 148, 81, 102] not to advise radiotherapy in the treatment of hypernephroma, whereas others regard it as an established part of the treatment [115, 122, 2, 80, 141].

In curative therapy, nephrectomy with radical excision of the regional lymph nodes is a basic necessity. Due to the growth characteristics of hypernephroma and the topographic anatomy of the kidney and neighboring organs, radical excision often cannot be achieved. Postoperative radiotherapy is directed at possible residual tumor in those areas from which relapses might develop. CAVANAUGH [23] and SIGEL et al. [133] recommend postoperative radiotherapy for all cases except those from whom there is evidence of complete removal of all lymph nodes from the diaphragm to the aortic bifurcation and who are histologically demonstrable as being free of disease. Irradiation may also be withheld when the tumor is very small and when there is no histological evidence of its invasion into blood vessels or the renal capsule. Obesity, debilitation, or old age may be reasons to refrain from radiotherapy, but with megavoltage therapy, obesity is no longer a problem.

Local recurrences after surgery can successfully be reduced or prevented by postoperative radiotherapy [73]. No recurrence was seen in the irradiated regions of GAUWERKY's patients [37]. RAFLA [108] observed 24 (25%) cases of local recurrence in 96 patients who had been treated with surgery alone and 7 cases (7.4%) in 94 patients who had also been irradiated postoperatively.

Recent studies [115, 80, 45, 122, 47, 141] show unanimously that local recurrence after postoperative irradiation appears in only 2%–3% of patients. Without radiotherapy, as much as 10% local recurrence must be expected [119]. A higher than average risk of local recurrence has been determined for those patients whose tumors penetrate beyond the renal capsule and for those with evidence of diseased lymph nodes at operation [97, 144, 88]. Distant metastases or local tumor spread may develop from the recurrence, or from residual tumor (after incomplete surgery or insufficient irradiation of the lymphatic region), hence the unfavorable prognosis of such cases.

Frequently, however, distant metastases are already present at the beginning of therapy. The 5-year survival rate after surgery alone varies between 33% and 48% [27–28]. Prognosis is improved by postoperative radiotherapy [31, 16, 20] especially in advanced local hypernephroma. RINGLEB and ROMMEL [116] found that postoperative radiotherapy increased the 5-year survival rate from 29.9% to 55.5%.

Invasion of the renal capsule by tumor is a bad prognostic sign. Without postoperative radiotherapy 28% of RAFLA'S [108] patients with this finding survived for 5 years. However, after postoperative radiotherapy, survival increased to 57%.

Tumor invasion of the renal vein is regarded as evidence of hematogeneous spread of the cancer, and radiotherapy has often been omitted in these cases. However, even in these seemingly unfavorable cases, postoperative radiotherapy improved the 5-year survival rate from 21% to 39% [73]. Studies confirming these encouraging results have yet to be published.

Initial suggestions of the usefulness of preoperative radiotherapy were made as long as 50 years ago [147]. It appears from further studies [10, 38, 142, 77] that today preoperative radiation therapy is an established treatment modality in otherwise inoperable hypernephromas [18, 19, 73]. The number of inoperable cases could thus be reduced to a minimum [17, 95], and the operation itself can be performed more radically after irradiation [151–152, 73, 2].

Tumor reduction results from resorption of radiosensitive destructed cells, decrease of inflammation, and shrinkage of tumor vessels, e.g. the renal capsule veins.

There are two methods of radiation fractioning, namely long-term and short-term preoperative irradiation. Long-term preoperative irradiation is based on the report by WATERS et al. [143] and was confirmed by SAKSELA et al. [126] who demonstrated that conventional preoperative radiotherapy reduced the cellular proliferation rate in kidney tumors. Its aim is to shrink the tumor in order to facilitate the operation.

Usually, 30 Gy (3,000 rads) tumor dose is given over 3 weeks [114, 37, 17, 151, 123]. Surgery is performed 3–4 weeks later [114, 17, 73, 2]. HUDGINS and COLLINS [52] recommend a longer interval of 4–6 weeks between the end of preoperative irradiation and surgery. Others favor shorter intervals, which, however, should not be shorter than 1 week, because the edematous reaction of the tumor and neighbouring tissue makes surgery more difficult [114].

In 1973, VAN DER WERF-MESSING [151] reported results of a randomized prospective study of preoperative radiotherapy. She found that patients who were irradiated preoperatively had a lower incidence of distant metastases and that there were also fewer local recurrences in the group of patients with advanced hypernephroma. There was, however, no difference between the survival rates of pre- and postoperatively irradiated patients. Since then, the value of preoperative radiotherapy has been controversial. Discussion in the literature is often based on small – sometimes not even significant – numbers of patients. KOB et al. [67] found, in a group of 71 patients who had been preoperatively irradiated with 30–40 Gy, an increase in the 5-year survival rate of 9.9% and a reduction in the frequency of metastases of 11.3%, compared to an untreated control group.

PACES et al. [95] carried out a prospective study on the value of long-term preoperative radiotherapy with 59 patients and found an increase in survival at 8 years of 29%, compared to 10.7% for the nonirradiated group.

ANDERSSON and EDSMYR [2] achieved an increase in the 5-year survival rate from 31% to 54% in a small group of 24 patients who were found to have poorly differentiated tumor tissue and who were pretreated in the target volume with a radiation dose of 35 Gy. However, in a group with fair to good tumor differentiation, conventional preoperative radiotherapy was not found to be of value. In another randomized study of 174 patients, published by HOP and VAN DER WERF-MESSING [48], it was found that preoperative irradiation did not change survival. Similarly, JUUSELA et al. [59] could not demonstrate an influence of preoperative irradiation on survival.

Although long-term preoperative radiotherapy of hypernephroma does not generally seem to influence the course of the disease, the suspicion remains that in special cases (large tumor mass, high degree of malignancy, positive lymph nodes), this procedure may have certain advantages. Therefory, many authors [151, 77, 67, 2] have suggested the need for a prospective clinical trial.

The advantages of short-term preoperative irradiation have been pointed out by HUG [55]. The mass of vital and proliferative tumor cells is reduced by a rapid sequence of sufficiently high single doses just before surgery, so that the probability of an intraoperative dissemination of tumor cells can be significantly reduced. GAUWERKY and ADAM [37] recommended a tumor dose of 20 Gy (2,000 rad) in 4 days, and VON LIEVEN et al. [74] a dosage of 12–16 Gy (1,200–1,600 rad) in 2 days, followed by surgery 1 day later.

CARL et al. [22] could demonstrate on the basis of autoradiography that radiation pretreatment with 16 Gy (1,600 rad) in 2–3 days considerably reduced the rate of DNA synthesis of 11 tumor specimens obtained from 5.4 patients. However, there were some cells at the margins of necrotic areas which continued to synthesize DNA. The experiments of VAN LIEVEN et al. [74] with eight tumors showed that a radiation pretreatment of 12–16 Gy (1,200–1,600 rad) over 2 days led to a reduction of the proliferating cells to below 2‰. After irradiation, the tumors did not produce in-vitro colonies.

Depending upon the situation found at the operation site, irradiation may be continued postoperatively. Bearing in mind the dose-dependence of side effects, a total dose of 50 Gy (5,000 rad) should not be exceeded [66, 122]. In some cases of advanced hypernephroma with invasion of the capsule, venous infiltration, and regional lymph node metastases, preoperative irradiation was supplemented by postoperative irradiation. The 3-year survival rate could be raised to 62% (13 of 21) compared to 25% (3 of 12) in an earlier patient group which had been only postoperatively irradiated [77].

Radiotherapy alone is only given when surgery is impossible for technical or medical reasons, or when the prognosis is very poor. Such palliative radiotherapy can stop hemorrhages or reduce pain caused by tumor growth. In individual cases it may prolong a patient's life.

NICKOLISEN and FALLON [88] reported two patients with primary tumors treated with radiotherapy and tumor embolization. Both patients, who had no evidence of distant metastases, developed a local recurrence 1 year after nephrectomy. Following local radiotherapy, the residual tumor was embolized selectively through a lumbar artery. Both these patients were alive and well 3 years later.

Palliative radiotherapy is indicated for local recurrence, even in the stage of tumor dissemination, as is the local irradiation of pulmonary, skeletal, and lymph node metastases, and of symptomatic metastases of the brain. A dosage of 30 Gy (3,000 rad) over 2–3 weeks will be sufficient to alleviate symptoms. Higher doses do not generally improve the results and should not be administered [32, 41, 111]. After irradiation of the whole brain with this dosage, plus simultaneous decadrone phosphate medication, a positive response can be achieved in 30% of cases [41].

The analgesic and stabilizing effects of radiation therapy on skeletal metastases are to be especially emphasized. A subjective response is reported by about 80% of all patients, although an objective response can be demonstrated in only about 50% [32, 13, 41].

In certain cases with, for example, solitary brain or bone metastases, a local saturation with up to 45 Gy can be justified.

Occasionally, a compression fracture of a vertebra and impending paralysis can be prevented. In addition, analgesic medication can be reduced to a minimum.

In this context it should be pointed out that patients with only bone metastases have a higher survival rate than those with visceral metastases [111]. When skeletal metastases alone are present, an aggressive schedule is justified, with surgical removal of metastases and possibly palliative nephrectomy with subsequent radiotherapy [69, 111, 14]. Rapid and prolonged relief of pain in patients with multiple skeletal metas-

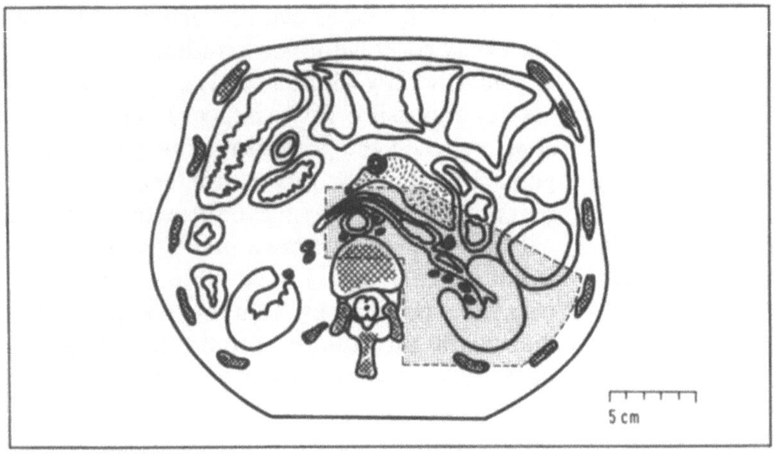

Fig. 1. Target volume for postoperative radiotherapy of renal cell carcinoma (ABBATUCCI et al. 1976). The *shaded* area indicates the target volume

tases has been achieved with endosteal radiostrontium therapy [29].

Adjuvant radiotherapy in hypernephroma should only be performed under megavoltage conditions. Fixed beam techniques [37, 27, 28, 66, 79, 122, 47, 109, 141] and rotational techniques [130, 37, 53, 115, 76, 80, 110] as well as a combination of both [145, 138] have been described.

In radiotherapy for hypernephroma, the topographic anatomy of the kidney and the difficulty of homogeneously irradiating the tumor bed and the regional lymph nodes without damaging the neighbouring organs have to be considered. The target volume includes the bed of the tumor, the renal pedicle, and the para-aortic and paracaval lymph drainages (TH 11–L 3).

According to the clinicopathological studies of NOECKER [89] and HERRLINGER et al. [43], the target volume should include not only the ipsilateral lymph nodes but also the contralateral and prevertebral nodes and should thus extend 1.5 cm beyond the midline. The surgical incision should also lie within the irradiation field. An exact individual therapy plan is established with the help of a CT-scanner. The advantages of this form of therapy planning have been described by HÜBENER and JUNKER [54]. They found, comparing CT edit planning to the more conventional method, that the former led on average to an increase in the target volume of 53%.

The CT films are fed into a calculator which simulates the various irradiation techniques and determines both the isodose patterns at different levels, and the radiation dosage of certain critical organs (spinal cord colon, contralateral kidney) (Figs. 1 and 2). In this way it is possible to construct a three-dimensional irradiation plan [76]. The intraoperative use of metal clips for denoting the volume to be irradiated should no longer be made, since these clips lead to artefacts in the CT films.

The dosage tolerance of the neighboring organs is an important factor in the irradiation planning of hypernephroma treatment. Special attention must be paid to the remaining healthy kidney, which must not receive more than 20 Gy (2,000 rad). Otherwise, following the early clinical signs of proteinuria, anemia, and hypertension, irreversible damage to the organ can be expected [121]. The mortality of radiation nephritis is 42% [128].

Radiogenic myelitis and irreversible damage to the spinal cord may develop if the radiation dosage is too high. The critical dosage is 30–40 Gy (3,000–4,000 rad) [16, 140]. In the case of pronounced kyphosis or lordosis of the vertebral column, attention must be paid to the increased danger to the spinal cord [54].

Although the radiation tolerance of the liver appears to be comparatively high, only a small section of it should be irradiated with a dosage over 25 Gy (2,500 rad), and the larger part of the parenchyma should not receive more than 20 Gy (2,000 rad) [105]. Due to its high capacity for regeneration, the remainder of the liver is able to compensate for the loss of function caused by fibrosis in the intensively irradiated area. ANDERSSON and EDSMYR [2] observed that for some patients with tumors of the right abdomen who were postoperatively irradiated with

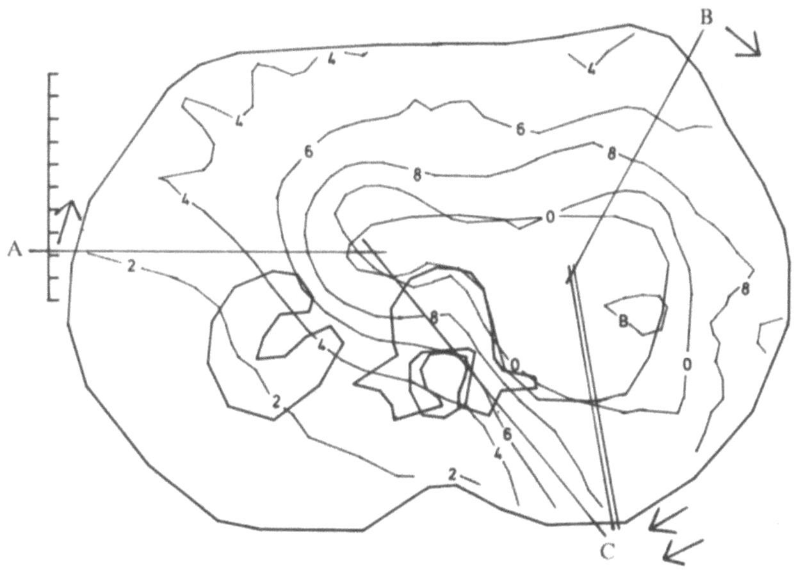

Fig. 2. Technique of biaxial rotation and an additional dorsal field. Isodose pattern using CT scanner and calculator. Point *C* marks the final position of the first rotation sequence starting at point *A* and the second rotation sequence starting at point *B*

50 Gy in the target volume, a temporary increase occurred in the serum hepatic enzyme values, normalizing in all cases after some time.

The radiation tolerance of the gastrointestinal tract is rather low [143]. A radiation dosage of more than 45 Gy (4,500 rad) may lead to irreversible damage, such as strictures, scars, ulcers, or even perforation of the intestine. Between the end of the radiation therapy and the presentation of these complications, a symptomfree interval of months or years may occur, so that often the connection between the causative irradiation and the symptoms is not recognized [124, 149]. The radiation tolerance of the intestinal tract is reduced if postoperative intestinal adhesions occur, fixing parts of the intestine permanently within the field of irradiation [45].

With a tumor dose of 56–60 Gy (5,600–6,000 rad), intestinal complications needing operative treatment can be expected in 10% of cases [122]. For irradiation of hypernephroma, a total tumor dose of 46–50 Gy (4,600–5,000 rad), with a maximal weekly dosage of 5 × 2 Gy (1,000 rad), appears to be appropriate.

3 Chemotherapy

Despite the recent general advances in the chemotherapy of malignant tumors, hypernephroma has remained one of the least susceptible to this approach. Because of the low therapeutic ratio of cytotoxics in the treatment of this disease, their use as an adjuvant therapy after surgical treatment has not been propagated [92]. Justification for treatment with chemotherapy exists only for patients with metastases at presentation and patients who develop metastases despite radical local treatment. Almost 50% of all patients with hypernephroma fall into one of these categories [64].

There have been many clinical studies on the use of chemotherapy in hypernephroma, but because of the many criteria for selection of patients, variety of drug dosage schemes, and differing evaluation of response, they are not easily comparable. In particular, the evaluation of response merits critical consideration because it is well known that during the course of this disease, even when untreated, spontaneous remissions may occur [33, 64]. This makes the objective assessment of therapy difficult.

Many clinical studies reviewed by Poster et al. [104] reported a response rate to chemotherapy of 10%–15%. Whereas the results with antimetabolites and alkylating agents were disappointing, vinblastine, with a response rate of up to 25%, seemed to be the most effective substance [49, 11, 82]. At the same time, a close correlation between dosage and tumor mass reduction was observed. Most useful appeared to be relatively high single weekly doses of 0.2–0.3 mg/kg [11, 63].

The prematurely optimistic reports on the use of CCNU [49] have, partly because of the considerable side effects, subsequently proved to be disappointing [120, 21]. Tumor remission rates of up to 13% have been reported for iphosphamide [68]. The results with methyl-GAG were similarly disappointing [65].

Polychemotherapy regimens have not proved to be superior to monotherapy [11, 33, 49], but those containing vinblastine seem to be more effective [64].

There have been many attempts to improve this disappointing situation. Worth mentioning in this context are the in vitro assays already developed for pretherapeutic testing of cytotoxics [72, 46, 25]. Here, the major advantage is the prediction of ineffective substances, thus excluding unnecessary toxic treatment. More recently, it has been possible to show with experiments using nude mice that vinblastine is dose-dependently more effective in tumors with a high proliferation rate and rapid growth [94].

Because of the particular tumor biology of slow-growing tumors, GARNICK [36] developed a model for the continuous infusion of cytotoxics using an implanted pump, thus hopefully leading to more effective and perhaps less toxic therapy. Finally, the increased effectiveness of the combination of chemo-, hormone-, and immunotherapy [62, 56, 82] gives rise to the hope of future advancements in the treatment of hypernephroma with drugs.

4 Hormone Therapy

Hormonal treatment of hypernephroma is based on results of animal experiments suggesting that tumor growth may be influenced by female as well as by male sex hormones [9, 127, 10].

It could be shown with male Syrian gold hamsters that renal carcinomas could be induced with high estrogen treatments and this induction could be inhibited with progesterone or testosterone [8].

The gestagens medroxyprogesterone acetate (MPA) and hydroxyprogesterone caproate, testosterone in the form of testosterone cyclopentyl propionate, and the anti-estrogens tamoxifen and naphoxidin were used [103, 100]. Clinical experience has been obtained mostly with MPA. POSSINGER et al. [103] showed in a review of the literature, that rates of remission claimed to be from 7% to 33% in studies between 1967 and 1973 could not be accepted. Critical analysis of these earlier studies suggested a more probable remission rate of 6% [131, 103, 99].

Experimental work from PEARSON et al. [100], PIZZOCARO et al. [101], and WEISSMÜLLER et al. [153] found that only 8%–24% of all hypernephromas demonstrated progesterone receptors. PIZZOCARO et al. [101] found in accordance with MCDONALD et al. [82], a higher proportion of progesterone and estrogen receptors in healthy kidney tissue than in the tumor itself. There does not seem to be a connection between the degree of differentiation and the receptor density [150, 87]. Thus, at present, the morphology gives no indication of the susceptibility of the tumor to hormone therapy.

Data showing the influence of hormonal treatment on total recurrence, rate of metastasis and survival are somewhat different and based on studies of very few patients: In the preliminary results of a prospective randomized trial published by PIZZOCARO et al. [101], the group which had been treated with MPA had a local recurrence rate of 13% compared to the untreated group with 28%. No connection was found between receptor status and recurrence rate. This study contained 83 patients and, because of the disappointing results, was prematurely terminated.

SATOMI et al. [129] compared a group of 35 patients with no evidence of distant disease, who were treated postoperatively with adjuvant MPA at a dose of 40–100 mg over 8 weeks, to an untreated group of 45 patients, similarly free of distant disease. After 3 years the metastases rate of the hormone-treated group was 25% less than the control group, but the 5-year-survival rate showed no significant difference between them. However, NAKANO et al. [87] obtained more favorable results using hormone therapy with 17 patients in an advanced stage of the disease. The group with positive receptor status showed a significantly longer survival than the group with negative receptor status. Both these groups of patients received 100 mg MPA daily, but, disappointingly, none of the patients so treated demonstrated a partial or complete tumor regression.

Ten patients with distant metastases observed by PEARSON et al. [100] received different forms of hormone therapy. None of these patients showed an objective response to the hormone treatment.

Despite the difficulty of assessing these low remission rates, the most effective dosage used in MPA treatment is suggested to be 160 mg daily [64, 104]. The poor response to hormone therapy is partly attributed to the low level of receptor concentration in hypernephroma. It is lower than that in cases of breast cancer, and also lower than that of experimentally estrogen-induced renal cell adenocarcinomas of male Syrian gold hamsters [100].

A radiosensitizing effect of MPA in laboratory experiments on endometrial carcinoma with positive progesterone receptor status could be demonstrated [51]. This effect has been attributed to an MPA-induced prolongation of the radiosensitive G_2 phase of the cell cycle. These findings may open new perspectives for combined therapy treatment with radiation and hormones, and will surely stimulate further experimental work in this direction.

Serious side effects due to hormone therapy are rare. Isolated cases of liver damage, drug-induced fever, and secondary amenorrhea have been described [129]. Before final judgement of the effectiveness of hormone therapy, it is necessary that further results from comparable studies, with particular reference to receptor status and long-term survival data, should be available.

Immunological treatment, another possible nonoperative treatment, is discussed elsewhere.

References

1. Abbatucci J-S, Quint R, Bloquel J, Roussel A, Urbajtel M (1976) Techniken der kurativen Telekobalttherapie. Enke Stuttgart
2. Andersson L, Edsmyr F (1982) Pre- and postoperative radiotherapy, influence on prognosis. Prog Clin Biol Res 100:609
3. Andreew A, Ranft R, Templin R (1971) Auswertung von 75 Patienten mit einem hypernephroiden Nierenkarzinom. Zentralbl Chir 43:1487
4. Arner O, Blanck C, von Schreeb T (1965) Renal adenocarcinoma: morphology – grading of malignancy – prognosis. Acta Chir Scand 346 (Suppl):1
5. Baisch H (1984) Flußzytometrische Untersuchungen des DNA-Gehaltes und der Proliferationskinetik menschlicher Tumoren. Strahlentherapie 160:431
6. Bennington JL, Kradjian RM (1967) Renal carcinoma. Saunders, Philadelphia
7. Bischoff W, Sommerkamp H (1977) Zur Problematik der operativen Therapie maligner Nierentumoren. Schweiz Med Wochenschr 107:699
8. Bloom HJG, Baker WH, Duke CE, Mitchley BC (1963) Hormone dependent tumors of the kidney. II. Effect of endocrine ablation procedure on the transplanted estrogen-induced renal tumors of the Syrian hamster. Br J Cancer 17:646
9. Bloom HJG, Roe F, Mitchley B (1967) Sex hormones and renal neoplasia. Inhibition of tumor of hamster-kidney by an estrogen antagonist. An agent of possible therapeutic value in man. Cancer 20:2118
10. Bloom HJG, Wallace DM (1971) Tumors of the urinary tract. In: Zuppinger A, Krokowski E (eds) Handbuch der medizinischen Radiologie. Spezielle Strahlentherapie maligner Tumoren, vol 19, part 3. Springer, Berlin Heidelberg New York, p. 399
11. Bodey CP (1979) Current status of chemotherapy in metastatic renal carcinoma. In: Johnson DE, Samuels MC (eds) Cancer of the genitourinary tract. Raven, New York
12. Boeminghaus F, Greipel V, Schwartmann KP (1982) Analyse der Langzeitergebnisse nach Nephrektomie wegen Hypernephrom anhand von 442 Fällen. Urologe A 21:201
13. Bostel F, Kuhne-Velte HJ, Wöllgens P (1983) Wertigkeit der Strahlentherapie bei Metastasen des hypernephroiden Karzinoms. Strahlentherapie 159:404
14. Bostel F, Kuhne-Velte HJ, Wöllgens P (1984) 12 Jahre Überlebenszeit eines Patienten mit metastasiertem Hypernephrom unter palliativer Schmerztherapie. Akt Urol 15:88
15. Boxer RJ, Waisman J, Lieber MM, Mampaso FM, Skinner DG (1979) Renal carcinoma: computer analysis of 96 patients treated by nephrectomy. J Urol 122:598
16. Bratherton DG (1964) Tumours of the kidneys and suprarenals. III. The place of radiotherapy in the treatment of hypernephroma. Br J Radiol 37:141
17. Brosig W, Baumgärtel H, Oeser H (1971) Die präoperative Bestrahlung der Nierentumoren aus chirurgisch-urologischer Sicht. In: Hug O (ed) Präoperative Tumorbestrahlung. Vorträge vom Deutschen Röntgenkongreß 1970. Sonderbände zur Strahlentherapie, vol 71. Urban and Schwarzenberg, München, p 84
18. Brühl P, Scheef W, Albert H, Bücheler E (1975) Therapie und Prognose des hypernephroiden Nierenkarzinoms. Med Klin 70:873
19. Brühl P, Vahlensieck W, Höfer-Janker H, Scheef W, Thelen M (1976) Das hypernephroide Nierenkarzinom. Aktuel Nephrol 1:97
20. Buschke F, Parker RG (1972) Radiation therapy in cancer management. Grune and Stratton, New York
21. Callahan SK, Knight WA, Murphy A (1981) A phase II trial of methyl-glyoxal bisguanylhydrazone (MGBG, methyl GAG) in renal carcinoma. Proc Am Assoc Cancer Res Am Soc Clin Oncol, (Abstract 649) 22:164
22. Carl P, Rabes H, Eisenberger F, Schmidt P (1974) Autoradiographische Untersuchungen zur DNS-Synthese bestrahlter und nichtbestrahlter Nierenkarzinome bei normothermer Perfusion. Verh Dtsch Ges Urol, 26. Tagung. Springer, Berlin Heidelberg New York, p 176
23. Cavanaugh PJ (1967) Adjunctive radiotherapy in renal carcinoma of adults. In: King JS (ed) Renal neoplasia. Little and Brown, Boston, p 559
24. Cinqualbre J, Goldschmidt P, Bollack C (1982) Le can-

cer du rein. A propos d'une serie de 230 cas. Sem Hop Paris 58:812
25. Day JW, Shrivastav S, Lin G, Bonar RA, Paulson DF (1981) In vitro chemotherapeutic testing of urologic tumors. J Urol 125:490
26. Egger B, Hartung R, Pollak E (1979) Staging und therapeutische Ergebnisse bei 288 hypernephroiden Nierenkarzinomen. Med Welt 30:920
27. Finney R (1973) The value of radiotherapy in the treatment of hypernephroma – a clinical trial. Br J Urol 45:258
28. Finney R (1973) An evaluation of postoperative radiotherapy in hypernephroma treatment – a clinical trial. Cancer 32:1332
29. Firusian N (1978) Endoossale Isotopentherapie maligner Skeletterkrankungen. Z Krebsforsch 91:143
30. Flamm J, Wöber L (1981) Der maligne Nierentumor. Wien Med Wochenschr 23/24:579
31. Flocks RH, Kadesky MC (1958) Malignant neoplasms of the kidney: an analysis of 353 patients followed five years or more. J Urol 79:196
32. Fossa SD, Kjolseth I, Lund G (1982) Radiotherapy of metastases from renal cancer. Eur Urol 8:340
33. Freed SZ, Halperin JP, Gordon M (1977) Idiopathic regression of metastases from renal cell carcinoma. J Urol 118:538
34. Fuhrmann SA, Lasky LL, Limas L (1982) Prognostic significance of morphologic parameters in renal cell carcinoma. Am J Surg Pathol 6 (7):655
35. Fuselier HA, Guice SL, Brannan W, Ochsner MG, Sangisetty KV, Beckman EN, Barnes CA (1983) Renal cell carcinoma: the Ochsner Medical Institution experience (1945-1978). J Urol 130:445
36. Garnick MB (1981) Advanced renal cell cancer (nephrology forum). Kidney Int 20:127
37. Gauwerky F, Adam K (1971) Die Rolle der Radiotherapie bei der Behandlung der malignen Nierentumoren Erwachsener. Strahlentherapie 142:629
38. Gauwerky F (1973) Strahlenhandlung von Nierentumoren Erwachsener. Dtsch Aerztebl 70:275
39. Giuliani L, Martorana G, Giberti C, Pescatore D, Magnani G (1983) Results of radical nephrectomy with extensive lymphadenectomy for renal cell carcinoma. J Urol 129:664
40. Grawitz PA (1883) Die sogenannten Lipome der Niere. Arch Pathol Anat 93:39
41. Halperin EC, Harisiadis L (1983) The role of radiation therapy in the management of metastatic renal cell carcinoma. Cancer 51:614
42. Hermanek P, Sigel A, Chlepas S (1976) Histological grading of renal cell carcinoma. Eur Urol 2:189
43. Herrlinger A, Sigel A, Schrott KM (1982) Die Bedeutung der lymphogenen Metastasierung des Nierencarcinoms für das Vorgehen bei der radikalen Tumornephrektomie. Verh Dtsch Ges Urol 34. Tagung. Springer, Berlin Heidelberg New York, p 104
44. Herrlinger A, Sigel A, Giedl J (1984) Methodik der radikalen transabdominalen Tumornephrektomie mit fakultativer oder systematischer Lymphdissektion und deren Ergebnisse an 381 Patienten. Urologe A 23: 267
45. Higer HP (1981) Risikofaktoren für Folgeerkrankungen der Hypernephromtherapie. Strahlentherapie 157:633
46. von Hoff DD, Casper J, Bradley E, Sandbach J, Makuch R (1981) Association between human tumor colony-forming assay results and response in individual patient's tumor to chemotherapy. Am J Med 70:1027
47. Hohenberg G (1983) Postoperative Radiotherapie beim hypernephroiden Karzinom – Auswertung von 63 Fällen. Urologe B 23:323
48. Hop WCJ, van der Werf-Messing BHP (1980) Prognostic indexes for renal cell carcinoma. Eur J Cancer 16:833
49. Hrushesky WJ, Murphy GP (1974) Evaluation of chemotherapeutic agents in a new murine carcinoma model. J Natl Cancer Inst 52:1117
50. Hrushesky WJ, Murphy GP (1977) Current status of the therapy of advanced renal carcinoma. J Surg Oncol 9:277
51. Huber H, Husslein P, Michalica W, Wagenbichler P (1984) Radiosensitizing effect of medroxyprogesterone acetate on endometrial cancer cells in vitro. Cancer 54:999
52. Hudgins PT, Collins VP (1966) Radiotherapy for renal adenocarcinoma. Am J Roentgenol 96:620
53. Hübener K-H, Eibach E (1977) Strahlentherapie des Nierenkarzinoms – Untersuchungen und Ergebnisse. Strahlentherapie 153:726
54. Hübener K-H, Junker A (1979) Vergleichende Bestrahlungsplanung mit konventioneller röntgendiagnostischer und computertomographischer Technik bei Nieren- und Harnblasenkarzinomen. Strahlentherapie 155:376
55. Hug O (1971) Strahlenbiologische Begründung, Methoden und Aussichten einer präoperativen Tumorbestrahlung. Zusammenfassung und Schlußwort. In: Hug O (ed) Präoperative Tumorbestrahlung. Vorträge vom Deutschen Röntgenkongreß 1970. Sonderbaende zur Strahlentherapie, vol 71. Urban and Schwarzenberg, München, p 115
56. Ishmael DR, Burpo LJ, Bottomley RH (1978) Combined therapy of advanced hypernephroma with medroxy-progesterone, BCG, adriamycin and vincristine. Abstract Proc Amer Soc Clin Oncol 19:407
57. Javadpour N (1984) Surgical management of renal cancer. In: Javadpour N (ed) Cancer of the kidney. Thieme-Stratton, New York, p 69
58. Jones GW (1982) Renal cell carcinoma. CA 32:280
59. Juusela H, Malmio K, Alfthan O, Oravisto KJ (1977) Preoperative irradiation in the treatment of renal adenocarcinoma. Scand J Urol Nephrol 11:277
60. Juusela H (1978) Renal adenocarcinoma: clinical features and factors correlating to survival in 173 patients. Ann Chir Gynaecol Fenniae 67 suppl 193:1
61. Kantor AF (1977) Current concepts in the epidemiology and etiology of primary renal cell carcinoma. J Urol 117:415
62. Katakkar SB, Franks CR (1978) Chemo-hormonal therapy for metastatic renal cell carcinoma with adriamycin, hydroxyurea, vinblastine and medroxy-progesterone acetate. Cancer Treat Rep 62:1379
63. de Kernion JB, Berry D (1980) The diagnosis and treatment of renal cell carcinoma. Cancer 45:1947
64. de Kernion JB (1983) Treatment of advanced renal cell carcinoma – traditional methods and innovative approaches. J Urol 130:2
65. Knight WA, Livingston RB, Fabian C, Costanzi J (1979) Methyl-gloxal bis-guanylhydrazone (methyl GAG, MGBG) in advanced human malignancy. Proc Amer Ass Cancer Res Amer Soc Clin Oncol (Abstract C-115) 20:319

66. Kob D, Arndt J, Klötzer K-H, Stecher M, Kriester A (1974) Ergebnisse der Therapie von bösartigen Nierentumoren mit der ultraharten Bremsstrahlung eines 30-MeV-Betatron. Radiobiol Radiother (Berl) 15: 669
67. Kob D, Klötzer K-H, Arndt J, Stadie G (1980) Klinische Untersuchungen zum Problem der Vor- und Nachbestrahlung maligner Nierentumoren. Radiobiol Radiother (Berl) 21:729
68. König HJ, Hartwich G (1980) Zytostatische Therapie des hypernephroiden Nierenkarzinoms. Dtsch Med Wochenschr 105:1810
69. Kurth KH, van der Werf-Messing B, Maksimovic PA (1983) Nierenkarzinom: Lokale Radiotherapie von Metastasen in der Wirbelsäule. Verh Dtsch Ges Urol 34. Tagung. Springer, Berlin Heidelberg New York, p 64
70. Lack EE, Cassady JR, Sallan SE (1985) Renal cell carcinoma in childhood and adolescence: a clinical and pathological study of 17 cases. J Urol 133:822
71. Lieber MM, Tomera FM, Taylor WF, Farrow GM (1981) Renal adenocarcinoma in young adults: survival and variables affecting prognosis. J Urol 125:164
72. Lieber MM, Kovach JS (1981) Soft agar clonogenic assay for primary human renal cell carcinoma: in vitro chemotherapeutic drug-sensitivity testing. Invest Urol 19:111
73. von Lieven H, Lissner J (1977) Strahlentherapie beim Adenokarzinom der Niere. Strahlentherapie 153:245
74. von Lieven H, Trott K-R, Sintermann R (1978) Experimentelle Ergebnisse der präoperativen Bestrahlung des renalen Adenokarzinoms. Strahlentherapie 154:299
75. von Lieven H, Meister P, Keiditsch E (1978) Die Bedeutung des Differenzierungsgrades beim Adenokarcinom der Niere. MMW 120:729
76. Lindner H (1981) Bestrahlungsplanung beim Nierenkarzinom. In: Schmiedt E, Bauer H-W (ed) Diagnostik und Therapie des Nierenkarzinoms. Zuckschwerdt, München, p 166
77. Lissner J (1974) Strahlentherapie bei Nierentumoren. Verh Dtsch Ges Urol 26. Tagung. Springer, Berlin Heidelberg New York, p 150
78. Ljungberg B, Stenling R, Roos G (1985) DNA content in renal cell carcinoma with reference to tumor heterogeneity. Cancer 56:503
79. Maentylae M, Nordman E, Minkkinen J (1977) Postoperative radiotherapy of renal adenocarcinoma. Ann Clin Res 9:252
80. Mau S, Rießbeck K-H, Mandel L, Coblenz R (1980) Ergebnisse der Kombinationstherapie maligner Nierentumoren. Radiobiol Radiother (Berl) 21:271
81. McDonald MW (1982) Current therapy for renal cell carcinoma. J Urol 127:211
82. McDonald MW, Diokno AC, Seski JC, Menon KM (1983) Measurement of progesterone receptor in human renal cell carcinoma and normal renal tissue. J Surg Oncol 22:164
83. McNichols DW, Segura JW, DeWeerd JH (1981) Renal cell carcinoma: long-term survival and late recurrence. J Urol 126:17
84. Meister P (1981) Nierenkarzinom: Pathologische Anatomie. In: Schmiedt E, Bauer H-W (ed) Diagnostik und Therapie des Nierenkarzinoms. Zuckschwerdt, Muenchen, p 1
85. Murphy GP, Schirmer HK (1963) The diagnosis and treatment of hypernephroma. Geriatrics 18:354
86. Murphy GP, Mostofi FK (1965) The significance of cytoplasmic granularity in the prognosis of renal cell carcinoma. J Urol 94:48
87. Nakano E, Tada Y, Fujioka H, Matsuda M, Osafune M, Kotake T, Sato B, Takaha M, Sonoda T (1984) Hormone receptor in renal cell carcinoma and correlation with clinical response to endocrine therapy. J Urol 132:240
88. Nickolisen R, Fallon B (1985) Locally recurrent hypernephroma treated by radiation therapy and embolisation. A report of two cases. Cancer 56:1049
89. Noecker D, Hobrecker M (1976) Therapieplanung und Prognosebeurteilung bei bösartigen Nierengeschwuelsten. Strahlentherapie 152:498
90. Nurmi MJ (1984) Prognostic factors in renal carcinoma. An evaluation of operative findings. Br J Urol 56:270
91. Ochsner MG, Brannan W, Pond HS, Goodier EH (1973) Renal cell carcinoma: review of 26 years of experience at the Ochsner Clinic. J Urol 110:643
92. Olver IN, Leavitt RD (1984) Chemotherapy and immunotherapy of disseminated renal cancer. In: Javadpour N (ed) Cancer of the kidney. Thieme-Stratton, New York
93. Otto U, Baisch H, Huland H, Klöppel G (1984) Tumor cell deoxyribonucleic acid content and prognosis in human renal cell carcinoma. J Urol 132:237
94. Otto U, Huland H, Baisch H, Kloeppel G (1984) Transplantation of human renal cell carcinoma into NMRI NU NU mice. II. Evaluation of response to vinblastine sulfate monotherapy. J Urol 131:134
95. Paces V, Poleckova V, Zamecnik J (1978) Preoperative irradiation of renal cell carcinoma in adults (controlled clinical trial). Int Urol Nephrol 10 (2):77
96. Palma LD, Kenney GM, Murphy GP (1970) Childhood renal carcinoma. Cancer 26:1321
97. Parienty RA, Richard F, Pradel J, Vallancien G (1984) Local recurrence after nephrectomy for primary renal cancer: computerized tomography recognition. J Urol 132:246
98. Patel NP, Lavengood RW (1978) Renal cell carcinoma: natural history and results of treatment. J Urol 119:722
99. Paulson DF, Perez CA, Anderson T (1985) Cancer of the kidney and the ureter. In: DeVita VT Jr, Hellman S, Rosenberg SA (eds) Cancer, principles and practice of oncology. Lippincott, Philadelphia, p 732
100. Pearson J, Friedmann MA, Hoffman PG (1981) Hormone receptors in renal cell carcinoma. Their utility as predictors of response to endocrine therapy. Cancer Chemother Pharmacol 6:151
101. Pizzocaro G, DiFronzo G, Piva L, Salvioni R, Ronchi E, Cappelleti V, Giongo A, Mastroberadino E, Cozzoli C, Dormia E, Minervini S, Zanollo A, Fontanella U, Giannoni R, Maggioni A, Lasio E (1983) Adjunctive medroxyprogesterone acetate to radical nephrectomy in category MO renal cell carcinoma. Eur Urol 9:202
102. Pontes JE (1983) Adjunctive treatment of renal cell carcinoma. Int Adv Surg Oncol 6:309
103. Possinger K, Hartenstein R, Ehrhart H (1981) Chemotherapie des Adenokarzinoms der Niere. In: Schmiedt E, Bauer H-W (eds) Diagnostik und Therapie des Nierenkarzinoms. Zuckschwerdt, Muenchen, p 183
104. Poster DS, Bruno S, Penta J, Pirna K, Vilk P, Macdonald J (1982) Current status of chemotherapy, hormonal therapy and immunotherapy in the treatment of renal cell carcinoma. Am J Clin Oncol 5:53

105. Prignitz J, Popp FA, Scholz H (1973) Zur Optimierung der Bestrahlungsplanung in der 60-Co-Tiefentherapie. Überlegungen zur Einstelltechnik bei Nierenmalignomen. Strahlentherapie 145:378
106. Rabes HM, Carl P, Meister P, Rattenhuber KU (1979) Analysis of proliferative compartments in human tumors. Cancer 44:799
107. Rabes HM (1981) Zellkinetik des Nierenkarzinoms. In: Schmiedt E, Bauer H-W (eds) Diagnostik und Therapie des Nierenkarzinoms. Zuckschwerdt, München, p 15
108. Rafla S (1970) Renal cell carcinoma. Natural history and results of treatment. Cancer 25:26
109. Rafla S, Parikh K (1984) The role of adjuvant radiotherapy in management of renal cell carcinoma. In: Javadpour N (ed) Cancer of the kidney. Thieme-Stratton, New York
110. Rahn H, Keiner P, Pinsler G (1982) Bestrahlungstechniken zur postoperativen Bestrahlung des Nierenkarzinoms. Radiobiol Radiother (Berl) 23:551
111. Rhomberg W (1983) Zur Klinik und Strahlensensibilitaet von Knochenmetastasen bei Nierenkarzinomen. Strahlentherapie 159:610
112. Riches EW (1966) The place of radiotherapy in the management of parenchymal carcinoma of the kidney. J Urol 95:313
113. Riches EW (1968) Cancer of the urogenital tract: kidney. Localized renal adenocarcinoma. The place of irradiation. JAMA 204:230
114. Riches EW (1970) Preoperative irradiation of carcinoma of the kidney. In: Riches EW (ed) Modern trends in urology, vol 3. Butterworths, London, p 216
115. Richter E, Bohndorf W (1979) Behandlungsergebnisse bei hypernephroiden Karzinomen unter besonderer Berücksichtigung des Metastasenproblems. Strahlentherapie 155:607
116. Ringleb D, Rommel K (1963) Zur radiologischen Klinik der Nierengeschwuelste Erwachsener. Strahlentherapie 121:323
117. Ritchie AW, Kemp IW, Chisholm GD (1984) Is the incidence of renal carcinoma increasing? Br J Urol 56:571
118. Robson CJ, Churchill BM, Anderson W (1969) The results of radical nephrectomy for renal cell carcinoma. J Urol 101:297
119. Robson CJ (1982) Results of radical thoraco-abdominal nephrectomy in the treatment of renal cell carcinoma. Prog Clin Biol Res 100:481
120. Rodriguez LH, Johnson DE (1978) Clinical trial of cisplatinum (NSC 119875) in metastatic renal cell carcinoma. Urology 11:344
121. Röder K, Theuring F (1981) Strahlenbiologische Aspekte und morphologische Befunde nach Nierenvorbestrahlung. Radiobiol Radiother (Berl) 22:609
122. Rohloff R, von Lieven H (1981) Die Rolle der Strahlentherapie bei der Behandlung des Adenokarzinoms der Niere. In: Schmiedt E, Bauer HW (ed) Diagnostik und Therapie des Nierenkarzinoms. Zuckschwerdt, München
123. Rost A, Brosig W, Ernst H (1976) Die präoperative Bestrahlung beim hypernephroiden Karzinom. Helv Chir Acta 43:309
124. Rübe W, Seegelken K (1974) Dickdarmstenosen nach Bestrahlung von Nierentumoren. Strahlentherapie 147:63
125. Saitoh H, Hida M, Nakamura K, Shimbo T, Shiramizu T, Satoh T (1982) Metastatic processes and a potential indication of treatment for metastatic lesions of renal adenocarcinoma. J Urol 128:916
126. Saksela E, Alfthan O, Malmio K (1973) Effect of preoperative radiotherapy on the growth of human renal carcinoma tissue in vitro. Scand J Urol Nephrol 7:181
127. Samuels ML, Sullivan P, Howe CD (1968) Medroxyprogesterone acetate in treatment of renal cell carcinoma (hypernephroma). Cancer 22:525
128. Sarre H, Moser F (1961) Bestrahlungsfibrose, Bestrahlungsnephritis und isolierte Hypertonie nach Röntgenbestrahlung der Niere. Dtsch Med J 12:232
129. Satomi Y, Takai S, Kondo J, Fukushima S, Furuhata A (1982) Postoperative prophylactic use of progesterone in renal cell carcinoma. J Urol 128:919
130. Scherer E (1980) Strahlentherapie, 2nd edn. Springer, Berlin Heidelberg New York
131. Schmidt CG (1976) Metastasierendes hypernephroides Nierenkarzinom. Dtsch Med Wochenschr 101:347
132. Selli C, Hinshaw WM, Woodart BH, Paulson DF (1983) Stratification of risk factors in renal cell carcinoma. Cancer 52:899
133. Sigel A, Chlepas S, Hermanek P, Herrlinger A (1981) Stagnation in der Therapie der Nierentumoren – Chancen einer Besserung. In: Schmiedt E, Bauer HW (eds) Diagnostik und Therapie des Nierenkarzinoms. Zuckschwerdt, München, p 109
134. Skinner DG, Colvin RB, Vermillion CD, Pfister RC, Leadbetter WF (1971) The diagnosis and management of renal cell carcinoma. A clinical and pathologic study of 309 cases. Cancer 28:1165
135. Skinner DG, Vermillion CD, Colvin RB (1972) The surgical management of renal cell carcinoma. J Urol 107:705
136. Smith RB, DeKernion JB, Ehrlich RM, Skinner DG, Kaufmann II (1984) Bilateral renal cell carcinoma and renal cell carcinoma in the solitary kidney. J Urol 132:450
137. Sparwasser C, Bach D, Sparwasser H, Altwein JE (1984) Das bilaterale Hypernephrom. Kritische Übersicht und eigenes Therapiekonzept. Akt Urol 15:312
138. Standke E, Ölßner W, Melzer R (1984) CT-gestützte Bestrahlungsplanung der Nierentumoren. Radiobiol Radiother (Berl) 25:361
139. Steinberg SM, Brodovsky HS, Goepp CE (1972) Renal carcinoma in mother and daughter. Cancer 29:222
140. Stender HS, Berndt G (1968) Strahlenbehandlung von Tumoren der Nieren und des Nierenbeckens. Röntgenblätter 21:69
141. Strietzel M, Ziegler P-G, Hamann D, Kittner KH, Hildebrandt K-H, Bast R (1984) Beitrag zur Strahlenbehandlung maligner Nierentumoren. Radiobiol Radiother (Berl) 25:383
142. Väth JM (1973) Cancer of the kidney – radiation therapy and its indications in non-Wilms' tumors. Cancer 23:1053
143. Vergau W, Buerkle G, Herzer R, Sadowski P (1972) Dünndarmschädigung der Telekobalt-Pendelbestrahlung der Nierenregion. Strahlentherapie 144:697
144. Vermillion CD, Skinner DG, Pfister RC (1972) Bilateral renal cell carcinoma. J Urol 108:219
145. Voss AC, Wöllgens P, Klöckner D (1974) Das hypernephroide Karzinom. Methodik und Ergebnisse der postoperativen Radiotherapie bei 223 Patienten. Strahlentherapie 147:447
146. Wagle DG, Moore RH, Murphy GP (1975) Secondary carcinomas of the kidney. J Urol 114:30–32

147. Wagle DG, Scal DR (1970) Renal cell carcinoma – a review of 256 cases. J Surg Oncol 2:23–32
148. Waters CA, Lewis LG, Frontz WA (1934) Radiation therapy of renal cortical neoplasms, with special reference to preoperative irradiation. South Med J 27:290
149. Waters WB, Richie IP (1979) Aggressive surgical approach to renal cell carcinoma. Review of 130 cases. J Urol 122:306
150. Wehbe S (1978) Duodenalstenosen nach Bestrahlung der Nierenregion wegen Malignom. Fortschr Geb Roentgenstr 129:421
151. Weissmüller J, Herrlinger A, von Maillot K (1983) Wert der Rezeptor-Bestimmung und der Hormontherapie beim metastasierenden Hypernephrom. Verh Dtsch Ges Urol, 34. Tagung. Springer, Berlin Heidelberg New York
152. van der Werf-Messing B (1973) Carcinoma of the kidney. Cancer 32:1056
153. van der Werf-Messing B (1974) La place de la radiotherapie dans le traitement du cancer du rein et du cancer de la prostate chez l'adulte: Carcinome du rein. Un essai therapeutique. J Radiol Electrol 55:785

Prenatal Wilms' Tumor

H. Chr. Dominick and K.-D. Bachmann

1 Introduction

In the field of oncology, prenatal malignant tumors appear to be a rather unusual phenomenon. The first comprehensive publication describing these astonishing "inborn" tumors was written by Wells [50] who gathered 255 observations. Although this important paper touches a very interesting biologic problem, it has not yet received much interest. Influenced by our own six cases of newborns with neuroblastoma and three newborns with Wilms' tumors, Bachmann tried – utilizing the cases described in the literature – to crystallize the general trend of this disease by analyzing its course in individuals. The definition of prenatally developed tumors follows an earlier description [4]:

1. A *definitely prenatally* developed tumor is one that was diagnosed clinically and/or histologically in newborns, prematures, or fetuses up to the 14th day of life.
2. A *probably prenatally* developed tumor is one that was diagnosed after the 2nd week of life up to the 3rd month.
3. A *possibly prenatally* developed tumor is one that was diagnosed clinically between the 4th and 12th months life.

We do not know much about the incidence of tumors developing in the prenatal period. Reviewing death certificates (1960–1964) Fraumeni and Miller [18] found that within the first 28 days of life, 6.24 deaths due to inborn tumors were found in 1 million live births. Table 1 shows the incidence of the various tumors. Over 50% of these deaths occurred in the 1st week, and one-third within the 1st day of life.

Despite these facts the true incidence of inborn tumors will remain obscure as death may occur – depending on the growth rate of the individual tumor – in the intrauterine or newborn period. On the other hand a slow spread of the tumor may allow life until the infant period. There also are indications of the existence of so-called clinically silent tumors (neuroblastoma in situ) [6], and for spontaneous regression of tumors due to maturation or regression of the malignant cells (e.g., neuroblastoma). Finally, there may be ill-defined biologic and immunologic peculiarities influencing therapeutic success within the first 6 or even 12 months of life.

The pathogenesis of the prenatal tumor has not yet been satisfactorily elucidated. Various observations exist that suggest certain conclusions or start general discussions. It seems to be very rare for a mother carrying a tumor to transfer that malignancy to her fetus via the placenta. Seven carcinomas, nine melanoblastomas, and two sarcomas were described by Hermann et al. [24]. There were two newborns with the same disease as their mothers, namely, Hodgkin's disease [28]. Interestingly enough, placental choriocarcinoma which originates from the trophoblast and, hence, is a tumor of the fetus, usually spreads to the mother, but in rare cases may involve the fetus, as has been occasionally described (53, 32).

Anders et al. [2] feel that the transfer of neuroblastoma cells from the fetus to the mother did not cause any problems. In one case numerous tumor emboli and fetomaternal erythrocyte

Table 1. Incidence of various tumors found within the first 28 days of life [18]

Leukemia	2.10
Neuroblastoma	1.30
Brain tumor	0.34
Wilms' tumor	0.43
Primary liver carcinoma	0.48
Teratoma	0.43
Sarcoma	0.58
Miscellaneous	0.58
Total per 10^6 live births	6.24

transfusion were found in the villi and vessels of the placenta. This newborn died on the 17th day of life from a neuroblastoma of the right adrenal gland. The mother remained clinically and biochemically normal when followed up for 1 year. STRAUSS and DRISCOLL [47] reported two newborns in whom tumor cells were found in almost all villi of the large placentas. Both mothers remained clinically neuroblastoma-free. There are no reports of spread of neuroblastoma cells into the maternal circulation (intervillous space of placenta) or evidence of metastases in the mother [45]. Prenatal tumor induction during pregnancy by stilbestrol, which after an interval of 14–22 years may lead to the development of vaginal adenocarcinoma in female offspring [23] is a classic example of carcinogenesis due to diaplacental transfer of chemical substances from the mother to the unborn child. Alcohol has also been incriminated to induce tumors prenatally; a few children with fetal alcohol syndrome developed embryonal tumors, e.g., nephroblastoma, neuroblastoma, and hepatoblastoma [29].

In patients with Down-, Fanconi-, Bloom-, Wiskott-Aldrich-, or Louis-Bar-syndrome and with inborn immunopathies, a disposition towards leukemia and non-Hodgkin's lymphoma leads to the conclusion that constitutional factors play a role in the development of malignancies. Whereas siblings and dizygotic twins of patients with leukemia have only a slightly greater risk than normal of developing leukemia, in monozygotic twins this risk is as high as 25% and is often found within a few weeks or months in the second twin after the diagnosis was made in the first twin. The concordance rates for leukemia diminish in identical twins from 100%, when the first twin is affected under 1 year of age, to no increase above that for siblings in general when the first twin is affected after age 6 [37]. A rare familiar disposition should be mentioned, in which a similar type (retinoblastoma) or localization of tumor is found in different generations of various family members.

Finally, the coincidence between hemihypertrophy and aniridia in patients with Wilms' tumor, and between neurofibromatosis (von Recklinghausen) and pheochromocytoma may give a possible explanation for the interrelationship between congenital abnormalities and tumor development. This is also based on animal experiments in which the same toxic substance that leads to congenital abnormalities in the 10th–18th week of pregnancy leads to the development of carcinoma at a later date of gestation [38].

2 Development of Prenatal Wilms' Tumor

The incidence of Wilms' tumor is approximately 5%–10% of all malignancies in children: 50% are diagnosed before the 3rd year of life and 80% by the 5th year. Although among 181 patients with neuroblastoma 20 were newborns and infants of the age group 0–90 days (11%), only 5 newborns (2.9%) were found among 168 patients with Wilms' tumor [21]. In our material, we have three newborns with a definitely prenatally developed Wilms' tumor.

Pathologico-anatomically, Wilms' tumor develops like normal kidney tissue from the metanephros as well as the ureteral bud. It is proposed that the malignant transformation of the tissue is induced by a substance resulting from ureteral budding [14]. Nodular renal blastema occurs in clusters in the renal cortex and deep within the renal substance. It has been associated with, and has progressed into, bilateral nephroblastomatosis. In addition these blastemic cells have been identified in kidneys also containing a Wilms' tumor, suggesting that it may be a precursor lesion of the tumor [5]. There are more than 20 cases of extrarenal Wilms' tumors [1, 35].

The macroscopic extension of the tumor as described in the staging of the National Wilms' Tumor Study Group is important for the prognosis of the tumor and is now used by most authors [3, 10, 11, 15]. The histologic differentiation (grading) also may have prognostic significance, especially in Wilms' tumors in which epithelial elements dominate. They seem to metastasize less often than tumors with undifferentiated spindle cells (see Havers, this volume).

Genetic factors probably play a role in the etiology of Wilms' tumor. Analyzing 58 cases of familial Wilms' tumors [31], 21% of patients with bilateral Wilms' tumor were found, compared with 3%–11% with nonfamilial Wilms' tumor [10, 11]. Also, the age at the time of diagnosis in familial Wilms' tumor was 2 years compared with 3–4 years in the nonfamilial group. These observations are explained by the authors through a two-step mutational process, the first mutation occurring in the germ cell and the second one in the somatic cell. This may lead to the hereditary form of bilateral Wilms' tumor. Alternatively, when both mutations occur in a somatic cell, a nonhereditary tumor may develop at a later age, which will invariably be a tumor on one side. The tumor then occurs as an autosomal dominant trait with a penetrance of approximately 63%, which means that only 37% of the gene carriers do not develop a tumor [30, 31]. Another indication of a possible genetic determination of some Wilms' tumors may be the high coincidence of nephroblastoma and genetically determined photostimulated convulsions under EEG [16].

In one newborn with bilateral Wilms' tumor, a B–C chromosome translocation was demonstrated [19]. Another important observation was that of a mother with congenital hemihypertrophy. Her three children were found to have Wilms' tumors at the ages of $2^1/_2$, 6, and 5 years [34]. Finally, there is a report on a Wilms' tumor in a $2^{11}/_{12}$-year-old girl who developed an adrenal cortical carcinoma 4 years after radical operation and irradiation (3,000 rad) and 2 years after termination of cytostatic therapy (total of 16 mg actinomycin D) at the age of $7^1/_2$ years. Hemihypertrophy of the left half of the tongue and the left leg as well as capillary hemangiomas on the back of the head and the left forearm had existed since birth [36].

The incidence of Wilms' tumors in children with hemihypertrophy, Wiedemann-Beckwith syndrome, aniridia, anomalies of the urinary tract, and trisomy 18 has increased. Several patients with Wilms' tumor have been described who, in addition to aniridia, anomalies of the urinary tract, and mental retardation, had an interstitial deletion on chromosome 11 [40, 54]. Another coincidence with a fatal course is Wilms' tumor, interstitial nephritis, and pseudohermaphroditism [46].

3 Diagnosis

The clinical picture of the definitely congenital Wilms' tumor is often dominated by a "large abdomen" with a tumor on palpation. In five newborns this large intra-abdominal tumor caused difficulties during delivery, leading to an embryotomy in two children [25, 39]. The three other children were delivered vaginally [13, 26, 44]. Problems with feeding, vomiting, and abdominal pain are nonspecific symptoms due to the large intra-abdominal tumor. Hematuria may also be a symptom pointing to the urogenital tract. Our three cases of newborns with definitely prenatally developed Wilms' tumor demonstrate these general symptoms and the individual course of the disease very clearly.

3.1 Case 1

Patient U.S., born 21 January 1966, male, started suffering from constant vomiting at the age of 8 days. A large right-sided abdominal tumor was palpated and removed surgically. At the same time, a pylorus hypertrophy was treated by the Weber-Ramstedt method. At the age of 5 months, radiation treatment with 2,340 rad was initiated. Follow-up examination $7^9/_{12}$ years later showed a completely healthy boy without any signs of irradiation damage.

3.2 Case 2

Patient A.G., born 4 August 1965, female, was admitted to the hospital on the 2-nd day of life with a palpable left-sided abdominal tumor. X-rays, including thorax, abdomen, and gastrointestinal tract, and urogram led to the diagnosis of vitium cordis with general enlargement of the heart, shifting of the intestine to the right, and a cystic tumor of the kidney (Fig. 1). As the child became more and more cyanotic, the tumor was punctured twice, and 100 and 70 ml respectively of a brownish fluid were evacuated. No tumor cells were found in the fluid. On the 10th day of life, when the child was in a better general condition, surgery was performed. An adenosarcoma of the left kidney was found, with occlusion of the ureteropelvic junction by the tumor, which also filled out the hydronephrotic collecting system. Radiation treatment with 2,200 rad in three series was started on the 10th postoperative day. At the age of 7 years and 8 months, an invaginated piece of small

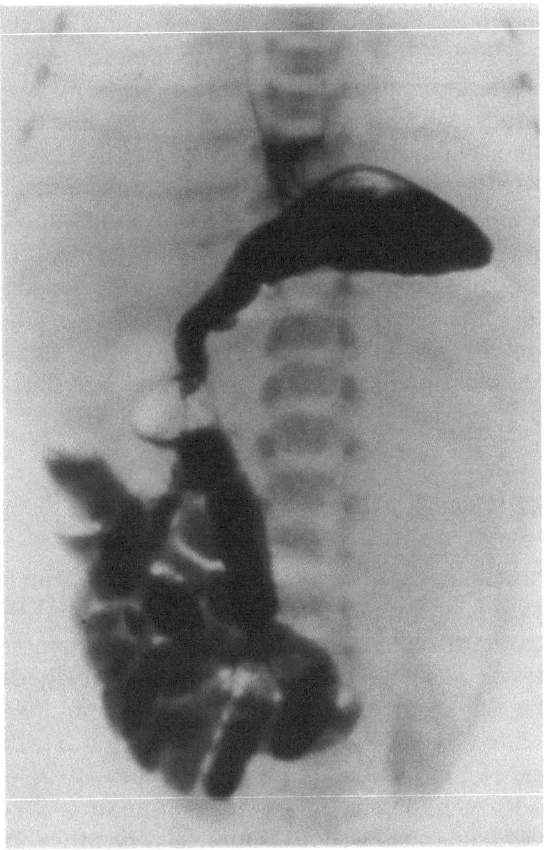

Fig. 1. Case 2. General view of abdomen and gastrointestinal passage in a newborn with left-sided Wilms' tumor. Displacement of the intestinal loop to the right with a suspected left-sided cystic renal tumor

bowel was resected. At 8 years old she appeared to be cured although she developed a slight scoliosis in the radiation field.

3.3 Case 3

Patient B.H., born 30 July 1957, had intermittent voiding difficulties since the 6th day of life. Edema of both legs and a large left-sided abdominal tumor were present. Surgery was performed at the age of 4 weeks; at that time the tumor appeared to be inoperable. Histologically, there was a spindle cell sarcoma of the left kidney arising from a Wilms' tumor. The child died on the 3rd postoperative day. There was no evidence of metastases.

The histologic slides were reviewed using rigid histologic guidelines. All three patients had true Wilms' tumors although the mesenchymal tissue was partly dominant.

4 Related Disorders

One group of prognostically very favorable congenital Wilms' tumors should be regarded separately. This includes the histologically separate group of benign renal tumors also called "congenital mesoblastic nephroma" [8] sometimes referred to as "fetal mesenchymal hamartoma" [51], or "leiomyomatous hamartoma" [7]. This benign tumor is the most common form of congenital renal neoplasia. In the past it was often misdiagnosed as "congenital Wilms' tumor", which explains the unusually good prognosis of this tumor in earlier publications [4]. Nephrectomy is the treatment of choice. If in rare cases the tumor behaves very aggressively (infiltration of the ureter, hypertension) and if new tumor growth appears [27], additional radio- and chemotherapy are indicated.

Another group of congenital and infantile congeners of Wilms' tumor are the well-differentiated epithelial nephroblastomas (two forms: monomorphic epithelial Wilms' tumor and cystic Wilms' tumor). These are also relatively benign.

A third important type of congenital renal disease has been recognized that is referred to as a nephroblastomatosis or nodular renal blastema. It is generally viewed as intermediate between malformation and true neoplasia. These nodules, often microscopic, has been found in 1 of 200–400 pediatric autopsies of patients under 4 months of age. After this age, they are generally no longer found at autopsy, suggesting that many of them regress [9].

5 Therapy and Complications

The new possibilities of differentiating, congenital and infantile congeners of Wilms' tumor lend themselves to a more individualized therapy. In most cases radical tumor nephrectomy can be expected. Occasionally, a very large tumor may be irradiated preoperatively to make surgery technically feasible. Radiation and cytostatic treatment, which are established modes of therapy in older children with Wilms' tumors [33, 20], should be discussed in each individual case. If any doubt exists whether the tumor has been removed radically, or in the case of extension of the tumor into neighbouring tissue, radiation and chemotherapy should be employed. The risk of therapy in definitely and probably prenatally developed Wilms' tumors is documented by the following observations. Five of thirteen newborns who were irradiated developed a more or less severe scoliosis of the spine [49, 51]. One infant died of radiation enteritis at 3 weeks of age [7]. Another four children developed sarcoma in the ribs and vertebrae of the irradiated fields [42]. Another five children developed fatal leukemia 4–16 years after successful Wilms' tumor therapy (two acute lymphatic, two acute myeloid, and one chronic myeloid leukemia) [43]. SABIO et al. [41] describe a case of an infant who was irradiated at 5 months of age with 2,100 rad because of Wilms' tumor. The boy developed from a colonic carcinoma when 12 years old. The possibility of growth retardation of the spine, maldevelopment of the blood vessels, and radiation nephritis [12, 17, 22, 48] should evoke a very restrictive indication for irradiation in newborns.

6 Prognosis

The prognosis of Wilms' tumor is definitely influenced by three factors:

1. The patient's age at the time of diagnosis
2. The spread and stage of the tumor ("staging")
3. The histologic differentiation of the tumor ("grading").

For definitely and probably prenatally developed Wilms' tumors, young age as well as the histologic differentiation may lead to a favorable prognosis. This should be taken into consideration when comparing the risk of treating newborns and young infants with radiologic and chemotherapeutic modalities, which in older children have proved successful but may lead to long-term side effects in the younger age group.

Acknowledgement

We would like to thank Prof. Dr. E. Grundmann, Director of the Institute of Pathology, University of Münster, for reviewing the slides.

References

1. Akhtar M, Kott E, Brooks B (1977) Extrarenal Wilms' tumor. Report of a case and review of the literature. Cancer 40:3087
2. Anders D, Frick R, Kindermann G (1970) Metastasierendes Neuroblastom des Feten mit Aussaat in die Placenta. Geburtshilfe Frauenheilkd 30:969
3. Bachmann K-D, Goldschmidt H (1974) Diagnose des Wilms-Tumors. Dtsch Med Wochenschr 99:358
4. Bachmann K-D, Kröll W (1968) Über das praenatal entstandene Neuroblastoma sympathicum. Z Kinderheilkd 103:61
5. Beckwith JB (1983) Wilms' tumor and other renal tumors of childhood: a selected review from the National Wilms' Tumor Study pathology center. Human Pathol 14:481
6. Beckwith JB, Perrin E (1963) In situ neuroblastomas; a contribution to the natural history of neural crest tumors. Am J Pathol 43:1089
7. Bogdan R, Taylor DEM, Mostofi FK (1973) Leiomyomatous hamartoma of the kidney. Cancer 31:462
8. Bolande RP, Brough AJ, Izant RJ (1967) Congenital mesoblastic nephroma of infancy. A report of eight cases and the relationship to Wilms' tumor. Pediatrics 40: 272
9. Bolande RP (1977) Childhood tumors and their relationship to birth defects. In: Mulvihill JJ, Miller RW, Fraumeni JF (eds) Genetics in human cancer. Raven Press, New York
10. Bond JV (1975) Bilateral Wilms' tumor. Age at diagnosis, associated congenital anomalies, and possible pattern of inheritance. Lancet I:482
11. Bond JV (1975) Prognosis and treatment of Wilms' tumor at Great Ormond Street Hospital for Sick Children, 1960–1972. Cancer 36:1202
12. Cassidy JR, Tefft M, Filler RM, Jaffe N, Paed D, Hellman D (1973) Consideration in the radiation therapy of Wilms' tumor. Cancer 32:598–609
13. v. Copeland L, Welburn JC, West OT (1958) Dystocia caused by Wilms' tumor. Am J Obstet Gynecol 76:1329
14. Croker JFS, Vernier RL (1972) Congenital nephroma of infancy: induction of renal structures by organ culture. J Pediatr 80:69
15. D'Angio GJ, Evans A, Breslow N, Beckwith B, Bishop H, Farewell V, Goodwin W, Leape L, Palmes N, Sinks L, Sutow W, Tefft M, Wolff J (1981) The treatment of Wilms' tumor. Results of the Second National Wilms' Tumor Study. Cancer 47:2302
16. Dieterich E, Gutjahr P (1978) Photosensibilität bei Kindern mit malignen Tumoren. EEG EMG 9:43
17. Diethelm L, Neidhardt M (1969) Die Therapie der Nierentumoren im Kindesalter. Radiobiol Radiother 10:511
18. Fraumeni JF, Miller RW (1969) Cancer deaths in the newborn. Am J Dis Child 117:186
19. Giangiacomo J, Penchansky L, Monteleone PL, Thompson J (1975) Bilateral neonatal Wilms' tumor with B–C chromosomal translocation. J Pediatr 86:98
20. Green DM (1985) The diagnosis and management of Wilms' tumor. Pediatr Clin North Am 32:735
21. Gutjahr P (1977) Solide bösartige Geschwülste im Kindesalter. Bericht über 1053 Fälle. Arbeitsgemeinschaft „Tumoren im Kindesalter" Monatsschr Kinderheilkd 125:454

22. Heaston DK, Libshitz HI, Chan RC (1979) Skeletal effects of megavoltage irradiation in survivors of Wilms' tumor. AJR 133:389
23. Herbst AL, Ulfelder H, Poskanzer DC (1971) Adenocarcinoma of the vagina: association of maternal stilbestrol therapy with tumor appearance in young women. N Engl J Med 284:878
24. Hermann G, Lemtis H (1965) Zur Frage der diaplazentaren Metastasierung maligner Blastome der Mutter. Z Geburtshilfe Gynekol 164:129
25. Jacobi H (1885) Primary sarcoma of the foetal and infant kidney. Kongreßverhandlungen. Pediatrie, Kopenhagen
26. Joseph C (1949) Embryoma of the kidney with symptoms at birth. Arch Dis Child 24:312
27. Joshi VV, Kay S, Milstein R, Koontz WW, Mc Williams NB (1973) Congenital mesoblastic nephroma of infancy: report of a case with unusual clinical behavior. Am J Clin Pathol 60:811
28. Kasdon SC (1949) Pregnancy and Hodgkin's disease. Am J Obstet Gynecol 57:282
29. Kiess W, Linderkamp D, Hadorn HB, Haass R (1984) Fetal alcohol syndrome and malignant disease. Eur J Pediatr 143:160
30. Knudson AG (1975) The genetics of childhood cancer. Cancer 35:1022
31. Knudson AG Jr, Strong LC (1972) Mutation and cancer: a model for Wilms' tumor of the kidney. JNCI 48:313
32. Krusemann ACN, van Lent M, Blom AH, Lauw GP (1977) Choriocarcinoma in mother and child, identified by immunoenzyme histochemistry. Am J Clin Pathol 67:279
33. Lemerle J, Tournade MF, Sarazin D, Valyer J (1975) Tumors of the kidney. In: Bloom HJG, Lemerle J, Neidhardt MK, Voute PA (eds) Cancer in children. Springer, Berlin Heidelberg New York
34. Meadows AT, Lichtenfeld JL, Koop CE (1974) Wilms' tumor in three children of a woman with congenital hemihypertrophy. N Engl J Med 291:23
35. Mc Caunley RG, Safaii H, Crowley CA et al. (1979) Extrarenal Tumor. Am J Dis Child 133:1174
36. Müller S, Gadner H, Weber B, Vogel M, Riehm H (1978) Wilms' Tumor and adrenocortical carcinoma with hemihypertrophy and hamartomas. Eur J Pediatr 127:219
37. Nance WE (1977) Relevance of twin studies in cancer research. In: Mulvihill JJ, Miller RW, Fraumeni JF (eds) Genetics of human cancer. Raven, New York
38. Napalkov NP (1973) Some general considerations on the problem of transplacental carcinogenesis. In: Tomahs L, Mohr U, Davis W (eds) Transplacental carcinogenesis. International Agency for Research on Cancer Scientific, p 1 (publication no 4)
39. Porter L, Carter WE (1920) Observations on tumor of kidney of children. Am J Dis Child 20:323
40. Riccardi VM, Sujansky W, Smith AC, Franke U (1978) Chromosomal imbalance in the aniridia-Wilms' tumor. Association: 11 p interstitial deletion. Pediatrics 61:604
41. Sabio H, Teja K, Elkon D, Sabio H, Teja K, Elkon D, Show A (1979) Adenocarcinoma of the colon following the treatment of Wilms' tumor. J Pediatr 95:424
42. Salmon JCM, Coignet R, Raybaud Cl et al. (1970) Succession d'un nephroblastome et d'un sympathoblastome chez un nourrisson. Pediatrie 25:337
43. Schwartz AD, Lee H, Baum ES (1975) Leukemia in children with Wilms' tumor. J Pediatr 87:374
44. Silver HK (1947) Wilms' tumor. J Pediatr 31:643
45. Smith CR, Chan HSL (1981) Placental involvement in congenital neuroblastoma. J Clin Pathol 34:785
46. Spear GS, Hyde TP, Gruppo RA, et al. (1971) Pseudohermaphroditism, glomerulonephritis with the nephrotic syndrome, and Wilms' tumor. J Pediatr 79:677
47. Strauss L, Driscoll SG (1964) Congenital neuroblastoma involving the placenta. Report of two cases. Pediatrics 34:23
48. Strietzel M, Eberhardt WJ (1970) Spätschäden nach Strahlentherapie bösartiger Tumoren im Kindesalter. Radiobiol Radiother 11:251
49. Uson AC, Wolff JA, Tretter P (1970) Current treatment of Wilms' tumor. J Urol 103:217
50. Wells HG (1940) Occurrence and significance of congenital malignant neoplasms. Arch Pathol 30:535
51. Wigger HJ (1969) Fetal hamartoma of kidney. Am J Clin Pathol 51:323
52. Wigger HJ (1976) Fetal rhabdomyomatous nephroblastoma – variant of Wilms' tumor. Hum Pathol 7:613
53. Witzleben CL, Bruninga G (1968) Infantile choriocarcinoma: a characteristic syndrome. J Pediatr 73:374
54. Zabel B, Gutjahr P, Baumann W (1980) Interstitielle Deletion am kurzen Arm des Chromosomes Nr. 11 bei einem Kind mit Aniridie and Wilms-Tumor. In: Spranger J, Tolksdorf M (eds) Klinische Genetik in der Pediatrie. Thieme, Stuttgart

Congenital Neuroblastoma

K.-D. BACHMANN and H. CHR. DOMINICK

1 Introduction

Neuroblastoma sympathicum represents 10%–15% of all malignant tumors in children. The annual incidence is estimated at 9 per million children under 15 years of age [9]. Although its appearance is scattered throughout childhood, diagnosis is made within the first 12 months of life in one-third of patients and in the 2nd and 3rd years of life in another one-third (Fig. 1).

The following observations are based on 6 of our own patients and 190 taken from the literature who were found to have a definitely prenatally developed neuroblastoma. In addition there are 169 patients with probably prenatally developed tumors, and 212 with possibly prenatally developed tumors in this review. General knowledge and results concerning prenatal tumor pathology have already been described (DOMINICK and BACHMANN: Prenatal Wilms' tumor, this volume).

During embryonal development, the sympathetic stem cells (sympathogonia) start migrating from the neural crest in a ventral direction and along the thoracic part of the spine from the sympathetic nervous system. During further growth cranially and caudally, sympathetic nerve cells and fibers are formed for visceral innervation. At that time sympathogonia migrate into the retroperitoneal space where the various sympathetic paraganglia (i.e., Zuckerkandl's organs) and the two adrenal glands develop. Of these sympathogonia the ganglion cells of the sympathetic nervous system and the chromaffin pheochromocytes start to differentiate at the 10th week of gestation (Fig. 1 DOMINICK and BACHMANN: Neuroblastoma, this volume). Postnatally, in the ganglion cells of the sympathetic nervous system as well as in the adrenal medulla, all stages of development starting from the stem cell up to the differentiated nerve and chromaffin cells (with and without mitoses) are still found. It is not before 2–3 years of age that the differentiation of the adrenal medulla is terminated anatomically [72]. In the newborn the very large paraganglia start to diminish in size.

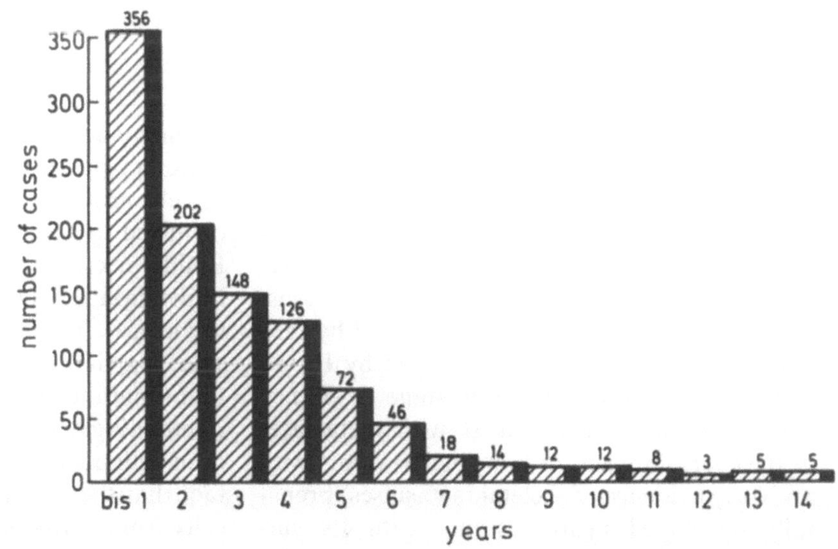

Fig. 1. Distribution by age of 1030 children suffering from sympathetic neuroblastoma [7]

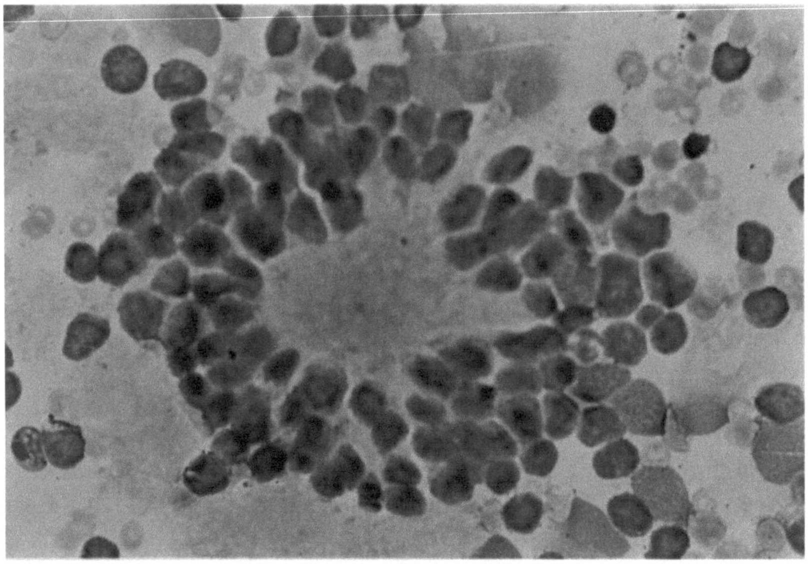

a

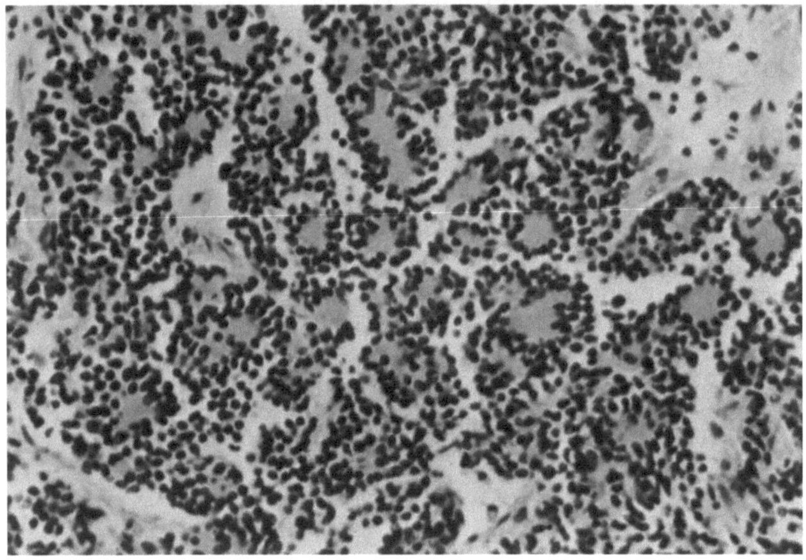

b

Fig. 2. a Bone marrow smear with rosette-like arrangement of the tumor cells. **b** Histologic section with rosette-like arrangement of the tumor cells in the case of a congenital neuroblastoma of the right adrenal gland (patient M.L., 1 day old)

Generally, neuroblastomas may arise anywhere ganglia of the sympathetic nervous system are found. Both the definitely and probably prenatally developed neuroblastomas as well as the postnatally developed tumors are very frequently found in the adrenal glands. Macroscopic staging of the tumor was initiated by PINKEL et al. [54] and further developed by EVANS et al. [24]. In this classification stage IV–S (i.e., primary tumor grade I or II with metastases of the liver, skin, and/or bone marrow only with no X-ray evidence of skeletal metastases) prenatally developed neuroblastoma with its surprisingly favorable prognosis is found quite frequently [6, 15, 43]. Histologically, the sympathogonias and sympathoblasts are found in the tumor to be arranged like rosettes (a grouping of cells around a tangle of young nerve fibers) or mixed in a very uncoordinated way (Fig. 2). Beside, necrosis, calcification, and lymphocytic infiltration especially at the border to normal tissue are frequently found. These "lymphocyte" barriers seem to be prognostically important (immune reaction?) [50, 10, 23]. The special immunologic potency of lymphocytes of children with neuroblastoma is demonstrated by the fact that they are able to stop their own tumor cells from forming colonies in-vitro. A similar blocking effect has also been demonstrated with the lymphocytes of mothers of children with neuroblastoma. This was not demonstrable in normal, unrelated control persons [35, 46].

It should also be mentioned that transfer of neuroblastoma cells from the embryo to the mother occurred without any consequences [2]. The villi of the placenta showed numerous tumor cell emboli, and a fetal-maternal transfusion could be demonstrated. The newborn clinically showing the picture of erythroblastosis died on the 17th day of life of a neuroblastoma of the right adrenal. The mother, however, was clinically and biochemically healthy at the 1-year follow-up examination. The mothers of the two other newborns in whom neuroblastoma cells were demonstrable in all villi of the placenta also remained tumor free [65].

For the discussion of histology and grading and their possible influence on the prognosis [38, 32] we refer the reader to the first chapter of this volume. It has been well demonstrated that maturation of the adrenal medulla is not completed before the 2nd or 3rd year of life, and therefore a variety of micromorphological pictures are found. These findings cast doubt on the "neuroblastoma in situ" concept inaugurated by Beckwith and Perrin [8]. These authors examined autopsy material of 30 children younger than 3 months in a very systematic fashion and found microscopically small areas of typical malignant tumors in otherwise microscopically normal adrenals 40 times more frequently than statistically expected. They drew the conclusion that such a neuroblastoma in situ could either develop into a clinically demonstrable tumor or most often regresses spontaneously.

Other studies, however, contradict these interpretations [67, 26]. They claim that these structures, found in an early stage of neuroblastoma, are supposed to be a more physiologic stage of maturation of the sympathetic stem cells. In all 169 adrenal glands from 92 fetuses examined, they found without exception neuroblastic nodules, with a peak incidence between the 17th and 20th week of gestation. On the other hand, when IKEDA and coworkers [39] analyzed the size of such fetal neuroblast nodules, they found those of neuroblastoma in situ were usually larger than fetal neuroblast nodules; the nuclear sizes were also significantly larger than those of the normal fetal cells. Thus, neuroblastoma in situ appears to be a true microscopic neoplasm that very often disappears after 3 months of age by spontaneous regression. Only in a few cases will it develop into neuroblastoma.

2 Case Studies

2.1 Case 1

M.S., female, born 1951. Eight days after discharge from the hospital, she presented with an enlarged abdomen and increased venous congestion on the skin. On the 14th day of life a subcutaneous node was found next to the scapula. At the time of admission the child was seriously ill, the liver was enlarged to the iliac crest, and pretibial edema was present. She had a rapid downhill course and died 4 days later. Neuroblastoma in both adrenal glands with large liver metastases and invasion of tumor into the paravertebral ribs were found at autopsy.

2.2 Case 2

J.N., male, born 1952. Two hours after home delivery, the child was sent to the hospital because of very pale skin; hemolytic disease of the newborn was suspected. On admission the child appeared moribund; anemia with a hemoglobin level of 10 wt% and 3.2 million erythrocytes was present. The abdomen was enlarged and the liver reached down to the iliac crest. There were hematomas and petechiae on the right side of the face, thorax, and abdomen. The child died 1 h after admission despite immediate treatment. Neuroblastoma of the left adrenal gland with multiple metastases in the liver was demonstrated at autopsy. The liver had ruptured, and the large intra-abdominal hemorrhage led to death.

2.3 Case 3

R.B., male, born 1964. On the 1st day of life an exploratory laparotomy was performed because of an enlarged abdomen. Neuroblastoma of the left adrenal with multiple metastases in the liver was found. No therapy was given, and the infant died on the 10th day of life.

2.4 Case 4

A.N., female, born 1966. At the age of 4 days, an enlarged abdomen was noticed. Neuroblastoma of a ganglion of the nervous system T12–L3 was detected. Therapy consisted of partial resection of the tumor, 2,500 rad radiation treatment, and administration of cyclophosphamide. In 1968 metastases to the right thigh were diagnosed.

2.5 Case 5

D.K., male, born 1966. A few hours after delivery the infant was admitted to the hospital because of postpartum asphyxia. On palpation of the abdomen no resistance was found. A plain film of the abdomen (Fig. 3) showed a onion-type calcification the size of a silver dollar, probably located in the retroperitoneal space. Dopamine excretion in the urine was elevated with 400 γ. At the time of surgery at the age of 14 days, a tumor of the right adrenal gland the size of a chestnut was removed in toto. A left-sided adrenal tumor the size of a hazelnut was removed from the normal kidney tissue at the age of 6 weeks. Histologic diagnoses of both tumors was sympathoblastoma. Besides postoperative radiation treatment with a total dose of 4,075 rad, cyclophosphamide therapy was initiated. No further growth of the neuroblastoma could be demonstrated during the further development of the child up to 12 years later. However, the boy is mentally retarded and has difficulties in finding and using words and so visits a special school. He sees and hears normally. He has enuresis and encopresis diurnally and nocturnally. Motorically he performs normally, and does not suffer from seizures.

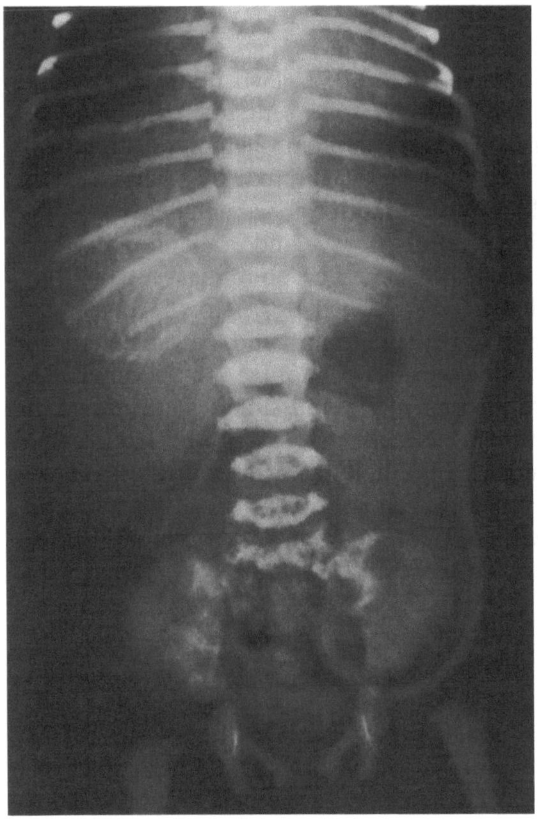

Fig. 3. Ring-shaped calcification in the case of a definitely prenatally developed neuroblastoma of the right adrenal gland (patient D.K., 2 days old)

2.6 Case 6

M.L., female, born 1970. On her 1st day of life, she was admitted to the hospital in a very poor condition with an enlarged abdomen and died shortly thereafter. Autopsy revealed neuroblastoma of the left adrenal gland with multiple liver metastases.

2.7 Cases in the Literature

In addition to our six cases, 184 further neuroblastoma cases in newborns diagnosed up to the 14th day of life were found in the literature. The localization of those definitely prenatally developed neuroblastomas is shown in Table 1.

As we have seen in older children with this tumor, prenatally developed neuroblastomas usually originate from the adrenals. Unusual lo-

Table 1. Localization of 190 definitively prenatally developed neuroblastomas

Adrenal	96
Retroperitoneal	28
Mediastinal	11
Spinal	17
Cervical	8
Sacral	4
Unknown	25
Unusual	1
	190

calization was found in a premature infant (1385 g) undergoing craniotomy because of hydrocephalus. Besides a ganglioneuroma of the adrenal gland and a neuroblastoma of the sympathetic chain, a fibroneuroma of the urinary bladder was found. Intra-abdominal neuroblastomas may sometimes hinder or prevent a normal birth [73]. In such a case, cesarian section may be necessary [30]. Rupture of the primary tumor in the adrenal glands during delivery accompanied by hemorrhage into the abdominal cavity similar to our second case of rupture of liver metastases was reported by KLEIN and PLÖCHL [41], FASANOTTI [25], BROCK and RICHETTS [12], and ANGERPOINTNER [3]. Massive adrenal gland hemorrhage caused by congenital neuroblastoma has been reported in only four cases [52, 63].

Among adrenal neuroblastomas, 33 were found on the right side, 29 on the left side, and 13 in both glands. In 21 patients the side was not mentioned. "Dumbbell" neuroblastomas have been reported in 22 newborns; in all infants partial or complete paralysis of both lower extremities was present at birth [37, 29]. The group of probably prenatally developed neuroblastomas encompasses 1 of our own cases and 158 infants between the 3rd and 12th week after birth.

Our own case was a 2-month-old male infant who presented with small nodes on the skin of the penis and scrotum extending to the thigh and abdomen. A tumor reaching from the left upper abdomen down into the pelvic area was palpable. The liver was palpable 3 cm below the right costal margin. The hemoglobin level measured 6.1 wt%. The catecholamine excretion in the urine was highly elevated: homovanillic acid 10.5 μg/day, 132 μg/mg creatinine; vanilmandelic acid 12.3 μg/day, 154 μg/mg creatinine. At surgery a retroperitoneal tumor as large as the head of a child was removed en bloc with the left kidney. The patient died 12 h later because of seizures that did not respond to any therapy. Multiple metastases to the liver, para-aortal lymph nodes, and pleura were found at autopsy in addition to skin metastases up to the size of a hazelnut.

Table 2 shows the site of the primary tumor in probably prenatally developed neuroblastomas. In this group the dominance of the adrenals as the primary site of the neuroblastoma is evident. The primary site of the tumor was the right adrenal gland in 24 cases, the left in 18 cases, and both glands in 11 cases. In 18 newborns the side was not mentioned. The five unusual locations concerned one neuroblastoma of the left testicle [62], one neuroblastoma possibly arising from the ganglion ciliare [57], one neuroblastoma of the posterior wall of the urinary bladder [33], one neuroblastoma of the abdominal wall [65], and one primary neuroblastoma of the skin [70].

The patterns of metastases showed a similar distribution in the definitively and probably prenatally developed neuroblastomas. In the 4–12 months age group of 270 patients (possibly prenatally developed neuroblastomas), 110 patients showed a deviation of the pattern of metastases. Only one-third of the children had solitary liver metastases (Pepper type), but 20% demonstrated skeletal metastases of the Hutchison type only. This type could only be demonstrated once (1%) in the group with definitively or probably prenatally developed neuroblastomas. A further 20% of the patients had metastases to the skeleton in combination with skin and/or liver metastases. DRESLER and coworkers [19] give a case report of a girl with congenital extra-adrenal neuroblastoma who died at 3 months of age with multiple parenchymal metastases of the brain and spinal cord, an extremely rare metastatic type (Table 3).

At the end of the first year of life, metastases to the skeleton are found three times more often than within the first 3 months of life. This relatively well-defined pattern – as far as time is concerned – is clinically significant. It seems to indicate that the biologic character of neuroblastomas or their growth and metastasizing behavior in the pediatric organism may change within the course of the first year of life! Metas-

Table 2. Localization of 169 probably prenatally developed neuroblastomas

Adrenal	71
Retroperitoneal	39
Mediastinal	16
Spinal	5
Sacral	5
Cervical	4
Unusual	5
Unknown	24
	169

Table 3. Metastases of 107 definitively, 97 probably, and 115 possibly prenatally developed neuroblastomas

	Definitively	Probably	Possibly
Liver metastases (Pepper type)	55	66	35
Skin metastases (Smith type)	16	12	13
Liver and skin metastases	13	4	4
Skin and bone metastases	6	3	3
Liver and bone metastases	–	4	21
Bone metastases (Hutchison type)	1	1	24
Lymph node metastases	–	7	12
Liver, bone, and skin metastases	1	–	2
No further data	15	–	1
	107	97	115

tases of the Pepper type (liver only) and Smith type (skin only) definitively have a better prognosis leading to a spontaneous clinical cure than metastases of the Hutchison type (skeleton only) which are found more often in older children.

The sex distribution of the 471 patients with neuroblastoma in the first year of life (definitively prenatal, 190; probably prenatal, 169; possibly prenatal, 112) shows 216 boys and 177 girls. No data were available for 78 patients.

Lee [47] reported one set of male monozygotic twins with neuroblastoma. Whereas one twin died of a right-sided adrenal neuroblastoma, the other one had a spontaneous cure without therapy (diagnostic biopsy of the left adrenal only). Monozygotic female twins both having a primary tumor in the right abdominal sympathetic chain leading to liver metastases died at the age of $9^1/_2$ and 11 months [14]. There are also reports on monozygotic twins among whom only one developed a neuroblastoma [64, 44].

Boyd [11] reported on dizygotic female twins. One had a neuroblastoma of the right adrenal with a spontaneous cure, although at exploratory laparotomy and biopsy it was found that this tumor was inoperable and no further therapy was given. The child was found to be healthy 12 years later. A familial increase in the incidence of neuroblastoma is, besides the above-mentioned twin case, also described in siblings [18, 13, 27, 31, 41, 73], between two generations [76, 75, 4], and in relatives [68, 31, 41, 42].

Although these are only scattered reports, they suggest a genetic disposition for a familial frequency of neuroblastomas. An autosomal dominant inheritance is suggested in numerous reports [49]. The two-step mutational model may explain how this tumor develops sporadically (the rule) as well as familially (seldom). The first mutational step may lead to dormant damage, increasing the person's susceptiblity to a tumor, while the second mutational step converts the already damaged sympathetic cell into a neuroblastoma cell [42, 58]. In familial neuroblastoma the first step is inherited in the germ cell line and will be present in all the cells of the body.

The clinical picture in prenatally developed neuroblastoma similar to that of the small and school-aged child is characterized by metastases. The most impressive main symptoms, besides the enlarged abdomen due to liver metastases and/or primary adrenal tumor, are nodular subcutaneous metastases. Hawthorne et al. [34] reported on a special type of subcutaneous neuroblastoma metastases in a newborn girl. She had firm blue subcutaneous nodules 0.5–1 cm in diameter spread all over the thorax, abdomen, and lower extremities. After palpation they became very erythematous for 2–3 min and even developed a 2–3 cm wide halo, which subsequently became pale and remained so for 30–60 min. Catecholamine granules and vesicles could be demonstrated by electron microscopy and histochemical fluorescent methods. This blanching of the nodular skin metastases was probably due to an excretion of catecholamine located within the granules of the neuroblastoma cells. Within 1 week after surgical removal of the left-sided adrenal neuroblastoma followed by a combination of chemotherapy with vincristine and cyclophosphamide, all skin metastases disappeared after the first injection of vincristine!

An unusual manifestation of congenital neuroblastoma is hydrops fetalis, reported in four cases [51]. Hypoglycemia due to nesidioblastosis or solitary islet adenoma is another rare symptom [68].

The diagnosis may be made more exactly by demonstrating an elevated excretion of catecholamines and/or catecholamine metabolites in the urine, neuroblastoma cells in the bone marrow, and also by biopsy (which possibly should include radical removal at the same time) of the primary tumor demonstrated radiologically. Before birth the diagnosis may be suspected by ultrasonography [40].

The increased fetal secretion of catecholamines accompanying a prenatally developed neuroblastoma led to similar symptoms in women during pregnancy: sweating, headache, tingling of fingers and toes, and episodes of blood pressure elevation [71, 69]. Six children had, either at birth or at the latest by the 9th month of age, a clinically symptomatic neuroblastoma. After delivery all symptoms disappeared in all mothers. In addition to these maternal symptoms a 28-year-old primipara developed coagulopathy and hepatorenal dysfunction. All symptoms are explained by the transplacental secretion of catecholamines by the fetal neuroblastoma [53].

The phenomena of paraneoplastic syndrome is more often found in older newborns and infants and consists of the infantile myoclonic encephalopathy (dancing eye, dancing feet, Kinsbourne syndrome). The incidence of these syndromes is not well known. Holschneider et al. [36] observed a myoclonic encephalopathy in 3 of 104 patients (2.9%). Four patients, however, with statomotoric retardation, known as a late symptom of myoclonic encephalopathy were also found. These authors as well as Senelick et al. [61] pointed out the high rate of neurologic late damage in patients with neuroblastoma (82% total, 63.5% of which had statomotoric retardation and 36.4% mental retardation). Roberts and Freemann [56] reported on a patient with cerebellar ataxia but without opsoclonia in a ganglioneuroblastoma of the mediastinum. Mostly the neurological symptomatology precedes the diagnosis of neuroblastoma; in only two cases was the diagnosis of neuroblastoma made before developing neurological signs [16, 59].

For the etiology of the combined development of neuroblastoma and myoclonic encephalopathy, an immune reaction of tumor antigens, viral infection, or toxicity of catecholamine metabolites are usually discussed. The formation of the para-O-methylated counterpart of homovanillinic acid, isohomovanillinic acid, which develops in neuroblastoma cells, is held responsible for the myoclonic encephalopathy syndrome [21].

The toxicity of catecholamine metabolites as a cause of myoclonic encephalopathy is seriously questioned in a paper by Delalieux et al. [16]. They reported on an 8-month-old female infant with a mediastinal ganglioneuroblastoma (vanilmandelic acid 33 μg/mg creatinine in urine) who after surgery and 2,000 rad irradiation treatment had a normal catecholamine excretion in urine and an uncomplicated statomotoric development (running without help at the age of 13 months). Nineteen months after surgery the parents noticed an insecure gait, and examination revealed ataxia and intention tremor with hyperreflexia of all four extremities and for the first time typical opsoclonia with tremor of the eyelids. The urinary excretion of homovanillic and vanilmandelic acid was normal. Even isohomovanillic acid could not be demonstrated despite the use of thin layer chromatography. The liquor was normal according to age.

Treatment may be successful with ACTH (40–80 units/day) or dexamethasone (0.3 mg/kg per day). Often, however, myoclonic encephalopathy is resistant to therapy. Seizure episodes, ataxia, opsoclonia, and corresponding mental and statomotoric retardation have been described as persisting as long as 7 years after treatment of the neuroblastoma [36]. The reviews by Senelick et al. [61], Lipinski et al. [48], and Rupprecht and Mortier [59] reported that of 83 patients, only 47 exhibited neuroblastoma. Comparison of the coincidence between opsoclonia and neuroblastoma in 28 patients revealed a very high survival rate, especially for the prognostically better stage IV-S as well as for five of seven patients in stage III–IV [1]. These authors discussed an unknown factor, possibly autoimmune in origin, which may stop growth and further extension of the tumor. There were also prognostically very favorable primary tumors: 16 thoracomediastinal, 9 abdominal but nonadrenal, 2 spinal, and 1 nonlocalized neuroblastoma. For planning treatment of prenatally developed neuroblastoma it should be especially noted that no other malignant tumor has as high a spontaneous cure rate as neuroblastoma: 1%–2% of all age

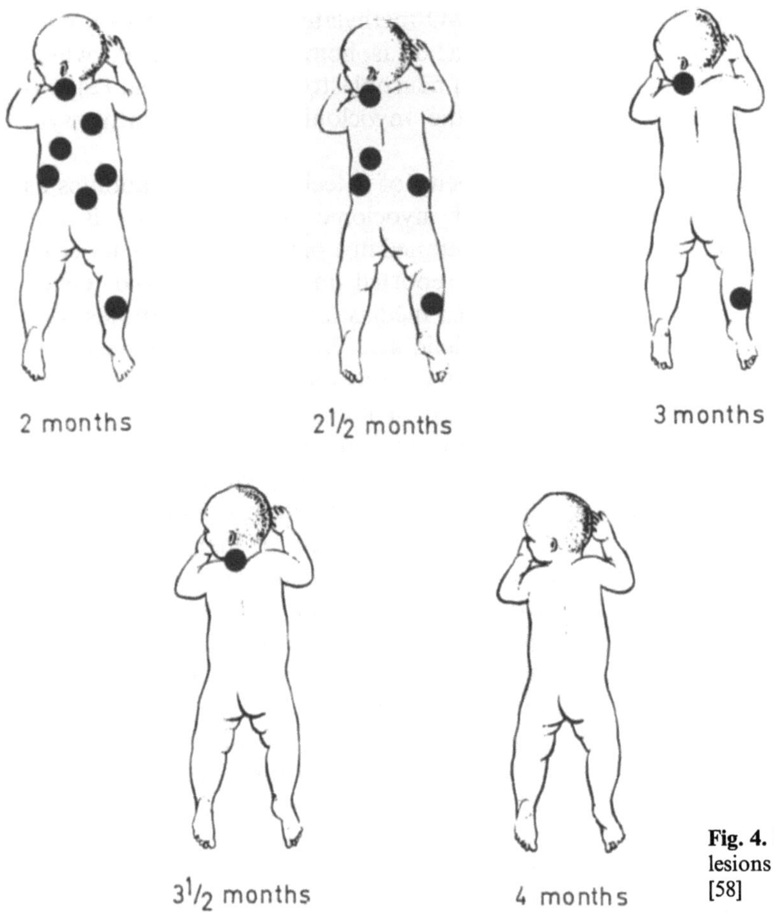

Fig. 4. Spontaneous regression of skin lesions of disseminated neuroblastoma [58]

groups [20] and 5%–10% of all diseases in newborns [17]. D'ANGIO et al. [15] as well as SCHWARTZ et al. [60] have had experiences similar to ours [5, 6]: newborns with isolated liver (Pepper type) and/or isolated skin metastases (Smith type) have an unexpectedly good prognosis as far as clinical cure is concerned.

SCHWARTZ et al. [60] described two patients 1 week and 3 months old who had significantly elevated catecholamine excretion in urine, normal intravenous pyelogram, and normal bone marrow. One patient demonstrated by scintigraphy hepatomegaly with abnormal uptake of the right lobe of the liver and the other had subcutaneous nodules, which histologically revealed neuroblastoma. Both patients were not treated but were supervised as outpatients; after 2–3 months (the 1-week-old newborn) and after 1 month (the 3-month-old infant), spontaneous regression of the tumor signs including normalization of the catecholamine metabolite excretion in the urine was observed (Fig. 4). DRUKKER [20] also reported on a 10-day-old boy with skin metastases who had a spontaneous cure without any therapy and still appears well 5 years later.

The patients treated by D'ANGIO [15] and EVANS [22] received an individual therapeutic regimen in which surgery, vincristine, and cyclophosphamide were combined with irradiation. This series includes 25 children of whom 21 (84%) survived. Of five patients, the left-sided neuroblastoma of the adrenal could be totally surgically removed in only one; in the other four only a biopsy was obtained. None of these five children received chemotherapy or irradiation treatment. Twenty children were younger than 13 months. All 25 children were stage IV–S [24]. Their prognosis is very favorable in comparison with stage IV in which of 131 patients treated by these authors, only 7 (5%) survived 2 years or longer. According to their experience gathered in Philadelphia, only surgical treatment (sometimes even partial resection) may lead to clinical cure in stage IV–S. Irradiation therapy is only recommended for liver metastases and mild chemotherapy in cases with bone marrow metastases [45]. This should be done in such a way that the immune suppression is kept as small as possible and the immunologic interaction between host and tumor is not completely wiped out [15, 22].

Among the 104 patients described by HOLSCHNEIDER et al. [36], 40 survived longer than 2 years after a combination of surgery, chemotherapy, and radiotherapy. However, only 11 of these patients (10.4%) failed to develop any late complications. In this connection one has to support the opinion of D'ANGIO and SCHWARTZ that therapy such as is administered to young children (0–6 months) with neuroblastoma and to those with a prognostically very favorable constellation (Pepper type, Smith type, extra-adrenal primary tumor) should only be initiated with extreme caution. On the other hand, there is no doubt that these treatment modalities should be applied in older children with neuroblastoma who have a much poorer prognosis. Few studies [45, 49] have shown that in stages III and IV of the disease no real improvement of the prognosis could as yet be obtained.

The difficulties that develop when discussing the therapeutic regimen may be outlined by the following case report by GRIFFIN and BOLANDE [27]. An 8-month-old female infant with neuroblastoma died following radiotherapy (bone marrow aplasia). The fifth child of the same family developed subcutaneous nodules directly after birth; this histologically demonstrated metastases from a neuroblastoma. The parents refused any treatment because of their previous experience. At 8 months the skin metastases became larger and the child had one bout of macrohematuria. After this the enlarged liver and skin metastases became smaller. Both at the age of 5 and 13 years, the child appeared normally developed and free of any signs of tumor. There are, however, 15–20 subcutaneous nodules palpable on various parts of the body. Excisional biopsy showed mature ganglion cells with collagenous material. This differentiation into a ganglioneurofibroma led the authors to discuss a possible relationship to neurofibromatosis.

This example may demonstrate the entire ambivalence of the situation: a prenatally developed neuroblastoma that becomes manifest during the 1st year of life should not – contrary to other tumors – be immediately treated surgically and medically. This should be saved for cases of large intra-abdominal or intrathoracic space-occupying lesions. First the patient should be observed without any therapy for weeks or months. It should be noted whether a regression or spontaneous cure is visible or whether a progression of the disease necessitates therapeutic interventions.

References

1. Altman AJ, Baehner RL (1976) Favorable prognosis for survival in children with coincident opsomyoclonus and neuroblastoma. Cancer 37:846
2. Anders D, Frick R, Kindermann G (1970) Metastasierendes Neuroblastom des Feten mit Aussaat in die Placenta. Geburtshilfe Frauenheilkd 30:969
3. Angerpointner TA (1985) Ein Fall von geburtstraumatisch rupturiertem, kongenitalem Neuroblastom. Monatsschr Kinderheilkd 133:241
4. Arenson EB, Hutter JJ Jr, Restuccia RD, Holton CHP (1976) Neuroblastoma in father and son. JAMA 236:727
5. Bachmann K-D (1962) Das Neuroblastoma sympathicum. Klinik und Prognose von 1030 Fällen. Z Kinderheilkd 86:710
6. Bachmann K-D, Kröll W (1968) Über das praenatal entstandene Neuroblastom sympathicum. Z Kinderheilkd 103:61
7. Bachmann KD (1971) Tumoren des sympathischen Nervensystems. In: Opitz H, Schmid F (eds) Handbuch der Kinderheilkunde (2nd ed.) Vol. 8: 328 Springer, Berlin Heidelberg New York
8. Beckwith J, Perrin E (1963) In situ neuroblastomas; a contribution to the natural history of neural crest tumors. Am J Pathol 43:1089
9. Berthold F (1985) Current concepts on the biology of neuroblastoma. Blut 50:65
10. Bill AH, Morgan A (1970) Evidence of immune reactions to neuroblastoma and future possibilities for investigation. J Pediatr Surg 5:111
11. Boyd W (1957) The spontaneous regression of cancer. J Can Assoc Radiol 8:45
12. Brock CE, Ricketts RR (1982) Hemoperitoneum from spontaneous rupture of neonatal neuroblastoma. Am J Dis Child 136:370
13. Chatten J, Voorhess ML (1967) Familial neuroblastoma. N Engl J Med 277:1230
14. Cochran W (1963) Neuroblastoma (sympathicoblastoma) in Northern Ireland: a review over a ten-year period. Ulster Med J 32:82
15. D'Angio GJ, Evans AE, Koop CE (1971) Special pattern of widespread neuroblastoma with a favourable prognosis. Lancet I:1046
16. Delalieux C, Ebinger G, Maurus R, Sliwowski H (1975) Myoclonic encephalopathy and neuroblastoma. N Engl J Med 292:46

17. De Lorimier AD, Bragg KU, Linden G (1969) Neuroblastoma in childhood. Am J Dis Child 118:441
18. Dodge HJ, Benner MC (1945) Neuroblastoma of adrenal medulla in siblings. Rocky Mt Med J 42: cited according to 13
19. Dresler St, Harvey DG, Levisohn PM (1979) Retroperitoneal Neuroblastoma widely metastatic to the central nervous system. Ann Neurol 5:196
20. Drukker A (1965) Neuroblastoma. Report of 3 cases with long-term survival. Acta Paedr Scand 54:397
21. Dziedzic S, Dziedzic L, Gitlow S (1973) Separation and determination of urinary homovanillic acid and iso-homovanillic acid by gas-liquid chromatography and electron capture detection. J Lab Clin Med 82:829
22. Evans AE (1977) Immunotherapy of neuroblastoma. Ninth meeting int. society paediatr. oncol (SIOP) Philadelphia, 20–24 September
23. Evans AE, Hummeler K (1973) The significance of primitive cells in marrow aspirates of children with neuroblastoma. Cancer 32:906
24. Evans AE, D'Angio GJ, Randolph J (1971) A proposed staging for children with neuroblastoma. Cancer 27:374
25. Fasanotti A (1948) Contributo albo studio dei tumori immaturi del simpatico. Pediatria 56:503
26. Finkelstein JZ (1976) Neuroblastoma: a unique solid tumor of childhood. In: Donaldson M, Seydel HG (eds) Trends in childhood cancer. Wiley, New York
27. Griffin ME, Bolande RP (1969) Familial neuroblastoma regression and maturation of ganglioneurofibroma. Pediatrics 43:377
28. Grotting JC, Kassel St, Dehner LP (1979) Nesidioblastosis and congenital neuroblastoma. Arch Pathol Lab Med 103:642
29. Haden MA, Keats TE (1983) Congenital intraspinal neuroblastoma with intraspinal calcification in the neonatal period: report of a case with a 32-year follow up. Pediatr Radiol 13:335
30. Hagstrom J (1930) Fetal dystocia due to metastatic neuroblastoma of the liver. Am J Obstet Gynecol 19:673
31. Hardy PC, Nesbit MF (1972) Familial neuroblastoma: report of a kindred with a high incidence of infantile tumors. J Pediatr 80:74
32. Harms D, Wilke H (1977) Pathologische Anatomie des Neuroblastoms. Z Kinderchirurg 22:122
33. Harvey F, Tennant R (1934) Primary neurogenic sarcoma of bladder. Am J Pathol 10:125
34. Hawthorne HC, Nelsen JS, Witzleben CL, Giangiacomo J (1970) Blanching subcutaneous nodules in neonatal neuroblastoma. J Pediatr 77:297
35. Hellström I, Hellström KE, Bill AH, Pierce GE, Young JPS (1970) Studies on cellular immunity to human neuroblastoma cells. Int J Cancer 6:172
36. Holschneider AM, Geiger H, Bolkenius N, Janka G, Lampert F (1977) Spätfolgen beim Neuroblastoma: Paraneoplastische Erkrankungen und Therapiefolgen. Monatsschr Kinderheilkd 125:69
37. Hrabovsky E, Jones B (1979) Congenital intraspinal neuroblastoma. Am J Dis Child 133:73
38. Hughes M, Mardsen HB, Palmer MK (1974) Histologic patterns of neuroblastoma related to prognosis and clinical staging. Cancer 34:1706
38. Ikeda Y, Lister J, Bouton JM (1981) Congenital neuroblastoma, neuroblastoma "in situ" and the normal fetal development of the adrenal. J Pediatr Surg 16:636
40. Janetschek G, Weitzel D, Stein W, Müntefering H, Alken P (1984) Prenatal diagnosis of neuroblastoma by sonography. Urology 24:397
41. Klein H, Plöchl E (1974) Familiäres Neuroblastom der Nebennieren beim Neugeborenen. Münch Med Wochenschr 116:1163
42. Knudson AG Jr, Meadows AT (1976) Developmental genetics of neuroblastoma. JNCI 57(3):675
43. Koop CE, Johnson DG (1971) Neuroblastoma: an assessment of therapy in reference of staging. J Pediatr Surg 6:515
44. Kushner B, Helson L (1985) Monozygotic siblings discordant for neuroblastoma. Etiologic implications. J Pediatr 107:405
45. Lampert F (1984) Neuroblastom. In: Kornhuber B (ed) Onkologie Pediatrie: Weiter- und Fortbildung. Springer, Berlin Heidelberg New York
46. Lampert F, Dietmair E (1973) Leukozyten-Adhärenz-Inhibition: Ein einfacher in vitro-Test zum Nachweis tumorspezifischer Immunität und blockierender Serumfaktoren bei Kindern mit Malignomen. Infection 1:17
47. Lee JAH (1967) Summer and death from neuroblastoma. Br Med J II:404
48. Lipinski C, Kratzer W, Daum R (1975) Die infantile myoklonische Encephalopathie – ein paraneoplastisches Syndrom bei Neuroblastom. Z Kinderchirurg 16:111
49. Lopez-Ibor B, Schwartz AD (1985) Neuroblastoma. Pediat Clin North Am 32:755
50. Martin RF, Beckwith JB (1968) Lymphoid infiltrates in neuroblastomas: their occurrence and prognostic significance. J Pediatr Surg 3:161
51. Moss ThJ, Kaplan L (1978) Association of hydrops fetalis with congenital neuroblastoma. Am J Obstet Gynecol 132:905
52. Murthy TVM, Irving IM, Lister J (1978) Massive adrenal hemorrhage in neonatal neuroblastoma. J Pediatr Surg 13:31
53. Newton ER, Louis F, Dalton ME, Feingold M (1985) Fetal neuroblastoma and catecholamine-induced maternal hypertension. Obstet Gynecol 65 [Suppl 3]:49S
54. Pinkel D, Pratt C, Holton C, James D, Wrenn E, Hustu O (1968) Survival of children with neuroblastoma treated with combination chemotherapy. J Pediatr 73: 928
55. Potter EL, Parrish JM (1942) Neuroblastoma, ganglioneuroma and fibroneuroma in a stillborn fetus. Am J Pathol 18:141
56. Roberts KB, Freemann JM (1975) Cellular ataxia and "occult neuroblastoma" without opsoclonus. Pediatrics 56:464
57. Rosta J, Gorcas L (1959) Malignant orbital tumor in a young infant. Ann Pediatr 193:304
58. Rüdiger HW (1978) Genetisch bedingte Risikofaktoren für maligne Tumoren beim Menschen. Dtsch Med Wochenschr 103:77
59. Rupprecht L, Mortier W (1975) Cerebelläre Bewegungsstörung und Neuroblastom. Monatsschr Kinderheilkd 123:392
60. Schwartz AD, Dadashzadeh M, Lee H, Swaney JJ (1974) Spontaneous regression of disseminated neuroblastoma. J Pediatr 85:760
61. Senelick RC, Bay PF, Lahey ME (1973) Neuroblastoma and myoclonic encephalopathy: two cases and a review of the literature. J Pediatr Surg 8:623
62. Smith J (1951) Case of ganglio-sympathicoblastoma of the testis in an infant. Br J Urol 23:39
63. Sober J, Hirsch M (1965) Unilateral massive adrenal hemorrhage in newborn infant. J Urol 93:430
64. Stadler HE, Worley RH (1955) Neuroblastomatosis in one of monozygotic twins. J Pediatr 47:485

65. Stewart FN, Copeland MM (1931) Neurogenic sarcoma. Am J Cancer 15:1235
66. Strauss L, Driscoll SG (1964) Congenital neuroblastoma involving the placenta. Report of two cases. Pediatrics 34:23
67. Turkel SG, Itabashi HH (1974) The natural history of neuroblastic cells in the fetal adrenal gland. Am J Pathol 76:225
68. Ullrich R (1970) Sympathicogoniome and Vererblichkeit maligner Geschwülste. Schweiz Med Wochenschr 100:749
69. van der Slikke JW, Balk AG (1980) Hydramnios with hydrops fetalis and disseminated fetal neuroblastoma. Obstet Gynecol 55:250
70. Vigorelli L (1962) Multiple subcutaneous sympathicoblastoma with favorable evolution. Minerva Pediatr 14:1219
71. Voute PA, Wadmann SK, van Putten WJ (1970) Congenital neuroblastoma symptoms in the mother during pregnancy. Clin Pediatr 9:206
72. Voute PA, van Putten WJ, Burgers JMV (1975) Tumors of the sympathetic nervous system. In: Bloom HJG, Lemerle L, Neidhard MK, Voute PA (eds) Cancer in children. Springer, Berlin Heidelberg New York
73. Wagget J, Aherne G, Aherne W (1973) Familial neuroblastoma: report of two sib pairs. Arch Dis Child 48:63
74. Weinberg T, Radman R (1943) Fetal dystocia due to neuroblastoma of adrenal with metastases to liver. Am J Obstet Gynecol 46:440
75. Wong KY, Hanenson SB, Lampkin BC (1971) Familial neuroblastoma. Am J Dis Child 121:415
76. Zimmermann J (1951) Ganglioneuroblastome als erbliche Systemerkrankung des Sympathicus. Beitr Pathol Anatol 111:335

Neuroblastoma

H. CHR. DOMINICK and K.-D. BACHMANN

1 Introduction

Neuroblastoma sympathicum is a tumor typically occurring during childhood. It derives from embryonic cells of the neural crest and frequently originates from the ganglion cells of the sympathetic chain and the adrenal medulla.

Although histologic examination leads to a classification distinguishing between sympathicogonioma, sympathicoblastoma, and ganglioneuroblastoma, the term neuroblastoma is widely accepted as the general term for this tumor (Fig. 1). Ganglioneuroma is a benign tumor. The other three, which differ in their histologic picture, are always malignant, although with different grades.

Approximately 10%–15% of all malignant tumors in childhood belong to the neuroblastoma group. Following Wilms' tumor, neuroblastoma is second in frequency among abdominal tumors. Neuroblastomas are found in all age groups although they are only rarely seen in adults [16, 51]. One-third of the children with neuroblastoma are younger than 12 months (including congenital neuroblastoma), and another one-third are between 2 and 3 years of age. For the last third, diagnosis is made after the 3rd year of life [3, 4]. Although the disease has sporadically been observed during childhood, an autosomal dominant inheritance has been discussed for some families [50].

2 Etiology

The etiology of neuroblastoma is unknown. Environmental factors are suggested by the fact that some epidemiologic studies and experimental data support the theory of a viral genesis [49, 60], and that the tumor is uncommon in children in certain geographic areas. It is nearly absent in black children in the Burkitt's lymphoma belt in Afrika and surrounding regions [55]. Analysis of abnormalities of chromosomes using banding techniques demonstrated that 15

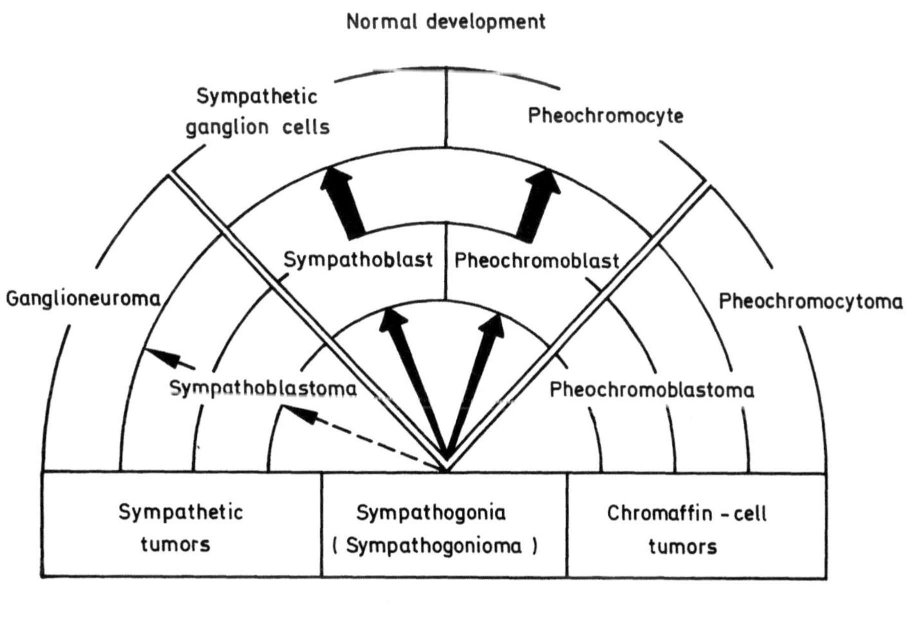

Fig. 1. Maturation and differentiation of sympathetic stem cells

of 24 neuroblastomas had abnormalities of the short arm of chromosome 1, with a deletion from *p* 32 to *pter* in 12 of the 15 cases. Partial monosomy for the short arm of chromosome 1 was the most consistent structural abnormality [10]. A deletion of the long arm of chromosome 11 also has been described [56]. PEGELOW and coworkers [59] give a fascinating case report of a newborn with congenital neuroblastoma who had two chromosomal abnormalities (balanced inversion of chromosome 11 and deletion of the short arm of chromosome 21) in his lymphocytes. One abnormality was found in each parent, each of whom by a previous marriage had had a child with neuroblastoma. By his earlier marriage the father had also had a phenotypically normal son whose wife later on delivered of a girl with congenital metastatic neuroblastoma lacking both abnormal chromosomes [30]. Neuroblastoma tumor cells may contain two additional cytogenetic abnormalities found also in solid tumors: extrachromosomal double minute chromatin bodies (DMs) and long, nonbanding, homogenously staining regions of chromosome (HSR) [7]. They are presumed to contribute to tumor progression [23].

A DNA segment closely related to the *myc* cellular oncogene and called *N-myc* has been found amplified 20- to 600-fold in 14 of 17 neuroblastoma cell lines [7]. The presence of amplification did correlate with the stage of the tumor, since no evidence of amplification was found in any of 15 patients with stage I or II, compared to 24 of 48 cases with stage III and IV without stage IV–S [11].

In a few patients with fetal hydantoin syndrome or fetal alcohol syndrome, a neuroblastoma has developed prenatally and also later on [2, 40]. Therefore it has been suggested that hydantoin and alcohol may be teratogenic as well as oncogenic.

3 Pathologic Anatomy

Neuroblastomas are nodular tumors of gray color. Only 10% are surrounded by a thin capsule that is very fragile, a factor that seems to be prognostically significant [71]. The tumor itself is mostly soft and fluctuant and liable to secondary changes of hemorrhagic necroses and calcification. Well-differentiated parts of the tumor are more solid and light in color. Histologically the tumor shows all grades of differentiation. There are extremely primitive cells, which lack cytoplasm and have small monomorphous and hyperchromatic nuclei, and foci of tumor cells, which are partially or completely differentiated into ganglioneuromatous cells. Pseudorosettes, which are important for making the diagnosis, do not seem to bear any prognostic significance [30]. The histologic grade of differentiation of the tumor varies within it and therefore different parts of the specimen should be examined. The grading of neuroblastoma as described by HUGHES, with its prognostically important different grades of malignancy, should be applied and is shown in Table 1. Grade I tumors have the most favorable prognosis. Besides the grade of differentiation, lymphocytic infiltration of the tumor seems to influence the prognosis [47].

Table 1. Grading of neuroblastoma (according to HUGHES et al. [32])

Grade I	Tumors showing a mixed pattern of undifferentiated cells and mature ganglion cells
Grade II	Tumors showing a mixed pattern of undifferentiated cells and some cells showing evidence of partial differentiation toward ganglion cells as indicated by any of the following: (a) vesicular nuclei, (b) presence of nucleoli, (c) increased cytoplasmic-nuclear ratio, (d) formation of cytoplasmic processes.
Grade III	Tumors consisting of undifferentiated cells without any evidence of maturation

Electron microscopy demonstrates a few granules in the cytoplasm of neuroblastoma cells. These granules, which are supposed to store the catecholamines produced by the tumor cells [78], are more often found in pheochromocytoma in which the cells are full of granules.

Neuroblastoma cells have also cytoplasmic structures consisting of neurofilaments and neurotubules. There is a correlation between the number of these dense core neurosecretory granules, the biochemical secretory pattern, and the clinical course, indicating that ultrastructural evaluation of undifferentiated neuroblastomas would appear to have prognostic value [68].

Reynolds and coworkers [64] found a rapid fluorescence assay for intracellular catecholamines to be positive in 81% of their neuroblastoma cases. They also used a tissue culture assay for neurite outgrowth that was positive in all 20 of the cases they studied.

Spontaneous regression of neuroblastoma is primarily seen in children before the age of 1 year. Even in the case of metastases, regression has been observed [13]; it is estimated that up to 10% of these children recover spontaneously [15]. Another very unusual feature of the neuroblastoma is its potential to go through a process of maturation and differentiation in vivo [54]. Spontaneous differentiation of neuroblastoma cells into ganglion cells could also be demonstrated with in-vitro cultures [57].

4 Immunology

Neuroblastoma cells probably possess a very pronounced antigenicity leading to stimulation of the cellular defense system and causing lymphocytic infiltration of the tumor. Hellström et al. [32] demonstrated this cell-mediated immunity against neuroblastoma cells utilizing the microcytotoxicity test. Studying the serum of patients with neuroblastoma, Lampert and Dietmair [45] were able to demonstrate the presence of factors that block the adherence of lymphocytes. No diagnostic or therapeutic consequences, however, can be derived from these findings. An increased lymphocyte count in the peripheral blood [8] or an increased level of lymphoblast cells in the bone marrow [17] may also be a sign of possible immunologic reactions.

A few cell surface antigens expressed by human neuroblastoma cells can be defined by heteroantisera which partly also have been found in normal neural cells [69]. These antigens may be of diagnostic and therapeutic value, as they can be operationally tumor specific [26].

5 Biochemistry

Neuroblastoma cells are capable of producing hormones. Approximately 80%–90% of the patients excrete increased amounts of catecholamines and/or catecholamine metabolites in the urine [37, 66]. The most frequently assayed urinary catecholamines are vanilmandelic acid (VMA) and homovanillic acid (HVA). If there is a doubtful result, other metabolites have to be determined, e.g., methoxytyramin, normetanephrine, dihydroxyphenylalanine, dopamine, noradrenalin, occasionally 3,4-dihydroxyphenylacetic acid (DOPAC), 3-methoxy-4-hydroxyphenylglycol (MHPG), and vanillin lactate acid (VLA). A common pattern of the catecholamines and their metabolites found in the urine, however, cannot be observed in patients with neuroblastoma. The VMA/HVA ratio has been shown to have prognostic significance, with a more favorable outcome associated with ratios greater than or equal to 1.5 [70]. Using high pressure liquid chromatography (HPLC), catecholamines and their metabolites also can be determined in serum [42]. Determination of catecholamines in urine is one of the most important aids for verification of neuroblastoma. It may also be a very important monitor of therapeutic intervention [64]. The most precise indicator of tumor recurrence is probably the increased production of dopamine and its metabolites and its excretion in urine [38].

Other biochemical markers have been described in patients with neuroblastoma. Cystathionine excretion in urine is increased and is suspected to correlate with a bad prognosis [46]. In some patients carcinoembryonic antigen is elevated in the serum [77], but this may reflect cross-reactivity with an antigen present in neuroblastoma tissue called the nonspecific cross-reacting antigen [73]. Elevated serum-ferritin levels appear to correlate well with the presence of active disease [29]. Its composition seems to be that of carcinofetal isoferritin. Increased levels of neuron-specific enolase have been described in neuroblastoma tissue and in the serum of patients. Values above 100 ng/ml at diagnosis are associated with a short survival [34]. The appearance of vanillin lactate acid and/or 3-dihydroxyphenylmandelic acid in the urine, however, seems to be a prognostically unfavorable sign [76]. Neuroblastomas without any endocrine activity probably represent a very undifferentiated tumor. The prognosis of these hormone-inactive neuroblastomas is generally poor [75].

6 Clinical Aspects

Patients with neuroblastoma demonstrate a wide spectrum of general and noncharacteristic clinical symptoms. These depend on the age of the patient and the site and extension of the primary tumor and its metastases. It is not unusual for a paraneoplastic syndrome to be the first hint leading to the diagnosis. Approximately 60% of the primary tumors are intra-abdominal, and in 30% the left or right adrenal gland is involved (Table 2). The intrathoracic primaries are found in the posterior mediastinum and may cause a pressure effect on the spinal cord. Primary intracranial neuroblastomas are very rare and mainly arise from the nervi olfactorii (esthesioneuroblastoma); the mass of the tumor is found inside the nasal cavity [27], and unilateral nasal obstruction and epistaxis are the most common clinical manifestations [1].

Another unusual primary tumor arises in the pancreas [52] or in the mandibula [12]. On initial examination 80% of the patients showed evidence of metastases or wide local involvement. Table 3 lists the first clinical signs found in 976 patients at the time of admission to the hospital. It can easily seen that in the majority of cases the clinical picture is based on the spread of the tumor. Besides general symptoms such as malaise, anemia, weight loss, and fever, there are signs of pressure effects by direct local extent of the tumor or metastases. In particular, spinal cord compression leads to very bizarre neurologic symptoms and may prevent early diagnosis [6, 25, 51]. The typical Horner syndrome occurs when the cervical and mediastinal sympathic chains are involved and is the only noticeable effect. This was observed in 8 of 30 patients. It is due to destruction of the cervical sympathetic ganglion by the tumor [35]. When the tumor arises in the ophthalmic sympathetic nerve, heterochromia iridis may result.

Among the paraneoplastic syndromes, the reversible stage following removal of the tumor should be distinguished from the irreversible stage. The reversible symptoms are fever, arterial hypertension, chronic diarrhea, myasthenia, ptosis, and a general hypotonia of the muscles [79]. Chronic diarrhea leads to a tremendous loss of electrolytes and fluids and may last for weeks. It is caused by a polypeptide (vasoactive intestinal peptide), which can be found in the serum and in the tumor itself [74, 65]. Hypotonia of the muscles can be an initial symptom, and therefore the disease may mimic myasthenia gravis [67]. Myoclonia and the myoclonus-opsoclonus-encephalopathy syndrome are paraneoplastic syndromes, which are not or only partially reversible, and whose symptoms include hypotonia of the muscles, tremor, and ataxia [9, 21]. In addition to these cerebellar symptoms, there may be a more or less pronounced mental retardation and even loss of speech. Although the primary tumor in neuroblastoma is mainly found in the abdomen, in the myoclonus-opsoclonus-encephalopathy syndrome the primary is located in the thorax [79].

Table 2. Site of primary tumor in 1580 children with neuroblastoma

	%
Head	2
Neck	5
Thorax	13
Abdomen	55
Adrenal gland	37
Sympathetic nerve chain	18
Pelvis	4
Other places	9
Unknown	12

Table 3. Clinical signs and symptoms in 976 patients with neuroblastoma

	%
General signs of tumor	25.5
Fever of unknown origin	23.1
Anemia	10.1
Local tumor signs	
Abdominal tumor	39.0
Hematuria	0.8
Metastases	
Skeleton	31.3
Lymph nodes	26.8
Skull	17.8
Liver	14.9
Exophthalmos	13.8
Lungs	10.9
Ecchymosis and ptosis	6.3
Skin	5.6
Kidney	2.4
Neurologic	5.1

7 Metastases

In neuroblastoma four different types of metastases can be found. They may be due to the age of the patient: (a) liver metastasis only (Pepper type); (b) skin metastasis only (Smith type); (c) isolated bone metastasis (Hutchison type); (d) generalized involvement of the liver, lymph nodes, and bones (especially skull, orbita, femur, and long bones). Although metastases to one organ are less frequent than generalized spread, the Pepper and Smith types are found in an increased proportion in congenital neuroblastomas and neuroblastomas in newborns in whom the diagnosis was made within the first 6 months. Patients with isolated liver metastases have a much more favorable prognosis than those with metastases to the skeletal system.

Compared with Wilms' tumor, lung metastases in neuroblastoma are extremely rare. The same can be said for the skull, where metastases are mainly localized in the bone or the meninges, and the brain itself commonly remains tumor free.

8 X-ray Findings

The plain film of the abdomen often already demonstrates suprarenal calcifications, which developed because of the typical regressive changes in neuroblastoma. The intravenous pyelogram shows both kidneys to be of normal length but displaced laterally and/or caudally. The collecting system appears normal. An aortogram occasionally helps in making the diagnosis and outlines the blood supply of the tumor. Cavography may, in rare instances, demonstrate an invasion of the tumor into the vena cava. The importance of ultrasonography for the early detection and sizing of abdominal neuroblastoma is nowadays undisputed. Usually it shows a solid mass with multiple internal echoes, sometimes greatly accentuated when the neuroblastoma contains calcium. Metastatic lymph node involvement may also be detected using that technique.

Intrathoracic neuroblastomas appear radiologically as large rounded tumors in the posterior mediastinum. At times, erosions of the intervertebral foramina or displacement of ribs and calcifications may also be seen.

The radiographically demonstrable anomalies of the skeleton are usually a sign of metastases. They are found primarily on the skull and the diaphyses of the long bones. Osteolytic areas of the skull with dehiscence of the suture line may also be typical [5], whereas the long bones (femur) show the characteristic symmetric "moth-eaten" foci with periosteal reaction.

Increased uptake of ^{99}Tc-diphosphate is often found weeks before lesions can be detected by radiography [72]. Kaufman et al. [39], however, reported false negative bone scans in two of nine patients with metastatic disease to bone localized at the end of the long bones. On radiographs small cystic lesions were demonstrated.

In six of seven patients with neuroblastoma the tumor was demonstrated by ^{131}I meta-iodobenzylguanidine scintigraphy; in three patients metastases also could be detected by this technique [41].

^{99m}Tc sulfur colloid bone marrow scanning is assumed to be useful in detecting bone marrow involvement [58]. Computed tomography renders possible the accurate determination of tumor localization, its size, and its infiltration into the surrounding tissues. Therefore it is used predominantly in the imaging of brain, thorax, and abdomen.

9 Differential Diagnosis

The differential diagnosis of neuroblastoma includes all diseases with general symptoms of fever, liver enlargement, joint pain, and lymph node enlargement, for example, rheumatic fever, Still's disease, hepatoblastoma, lymphosarcoma, histiocytosis X, and Hodgkin's disease. If the tumor is localized intrathoracically, a ganglioneuroma or teratoma located in the posterior mediastinum should be suspected.

Wilms' tumor is thought to be the most important differential diagnosis in retroperitoneal neuroblastoma. Hydronephrosis may also present as a palpable retroperitoneal tumor. With intra-abdominal tumors, one has to consider an enlarged liver or spleen or metastases to the lymph nodes and mesenterium, and ovarian cysts, also. Persistent diarrhea in conjunction with neuroblastoma should not be confused with the malabsorption syndrome. Metastases to the bone marrow may imitate an acute leukemia [63].

10 Diagnosis

If a neuroblastoma is suspected or has been diagnosed, the following additional steps should be taken:

(a) Detection of an abnormally high excretion level of catecholamine metabolites in the urine. With this method the diagnosis can be secured in 70%–90% of patients. The spot test by LA-BROSSE has not been found to be a very reliable screening test because of the frequent false positive and false negative results [18, 19, 36].
(b) A radiographic examination of the thorax, abdominal organs, and skeleton, and an intravenous pyelogram. Computed tomography of the chest or abdomen may be useful to determine the extent of the disease and lymph node involvement.
(c) Bone marrow aspiration to identify bone marrow involvement and rosette-forming tumor cells. Bone marrow involvement is present in more than 50% of patients, while rosettes are only seen in less than 2% of samples [22].
(d) Measuring serum ferritin and neuron-specific enolase may be of value because of their prognostic significance.

11 Therapy

The correct therapeutic procedure today takes into consideration the age of the patient and the stage of the disease based upon the classification by EVANS (Table 4).

In stage I and II radical surgical extirpation is the treatment of choice. There is no evidence that further therapy improves survival, even when macroscopic disease is left behind [50]. In patients with stage III, sometimes surgery is only possible as a second-look procedure after radiation and chemotherapy. The exact role of

Table 4. Staging of neuroblastomas (according to EVANS et al. [18, 19]

Stage I	Tumors confined to the organ or structure of origin
Stage II	Tumors extending in continuity beyond the organ or structure of origin but not crossing the midline; homolateral lymph nodes may be involved
Stage III	Tumors extending in continuity beyond the midline; bilateral regional lymph nodes may be involved
Stage IV	Dissemination with metastases in skeleton, organs, soft tissue, distant lymph nodes, etc.
Stage IV-S	Patients who would be in group I or II were it not for the fact that they show dissemination in liver, spleen, or bone marrow but without radiographic evidence of bone metastases

surgery in patients with stage IV has yet to be defined. For these patients chemotherapy is usually the initial treatment of choice. Radiation therapy only plays a role in palliative treatment to relieve osteoalgia. Predominantly in patients with stage III radiation therapy (2,000 rad to the tumor's bed) is indicated. In any radiation therapy the following side-effects should be taken into consideration:

(a) Disturbance of spinal growth
(b) Radiation damage to the liver and the kidneys, which either stops normal growth or leads to fibrosis of the liver, atrophy of the kidney, or irradiation myelitis
(c) Whereas testes can be shielded satisfactorily, the ovaries are at risk
(d) Retarded growth of the heads of the femur
(e) Development of secondary malignancies following irradiation

The development of multiple adenomas of the thyroid gland has been observed 24 years after radiotherapy of neuroblastoma of the neck [53].

Chemotherapy with cytostatic agents does not seem to improve the prognosis of neuroblastoma (chiefly stage IV) even with application of the newer drugs in combination therapy. At present cyclophosphamid in combination with adriamycin, vincristine, decarbazine (DTIC-Dome), VM-26 (Vumon), and cisplatinum appear to be useful in achieving a clinical response.

In 1971 D'ANGIO and coworkers described a special pattern of widespread neuroblastoma with a favorable prognosis (stage IV–S) in infants with a small primary tumor [14]. There are only a few patients with real stage IV–S in whom spontaneous regression occurred. In a retro-spective study only 17 out of 207 patients with neuroblastoma had a disease staged IV–S [20]; in 12 of the 17, an enlarged liver was the presenting sign. Treatment should only be directed at this symptom. Low dose irradiation (200 rad single dose to 600–1,200 rad over 1–2 weeks) or mild chemotherapy are effective. The differential diagnosis between stage IV and IV–S may be made measurement of serum ferritin, which is not increased in stage IV–S [28].

During the follow-up period regular control of catecholamine urinary excretion and blood counts should be made; depending on the site of the primary tumor or metastases, X-rays (thorax, abdomen, intravenous pyelogram, skeleton), evaluation of liver and kidney function, and bone marrow examination are necessary [43]. Recurrence of tumor may be indicated by an increased lactate dehydrogenase activity [62] and by enhanced serum ferritin level [29].

12 Prognosis

Analogous to the 5-year cure rate of cancer patients in the adult age group, a clinical cure in infants with neuroblastoma can be assumed if after 3 years no clinical or biochemical signs and symptoms are observed. A 100% cure rate can be assumed for stage I neuroblastoma, which has been radically removed; the prognosis is worse in stage II (86%) and stage IV (79%). A 68% survival rate is documented for children having stage IV and diagnosed between 0 and 12 months of age; in older children survival rate decreases down to 8% [44]. Even the combined treatment modalities with surgery, radiation, and polychemotherapy did not improve the survival rate, although neuroblastoma seems to be more responsive in the early phase. So far improvement of prognosis can only be achieved when the tumor is diagnosed early.

References

1. Albert RW (1981) Esthesioneuroblastoma. Ear Nose Throat J 60:522
2. Allen RW, Ogden B, Bentley F, Jung AL (1980) Fetal hydantoin syndrome, neuroblastoma, and hemorrhagic disease in a neonate. JAMA 244:1464
3. Bachmann K-D (1962) Das Neuroblastoma sympathicum. Klinik und Prognose von 1030 Fällen. Z Kinderheilkd 86:710
4. Bachmann K-D (1971) Tumoren des sympathischen Nervensystems. In: Opitz H, Schmid F (eds) Handbuch der Kinderheilkunde, vol 8, 2nd edn. Springer, Berlin Heidelberg New York
5. Bachmann K-D, Friedmann G (1967) Schädelmetastasen beim Neuroblastom mit bevorzugter Absiedlung im Nahtbereich. Fortschr Röntgenstr 106:422
6. Balakrishnan V, Rice MS, Simpson DA (1974) Spinal neuroblastomas. Diagnosis, treatment and prognosis. J Neurosurg 40:631
7. Berthold F (1985) Current concepts on the biology of neuroblastoma. Blut 30:65
8. Bill AH, Morgan A (1970) Evidence for immune reactions to neuroblastoma and future possibilities for investigation. J Pediatr Surg 5:111
9. Boltshauser E, Deonna Th, Hirt HR (1979) Myoclonic encephalopathy of infants or "dancing eyes syndrome". Helv Paediatr Acta 34:119
10. Brodeur GM (1982) Genetics and cytogenetics of human neuroblastoma. In: Pochedly C (ed) Neuroblastoma. Elsevier Biochemical, New York
11. Brodeur GM, Seeger RC, Schwab M, Varmus HE, Bishop JM (1984) Amplification of *N-myc* in untreated human neuroblastomas correlates with advanced disease stage. Science 224:1121
12. Burkes EJ, Kelly DE, Hill C (1980) Primary mandibular neuroblastoma. J Oral Surg 38:131
13. Carvalho L (1973) Spontaneous regression of an untreated neuroblastoma. Br J Ophthalmol 57:832
14. D'Angio GJ, Evans AE, Koop CE (1971) Special pattern of widespread neuroblastoma with favorable prognosis. Lancet I:1046
15. De Lorimier AD, Bragg KU, Linden G (1969) Neuroblastoma in childhood. Am J Dis Child 118:441
16. Dosik GM, Rodriguez V, Benjamin RS, Bodey GP (1978) Neuroblastoma in the adult. Cancer 41:56
17. Evans AE, Hummeler K (1973) The significance of primitive cells in marrow aspirates of children with neuroblastoma. Cancer 32:906
18. Evans AE, D'Angio GJ, Randolph J (1971) A proposed staging for children with neuroblastoma. Cancer 27:374
19. Evans AE, Blore J, Hadley R, Tanindi S (1971) The La Brosse spot test: a practical aid in the diagnosis and management of children with neuroblastoma. Pediatrics 47:913
20. Evans AE, Chatten J, D'Angio GJ, Gerson JM, Robinson J, Schnaufer L (1980) A review of 17 IV–S Neuroblastoma patients of the Children's Hospital of Philadelphia. Cancer 45:833
21. Förster C, Weinmann H (1971) Symptomatische infantile Polymyoclonie. Monatsschr Kinderheilkd 111:240
22. Franklin JM, Pritchard J (1983) Detection of bone marrow invasion by neuroblastoma is improved by sampling at two sides with both aspirates and trephine biopsies. J Clin Pathol 36:1215
23. Gilbert F, Balaban G, Brangman D, Herrmann N, Lister A (1983) Homogeneously staining regions and tumorigenicity. Int J Cancer 31:765
24. Gitlow StE, Dziedzic LB, Dziedzic StW (1982) Patterns of catecholamine metabolism in neuroblastoma. In: Po-

chedly C (ed) Neuroblastoma. Elsevier Biochemical, Amsterdam
25. Gordes W, Fischer V (1973) Intraspinales Neuroblastom im Kindesalter. Arch Orthop Unfallchir 77:236
26. Goldman A, Vivian G, Gordon Pritchard J, Kemshead J (1984) Immunolocalization of neuroblastoma using radiolabeled monoclonal antibody UJ 13 A. J Pediatr 105:252
27. Hamilton AE, Rubenstein LJ, Poole GJ (1973) Primary intracranial esthesioneuroblastoma (olfactory neuroblastoma). J Neurosurg 38:548
28. Hann HL, Evans AE, Cohen IJ, Leitmeyer BA (1981) Biologic differences between neuroblastoma stages IV-S and IV: measurement of serum ferritin and E-rosette inhibition in 30 children. N Engl J Med 305:425
29. Hann HL, Levy HW, Evans AE (1980) Serum ferritin as a guide to therapy in neuroblastoma. Cancer Res 40:1411
30. Harms D, Wilke H (1977) Pathologische Anatomie des Neuroblastoms. Z Kinderchirurg 22:122
31. Hecht F, Kaiserhecht B, Northrup SC (1982) Genetics of familial neuroblastoma: long range studies. Cancer Genet Cytogenet 7:227
32. Hellström I, Hellström KE, Bill AH, Pierce GE, Yong JPS (1970) Studies on cellular immunity to human neuroblastoma cells. Int J Cancer 6:172
33. Hughes M, Mardsen HB, Palmer MK (1974) Histologic patterns of neuroblastoma related to prognosis and clinical staging. Cancer 34:1706
34. Ishiguro Y, Kato K, Ito T, Nagaya M, Yamada N, Sugito T (1983) Nervous system specific enolase in serum as a marker for neuroblastoma. Pediatrics 72:696
35. Jaffe N, Cassady JR, Filler RM, Petersen R, Traggis D (1975) Heterochromia and Horner syndrome associated with cervical and mediastinal neuroblastoma. J Pediatr 87:75
36. Johnsonbough RE, Cahill R (1975) Screening procedures for neuroblastoma: false-negative results. Pediatrics 56:267
37. Käser H (1972) Biochemische Diagnostik des Phäochromozytoms, des Neuroblastoms und anderer neuro-ektodermaler Neoplasien. Helv Paediatr Acta [Suppl] 29:1
38. Käser H, Wagner HP, Zuppinger K, Zurbrügg R (1974) Zur biochemischen Tumordiagnostik im Kindesalter. Schweiz Med Wochenschr 104:642
39. Kaufman RA, Thrall JH, Keyes JW, Braun ML, Zakem JF (1978) False-negative bone scans in neuroblastoma metastatic to the ends of long bones. AJR 130:131
40. Kiess W, Linderkamp O, Hadorn H-B, Haas R (1984) Fetal alcohol syndrome and malignant disease. Eur J Pediatr 143:160
41. Kimmig B, Brandeis WE, Adolph J (1985) Diagnose und Therapiekontrolle des Neuroblastoms mit meta-Jod-Benzylguanidin. Dtsch Med Wochenschr 110:175
42. Krivit W, Mirkin BL, Freier E, Nesbit U, Cooper NJ (1980) Serum catecholamine metabolites in stage IV neuroblastoma. In: Evans AE (ed) Advances in neuroblastoma research. Raven, New York
43. Kurz R, Mutz J, Pichler E (1977) Neuroblastom: Diagnose, Therapie und Prognose an Hand von 56 Patienten. Wien Klin Wochenschr [Suppl 67] 89:16
44. Lampert F (1984) Neuroblastom. In: Kornhuber B (ed) Onkologie Pädiatrie. Weiter- und Fortbildung, p 89 Springer, Berlin Heidelberg New York
45. Lampert F, Dietmair E (1973) Leukozyten-Adhärenz-Inhibition: ein einfacher in vitro-Test zum Nachweis tumorspezifischer Immunität und blockierender Serumfaktoren bei Kindern mit Malignomen. Infection 1:17
46. Lang WE, Siegel SE, Shaw KNF et al. (1978) Initial urinary catecholamine metabolite concentrations and prognosis in neuroblastoma. Pediatrics 62:77
47. Lauder I, Aherne W (1972) The significance of lymphocytic infiltration in neuroblastoma. Br J Cancer 26:321
48. Leape LL, Lowmann JT, Loveland GC (1978) Multifocal nondisseminated neuroblastoma. J Pediatr 92:75
49. Lee JAH (1976) Summer and death from neuroblastoma. Br Med J II:404
50. Lopez-Ibor B, Schwartz AD (1985) Neuroblastoma. Pediatr Clin North Am 32:755
51. MacKay B, Luna MA, Butler JJ (1976) Adult neuroblastoma electron microscopic observations in nine cases. Cancer 37:1334
52. Margueritte G, Galifer RB, Pons JG (1982) Neuroblastoma of the pancreas in a two year old boy. In: Rayband G, Clement R, Lebrenil G (eds) Pediatric oncology. International congress series 570:66 Excerpta Medica, Amsterdam
53. McKenzie CG, Hope-Stone HF (1975) Multiple adenomas of the thyroid occurring 20 years after successful radiotherapy of neuroblastoma in the cervical lymphnodes. Br J Radiol 48:1028
54. McLaughlin JE, Urich H (1977) Maturing neuroblastoma and ganglioneuroblastoma: a study of four cases with long survival. J Pathol 121:19
55. Miller RW (1977) Ethnic differences in cancer occurrence: genetic and environmental influences with particular reference to neuroblastoma. In: Mulvihill JJ, Miller RW, Fraumeni JF Jr (eds) Genetics of human cancer. Raven, New York, p 169
56. Moorhead PS, Evans AE (1980) Chromosomal findings in neuroblastoma patients and families. In: Evans AE (ed) Advances in neuroblastoma research. Raven, New York, p 132
57. Murray MR, Stout AP (1948) Sympathetic ganglioneuroblastoma cultivated in vitro. Cancer 1:242
58. Oseas RS, Siddiqui AS, Wellman HN et al. (1982) Usefullness of bone marrow imaging in childhood malignancies. J Pediatr 101:206
59. Pegelow GH, Ebbin AJ, Powars D, Towner JW (1975) Familial neuroblastoma. J Pediatr 87:763
60. Prasad KN, Zambernard J, Lasher R, Vanwoert MH (1970) Transmission of mouse neuroblastoma by a cell-free extract. Nature 228:997
61. Punt J, Pritchard J, Pincott JR, Till K (1980) Neuroblastoma: a review of 21 cases presenting with spinal cord compression. Cancer 45:3095
62. Quinn JJ, Altmann AJ, Frantz CN (1980) Serum lactic dehydrogenase, an indicator of tumor activity in neuroblastoma. J Pediatr 97:89
63. Raney RB, Lyon GM, Porter FS (1976) Neuroblastoma simulating acute leukemia. J Pediatr 89:433
64. Reynolds CP, Smith RG, Frenkel EP (1981) The diagnosis dilemma of the "small round cell neoplasm". Cancer 48:2088
65. Ricour C, Duhamel JF, Lesec G, Schweisguth O (1977) Diarhee choleriforme dans un cas de ganglioneuroblastome. Arch Franc Pediatr 34:552
66. Robinson R (1980) Tumors that secrete catecholamines. Wiley, Chichester
67. Robinson MJ, Howard RN (1969) Neuroblastoma presenting as myasthenia gravis in a child aged 3 years. Pediatrics 43:111

68. Romansky SG, Crocker DW, Shaw KNF (1978) Ultrastructural studies of neuroblastoma. Evaluation of cytodifferentiation and correlation of morphology and biochemical and survival data. Cancer 42:2392
69. Seeger RC (1982) Immunology of neuroblastoma. In: Pochedly C (ed) Neuroblastoma. Elsevier Biochemical, New York
70. Siegel SE, Lang WE, Hanlow PJ et al. (1980) Patterns of urinary catecholamine excretion in neuroblastoma. In: Evans AE (ed) Advances in neuroblastoma research. Raven, New York, p 25
71. Stowens D (1957) Neuroblastoma and related tumors. Arch Pathol 63:451
72. Sty JR, Kun LE, Casper JT (1980) Bone imaging as a diagnostic aid in evaluating neuroblastoma. Am J Pediatr Hematol Oncol 2:115
73. Sugimoto T, Sawada T, Kusunoki T (1979) Immunological and biochemical studies on the carcinoembryonic antigen-like substance in human neuroblastoma. Pediatr Res 13:91
74. Trump DL, Livingston JN, Baylin SB (1977) Watery diarrhea syndrome in an adult with ganglioneuroma-phaeochromocytoma. Cancer 40:1526
75. Voute PA, Voss A, Delemarre JFM et al. (1980) The persistent challenge of neuroblastoma. In: Van Eys J, Sullivan MP (eds) Status of curability of childhood cancer. Raven, New York, p 145
76. Voute PA, van Putten WJ, Burgers JMV (1975) Tumors of the sympathetic nervous system. In: Bloom HJG, Lemerle J, Neidhardt MK, Voute PA (eds) Cancer in children. Springer, Berlin Heidelberg New York, p 138
77. Weng JJ, Sinks LF, Chu TM (1974) Carcinoembryonic antigen in patients with neuroblastoma. J Surg Oncol 6:211
78. Williams ThE, Donaldson MH (1973) Neuroblastoma. In: Sutow WW, Vielti TJ, Fernbach DJ (eds) Clinical pediatric oncology. Mosby, St. Louis, p 506
79. Winkler K (1976) Paraneoplastische Symptome bei Neuroblastom. Monatsschr Kinderheilkd 124:527

Nonsurgical Management of Wilms' Tumor

W. HAVERS

1 Introduction

The extraordinary improvement in the results of treatment of Wilms' tumor in the last 20 years is demonstrated by the fact that it has one of the highest cure rates of all malignancies in children. Even with the presence of metastases at the time of diagnosis, or in the case of bilateral Wilms' tumor, promising therapeutic regimens have been reported [39, 7, 4]. Advances in treatment in the past decade have also improved the survival rate for patients with Wilms' tumor. Actinomycin D and vincristine were introduced as chemotherapeutic agents, and the importance of combined surgical, radiotherapeutic, and chemotherapeutic regimens was recognized. The reason for this therapeutic progress may be summarized as follows: (a) Radical, transperitoneal nephrectomy; (b) radiotherapy to destroy residual tumor; (c) adjuvant polychemotherapy to eradicate micrometastases.

The difference between the survival rate in children with Wilms' tumor in 1920 and today (Table 1) is not only due to more aggressive therapy. The studies and results of the National Wilms' Tumor Study Group (NWTS) and the clinical trial conducted by the International Society of Pediatric Oncology (SIOP) enlarged the knowledge about this malignant tumor in children and reached more people interested in this disease [25, 26, 27, 1, 4]. Today, the therapy of a child with Wilms' tumor is highly individualized according to several factors present at the time of diagnosis. In early stages of the disease, treatment can be reduced without jeopardizing tumor control.

Table 1. Survival of patients with Wilms' tumor

Author	*n*	Period	Survival (%)	Therapy
[19]	27	1914–1930	15	OP
	31	1931–1939	32	OP
	38	1940–1947	47	OP + RAD
[42]	46	1936–1960	39	OP + RAD
[25, 26]	248	1952–1967	54	OP + RAD (+AMD)
[45]	53	1964–1968	75	OP + RAD + AMD
[22]	49	1969–1974	81	OP + RAD + AMD/VCR

OP, operative; RAD, irradiation; AMD, actinomycin D; VCR, vincristine; *n*, number of patients

2 Prognostic Factors Influencing the Treatment Plan

When the diagnosis of Wilms' tumor is supported by radiological and clinical evidence, the primary tumor will generally be removed by nephrectomy. Further treatment is influenced by surgical findings and the pathologic examination. A variety of factors have been described which determine the prognosis of a child with Wilms' tumor. Using a multivariate analytical technique, only a few factors were identified as predicting the likelihood of relapse-free survival [9, 6, 16]: (a) extent of disease, e.g., evidence of hematogeneous metastases, tumor weight greater than 250 g, involvement of lymph nodes; (b) age of patient at the time of diagnosis; (c) tumor histology. A staging system based on the extent of disease has been proposed by the present National Wilms' Tumor Study [16] as shown in Table 2.

The results of the first NWTS demonstrated that age influenced the prognosis of stage I patients. In children younger than 24 months, a 2-year tumor-free survival was found in 89%, compared with 67% in the group of children older than 2 years of age [1]. The mortality rate

Table 2. National Wilms' Tumor Study Staging System

Stage I	Tumor limited to the kidney and completely excised
Stage II	Tumor extends beyond the kidney but is completely excised. The vessels outside the kidney substance are infiltrated or contain tumor thrombus. The tumor may have been biopsied, or there has been local spillage of tumor confined to the flank
Stage III	Residual nonhematogenous tumor confined to the abdomen. Lymph node involvement in the abdomen. Diffuse peritoneal contamination by spillage or tumor growth that has penetrated through the peritoneal surface
Stage IV	Hematogenous metastases. Deposits beyond stage III, e.g., lung, liver, bone, and/or brain
Stage V	Bilateral renal involvement at diagnosis

of all patients under 2 years who entered the first NWTS was significantly lower compared with those over 2 years of age if histology was favorable [6]. Age yields no benefit to those with an unfavorable histologic pattern.

The most important factor influencing the prognosis of the patient is the histologic type of Wilms' tumor. Sarcomatous-clear cell, rhabdoid, and anaplastic tumor morphology indicates a poor prognosis. Thus, of the 49 patients with either a predominantly sarcomatous stroma or an anaplastic pattern, 28 (57.1%) died of it [6]. These two variants are now referred to as Wilms' tumors with unfavorable histology. Differentiation of tumor cells in tubular, glomerular, and microcystic structures occurs in about 90% of Wilms' tumors and indicates a favorable prognosis.

Some authors have suggested that the degree of epithelial differentiation is of prognostic significance [25, 26, 11], but using multivariate analyses, no influence of differentiation could be demonstrated [9].

3 Radiation Therapy

Gross and Neuhäuser [19] reported their results of treatment of Wilms' tumor utilizing postoperative irradiation of the renal fossa. The survival rate of 47% was, at that time, the highest ever reported. Since then, abdominal irradiation has become a cornerstone of treatment in Wilms' tumor, although indications for postoperative irradiation have changed considerably.

Few controlled data regarding the necessity for postoperative irradiation have been available until now. Analysis of its effect on relapse-free survival is often hampered by failure to compare and/or analyze important factors, such as the treatment volume, the elapsed time from nephrectomy to the start of irradiation, the combination with chemotherapy, and the radiation dose.

Cassedy et al. [10] reported on patients with recurrence in the abdominal cavity and concluded that the entire abdomen should be irradiated. Data from the NWTS, however, suggested that flank irradiation is sufficient for those children who had tumor spill confined to the flank. Only when contamination of the entire abdomen had occurred did whole abdomen irradiation seem to be necessary [36]. In the first and second NWTS, it was shown that a delay of more than 10 days from laparotomy to the start of irradiation adversely affected the outcome of therapy [2, 37]. A randomized study among children with stage I tumors, in which half the children were treated with actinomycin D and postoperative irradiation, and the others with actinomycin D only, was conducted by the NWTS. Flank recurrences occurred more frequently in the group without irradiation, but the difference was not statistically significant [3]. The relationship between the radiation dose and the rate of local recurrence has been examined by several investigators. If administered with adjuvant chemotherapy, the rate of local control did not improve when doses in excess of 24 Gy were employed [22, 2, 21, 37]. Doses below 20 Gy may be sufficient for those patients who require postoperative irradiation and chemotherapy on account of residual microscopic disease [5].

The flank irradiation field encompasses the tissues in which the involved kidney was located. Especially in stage III patients, radioopaque chips placed at the margin of the tumor at the time of nephrectomy help to delineate conveniently the field of irradiation. The medial border of the radiation beam includes both epiphyseal growth centers of the vertebra but does not extend further into the contralateral hemiabdomen. Thus, direct irradiation of the contralateral kidney is avoided. When whole abdomen irradiation is required, the remaining kidney must be shielded.

4 Chemotherapy

An important achievement made in the treatment of Wilms' tumor is the role chemotherapy plays in postoperative systemic therapy even when no metastases are present. FARBER [15] was the first to pioneer the use of actinomycin D as adjuvant treatment. When the substance was given in a single course immediately after the nephrectomy, the recurrence rate was 52%. It could be lowered to 14% when actinomycin D was administered in several additional courses over a longer period of time [44]. Six years later, the same patients showed recurrence rates of 57% and 28%, respectively, although no significant difference in survival rate could be demonstrated. Two subsequent studies failed to show any beneficial effect of multiple versus a single course of actinomycin D on relapse-free survival rates [25, 26, 18], but these studies did not consider other factors now known to be significant in determining the risk of recurrence.

SUTOW introduced vincristine in the mid-1960s for the treatment of Wilms' tumor. The results with adjuvant therapy using vincristine were similar to those obtained with actinomycin D therapy [33]. It was the NWTS that demonstrated the advantage of combination therapy using both substances, compared with using one drug alone [4]. In advanced Wilms' tumor (stages II and III), the 4-year tumor-free survival rate of patients receiving combination chemotherapy was 79%, significantly higher than in patients treated with either vincristine or actinomycin D alone.

In another study conducted by the NWTS, children with stage I tumors did not receive postoperative irradiation, and were randomly given either 6 or 15 months of adjuvant chemotherapy with the two drugs. The relapse-free survival rate was more than 90% in both groups, and the difference was not statistically significant. Thus, children with stage I tumors have an excellent prognosis when treated with adjuvant combination therapy without postoperative abdominal irradiation.

In the second NWTS, started in 1974, it could be demonstrated that stages II and III patients with a favorable histology had a considerably better relapse-free survival rate when treated with actinomycin D, vincristine, and adriamycin than when treated with the first two alone. The benefit may be due to the greater intensity of the three-drug regimen rather than the addition of a third agent. In fact, preliminary results of a subsequent study suggest that intensive treatment with vincristine and actinomycin D is equivalent to the three-drug regimen [5].

The chemotherapy protocol in our clinic is based on that of the NWTS (Fig. 1). Chemotherapy starts in the first days after nephrectomy in children with stages I, II, and III tumors with favorable histology. All patients who demonstrate tumors with unfavorable histology are treated with a four-drug regimen (cyclophosphamide, vincristine, adriamycin, and actinomycin D), like that used for patients with soft tissue sarcoma. The toxicity of chemotherapy is primarily due to the potentiation of irradiation by actinomycin D and the disturbance of bowel motility caused by vincristine in the postoperative phase. Mucositis of the entire gastrointestinal tract due to actinomycin D increases the rate of infection expecially with fungi. The NWTS reported that 10 of 359 children died because of the toxic effect of the treatment, or

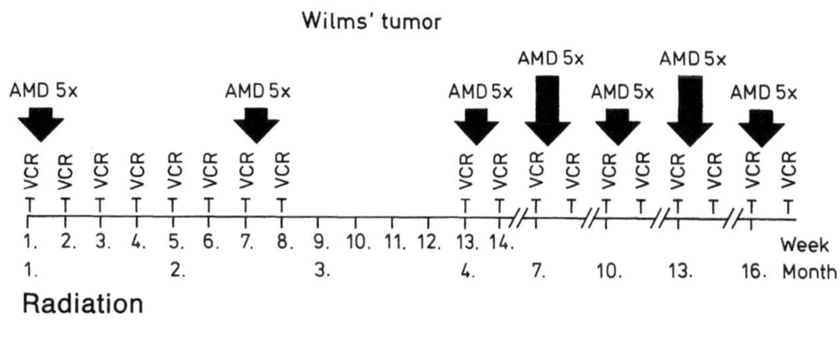

Fig. 1. Schedule for radiation and chemotherapy. AMD, actinomycin D (0.015 mg kg^{-1} d^{-1} i.v. or 0.450 mg m^{-2} d^{-1} i.v.); VCR, vincristine (1.5 mg m^{-2} d^{-1} i.v.)

because of infection during therapy; five of these had no residual tumor [1].

5 Planning Patient Treatment

Tumor nephrectomy should be the first therapeutic step in patients with Wilms' tumor. Excluded are those patients with bilateral disease and those with hematogeneous metastases, who may require specific therapy prior to nephrectomy. Results gathered by the SIOP Wilms' tumor trial and study have shown that there is no improvement in survival rates after preoperative irradiation [25, 26]. The administration of preoperative chemotherapy has been proposed for all children with a presumptive diagnosis of Wilms' tumor [27]. As the risk of erroneous preoperative diagnosis of Wilms' tumor was about 8% in patients entering the NWTS and SIOP trials, pretreatment with irradiation or chemotherapy should only be performed in special situations.

Table 3. Indications for therapeutic modalities in Wilms' tumor according to stage and age (only tumors with favorable histology)

Therapeutic modality	stage I, age <1 year	stage I, age >1 year	II	III	IV
Nephrectomy	+	+	+	+	+
Postoperative irradiation	–	–	(+)	+	(+)
Chemotherapy	(+)	+	+	+	+

For all patients without visible metastases or bilateral disease at diagnosis, it is only after nephrectomy and histologic examination of the tumor that an individual therapeutic regimen can be proposed according to ages as shown in Table 3. Patients with unfavorable histology are excluded from the normal treatment plan. More aggressive chemotherapy and postoperative abdominal irradiation have to be administered in an effort to improve the outlook of those known to have a poor prognosis.

In stage I patients who are younger than one year, tumor nephrectomy is the sole therapeutic modality, providing there has been a detailed description of the operation and an exact gross and microscopic pathologic examination of the specimen. In children older than 1 year, a shortened chemotherapy protocol ending after 6 months is used in our clinic. All patients with stages II–IV tumors receive chemotherapy with vincristine and actinomycin D. In individual stage II patients younger than 12 months, we may abstain from radiotherapy because of severe side effects in this age group. Although it is possible that some patients in stages I and II may be overtreated, combination therapy with all three modalities in stage III is unquestionably advisable. In patients with hematogeneous metastases, we plan irradiation of the renal fossa according to the abdominal extension of the tumor.

Figure 2 shows the relapse-free survival rate of children with Wilms' tumor diagnosed at the

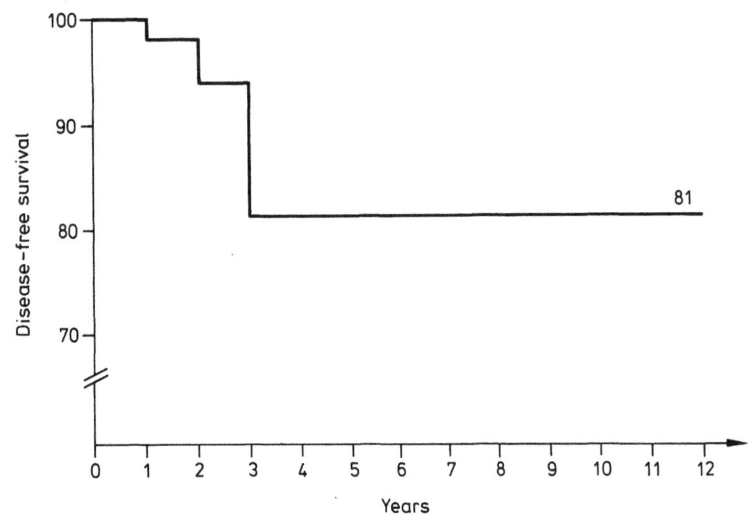

Fig. 2. Disease-free survival of 51 patients with Wilms' tumor treated in Essen since 1972. Stage I, n=17; II, n=12; III, n=16; IV, n=4; V, n=2

University Hospital of Essen up to 1984. Since 1972, we have treated patients according to the treatment plan presented above. A few patients initially received only actinomycin D; however, this did not influence the relapse-free survival rate, which is now 81%.

6 Treatment of Bilateral Wilms' Tumor

The incidence of bilateral Wilms' tumor is estimated to be between 3% and 12% [8, 7, 17, 40]. The bilateral tumor usually presents in both kidneys at once. A lot of children with bilateral disease are diagnosed not on the basis of physical examination or intravenous urography, but at the time of abdominal exploration [7]. Ultrasonography and computerized tomography will facilitate the detection of bilateral Wilms' tumor before laparotomy. Bilateral disease appears to differ from unilateral disease. The children are usually younger than the average patient with Wilms' tumor, and have a greater incidence of associated anomalies [8].

The treatment of patients with bilateral renal involvement must be highly individualized. During surgery, an attempt should always be made to remove both tumors if possible, and preserve enough residual tissue for adequate renal function. Most investigators propose removal of the most-involved kidney and a partial removal of the less-involved kidney. Like other authors [43, 20] we prefer bilateral partitial nephrectomies whenever possible. If primary resection of the tumor is technically impossible, tumor reduction with chemotherapy is indicated to find out whether an organ is worthy of surgical intervention.

Postoperative irradiation with a reduced dose is required to destroy possible residual tumor in the kidney and to decrease the risk due to the iatrogenic "rupture" of the renal capsule. Adjuvant combination chemotherapy should be carried out at the same time. Residual tumor in remaining kidney tissue may be one of the main reasons for unsuccessful therapy, but in a series of 30 children with bilateral Wilms' tumor, local control was achieved in 90% [7].

Many other therapeutic modalities, including bilateral nephrectomy with subsequent dialysis and allotransplantation, have been proposed in the treatment of bilateral Wilms' tumor [28, 14]. The survival rate of children treated with transplantation may be inferior to that achieved with other treatment modalities [29]. According to a literature review, the average survival rate for children who present with bilateral Wilms' tumor is about 60%.

7 Treatment of Metastases at Diagnosis

Metastatic disease in patients with Wilms' tumor is mainly seen in the lungs. The incidence of pulmonary metastases at diagnosis reported by several studies was about 3%–15%.

Children who present with pulmonary metastases should be treated with curative intention. The treatment plan should be based upon the situation of the individual patient. Most often it has been proposed to start with exploratory laparotomy and nephrectomy. We prefer preoperative chemotherapy for all patients, followed by nephrectomy and individual treatment for the metastases. A limited number of pulmonary metastases should be removed surgically. If no further tumor is found during surgery, we only use combination chemotherapy postoperatively. Children with diffuse pulmonary metastases have been treated with chemotherapy and whole lung irradiation. Doses between 14 Gy in 7–10 fractions, five treatments per week [36], and 20 Gy in 20 fractions [22] are proposed. Residual tumor after irradiation of the entire lung could be treated with a higher dose, focusing on the tumor.

Only 10% of patients survived when whole lung irradiation was employed without chemotherapy. Following treatment with surgery, whole lung irradiation, and combination chemotherapy, about 50% of patients who present with pulmonary metastases will survive [17, 4, 23].

The liver is the second most common organ involved by Wilms' tumor, either by direct extension of the renal tumor or by hematogeneous spread. In the NWTS, 5.1% of patients had liver involvement at diagnosis [24]. Rarely, metastases are found in brain, bone, bone marrow, and other unusual sites. Chemotherapy and irradiation, with or without surgical removal of the metastases, have been successfully administered. Because of the high risk involved, treatment should only be performed in a center with adequate experience in pediatric oncology.

8 Treatment of Recurrent Disease

Wilms' tumor may recur in several organs, including the opposite kidney and other intra-abdominal sites, the lung, bone, and brain. The most common site of recurrence is the lung. Therefore, chest X-rays should be done every 6–8 weeks during the first year after diagnosis and periodically later on. Most recurrences are diagnosed within the first 2 years of observation.

The treatment of children who develop only pulmonary metastases depends upon the same considerations as described for patients with metastatic disease at diagnosis. All such children should be approached with curative intent. The chemotherapy recommended for metastatic Wilms' tumor in previously treated children is vincristine, actinomycin D, and cyclophosphamide, with or without adriamycin [31, 13]. Successful treatment of metastases in sites other than the lung has been reported for children with metastases in the liver [41, 32], and even for brain metastases [38, 30, 12].

9 Outlook for Further Development in the Treatment of Wilms' Tumor

As a combination of good surgical skills, postoperative radiotherapy, and adjuvant chemotherapy increased the survival rate to over 80%, it should be demanded that new therapeutic regimens be introduced only very cautiously. It is vital to individualize the treatment of each patient to avoid unnecessary additional therapeutic modalities with acute and/or long-term morbidity. For children with stage I tumor, current research is attempting to define the minimal necessary treatment. On the other hand, we must devise more effective treatment programs for patients with tumors of unfavorable histology. At present, the diagnosis and treatment of Wilms' tumor, with its life-threatening course, exert a tremendous influence on the life of the child and his family. We should consider this aspect of the disease despite the therapeutic progress. It may be possible, with even more individualized treatment, to offer better help towards successful physical and emotional rehabilitation.

References

1. D'Angio GJ, Evans AE, Breslow N, Beckwith B, Bishop H, Feigl P, Goodwin W, Leape LL, Sinks LF, Sutow W, Tefft M, Wolff J (1976) The treatment of Wilms' tumor. Cancer 38:633–646
2. D'Angio GJ, Tefft M, Breslow N, Meyer JA (1978) Radiation therapy of Wilms' tumor – results according to dose, field, post-operative timing and histology. Int J Rad Oncol Biol Phys 4:769–780
3. D'Angio GJ, Beckwith JB, Breslow NE, Bishop HC, Evans AE, Farewell V, Fernbach D, Goodwin WE, Jones B, Leape LL, Palmer NF, Tefft M, Wolff JA (1980) Wilms' tumor: an update. Cancer 45:1791–1798
4. D'Angio GJ, Evans AE, Breslow N, Beckwith B, Bishop H, Farewell V, Goodwin W, Leape LL, Palmer N, Sinks LF, Sutow W, Tefft M, Wolff J (1981) The treatment of Wilms' tumor: results of the second national Wilms' tumor study. Cancer 47:2302–2311
5. D'Angio GJ, Evans AE, Breslow N, Beckwith JB, Baum E, DeLorimier A, Fernbach D, Hrabovsky E, Jones B, Kelalis P, Otherson HB, Tefft M, Thomas P (1984) Results of the third national Wilms' tumor study (NWTS-3) – a preliminary report. Proc Am Assoc Cancer Res 25:183 (abstract)
6. Beckwith JB, Palmer NF (1978) Histopathology and prognosis of Wilms' tumor, Cancer 41:1937–1948
7. Bishop HC, Tefft M, Evans AE, D'Angio GJ (1977) Survival in bilateral Wilms' tumor – review of 30 national Wilms' tumor study cases. J Pediatr Surg 12:631–638
8. Bond JV (1975) Bilateral Wilms' tumor. Lancet 2:482–484
9. Breslow NE, Palmer NF, Hill LR, Buring J, D'Angio GJ (1978) Wilms' tumor: prognostic factors for patients without metastases at diagnosis. Cancer 41:1577–1589
10. Cassady JR, Tefft M, Filler RM, Jaffe N, Hellman S (1973) Considerations in the radiation therapy of Wilms' tumor. Cancer 32:598–608
11. Chatten J (1976) Epithelial differentiation in Wilms' tumor: a clinicopathologic appraisal. Perspec Pediatr Pathol 3:225–254
12. Deutsch M, Albo B, Wollman MR (1982) Radiotherapy for cerebral metastases in children. Int J Rad Oncol Biol Phys 8:1441–1446
13. Dunger DB, Malpas JS, Graham-Pole JR, Sandland MR, Stansfeld AG, Freeman JE (1981) The use of four-drug combination chemotherapy (D.A.V.E.) in the treatment of advanced Wilms' tumor. Cancer Chemo Pharmacol 5:211–215

14. Ehrlich RM, Goldman R, Kaufman JJ (1974) Surgery of bilateral Wilms' tumors: the role of renal transplantation. J Urol 111:277–281
15. Farber S (1966) Chemotherapy in the treatment of leukemia and Wilms' tumor. JAMA 198:826–836
16. Farewell VT, D'Angio GJ, Breslow N, Norkool P (1981) Retrospective validation of a new staging system for Wilms' tumor. Cancer Clin Trials 4:167–171
17. Green DM, Jaffe N (1978) Wilms' tumor – model of a curable pediatric malignant solid tumor. Cancer Treat Rev 5:143–172
18. Green DM, Jaffe N (1979) The role of chemotherapy in the treatment of Wilms' tumor. Cancer 44:52–57
19. Gross RE, Neuhauser EBD (1950) Treatment of mixed tumors of the kidney in childhood. Pediatrics 6:843–852
20. Gruner M, Chaouachi B, Bitker M (1982) Surgical aspects of simultaneous bilateral Wilms' tumors. Prog Clin Biol Res 100:155–164
21. Jeal PN, Jenkin RDT (1980) Abdominal irradiation in the treatment of Wilms' tumor. Int J Rad Oncol Biol Phys 6:655–661
22. Jenkin RDT (1976) The treatment of Wilms' tumor. Pediatr Clin North Am 23:147–160
23. de Kraker J, Voûte PA, Lemerle J (1982) How to treat nephroblastoma stage IV patients. In: Raybaud C et al. (eds) Pediatric oncology. Proceedings of the XIIIth Meeting of the International Society of Pediatric Oncology. Marseilles, September 15–19, 1981. Excerpta Medica, Amsterdam, pp 292–294
24. Leape LL, Breslow NE, Bishop HC (1978) The surgical treatment of Wilms' tumor: results of the national Wilms' tumor study. Ann Surg 187:351–356
25. Lemerle J, Tounade M-F, Gerard-Marchant R, Flamant R, Sarrazin D, Flamant F, Lemerle M, Jundt S, Zucker J-M, Schweisguth O (1976) Wilms' tumor: natural history and prognostic factors. Cancer 37:2557–2566
26. Lemerle J, Voûte PA, Tournade MF, Delemarre JFM, Jereb B, Ahstrom L, Flamant R, Gerard-Marchant R (1976) Preoperative versus post-operative radiotherapy, single versus multiple courses of actinomycin D in the treatment of Wilms' tumor. Cancer 38:647–654
27. Lemerle J, Voûte PA, Tournade MF, Rodary C, Delamarre JFM, Sarrazin D, Burgers JMV, Sandstedt B, Mildenberger H, Carli M, Jereb B, Moorman-Voestermans CGM (1983) Effectiveness of preoperative chemotherapy in Wilms' tumor: Results of an International Society of Paediatric Oncology (SIOP) clinical trial. J Clin Oncol 1:604–609
28. de Lorimier AA, Belzer FO, Kountz SL, Kushner JH (1968) Simultaneous bilateral nephrectomy and renal allotransplantation for bilateral Wilms' tumor. Surgery 64:850–855
29. de Maria JE, Hardy BE, Brezinski A, Churchill BM (1979) Renal transplantation in patients with bilateral Wilms' tumor. J Pediatr Surg 14:577–579
30. Morgan SK, Buse MG (1976) Survival following brain metastases in Wilms' tumor. Pediatrics 58:130–132
31. Ortega JA, Higgins GR, Williams KO, Wald BR, Isaacs H, Siegel SE (1986) Vincristine, dactinomycin and cyclophosphamide (VAC) chemotherapy for recurrent metastatic Wilms' tumor in previously treated children. J Pediatr 96:502–504
32. Price JB Jr, Schullinger JN, Santulli TV (1982) Major hepatic resections for neoplasia in children. Arch Surg 117:1139–1141
33. Sullivan MP, Sutow WW (1969) Successful therapy for Wilms' tumor. Texas Med 65:46–50
34. Sutow WW, Thurman WG, Windmiller J (1963) Vincristine (leurocristine) sulfate in the treatment of children with metastatic Wilms' tumor. Pediatrics 32:880–887
35. Tefft M (1976) The role of radiation therapy in the management of Wilms' tumor. In: Pochedly C et al. (eds) Wilms' tumor. John Wiley & Sons, New York, pp 189–202
36. Tefft M, D'Angio GJ, Grant W III (1976) Postoperative radiation therapy for residual Wilms' tumor. Cancer 37:2768–2772
37. Thomas PRM, Tefft M, Farewell VT, Norkool P, Storer B, D'Angio GJ (1984) Abdominal relapses in irradiated second national Wilms' tumor study patients. J Clin Oncol 2:1098–1101
38. Traggis D, Jaffe N, Tefft M, Vawter G (1975) Successful treatment of Wilms' tumor with intracranial metastases. Pediatrics 56:472–473
39. Wara WM, Margolis LW, Smitz WB, Kushner JH, de Lorimier AA (1974) Treatment of metastatic Wilms' tumor. Radiology 112:695–697
40. Wasiljew BK, Besser A, Raffensperger J (1982) Treatment of bilateral Wilms' tumors – a 22-year experience. J Pediatr Surg 17:265–268
41. Wedemeyer PP, White JG, Nesbit ME, Aust JB, Leonard AS, D'Angio GJ, Krivit W (1968) Resection of metastases in Wilms' tumor: a report of three cases cured of pulmonary and hepatic metastases. Pediatrics 41:446–451
42. Westra P, Kieffer SA, Mosser DG (1967) Wilms' tumor. Am J Roentgenol 100:214–221
43. Wiener ES (1976) Bilateral partial nephrectomies for large bilateral Wilms' tumors. J Pediatr Surg 11:867–869
44. Wolff JA, Krivit W, Newton WA Jr, D'Angio GJ (1968) Single versus multiple dose dactinomycin therapy of Wilms' tumor. New Engl J Med 279:290–294
45. Wolff JA, D'Angio GJ, Hartmann J, Krivit W, Newton WA Jr (1974) Long-term evaluation of single versus multiple courses of actinomycin D therapy of Wilms' tumor. New Engl J Med 290:84–86

Immunologic Aspects of Malignant Renal Disease

R. Ackermann

1 General Immunologic Considerations

The biology of human renal cell carcinoma (RCC) has long been considered to be influenced by the immune system of the tumor host. The observation of occasional spontaneous regression of metastases, their erratic growth, or their occasional late occurrence following nephrectomy were thought to be strong clinical arguments for this assumption. Ljunggren et al. (1959), reporting on a case of histologically proven spontaneous regression of lung metastases, already suggested "antibody actions" as a possible explanation for such a phenomenon. Although these clinical findings are exceedingly rare and in many cases not substantiated by histology, there is definite proof that spontaneous regression of lung metastases, rather than those at other organ sites, occurs in RCC.

There are a number of experimental models which support the hypothesis that the mechanism underlying spontaneous regression of metastases is immunological in nature.

The classic experiments conducted by Prehn and Main (1957) were based on the existence of a tumor-specific transplantation antigen expressed by the methylcholanthrene-induced tumors which were transplanted in syngeneic mice. The tumor grafts were later removed when the transplant became palpable. When these animals were subsequently challenged with a graft of the same tumor, they showed a high degree of immunity. Since these mice accepted skin grafts but rejected tumor transplants from other animals, it was concluded that the tumor had been recognized as "nonself." The mode of action required for this is the presence of a tumor-specific transplantation antigen and its recognition by the host, which in turn stimulates the formation of specifically sensitized cytotoxic effector cells (T cells).

In the recent past evidence has accumulated both in vivo and in vitro that apart from this immunological mechanism tumor cell lysis can occur without deliberate sensitization of the tumor-bearing host. Natural killer (NK) cells have been recognized as being responsible for the spontaneous cytotoxicity. Haller et al. (1977) inoculated semisyngeneic tumor cells in F1 hybrids of mice exhibiting low NK cell activity and in mice with high NK cell activity. Tumor development was observed only in animals with low NK cell activity. Similar experiments have been reported by other investigators (Kasai et al. 1979; Cheever et al. 1980). Talmadge et al. (1980) inoculated melanoma B 16 cells in NK cell deficient "beige" mice. Again this resulted in a significantly higher incidence of tumors and metastases than with the inoculation of the same tumor cell in syngeneic heterozygous C 57/B 1/6 mice which possess normal NK cell activity.

Although we still do not know which of the basic mechanisms underlying these experiments may be effective in man and to which extent, the rapid progress in the field of immunology has provided a vast body of evidence that an immunogen such as a tumor cell can be eliminated by the organism. In general two distinct immunological effector mechanisms are capable of eliminating an immunogen and for this purpose must be able to recognize it as nonself. The humoral immune response is mediated by antibody-producing B-lymphocytes. The cellular effector mechanisms can be mediated by T cells, NK cells, K cells, and macrophages. Both arms of the immune system depend on each other, inasmuch as antibodies may inhibit or amplify cell-mediated immune reactions. Antibodies are essential for the recognition of tumor cells by K cells (antibody-dependent cellular cytotoxicity).

The facts that experimental tumors induced in animals are not comparable to spontaneously developing tumors in man and that many of the basic principles of immunological defence are elaborated from animal experiments must be kept in mind in a review of our current immunological understanding of human renal cell cancer. The foremost problem for studying the immunological nature of host-tumor interactions consists in defining the antigenicity of malignant renal cells. Since transplantation experiments in syngeneic inbred populations, such as have been used successfully to identify tumor-associated antigens in experimental tumor systems, meet ethical and genetic limitations in humans, the search for such antigens is mainly focused on in vitro investigations. As described in Sect. 2, analyses of the antigenicity of tumor cells were mainly based on the evaluation of the specificity of reactions in which tumor cells were lysed in vitro, mediated by either humoral factors or effector cells. The recently developed technique of cell hybridization, which allows the production of monoclonal specific antibodies, is now extensively applied to identify antigens on tumor cells. Such antigens may be of utmost relevance to improving both the diagnosis and the treatment of RCC (KÖHLER and MILSTEIN 1975).

2 Humoral Immunity in Renal Cell Carcinoma

Immunodiffusion, immunofluorescence (IF), complement fixation, and microcytotoxicity assays have been applied to investigate antibody formation against a possibly existing tumor-specific transplantation antigen of RCC. RAVITZ et al. (1972) have tested, in a limited study, sera of five patients with RCC for tumor-directed antibodies on frozen autochthonous and allogeneic tumor sections, applying the indirect immunofluorescence technique. Since fluorescence of the tumor cell surface and cytoplasm indicating a possible tumor-specific antigen was observed with four of five sera only in autologous situations, the authors concluded that RCCs may not share a common tumor-specific or tumor-related antigen. However, the experiments provided evidence that any given RCC may have its own specific antigenic marker, as only one of four antibody-positive sera reacted on sections of autochthonous normal kidney tissue. The lack of very important additional controls in this study, such as testing sera of a group of healthy volunteers and of patients with cancers of various other organ sites, led to an extended investigation. The search for tumor-directed antibodies was carried out for 288 sera obtained from patients with various types of malignancies, including tumors of the urogenital system, with 138 sera of normal subjects and 79 sera from patients with nonmalignant diseases using the IF technique on allogeneic frozen sections of RCC. Although the highest rate of positive IF reactions (29.6%) occurred with sera from patients with RCC (8/27 sera), positive reactions were also obtained with sera from patients suffering from other types of cancer, such as malignant melanoma or Hodgkin's disease, and even with a single serum from a healthy individual as well as with sera of three patients with noncancerous diseases (ACKERMANN 1975). These data indicate that the antibodies found may well be tumor-associated, but they appear to differ from the conventionally expected specificity classifications inasmuch as they are not specific for a given type of cancer, e.g., RCC, melanomas, etc.

In two other studies, microcytotoxicity assays were applied to the search for tumor-directed antibodies (CUMMINGS et al. 1974; HAKALA et al. 1974). In both investigations, it was clearly demonstrated that some sera of patients with RCC were cytotoxic in the presence of complement to explanted RCC tumor cells, whereas only one of five sera of healthy subjects exhibited a complement-dependent killing of the RCC target cells. The immunologic nature and the tumor specificity of the reactions have been proved since cytotoxicity could be absorbed with fresh frozen autochthonous tumorous tissue but not with fresh frozen autochthonous nontumorous kidney. Furthermore, cultured nontumorous kidney cells were affected by the antibodies only to a minor degree compared to their malignant counterparts. This suggests not only an antigenic difference between tumorous and nontumorous kidney tissues, but also that this different antigenicity is partially maintained in culture. In addition, these experiments ruled out the possibility that the identified cytotoxic antibodies were directed against normal transplantation antigens (HL-A). In a more recent investigation by DeKernion et al. (1979), anti-RCC antibodies were detected quantitatively with a microcomplement fixation technique in 94% of the sera from a total of 75 patients. However, 20% of the sera of healthy subjects also contained antibodies directed against RCCs but in a significantly lower titer. These authors showed that sera of RCC patients also reacted to normal kidney cells. However, absorption of these sera with pooled kidney cells resulted in a complete removal of these non-tumor-related antibodies, whereas a reduced titer of anti-RCC antibodies remained. It is unknown whether the antibodies have to be considered only as an indication of a tumorous lesion or whether they have any impact on the tumor growth. However, there is strong evidence that the antibody titer correlates with the extent of the tumor lesion and decreases invariably in an advanced stage of the disease. Furthermore, disappearance of these antibodies within 1 year following nephrectomy has been noticed in nine of ten tumor-free patients, whereas an antibody titer greater than 1:4 and its increase may indicate, prior to any other clinical detection, either tumor persistence or recurrence. Using an autologous system Ueda and associates (1979) detected three classes of surface antigens on renal carcinoma cells. They detected antibody reactivity in sera of 28 patients with immune adherence, protein A, and C 3 hemadsorption assays against class 1 antigens restricted to autologous renal cancer cells, against class 2 antigens present on certain allogeneic renal and nonrenal cancer cells and against class 3 antigens expressed on various normal and malignant cells.

These various reports on tumor-directed antibody formation in patients with RCC differ from each other not only with regard to the technique applied but also considerably with regard to the selection of controls, which are of paramount importance. Thus, it is difficult to compare the data obtained in these different experiments. However, they indicate that it is most likely that, apart from differentiation antigens, tumor-related antigens in RCC are expressed, although serologic techniques failed to identify them unequivocally.

3 Cell-Mediated Immunity in Renal Cell Carcinoma

It is fairly well established that the cellular component of a tumor-directed immune response is most relevant for the destruction of proliferating tumor cells. This can be demonstrated by the observation that tumor immunity can be transmitted from one animal to another only by transfer of immune cells but not by transfer of humoral factors with the serum.

In vitro techniques developed to evaluate the degree and the specificity of cell-mediated immune reactions are mainly microcytotoxicity assays, leukocyte migration techniques, and stimulation of lymphocytes (mixed lymphocyte target cell interaction, MLTI) with purified TAA or whole tumor cells.

Data obtained from several investigations using a microcytotoxicity assay described by Takasugi and Klein (1971) are limited with regard to the total number of only 75 patients tested so far (Bubenik et al. 1971; Cole et al. 1976; Cummings et al. 1973; Daly et al. 1974; Elhilali and Nayak 1975; Hellström et al. 1971; Montie et al. 1976). Since mononuclear cells isolated from venous blood by different methods and cell lines derived from different renal cell carcinomas were used in the experiments, the comparability of the results should be expected to be extremely limited. However, it is remarkable that several authors reported similar observations. Lymphocytes from some patients with RCC were cytotoxic in vitro (Bubenik et al. 1971; Daly et al. 1974; Elhilali and Nayak 1975; Hellström et al. 1971; Montie et al. 1976), whereas effector cells from patients with other types of malignancies and those from healthy volunteers reacted to a significantly lower degree. Furthermore, lymphocytes that were able to kill renal carcinoma cells did not affect fibroblasts of the tumor target cell donor (Daly et al. 1974). However, there exists considerable disagreement with regard to a correlation between the clinical stage of the tumor and the occurrence or absence of cell-mediated cytotoxicity. On the one hand, Montie et al. (1976), studying 25 patients, did not observe any correlation but noticed an increase in cytotoxicity when nephrectomy was performed. On the other hand, Bichler et al. (1975), using a ^{51}Cr release assay for estimating cell-mediated cytotoxicity, demonstrated that in patients with tumor lesions in progression cytotoxicity disappeared significantly.

In some tests it has been demonstrated that either autochthonous or allogeneic serum of patients with RCC, when added to the lymphocytes, may block cell-mediated cytotoxicity. This has been explained by the occurrence of blocking antibodies or antigen-antibody complexes in such sera, which may thus enhance the tumor growth (HELLSTRÖM et al. 1971). Although there have been reports that these factors cannot be identified in tumor-free patients (COLE et al. 1976), others claim that they occur both in the presence and in the absence of tumor (ELHILALI and NAYAK 1975). Because they appear in the serum of most patients with advanced disease, the definite significance of these observations is yet to be determined.

KJAER (1974, 1975) and KJAER and THOMSEN (1976) have contributed much to the understanding of cell-mediated immunity in patients with RCC. Their investigations have clearly underlined the observation that there is a tumor-directed, cell-mediated hypersensitivity in this type of cancer. Six of 11 patients showed either a stimulation or inhibition in a leukocyte migration assay when tested with autologous tumor extract. This did not occur when the same group was tested using extracts of autochthonous normal renal tissue. These data have been confirmed in an independent study by PAPPAS and SCHWARZE (1974). In addition, some patients with RCC seem to exhibit a cell-mediated hypersensitivity towards fetal kidney extracts. The kidney antigen(s) identified in this experiment were expressed in the third trimester of gestation. Pre- and postoperative evaluation of cell-mediated hypersensitivity and thorough clinical staging of all patients has produced evidence that a decrease in the tumor-directed, cellular hypersensitivity goes along with tumor spread beyond the immunologic barrier of the regional lymph nodes. Since this observation would be of great clinical interest, the test conditions have been improved and more precisely defined by the authors.

To obtain more accurate results with higher reproducibility, further purification of the tumor-related antigenic material contained in tumor extracts is needed. A promising step towards the goal has been accomplished by WRIGHT et al. (1977), who subjected crude 3 MKCl extract of fresh RCC to fractionation by preparative gradient acrylamide gel electrophoresis. One fraction still contaminated with albumin yielded positive leucocyte migration inhibition tests with leukocytes from five of seven RCC patients, whereas leukocytes from none of the controls reacted positively. It would be of great interest to study the specificity of this antigen in other test systems, e.g., by in vitro stimulation of lymphocytes. In this context, it should be mentioned that lymphocytes can be stimulated by autochthonous renal cells (STJERNSWÄRD et al. 1970). This observation was extended by the finding that peripheral blood lymphocytes can be stimulated more intensively with partially purified hypernephroma plasma membranes than with plasma membranes obtained from adjacent normal kidney (HEMSTREET et al. 1978).

Whether the specific positive reactions in leukocyte migration assays and the specific lymphocyte stimulation in vitro is due to a tumor-related antigen or to a fetal antigen that may be expressed on RCC remains unclear. There is at least some evidence that fetal antigens may play a role in these reactions. Some patients with RCC seem to exhibit a cell-mediated hypersensitivity towards fetal kidney extracts.

Most of the data on cell-mediated immunity in patients with RCC seem to indicate that tumor-associated antigens exist on human RCC. However, one has to realize that many questions remain unsolved. Effector cells that are responsible for the target cell destruction in a microcytotoxicity assay have not yet been determined. Since crude preparations of mononuclear cells, rather than purified T-lymphocytes, have been used, it is most likely that many if not all of the cytotoxic reactions were mediated by NK cells. The first evidence that false conclusions may have been drawn from such studies was produced by TAKASUGI et al. (1973), who demonstrated that the reactivity of lymphocytes from normal persons against a variety of cultured human tumor cells was significantly stronger than that of lymphocytes obtained from patients with malignant disease of the same histological type. Since it is generally accepted that interleukin 2 augments NK cells through the production of gamma interferon,

NAKANO et al. (1985) tested the cytotoxic activity of peripheral mononuclear cells exposed to interleukin 2 against autologous renal tumor cells. In five of seven patients peripheral blood lymphocytes grown in interleukin 2 were capable of lysing autologous tumor cells whereas no cytotoxic reactivity was seen with the unexposed effector cells. Although tumor-associated antigens for carcinoma of the kidney could not be defined with these experiments, they are of potential therapeutic value, e.g., by reinfusing in the patient large numbers of separated, in vitro interleukin 2 treated peripheral blood lymphocytes.

4 Renal Carcinoma Antigens Defined by Monoclonal Antibodies

Soon after KÖHLER and MILSTEIN (1975) published their paper on "Continuous Cultures of Fused Cells Secreting Antibody of Predefined Specificity," the hybridoma technique developed by these authors has been widely applied to produce monoclonal antibodies. Due to their high specificity, these can identify antigens on malignant cells which are not expressed on their normal counterparts.

UEDA and his coworkers (1983) derived 17 monoclonal antibodies from fusions with spleen cells from mice immunized with established cell cultures from renal carcinomas. The antibodies identified antigenic determinants restricted to both normal and malignant renal cells. They were thus directed against differentiation antigens of the kidney. Among others (HESS et al. 1982; SCHERBERICH et al. 1983; JÜRGENLIEMK et al. 1983), BANDER et al. (1985) reported on additional nine antibodies specific for differentiation antigens of the kidney such as antigenic determinants expressed on the glomerular basement membrane, on glomerular and proximal tubular epithelial cells, and on cells of the proximal tubule and portions of Henle's loop. OOSTERWIJK and coworkers (1984) obtained antibodies with similar specificity. One of the antibodies which did not react with carcinomas of different origin, sarcomas, and melanomas, detected antigeneic determinants in 75% of primary renal cancers but only in 16% on metastatic lesions. The fact that metastases usually consist of more dedifferentiated cells may account for the lower expression of differentiation antigens on metastatic lesions. This finding further supports the assumption that the expression of differentiation antigens of the kidney may correlate with the malignant potential of the tumor (BANDER et al. 1983). The identification of antigenic determinants of the proximal tubule in almost all renal cancers is consistent with earlier biochemical and ultrastructural findings that indicate that the origin of carcinoma of the kidney is from cells of the proximal tubule of the nephron. Further analysis of the specificity of six monoclonal antibodies directed against cell surface antigens of renal carcinoma revealed one particular antigenic phenotype among seven which was found in 15 out of 20 tumors. In this study one antigen (S 22) was not detected on any normal fetal or adult tissue but was identified on a subset of renal carcinomas (FINSTAD et al. 1985). Apart from this antibody, which may be directed against tumor-specific antigenic determinants, SCHÄRFE and his coworkers (1985) have obtained four additional monoclonal antibodies which were highly reactive on over 90% of 97 different specimens of RCCs but did not react with normal tissue and tumor tissue of other origin. Although these antibodies may be tumor-specific, it is also conceivable that due to a less sensitive test system only quantitative differences in the expression of differentiation antigens between normal and malignant tissue may reflect a presumable tumor specificity.

Despite the fact that most of the monoclonal antibodies are directed against differentiation antigens, they are a promising tool for the evaluation of the malignant potential of RCCs from an immunological point of view. The ultimate proof of the tumor specificity of some of the antibodies reported is urgently needed since both diagnostic and therapeutic improvements are then conceivable. Similar to the earlier work reported by BELITSKY and his coworkers (1978a, b) these antibodies can be conjugated to radioactive tracers for the identification of primary and metastatic lesions by radionuclide imaging. Conjugation of cytotoxic agents and radioisotopes are therapeutic perspectives which are currently under study.

5 Immunotherapy

Application of immunotherapeutic principles in the management of patients with RCC was probably first attempted by NAIRN et al. (1963), who injected allogeneic microsomal material from RCC in a woman also suffering from a metastatic RCC. Although specific antitumor precipitin formation developed, there was no indication that the immunization procedure had any effect on the tumor growth or the clinical course.

In some pilot studies nonspecific immunostimulation with Bacille Calmette-Guèrin (BCG) has been investigated as adjuvant therapy in patients with or without disseminated renal cancer. Although various immune parameters (e.g., delayed cutaneous hypersensitivity, peripheral lymphocyte counts, number of T and B cells, and the mitogenic stimulation index) improved following BCG stimulation, objective clinical responses were rare and of transitory nature (MORALES and EIDINGER 1976; MINTON et al. 1976). In another study, comprising 10 patients with advanced renal cell carcinoma who received BCG immunostimulation and 12 patients without immunotherapy, no significant difference in survival was recorded (BROSMAN et al. 1975). In addition a combination of adjunctive nephrectomy and adjuvant stimulation with BCG did not improve the survival of these patients compared to those who had been treated by nephrectomy alone (MORALES et al. 1982). Similar disappointing observations have been published for patients with advanced carcinoma of kidney treated with transfer factor following nephrectomy. Although transitory stabilization of metastatic growth has been recorded, complete remission has not been achieved (MONTIE et al. 1977). In an up-dated report of this study including 31 patients with metastatic RCC, treated either with transfer factor alone or in combination with BCG, a complete response has been noticed in only one patient. Due to the lack of effective responses in almost all patients, both BCG and transfer factor are regarded as an obsolete immunotherapeutic approach.

Specific passive immunotherapy with xenogeneic immune RNA has been investigated in a number of patients with metastatic disease or with minimal tumor burden following nephrectomy. This modality is based on the assumption of the transfer of an allegedly specific antitumor activity by ribonucleic acid (RNA) extracted from animals immunized with extracts of RCCs. In a phase I trial, including 12 patients with renal cancer of different stages, no toxic reactions after application of xenogeneic immune RNA have been seen (SKINNER et al. 1976). The efficacy of this type of immunotherapy has been investigated on 20 patients with metastatic carcinoma and nine patients with minimal residual disease. The survival of these patients was significantly greater than that of a matched group of patients (86 consecutive cases with RCCs treated by nephrectomy alone). Although none of the nine patients with minimal residual disease developed recurrence within a mean follow-up of 18 months, complete regression did not occur in patients with metastatic disease. In a later report from the same institution, long-term observation for up to 4 years confirmed the limited efficacy of xenogeneic immune RNA in metastatic renal carcinoma since most of the patients treated with this modality had died within this period of time. Although the mode of action of xenogeneic immune RNA is not fully understood, experimental observations indicate that xenogeneic immune RNA may possess adjuvant activity that may magnify a tumor-directed immune response (WHITE 1974) or may act as an antigen RNA complex containing the antigen which has been used for the immunization (ASKONAS and RHODES 1965). These presumable effects may be abolished by degradation of the intradermally injected material by tissue ribonucleases. RICHIE and associates (1981) have tried to avoid this problem by exposing the patients' isolated peripheral mononuclear cells in vitro to xenogeneic immune RNA which had been raised against his tumor. The mononuclear cells were then reinfused in the patient. One out of six patients with metastatic renal cancer had a complete regression and was alive 24 months after therapy. The efficacy of this approach remains to be determined in randomized clinical trials.

This is also true for various forms of active specific immunotherapy, which consist either in the immunization of the patient with its own lethally irradiated tumor cells, usually in combination with an adjuvant like *Corynebacterium parvum* (McCune et al. 1981) or candida antigen (Schärfe et al. 1986) or in the intradermal injection of a soluble tumor fraction in combination with purified protein derivative or candida antigen. The soluble tumor fraction is obtained by hypotonic tumor cell lysis, subsequently polymerized to small particles with ethylchloroformiate (Tykkä 1981). The latter approach has been investigated in 71 patients with advanced RCC (Tallberg et al. 1985). Although the study was not assigned as a prospective randomized trial, the statistical calculated life expectancy of this group of patients was significantly higher than that of a control group of 56 patients with metastatic disease who did not receive adjuvant immunotherapy. The survival rate in the follow-up time ranging from 3–13 years was 18.3% for the immunotherapy group as compared to 5.4% for the control group. However, these promising results have recently been doubted (Fowler 1986). The lack of complete responses in 16 patients with metastatic RCC included in this study may be due to the extremely poor status of these patients with metastases at multiple organ sites rather than with metastases confined to the lungs. This is further supported by the observation of two complete responses in the series reported by Neidhart and associates (1980). Although active specific immunotherapy seems to be effective only in a limited proportion of patients with advanced RCC, further prospective randomized trials may allow us to define those patients who may benefit from this type of therapy. However, the situation may become more complicated as the various forms of active specific immunotherapy may have to be compared with each other with regard to their efficacy. Currently one phase III trial compares the standard therapy with a specific immunotherapeutic regimen using autologous tumor cells and *C. parvum* (DeKernion 1983).

Although it remains to be determined whether the antitumoral effect of interferon (IFN) is mediated by modulation of the patient's immune system or by its antiproliferative activity, it appears to be reasonable to discuss the results obtained with IFN treatment in advanced renal cancer in the context with the immunotherapeutic approaches described above. Again as in most other studies, the number of patients treated with IFN is small. In addition, several types of interferons have been used, which limits the evaluation of this type of therapy. Apart from isolated examples of interferon activity against RCC with a partial response in one out of 13 patients (Queseda et al. 1983) a complete response in one out of 13 patients (Retsas et al. 1983) and an additional complete response in each of two other studies with a total of 70 patients (DeKernion 1983; Kirkwood et al. 1983), the therapeutic effect of IFN-alpha at least remains questionable. More recently, immune interferon (IFN-gamma) has been investigated for use as an adjuvant measure in advanced renal cancer. In a pilot study Otto and associates (1986) treated 16 patients with metastatic RCC with recombinant IFN-gamma. Patients received IFN-gamma at a dosage of 100 $\mu g/m^2$ in a 4-h infusion three times a week every second week for 3 months. In cases either with stabilization after this period of time or with tumor progression under therapy, treatment has been changed to a high dosage protocol consisting of 24 h infusion with 500 $\mu g/m^2$ on 5 days every second week. Four of 16 patients showed partial regression under low dose IFN-gamma therapy, which lasted from 2.5 up to 24 months. In one patient with a high dose regimen complete regression has been observed. More recently Garnick and associates (1986) reported their experience with IFN-gamma in patients with advanced renal cancer. Of 58 patients, 38 were evaluable for response to therapy. Although the dose schedule differed significantly from the above-mentioned study, the number of complete and partial responses was similar to that reported by Otto et al. (1986). The high dose regimen resulted in dose-related side effects with nausea and vomiting in 49% of the patients, proteinuria in 49%, hepatotoxicity in 40%, myelosuppression in 74%, and thrombocytopenia in 14%. Non-dose-related side effects consisted in fever, chills and rigors, anemia, lethargy, and headaches in 31%–94% of the patients depending on the symptom. Comparing the experience obtained with various interferons and different dose schedules, it is still unclear from which regimen patients may benefit most. Although the most effective dose, interval, and duration of therapy is not known, responses achieved with low dose regimen may be appropriate particularly as severe side effects can be avoided.

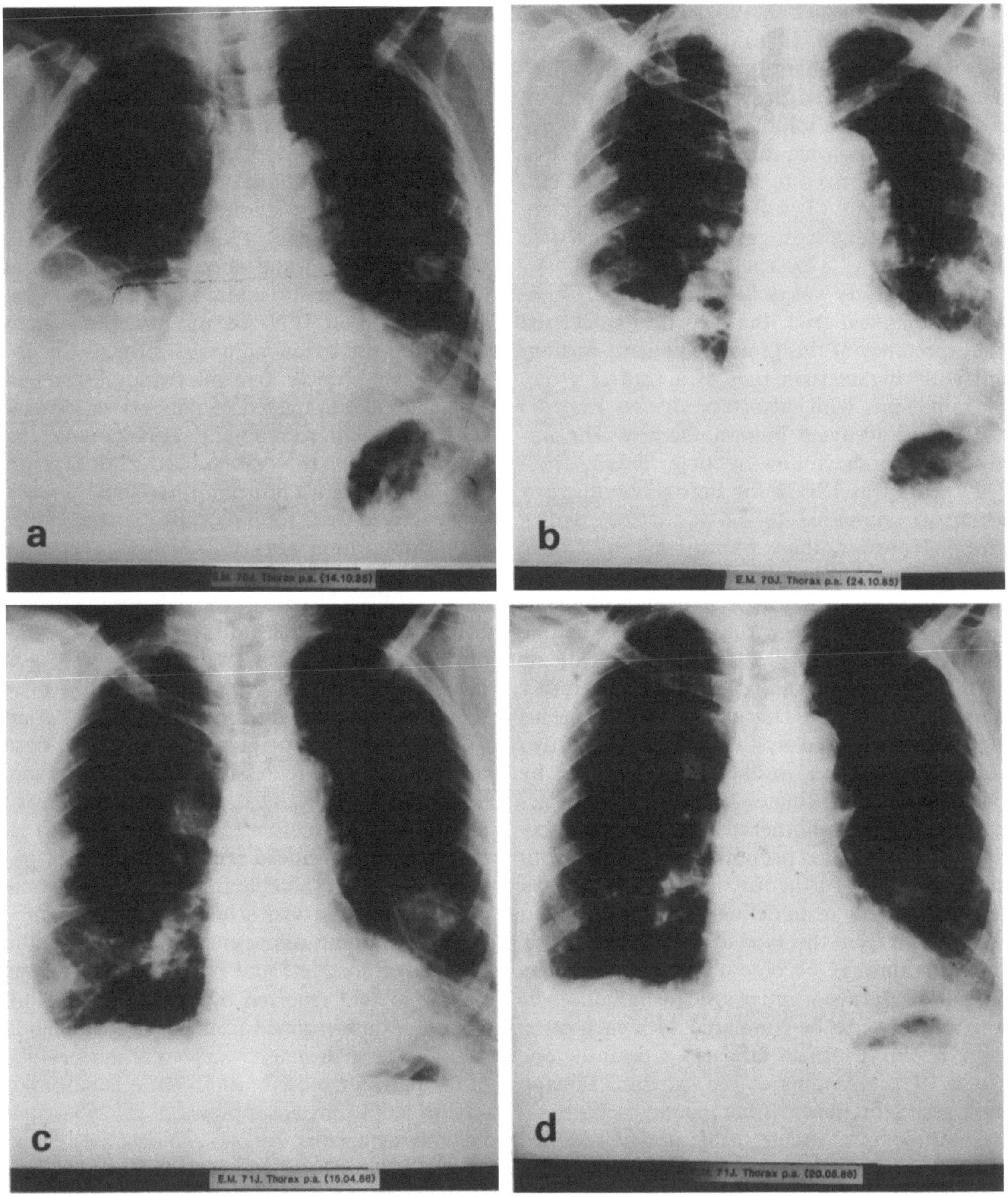

Fig. 1. **a** Chest X-ray 2 weeks following nephrectomy, **b** 3 weeks following nephrectomy, **c** 4 weeks after initiation of IFN-gamma treatment, and **d** 8 weeks after initiation of IFN-gamma treatment

Figure 1 shows a partial response of pulmonary metastases of a patient who has been treated with IFN-gamma at our institution. Following nephrectomy rapid growth of pulmonary metastases occurred within several weeks. Therapy with IFN-gamma has been initiated 4 months following nephrectomy. Although a marked objective response was detectable, there is still evidence of remaining tumor. Although side effects of any type of immunotherapy, in particular during treatment with interferon, are severe, this example along with similar observations also seen with other forms of immunotherapy should stimulate further efforts in the field of immunotherapy of RCC especially as long as effective alternative therapeutic regimens are not available.

References

1. Ackermann R (1975) Tumor-associated antibodies against renal cell carcinomas detected by immunofluorescence. Eur Urol 1:154–156
2. Askonas BA, Rhodes JM (1965) Immunogenicity of antigen-containing ribonucleic acid preparations from macrophages. Nature 205, 470–474
3. Bander NH, Whitmore WF, Old LJ (1983) Monoclonal antibody defined cell surface antigens of human renal cancer. 78th Meeting of the American Urological Association, Las Vegas, p 114
4. Bander NH, Cordon-Cardo C, Finstad CL, Whitmore WF, Vaughan ED, Oettgen HF, Melamed M, Old L (1985) Immunohistological dissection of the human kidney using monoclonal antibodies. J Urol 133:502–505
5. Belitsky P, Ghose T, Aquino J, Norvell ST, Blair AH (1978a) Radionuclide imaging of primary renal cell carcinoma by I-131-labelled antitumor antibody. J Nucl Med 19:427–430
6. Belitsky P, Ghose T, Aquino J, Tai J, MacDonald AS (1978b) Radionuclide imaging of metastases from renal-cell carcinoma by 131-I-labelled antitumor antibody. Radiology 126:515–517
7. Bichler KH, Ax W, Tautz CH (1975) Cell-mediated immunity in patients with renal adenocarcinoma. Eur Urol 1:231–234
8. Brosman S, Hausman M, Shacks S (1975) Studies on the immune status of patients with renal adenocarcinoma. J Urol 114:375–380
9. Bubenik J, Jakoubkova J, Krakora P, Baresova M, Helbich P, Viklicky V, Malaskova V (1971) Cellular immunity to renal carcinomas in man. Int J Cancer 8:503–513
10. Cheever MA, Greenberg PD, Fefer A (1980) Therapy of leukemia by nonimmune syngeneic spleen cells. J Immunol 124:2137–2142
11. Cole AT, Avis I, Fried FA, Avis F (1976) Cell-mediated immunity in renal cell carcinoma – preliminary report. J Urol 115:234–238
12. Cummings KH, Peter JB, Kaufman JJ (1973) Cell-mediated immunity to tumor antigens in patients with renal cell carcinoma. J Urol 110:31–35
13. Cummings KH, Peter JB, Kaufman JJ (1974) Cytotoxic serum factors in patients with renal cell carcinoma. J Urol 111:330–333
14. Daly JJ, Prout GR, Ahl CA, Lin JC (1974) Specificity of cellular immunity to renal cell carcinoma. J Urol 111:448–452
15. DeKernion JB (1983) Treatment of advanced renal cell carcinoma – traditional methods and innovative approaches. J Urol 130:2–7
16. DeKernion JB, Ramming KP, Gupta RK (1979) The detection and clinical significance of antibodies to tumor-associated antigens in patients with renal cell carcinoma. J Urol 122:300–305
17. Elhilali MM, Nayak S (1975) Immunologic evaluation of human renal cell carcinoma. Invest Urol 13:60–66
18. Finstad CL, Cordon-Cardo C, Bander NH, Whitmore WF, Melamed MR, Old LJ (1985) Specificity analysis of mouse monoclonal antibodies defining cell surface antigens of human renal cancer. Proc Natl Acad Sci USA 82:2955–2959
19. Fowler JE (1986) Failure of immunotherapy for metastatic renal cell carcinoma. J Urol 135:22–25
20. Garnick B, Reich SD, Richie JP (1986) Phase I/II study of recombinant interferon gamma (Immuneron TM) in advanced renal cell carcinoma (RCC). 81st Annual meeting of the American Urological Association (abstract no. 250). J Urol 135:166 A
21. Hakala TR, Castro AE, Elliott A, Fraley E (1974) Humoral cytotoxicity in human renal cell carcinoma. Invest Urol 11:405–410
22. Haller O, Hanson M, Kiessling R, Wigzell H (1977) Role of non-conventional natural killer cells in resistance against syngeneic tumor cells in vivo. Nature 270:609–611
23. Hellström I, Hellström KE, Sjögren HO, Warner GA (1971) Demonstration of cell-mediated immunity to human neoplasms of various histologic types. Int J Cancer 7:1–16
24. Hemstreet GP, Dawson JR, Seigler HF (1978) Tumor membrane lymphocyte stimulation assay in patients with renal cell carcinoma. Cancer Res 38:1447–1456
25. Hess H, Alheid U, Biermann S, Waks T, Scherberich JE, Mondorf AW, Schoeppe W, Senge T, Falkenberg FW (1982) Preparation and characterization of monoclonal antibodies against antigens of human renal adenocarcinoma. In: Peeters H (ed) Protides of the biological fluids, 29th colloquium 1981. Pergamon, Oxford, pp 903–905
26. Jürgenliemk I, Senge T, Scherberich JE, Falkenberg FW (1983) Detection of different morphological structures in human kidneys and kidney carcinomas by monoclonal antibodies. Immunobiol 165:288
27. Kasai M, Leclerc JC, McVai-Boudreau L, Shen FW, Cantor H (1979) Direct evidence that natural killer cells in nonimmune spleen cell populations prevent tumor growth in vivo. J Exp Med 149:1260–1264
28. Kirkwood JM, Harris JE, Vera R, Sandler S (1983) Randomized trial of two doses of leucocyte interferon in metastatic renal cell carcinoma. The American Society Collaborative Trial. In: Proceedings ASCO, Abstract 579, San Diego
29. Kjaer M (1974) In vitro demonstration of cellular hypersensitivity to tumor antigens by means of leucocyte migration technique in patients with renal carcinoma. Eur J Cancer 10:523–531
30. Kjaer M (1975) The dose-related effect of tumor extract on the in vitro migration of leucocytes from patients with renal carcinoma. Eur J Cancer 11:281–289
31. Kjaer M, Thomsen M (1976) General immunocompetence and tumor-directed, cell-mediated hypersensitivity in vitro in patients with renal carcinoma. Acta Pathol Microbiol Scand (C) 84:403–413
32. Köhler G, Milstein C (1975) Continuous cultures of fused cells secreting antibody of predefined specificity. Nature 256:495–497
33. Ljunggren E, Holm S, Karth B, Pompeius R (1959) Some aspects of renal tumors with special reference to spontaneous regression. J Urol 82:553–557
34. McCune CS, Schapira DV, Henshaw EC (1981) Specific immunotherapy of advanced renal carcinoma. Cancer 47:1984–1987

35. Minton JP, Pennline K, Nowrocki JF (1976) Immunotherapy of human kidney cancer. Proc Am Soc Clin Oncol 17:301
36. Montie JE, Straffon RA, Deodhar SD, Barna B (1976) In vitro assessment of cell-mediated immunity in patients with renal cell carcinoma. J Urol 115:239–242
37. Montie JE, Bukowski R, Deodhar S, Hewlett J, Stewart B, Straffon R (1977) Immunotherapy of disseminated renal cell carcinoma with transfer factor. J Urol 117:553–554
38. Morales A, Eidinger D (1976) Bacillus Calmette-Guérin in the treatment of adenocarcinoma of the kidney. J Urol 115:377–380
39. Morales A, Wilson JL, Pater JL, Loeb M (1982) Cytoreductive surgery and systemic Bacillus Calmette-Guerin therapy in metastatic renal cancer: A phase II trial. J Urol 127:230–235
40. Nairn RC, Philip J, Ghose T, Porteous IB, Fothergill JE (1963) Production of a precipitin against renal cancer. Br Med J I:1702–1704
41. Nakano E, Tada Y, Ichikawa Y, Fujioka H, Ishibasi M, Matsuda M, Takaha M, Sonoda T (1985) Cytotoxic activity of peripheral blood lymphocytes grown with interleukin 2 against autologous cultured tumor cells in patients with renal cell carcinoma. Preliminary Report. J Urol 134:24–28
42. Neidhart JA, Murphy SG, Hennick LA, Wise HA (1980) Active specific immunotherapy of stage IV renal carcinoma with aggregated tumor antigen adjuvant. Cancer 46:1128–1134
43. Oosterwijk E, Fleuren GJ, Jonas U, Zwartendijk J, te Velde J, Warnaar SO (1984) The expression of renal antigens in renal cell carcinoma. J Urol 2:156–158
44. Otto U, Huland H, Denkhaus H, Klosterhalfen H (1986) Therapie mit rekombinantem Alpha-2 oder rekombinantem Gamma-Interferon bei Patienten mit metastasierendem Nierenkarzinom. Verhandlungsbericht der Deutschen Gesellschaft für Urologie, 37. Tagung (1985). Thieme, Stuttgart
45. Pappas A, Schwarze G (1974) In vitro demonstration of cell-mediated immunity against human renal cell carcinoma assessed by the leucocyte migration assay. Z Immunitaetsforsch 148:142–150
46. Prehn RT, Main JM (1957) Immunity to methylcholanthrene-induced sarcomas. J Natl Cancer Inst 18:769
47. Queseda JR, Swanson DA, Trinoka A, Gutterman JK (1983) Renal cell carcinoma: anti-tumor effects of leucocyte interferon. Cancer Res 43:940–947
48. Ravitz G, Watne AL, Milam DF (1972) Autoantibodies to human renal cell carcinoma. J Urol 107:26–28
49. Retsas S, Priestman TJ, Newton KA (1983) Treatment of metastatic renal cell carcinoma with human lymphoblastoid interferon. A phase-II study. In: Proceedings ASCO, Abstract C-515, San Diego
50. Richie JP, Wang BS, Steele GD, Wilson RE, Mannick JA (1981) In vivo and in vitro effects of xenogeneic immune ribonucleic acid in patients with advanced renal cell carcinoma: a phase I study. J Urol 126:24–28
51. Schärfe T, Becht E, Kaltwasser R, Thüroff JW, Jacobi GH, Hohenfellner R (1985) Tumor-specific monoclonal antibodies for renal cell carcinoma. Eur Urol 11:1176–1120
52. Schärfe T, Becht E, Klippel KF, Jacobi GH, Hohenfellner R (1986) Active immunotherapy of stage IV renal cell cancer using autologous tumor cells. W J Urol 3:245–248
53. Scherberich J, Hess H, Alheid U, Falkenberg F, Mondorf W, Schoeppe W (1983) Immunological studies on membrane associated antigens from renal adenocarcinoma and human kidney cortex using poly- and monoclonal antibodies. In: Peeters H (ed) Protides of the biological fluids, proceedings of the 30th colloquium. Pergamon, Oxford
54. Skinner DG, DeKernion JB, Brower PA, Ramming KP, Pilch Y (1976) Advanced renal cell carcinoma: Treatment with xenogeneic immune ribonucleic acid and appropriate surgical resection. J Urol 115:246–250
55. Stjernswärd J, Almgard LE, Franzen S, Schreeb von T, Wadström LB (1970) Tumor-distinctive cellular immunity to renal carcinoma. Clin Exp Immunol 6:963–968
56. Takasugi M, KLein E (1971) The methodology of microassay for cell-mediated immunity (MCI) In: Bloom BR, Glade PR (eds) In vitro methods in cell-mediated immunity. Academic, New York
57. Takasugi M, Mickey MR, Terasaki PI (1973) Reactivity of lymphocytes from normal persons on cultured tumor cells. Cancer Res 33:2898–2902
58. Tallberg T, Tykkä H, Mahlberg K, Halttunen P, Lehtonen T, Kalima T, Sarna S (1985) Active specific immunotherapy with supportive measures in the treatment of palliatively nephrectomized, renal adenocarcinoma patients. A thirteen-year follow-up study. Eur Urol 11:233–243
59. Talmadge JE, Meyers KM, Prieur DJ, Starkey JR (1980) The role of NK cells in tumor growth and metastasis in beige mice. Nature 284:622–624
60. Tykkä H (1981) Active specific immunotherapy with supportive measures in the treatment of advanced palliatively nephrectomised renal adenocarcinoma. A controlled clinical study. Scand J Urol Nephrol (Suppl) 63:7–107
61. Ueda R, Shiku H, Pfreundschuh M, Takahashi T, Li LTC, Whitmore WF, Oettgen HF, Old LJ (1979) Cell surface antigens of human renal cancer defined by autologous typing. J Exp Med 150:565–579
62. Ueda R, Ogata SI, Morrissey DM, Finstad CL, Szkudlarek J, Whitmore WF, Oettgen HF, Lloyd KO, Old LJ (1983) Cell surface antigens of human renal cancer defined by mouse monoclonal antibodies: Identification of tissue-specific kidney glycoproteins. Proc Natl Acad Sci USA 78:5122–5126
63. White RG (1974) Workshop report. In: Brent L, Holborow J (eds) Progress in immunology II. North Holland, Amsterdam, vol 2, p 385
64. Wright GL, Schellhammer PF, Faulconer R (1977) Isolation of a soluble tumor-associated antigen from human renal cell carcinoma by gradient acrylamide gel electrophoresis. Cancer Res 37:4228–4232

Subject Index

MIX
Papier aus verantwortungsvollen Quellen
Paper from responsible sources
FSC® C105338

If you have any concerns about our products,
you can contact us on
ProductSafety@springernature.com

In case Publisher is established outside the EU,
the EU authorized representative is:
Springer Nature Customer Service Center GmbH
Europaplatz 3, 69115 Heidelberg, Germany

Printed by Libri Plureos GmbH
in Hamburg, Germany